D0898432

A Handbook for the Assessment of Children's Behaviours

Wiley Desktop Edition

This book gives you access to a Wiley Desktop Edition – a digital, interactive version of your book available on your PC, Mac, laptop or Apple mobile device.

To access your Wiley Desktop Edition:
- Find the redemption code on the front cover of this book and carefully scratch away the top coating of the label.
- Visit www.vitalsource.com/software/bookshelf/downloads to download the Bookshelf application.
- Open the Bookshelf application on your computer and register for an account.
- Follow the registration process and enter your redemption code to download your digital book.

A Handbook for the Assessment of Children's Behaviours

With Wiley Desktop Edition

Jonathan Williams and Peter Hill

WILEY-BLACKWELL

A John Wiley & Sons, Ltd., Publication

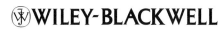

This edition first published 2012 © 2012 by John Wiley & Sons, Ltd.

Wiley-Blackwell is an imprint of John Wiley & Sons, formed by the merger of Wiley's global Scientific, Technical and Medical business with Blackwell Publishing.

Registered office: John Wiley & Sons, Ltd, The Atrium, Southern Gate, Chichester, West Sussex, PO19 8SQ, UK

Editorial offices: 9600 Garsington Road, Oxford, OX4 2DQ, UK
The Atrium, Southern Gate, Chichester, West Sussex, PO19 8SQ, UK
111 River Street, Hoboken, NJ 07030-5774, USA

For details of our global editorial offices, for customer services and for information about how to apply for permission to reuse the copyright material in this book please see our website at www.wiley.com/wiley-blackwell.

The right of the author to be identified as the author of this work has been asserted in accordance with the UK Copyright, Designs and Patents Act 1988.

Library of Congress Cataloging-in-Publication Data

Williams, Jonathan, 1959-
  A handbook for the assessment of children's behaviours / Jonathan Williams and Peter Hill.
    p. ; cm.
  Includes bibliographical references and index.
  ISBN 978-1-119-97589-2 (paper)
  1. Behavioral assessment of children. 2. Mental illness--Diagnosis. 3.
Psychodiagnostics. I. Hill, P. D. (Peter David) II. Title.
  [DNLM: 1. Child Behavior. 2. Behavioral Symptoms--diagnosis. 3.
Neurobehavioral Manifestations. WS 105]
  RJ503.5.W57 2012
  618.92'89--dc23
                              2011019732

A catalogue record for this book is available from the British Library.

This book is published in the following electronic formats: Wiley Online Library
9781119977452

Typeset in 8/12pt Times New Roman by Laserwords Private Limited, Chennai, India.
Printed and bound in Malaysia by Vivar Printing Sdn Bhd

First Impression 2012

Table of Contents

Symbols used in the book
(for abbreviations see glossary)

☼   These sections discuss general principles.

♠   Indicates *umbrella constructs* (e.g. ADHD, Autism) to
           emphasise their nonspecificity (see figure on p.385).

!!   Conditions that are potential emergencies.

👁   Important conditions that are particularly easy to miss.

‖sleepy   A heavy bar on the left indicates the most common causes
           in a list, which are often normality and misunderstanding.

List of behaviours

Questions arising in assessment

Conundrums

Photocopiable investigation planners

**These are provided for the symptoms that have many important
causes identifiable through laboratory testing**

Figures

Additional Tables

Acknowledgements

Much of this book is based on case discussions in the Children's Multispecialty Assessment Clinic in Barnet, London, to which the following colleagues have contributed enormously: Adriana Fernandez-Chirre and Juliet Pearce; Elaine Clarke, Imogen Newsom-Davis, and Leora Zehavi.

Special thanks to Chung Chan, Uttom Chowdhury, Rosemary Tannock, and Stephanie Vergnaud for advice and numerous other contributions.

Thanks also to Nirmal Arora, Niraj Arora, Stephen Baker, Tobias Banaschewski, Lourdes Berdasco, Mike Berger, Frank Besag, Dickon Bevington, Natalie Canham, Johanne Carstairs, Mark Carter, Nicola Feuchtwang, Traciy Fogarty, Danya Glaser, Jane Gilmour, David Hall, Sebastian Hendricks, Sally Hulin, Holly Hurn, Ilan Joffe, Tony Kaplan, Joel Khor, Bruce Kitchener, Su Laurent, Robin Miller, Michael Moutoussis, Michelle Moore, Geetha Nagendran, Dasha Nicholls, Libby Read, Melanie Rose, Simon Roth, Dominic Smith, Jackie Silverman, David Skuse, Eric Taylor, James Underhill and Cathy Wainhouse for their comments on sections of the book and/or help with difficult assessments. We are haunted by the worry that we have missed somebody.

Introduction

It is a standard task, and often straightforward, to produce an account of a child's behaviours in psychodynamic terms, or in terms of learning theory, or family functioning, or as a diagnostic category in DSM or ICD. In practice, which type of account is given usually depends on the training of the clinician, rather than on the child's behaviour[1326]. Yet there are many paths to the same behaviour. Whichever of these approaches is adopted, parents and professionals are often left wondering: Would a different perspective be more useful? Have underlying problems been missed? The purpose of this book is to help to answer these questions.

We aim to provide a behaviourally oriented little brother for Illingworth's *Common Symptoms of Disease in Children*[743] (or [371,611]), and Sims' *Symptoms in the Mind*[1487]. Symptoms that are mainly medical will be found in Illingworth, and detailed analyses of psychopathology in Sims.

The title has been interpreted loosely. Most of the behaviours in the book occur not just in pre-pubertal children, but also in adolescents or adults. We include not just voluntary actions, but also movements whose voluntary nature is questionable, as well as hobbies and preferences. Some of the symptoms lead to referral because they produce behavioural manifestations (e.g. *depression*, or *poor relationship with mother*). Overall, the book spans the behavioural, cognitive, social, and emotional problems of children [5,1172,1173,1342,1798]. We also include some behaviours because they are under-discussed, and some because they are intriguing.

Relationship to other aspects of diagnosis

This is a book about symptoms. Our approach addresses each individual symptom separately, describing it and listing factors that can contribute to or *cause* it (this term is discussed on p.393). The reader is thereby helped to decide whether the symptom merits attention (stage **B** in the figure below) and then invited to consider which of the causes are most likely, or which require further testing, even if they are unlikely (stage **C**). The approach is related to low-level checklists that probe for causes (e.g. of school refusal[823]) or for subtypes (e.g. of pedantry[558]).

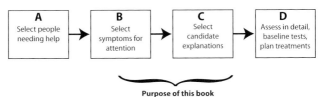

Purpose of this book

The approach is different from high-level diagnostic checklists (e.g. DSM[33], ICD[1797], Autism Diagnostic Interview[918]), that weigh symptom counts against a threshold to produce a "diagnostic code" or a probability. These systems generally require the user to have already decided on a potential diagnosis. Such an approach is useful at stage **D** in the above figure, *after* the long list of potential explanations in this book has been whittled down to a very small number. Some of the best such questionnaires, including several in the public domain, can be found in [565].

The approach of the current book is also distinct from wide ranging questionnaires designed to discover whether a child has a problem. Examples are the Strengths and Difficulties Questionnaire[592] and the Child Behavior Checklist[5]. These efficiently focus professional attention on the children most likely to need help, and on their most troublesome symptoms. These form stage **A** and part of **B** in the figure above, and rationally *precede* use of the current book to find underlying causes.

The description of each symptom

Discussion of each symptom starts with a definition and comments about how it usually presents. Common changes during childhood are described. Since normal children do almost anything at one time or another, we indicate the limit of frequency or severity, beyond which it is reasonable to consider the behaviour as abnormal. We describe some common misconceptions.

Due to space limitations, we could not include much information on each symptom. Further details can be found by following the links, and in the glossary (p.417); by reading the references, standard texts, SCAN[1796], DSM, ICD or online. For less well-studied problems, of which there are many in children's mental health[599], the symptom descriptions and the lists of causes are based on multidisciplinary discussion of many cases.

The choice of causes in each list

Research on evidence-based *treatments* is well under way for many disorders, but less is known about the process of *assessment*[684,1389]. Of necessity, therefore, this book assembles both research evidence and clinical experience. We have tried to combine clinical common sense and therapeutic utility, including what we judge to be the most solidly based traits, states, and other "hypothetical constructs" [989]. We are well aware that such judgments are subjective, and we welcome suggestions for improvements. Thousands of rare causes are omitted, but we hope to have most of the common ones, as well as many of the treatable rarities. We offer no apology for including rare causes: recognising them is an important professional goal.

Some categories of causation are only lightly covered. Most genetic/imaging research is not yet ready for clinical application, though this area is evolving fast (for constantly updated websites see p.383). Only the most common medication effects are included, because there are so many and they are quite easy to look up, as most children are on none or very few.

Levels of explanation

The causelists include patterns of learned behaviour and family dynamics, some specific genetic or medical syndromes, and broad DSM-IV syndromes. All these have their uses. Multiple contributory factors, on the same and different levels should be sought in all cases. Resources to help in this are provided in the appendices.

Identifying a pattern named in DSM-IV such as ADHD or ASD or ID (see glossary for abbreviations) is useful where it is a well-recognised shorthand, and as a link to high-quality research, to treatments that work in large groups, and to funding for care. It can also be reassuring, and even therapeutic[1603].

However, with the child and family in the room, and with detailed school reports and psychometric results, it is usually possible to identify causes of symptoms that are much more precise, are specific to the child (see p.385; or compare p.79 with p.383), and which can guide behavioural, cognitive, social and family interventions.

The order of each list

We considered several ways of ordering the lists. Illingworth's method of ordering them strictly by prevalence is difficult when the prevalence is not known, and when causation is multifactorial. Standard groupings of causation (e.g. genetic, adaptive, learned, social) did not make the lists clearer, to our surprise. Grouping by associated clinical signs or age helps in linking some tables to the diagnostic process, but unfortunately gives the impression of either/or choices rather than multifactoriality. In the end, we grouped and ordered each list in the way that seemed clearest.

When describing problems that occur in either sex, the words *he* and *she* are used interchangeably. The term *Intellectual Disability* is used to refer to global learning deficits (see p.498).

Single Symptoms

The appropriate table in this book can usually be found via the Table of Contents or the index. If your patient's symptom doesn't have a list, look for *similar* symptoms in the index. If the child has uncommon social or medical problems, you can also look these up in the index to see if they could be contributing to the current problem (i.e. you can work forwards or backwards to find the connections). The catalogue of causes (p.393) may trigger a useful association. Together, these methods usually provide adequate ideas for thinking about causes of your patient's symptom.

Ways to get sensitive information from a child or parent

This is crucial, because the most sensitive information has the greatest emotional impact and the greatest likelihood of influencing behaviour. Obtaining detailed information about the whole family's ideas, concerns, and expectations (p.13) will later enable them to believe you know them, and to accept difficult feedback. This is especially true if the feedback challenges the family's previous views or is painful (see pp.19,166).

Tears in children most often indicate anxiety. Tears in their parents (p.315) are sometimes a sign of low mood (p.309) but more often they are a sign of exhaustion, or exasperation, or that the person is trying to communicate the degree of their suffering. They are not something to be simply wiped away, but something to be met with overt sympathy and encouragement to talk: "I'm so sorry you're going through such a difficult time. Would you like to tell me about it?"

What to do

- Introduce yourself. Don't fidget or answer your mobile. Smaller rooms and easy chairs may help.

- In most cases interview the parents and the child together, at least for the first few minutes. Settle them, and orient them to the task in hand, mainly addressing the child: "I need to ask a lot of questions over the next [hour]. This is boring for you but fascinating for me because I'm a sad case. Let's make a list of what we've got to talk about – everyone chip in." If it's a contentious situation, interview family members individually then together. Sometimes it is useful to have other family members present too, e.g. all the children and a grandparent.

- Start your assessment with the problems that are foremost in their mind.

  As much as possible, follow the person's interest. If they say something surprising, ask for explanation then rather than later. Sometimes echo what the person said, and ask for more information.

- Take time (p.22). Don't interrupt, even if they need time to organise their thoughts. More than one session in a day, especially if punctuated by meals, or with tea, establishes a trusting atmosphere (p.23).

- Empathic understanding is an important part of a practitioner–patient relationship[1362]. It can be fostered by non-judgmentally trying to feel what patients feel, appearing interested and concerned, respecting the patients' views (as well as their good intentions and occasional lapses from them), paying attention to both verbal and non-verbal cues, and making them feel known personally[1527]. In fact occasionally achieving such a connection is one of the most important parts of treatment, for example if a child thinks he or she is weird and no one could ever understand them. The transfer of patients between clinicians often completely loses this connection; such loss can sometimes be reduced by transferring via a joint meeting.

- Don't press shy preschoolers. First get them in the habit of interacting, using yes/no questions (to reduce cognitive load and make expectations explicit). Or do a visual analogue scale with fingers drawing on the table and ask them to show where they or their feelings are. If they are talking, follow their lead, but if they are not, talk about friends, school, and home, starting with closed questions in the area they find easiest: "What's the name of your school?"

- With disgruntled teens: respect, talk to them first, and don't be overtly censorious. Especially with *older* teens, consider telling them you will not break their confidentiality unless someone is in danger. Another option is to wait, and if they say *this is confidential* say "yup, but I'll stop you if I think it shouldn't be." Confidentiality needs to be weighed against the child's interests, though usually confidentiality should win.

- Do pay attention to your *feelings* about the person, and your *initial reactions*, as the person probably often meets people with these reactions. To some extent your feelings will be shaped by your own experiences. For example, you are likely to moderate your criticism of a parent's failings if you are a parent yourself[1458].

- Vary your language to suit the listener, without being patronising.

- If you have to ask something difficult, prepare the person first, e.g. "I hope you don't mind my asking this, but…"

- If you cannot do it well, try to do most of your difficult assessments jointly with someone who is known to be excellent at it. Or consider matching interviewers to interviewees, by sex, age, and/or culture.

- Some families have *hidden information*, which they may or may not tell you as they get to know you better. It can be an agenda such as wanting help with an embarrassing rash, or housing, or legal reports or a marital row. Or the parents may conceal information about physical punishments of their child, or about their own health, for privacy or to avoid wasting your time. Less common are beliefs in demonic possession, unusual religions, and belief that the child has paranormal powers. The most common ways to discover any of these secrets are use of information from other sources (teacher, GP, previous professionals); and recognising inconsistency. Sometimes non-verbal signs can reveal the concealment: e.g. lack of involvement, hesitation before answering, or pressing the lips together. If you suspect concealment, consider whether the child is at risk; if so you need to involve other professionals (p.272). Motivational interviewing (p.355) and working through checklists in this book are non-confrontational ways of seeking more information.

Extending the history

For any problem, you need the following information, plus *severity* and *sequelae,* the *trend over time,* and the child's and parents' *ideas.* For an example of a more detailed list see p.139.

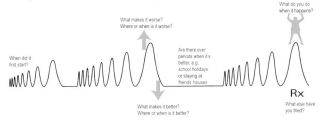

Figure 1. The history of each symptom is important.

A diary (prospective record) is much more reliable than memory (retrospective record). The school's report is crucial in assessments, because (a) it is peer-referenced and relatively impartial; (b) it helps you work out whether the problem occurs in all places (so is more likely to be in the child than in a particular environment).

The family's ideas

It is very useful to understand what the family think about the symptom[902]. This includes their *ideas* of what it is or what caused it, their *concerns* about what it may lead to, and their *expectations* of what you will do (giving the acronym ICE). Paying attention to I,C, E increases the family's concordance with treatments.

I: Very commonly, one or both parents (and teachers too) view a child's symptom as deliberate. This usually leads to a lot of criticism that worsens the child's self-esteem and also often worsens the behaviours (e.g. in tics and attention problems).

C: A minor behavioural problem may be interpreted by an anxious family as a sign that this child will turn out to have schizophrenia like another relative. The family will not be sure you are saying anything relevant, until you have addressed this concern.

E: If the family expects you to prescribe medicine, you need to explain why this is not the best or next step (if it isn't).

Asking the family about their ideas can sometimes give them the idea that you don't know what to do. This can be avoided by a relaxed manner, by being well informed, by offering choices, and by careful choice of words (http://www.gp-training.net/training/communication_skills/calgary/ice.htm).

Very few parents keep records, and even fewer keep reliable records. But even unreliable records are more reliable than the parents' memory.

Choosing causes from a list in this book

Within the lists, a few of the causes listed are ICD/DSM disorders. Many people view such terms as causes, though the idea of an umbrella is more accurate (see figure on p.385). If you can find more precise causes, these are more likely to lead to precisely targeted treatments.

If you cannot work out which of the entries in a table are most relevant, consider doing an ABC diary or a functional analysis (p.365).

In choosing which causes to consider further, keep in mind the need for a *full formulation* of the presenting problem and other notable findings (such as discrepancies or sensitive topics), for safety, reliability and persuasion; and the sometimes opposing requirement for the *simplest and most treatable* formulation. To some extent you will be driven by the family's request (e.g. for a diagnosis, an explanation, a rescue, advice on promoting development, or what to say to his brother). But if you try to do any of these without a full formulation you will be building on sand.

Multiple causes. The more people have already tried to help, and failed, the more likely it is that several causes are acting together. This is the sort of situation in which unnecessary disagreements arise, because individuals focus on just one contributory cause. A good place to start is to look for one or more current psychological motivations for a behaviour. On top of this, there are often longer-term causes such as genetic inheritance and upbringing, entrenched beliefs or family dynamics (see diagram, p.394). There may also be reasons why the normal inhibition against a behaviour fails to operate (p.261).

Hierarchical causes. Some of the lists refer to other lists. For example, the list for inattention shows that it can be caused by depression, and if you consider this a realistic possibility you need to then look up the causes of depression. This list suggests the possibility of child abuse, substance abuse, PANDAS, and even epilepsy, and if you think any of these is worth considering you are referred to separate sections on these.

Serial causes are frequently overlooked. A child may have moved through several stages, all of which need to be described in a full formulation. For example an inborn emotionality; then a learned/reinforced response to star charts; then learning that a demand for rewards can be used to control his or her parents; then feeling omnipotent and unsafe so talking about extreme feelings. For another example see *pervasive refusal*, p.527.

Symbolic causes lead a person to do something that represents something else (see also *symbols*, p.559). Symbols have several characteristics that are important clinically. They are learned; the meaning may only be in the mind of the child; they need to be translated; and they become more common with mental maturation. Obvious examples are a child wearing a jacket because he wants to be like his dad; or not using his arm because it is like his grandpa's arm that doesn't work; and religious and cultural practices from around the world. Symbolic explanations can be constructed for almost any presenting problem, but their vast explanatory power means their ability to account for a symptom *cannot* be used as confirmatory evidence. Occam's razor requires that they be adopted only as a last resort after looking for a neurologically simpler or demonstrably commoner explanation (for example, it is far more common to resist needles because they hurt, than because they symbolise illness). Symbolic explanations are more likely to be correct if other symbols with the same cognitive significance to the child have the same behavioural effect; and if symbols that are physically similar but without the same significance to the child do not. One needs to bear in mind that the child and family will often have already considered a symbolic cause.

Assessment hierarchies

Several factors govern the order in which one needs to think about the problems facing a child: *urgency, trust, reliability, importance to the family, general importance, exclusions,* and *logical dependence.*

- When booking an assessment, the following are indicators of *urgency*: escalating self-harm (or threats), escalating harm to others (or threats, especially to specific people), suspected abuse, suspected psychosis, escalating school exclusion, escalating dangerously impulsive or reckless behaviour, worsening function, worsening parental mental state.

- Demographic and uncontentious information should be sought first, and sensitive information later after the family have developed *trust.*

- Sometimes the whole assessment produces only vague or disputable problems. In such cases, build your thinking around the most solid facts (*reliable* facts with clear implications). These tend to be observations by staff (e.g. IQ; others on p.56) especially when the child is alone; family history; hard neurological signs (p.58); and physical investigations.

- In the session, you should first listen to the *concerns* of parents and teens; younger children's views are best sought later. Usually the parents' identification of the main problem is reasonable, but occasionally they are blind to a much bigger problem.

- Some issues have more *importance* or *influence* than others, because of dangerousness, severity, treatability, and the fact that some problems cause others. One should not spend much time on less important questions before the big issues are worked out. An assessment of the big issues is useful even if it defers consideration of smaller issues; but an assessment that focuses on small issues and ignores the big issues is often wrong and can be negligent. This is important in assessing causes (e.g. pp.14,131 and Maslow's pyramid, p.505).

- Some diagnoses have traditionally been thought to *exclude* others. This is sometimes shown as a pyramid (right), where each diagnosis trumps, or prevents, the diagnoses below it; for example DSM-IV specifies that ADHD ⬆ is not possible in autism ⬆. Such hierarchies have the benefit of focusing attention on the most enduring or severe conditions, but have the major disadvantage of removing attention from other conditions that people have simultaneously, that are sometimes even more disabling than the higher condition[153].

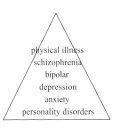

Figure 2. Diagnostic hierarchy (of exclusions).

- **Developmental** assessment, even if very brief, is first because it is needed for understanding symptoms. For example, the likely cause of children throwing things (p.103) or not attending school (p.217) depends very much on their mental age. More generally, short-term symptoms can often only be understood after longer-term difficulties are known. **Risk** is second: if risk is not adequately managed, the niceties of diagnosis are irrelevant. Risk includes the risk of untreated progressive physical illnesses, so these are considered here. You may need to reconsider risks again later after **processes** are better understood. This includes diagnoses, progression, interactions, etc. Resist the urge to focus the assessment on issues that you identify with, or are personally interested in, or on the basis of rarity, trauma, sympathy, interestingness, symbolism, or your background. These can all be given due attention later.

Diagnostic axes

The term *axis* implies that these areas of enquiry are independent of one another but this is generally not true (one level may simply restate another, or can cause or result from another[257]). Listing axes ensures that you have checked each one – but does not ensure that you have been sufficiently thorough with each. The most commonly used systems are:

Table 1. Multiaxial systems of diagnosis

	ICD-10 (modified)	DSM-IV
1	Behavioural and emotional disorders with onset usually occurring in childhood / adolescence	Clinical disorders
2	Developmental disorders	Personality disorders, Mental retardation
3	Intellectual level	General medical conditions
4	Medical condition	Psychosocial and environmental problems
5	Associated abnormal psychosocial situations	Global assessment of functioning

Another system, OPD-2 (p.519) distinguishes a patient's experience; relationships; conflicts; personality; plus ICD-10's axis 1 as shown in the table above[1194,1438].

Relating impairment criteria to single problems

(see also impairment with *multiple* problems, p.25).

For many disorders, DSM-IV requires "clinically significant distress or impairment in social, occupational, or other important areas of functioning." "Clinically significant distress" can obviously be interpreted in many ways. Definitions of *impairment* are much debated, but a fairly standard version is: any loss or abnormality of psychological, psychological, or anatomical structure or function (compare *disability*, p.452; *handicap*, p.476).

"Abnormality" is not defined, so there is a lot of room for the clinician's judgment. It can be relative to population norms, relative to how able the child would be if the disorder were suddenly taken away, relative to feasible alternatives (such as his or her level of function with medication or CBT) or to unfeasible alternatives (such as his level of function if provided with full time superb 1:1 supervision). In practice most clinicians try to estimate the second.

The fact that a child has been referred for assessment, and the parents have gone to the trouble of bringing the child, usually means that he or she has an impairment (for some exceptions see p.205). Some clinicians and health services are much more strict, operating an implicit triple filter: they exclude patients who are not impaired by some general measure; or who have symptoms less numerous than a DSM threshold; or whose (often familial) impairments prevent regular attendance and compliance.

There are other difficulties in DSM. One is the case of children who are obviously impaired while not satisfying any DSM diagnostic criteria [45,1254]. A more specific example is Tourette syndrome (p.101). This syndrome is *defined* in terms of tics, but it may be that the tics are just the most visible signs of the underlying disorder (less pathognomonic signs being ADHD-like and OCD-like matching behaviours). In this case, how could one be sure that the movements themselves were the main cause of social or emotional impairment? This is one of the reasons why impairment has slid in and out of the DSM criteria for this disorder.

Government and family thresholds differ

If a child has an IQ of 140 but is having difficulty keeping up with schoolwork due to inattentiveness, should the school adapt its lessons to keep him interested? Should it give him 1:1 attention for the same reason, bearing in mind this means a child at the opposite end of the IQ scale will be denied it? Should he be given medication for attention? Should he be eligible for any diagnosis at all? Many parents disagree with governments on these issues when their own child is affected.

Within children's health, state provision is relatively generous, so there is limited desire to "go private" either as a top-up or completely. There are also important (practical and emotional) difficulties in coordinating treatments between separate sites, so it is difficult to see a substantial future in public–private co-prescribing or talking therapies. However, families sometimes access private psychology assessments and second opinions. Some private practitioners become known for unusual clinical practice (e.g. using broader DSM categories, or not requiring population-normed impairment). This and the accusation of queue jumping sometimes make it easier for a patient to move from the state to private care than the reverse. Of course the wide disparities of clinical practice between state clinicians can lead to similar moves.

Unavoidable challenges in making a formulation

As humans, we habitually use heuristics (cognitive biases, p.534, or preferred ways of simplifying problems that usually help but sometimes hinder), that can interfere with clinical thinking[344,379]. The "representativeness" bias tries to match the patient against a prototype, or model patient, that we have in our head to represent each disorder. The "availability" bias favours easy-to-recall diagnoses. The "anchoring" bias makes us fixate too much on our first impressions, producing "premature closure" of thinking. The "fundamental attribution error" makes us overvalue long-term personality-based explanations for people's behaviour, and undervalue the effect of the situation they were in (see p.426).

Several strategies that help us to avoid these cognitive biases are combined in the "full integrative assessment" starting on p.22.

When is intuition useful?

Intuition is a belief based on instinct or feelings, without explainable reasoning to support it [1529]. It is always present, and sometimes has to be relied on, as when time constraints prevent full analysis of a situation. It is sometimes used as an excuse for not being thorough.

In judging risk: In the area of risk prediction, reliance on intuition can help clinicians (e.g. by making them feel they know what to do in a case of self-harm, thereby increasing efficiency or morale) but at the cost of strongly penalizing the tiny minority who, often using the exact same intuitions, fail to predict a disaster. There are also many examples of misguided professional intuition damaging families and children. The symbol ⊜ in this book indicates where risk is greatest, so intuition can be avoided.

In making diagnoses: Seniority, experience, and ability to cite precedents do not significantly increase reliability of predictions or diagnoses in the *psychological* arena[378]. So treasure people who make reliable judgments, whether they are experienced or not.

In making simple physical predictions: GPs tend to take a slightly more confident line regarding their intuition, but this is probably justified by their taking some objective measurements such as temperature, and their emphasis on predicting big issues (collapse, death) rather than more subtle things.

A sensible middle road is to allow intuition to make us more careful, but never less; and to use intuition more in the physical sphere (where things are relatively concrete) than in the psychological or social spheres.

Communicating the problems and treatments
(see pp.326-328 of [600])

To adolescents

- Talk about situations, problems and solutions from *their* point of view. Use themes they have mentioned are important to them, such as courage, dignity, integrity, tolerance or sacrifice[1172].

- Consider how much they already know, how much they will find out, and how much will help them, as opposed to upsetting or annoying them. If you decide to withold information from the teenager or the parent, make sure you discuss this privately with the other party first, otherwise there may be bafflement or awkward questions.

To parents

- Start your feedback with the problems that are foremost in their mind. Reach agreement on all the problems before discussing treatment. Tell them you will give them a written version so they don't worry about forgetting things. Consider telling them there are no bad surprises in the feedback, so they can relax and think better.

  - ► If the formulation is very complicated, you may well have made a mistake. Further discussion is needed. You will need to communicate a simple version to the family and other professionals. If the parents have ID, have a friend or counsellor present.

  - ► If part of the formulation is very unwelcome, e.g. the damaging effect of the parents' behaviour on the child, it can be presented as one of a list of possibilities, so it sounds non-judgmental and gets the parents thinking about causes – they may then "own" the decision about what the cause is. Consider asking the clinician with whom they were most comfortable to present their version of this. If the family get upset, remain calm and sympathetic, and offer a break or a follow-up session.

- Some explanations are more *acceptable* to parents than others, and this strongly affects how you discuss it with them. It is usually easier for parents to accept that their child has several specific learning disabilities, than that he has a general ID. Problems in the parents themselves usually require "re-framing" to be accepted, e.g. "we need to find a way of getting more food into Johnny".

Table 2. Hierarchy of acceptability of causes to parents

Problems in child	Problems in parents
Semantic pragmatic disorder (p.546)	Too-good parenting (p.190)
ADHD, Dyslexia	over-protectiveness
Specific Learning Disability	exhaustion
Pathological Demand Avoidance (p.527)	mental illness (p.191)
Most mental illnesses	unpredictability
Schizophrenia, Autism	intolerance / rigidity
General ID	
Cancer (p.569)	Munchausen's / abuse
Huntington's (p.482)	

> ▶ If the formulation is stigmatising it needs to be presented slowly, calmly, sympathetically and non-judgmentally.

> ▶ If the formulation involves a deteriorating prognosis, double-check your ideas, find a quiet place, and prepare them with your demeanour. Avoid shock by giving a warning combined with a link to what the person already knows: "I know you've been wondering what the cause is. What ideas have you had?" Most importantly, do not take away all hope. Offer a follow-up session.

- Remember that listing numerous problems may impress professional readers (or yourself) without being helpful to the patient. Minor diagnoses distract attention from major ones. A diagnosis you make may be unusable, wrong, woolly, obvious (e.g. if it applies to almost everyone), trivial, or even worse – distracting, or damaging to self-esteem or to professionals' relationship with the family. If you do list numerous problems, be clear about which one or two you see as most important.

- If a diagnosis has previously been made by another professional, you need to consider the parents' view of this, and the quality of that professional/formulation, before deciding what is the most useful formulation to present to the parents. For example, if the diagnosis of ADHD was made five years ago, and you are convinced that it was wrong, and that family chaos or abuse was the real cause, it may be best to leave the question of ADHD alone while you persuade the family that there is an *additional* problem that you have noticed and can help with. If you try to convince them that they were wrong, and the previous doctor was wrong, and you know better, all at the same time, you will need very strong interpersonal skills to convince them!

- Prioritise the treatments, based on importance to child and family; likelihood of treatment success; availability and acceptability of treatment, etc. In most cases you should be offering a selection of social, educational, psychological, systemic and medical treatments.

To other professionals

- Confidentiality. Information should be disclosed on a "need to know" basis (see p.413).

Multiple symptoms occurring together

If a child has multiple symptoms, look them all up, in the main causelists or the index. Occasionally there is a single simple explanation for all the symptoms, which can be identified by comparing the lists. More often there are multiple contributory factors. If the child has physical problems as well, look them up in the glossary to find the behavioural implications.

When a child's problems are numerous, they are less likely to just go away. When they are comorbid (p.442), complex, or persistent, they are far more likely to cause distress, to cause problems in peer relations, and to be referred[149,1792]. It is tempting to stop assessing as soon as a single diagnosis or other explanation is found – but the extreme tendency to comorbidity in child mental health means that your confirming one problem makes other problems *more* rather than *less* likely[775,1431]. For example, sexual abuse is much more likely to lead to presentation or admission, if the child has suffered other abuse as well, or has neurodevelopmental problems, or is not supported by a good relationship with her parents.

These diagrams illustrate the complex causal networks leading to presenting complaints (green dots) and their sequelae.

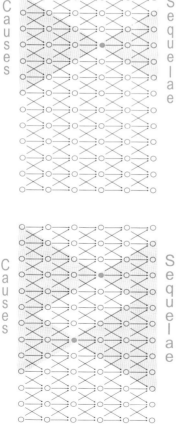

◀ Brief assessments focus on causes and sequelae of the presenting complaint. They are appropriate in:

- high-fliers (or previous high-fliers) who need less assessment because most aspects are likely to be OK, and as soon as you find a problem you have a fair chance that it is the only one

- emergency services, or hard-pressed services that have been reduced to fire fighting

- tier 1–2 services with few treatments available

- perhaps if you are just offering a second opinion which will be carefully considered by the referrer and family.

◀ Exhaustive assessment is justified if:

- there are multiple problems, as shown by the two green dots, with their causes and effects having potential to interact

- previous more focused assessments didn't produce a solution that worked

- a child has never functioned well (because they tend to have more things wrong with them)

- you are making decisions rather than recommendations.

Figure 3. Interacting difficulties require broader assessment.

Overview of a full integrative assessment

The following overall approach to assessment is safe for staff and patients, fun, logically sensible, and makes a considerable contribution to the team's intellectual development and interagency working. It also allows you to match team members to interviewees. More subtly, it also produces well-measured judgments of severity, priority and the weight given to the referrer's and parents' opinions.

1.   Getting started

- To do this really well requires multiple staff with different backgrounds and training, who have seen different conditions recently and who are involved in treatment as well. Ideally there will be biological, psychological and social participants, including at least one non-CAMHS staff, e.g. a paediatrician or teacher.

- Have a very recent broad-based informal school report. If the assessment has been triggered by specific episodes, make sure you have first-hand accounts of them. Also have all the previous reports available, not just because they save time and act as second opinions to your own, but also because they help work out when things started to go wrong. They can give you an idea of the best functioning a child is capable of, e.g. pre-regression; and also the opposite: autism symptoms tend to be most severe at age 4−6, so reports from that age may be diagnostically more clear-cut than later assessments. Don't look at all this information until you have spent an hour with the family, so you form an independent view (this is very useful for assessing yourself).

- If you don't feel confident about taking a medical and developmental history, ask the parents to complete a standard questionnaire before the appointment (e.g. the Child Neuropsychology Questionnaire[107]).

- Start taking the history with an open mind. Even forget everything you ever learned − at least the categories − while figuring out the pattern. You can categorise later.

2.   Information gathering

- Do the whole assessment in one block of time so the details are fresh in your mind.

- Being relaxed and sympathetic will reveal more information (p.11)

- Wide-ranging semi-structured interviews (using a proforma such as that in the appendix, p.399; or pp.30−34 of [600]) are fairly unnatural and time consuming, but they have the great benefit of being tried and tested ways of revealing the information that is likely to be useful. If you rely on the referrer, parent and your judgment to obtain all the relevant information you are taking a risk of missing something important, albeit a risk that reduces with experience. If we find a cause that could account for the child's current problem, we can permit ourselves an "aha" moment, but only a little one, because we need to continue looking for other contributory factors too: the first one we found may turn out to have been smaller or less remediable than others [1799]. This is especially important in Child Mental Health because many factors contribute to many different outcomes.

- Don't consider trying to assess the situation without spending time with the child, as some clinicians do (amazingly). For teenagers this will form the bulk of the assessment, and for preschoolers a lesser part. For many older children, the direction, "Tell me the things you didn't want to talk about in front of your mother" works better than an open question. (Remember also to ask a similar question of parents.)

If a child is not talking much, try non-spoken communication. For example, get him to join in preparing a glass of juice for himself, or a cup of tea for mum. Ask him to "give me five" (p.378) or to draw dad (p.56), or to write what his best friend would write about him (including his best friend describing his difficulties in a very kind way). The Beck Youth Inventory explores many symptoms in a checklist way. Also free play while you talk to mum, such as being left with a pile of toys or some crayons or a computer, will often reveal the child's interests and skills.

- Make a genogram of three generations (p.203).

- Ideally use multiple family members and multiple staff professions.

- Small rooms are good for quiet confidential discussions, but large rooms are better for observing behaviours, for seeing whole families, and for having multiple staff simultaneously assessing and observing. Passive observation of the entire family in a large room for several hours in a row (with breaks for food) is usually very revealing of personalities, degree of severity and habitual responses. It is useful to get the children thoroughly bored with an intentional shortage of toys, to see what they and the parents do. After this, toys can be introduced. The time can be productively passed by working through standard assessments with the parents in the corner of the room. This also makes the parents and children feel they are not being watched.

- Don't avoid embarrassing questions. Lists in this book can be openly worked through with parents so they realise you are not being wrongly intrusive or accusatory.

- **Make a brief list of 1−10 items that need explanation. This should include all the presenting complaints and any significant abnormalities or surprises (paradoxes, p.523) from the data trawl.**

3. Formulating

Once you have a broad range of information, try the following:

- *Simplify the task*: Don't consider confidentiality, practicality, or child's and parents' wishes in making your initial working formulation.

- You need an **array of diagnoses, categories, or processes**, to organise your thinking. The list of diagnoses in ICD/DSM is a good start, though there are many other sensible additions to this list, as shown in this book. Yet most individual child mental health professionals use only a small set of diagnoses in their day-to-day work, tending to "see" or recognise primarily behavioural or systemic or DSM or developmental categories of problems. These are determined by the degree of focus in our training, our own intellectual limitations, personal preferences in the ways we like to work, research interests, drug company advertising, and also by the mix of patients that we see. These factors are often far from benign, and contribute to a gradual *decline* in effectiveness through a clinician's career[292,378,758]. It is important to work in ways that stop us falling into these ruts, such as multidisciplinary working; seeing a broad range of referrals; continuing education (with active debating and speaking); using diagnostic tools that absorb new ideas automatically (e.g. patient-based literature searches); and assessing thoroughly before we treat.

- *However*, the question of how you work out whether a **particular diagnosis** applies to a particular child is more problematic. There are many symptom lists available (see [423]), of which the DSM and ICD are pre-eminent due to their usefulness in running randomised controlled trials and finding the results of these; they have quasi-legal roles in service organisation, education and in court. All the checklists are useful for ensuring that you have gathered enough information to consider the diagnosis. The checklist designers usually have superb clinical knowledge which can be gleaned from the lists (and supporting literature); and the scales are indisputably useful for tracking treatment progress. Unfortunately many parents, managers and even clinicians fall into the trap of believing that such **checklist diagnoses** are sufficient for understanding children:

  - Neither the DSM nor the other checklists adequately indicate how to judge what is normal, what is abnormal but more relevant to a different disorder, what is abnormal but not worrying, what is impairing (p.17), or how having one disorder affects the features of others (see Conundrums listed on p.5).

  - Cognitive bias (p.534) is created by focusing on just a few checklists. Many checklists measure little more than how right we were in choosing that particular list; and if we complete the checklist in full expectation of what we expect the outcome to be then the impression of impartiality is false. Such diagnoses then attract unjustified weight over other areas not explored in such detail.

  - The descriptions of symptoms in the checklists are less precise than they appear. Clinicians are expected to use experience to work out whether the child has the symptom in a way that is relevant to the disorder in question. Parents often produce different diagnoses from clinicians, sometimes by not considering alternative explanations (hence the cross- references from pp.387–391 to other parts of the book).

  - A few children are profoundly impaired by small numbers of symptoms yet they fail to meet the "number of symptoms" criteria in DSM/ICD [45,1254]. This is widely recognised in clinical practice, where thresholds to obtain treatment are determined more by impairment (p.17) than by symptom counts. You need to make a clinical judgment about whether this diagnosis is a sensible way to categorise the child, and to obtain appropriate help for him or her.You can write "this child essentially meets the criteria for xxx disorder" or similar.

  - DSM / ICD diagnoses provide useful links to evidence-based treatments for populations, but not for the particular child sitting in the consulting room. If a child's mood is lowered by bullying or inadequate sleep, those are the relevant issues, not the statistical associations between DSM/ICD categories and these or other factors [1123].

  - ICD is based on the notion of syndromes. It encourages the clinician to search for the best possible single diagnosis, i.e. it discourages diagnosis of comorbidity (p.442). However, the idea that you should distil the child's problems to one diagnosis is nonsense given the complexity of the brain, and the increased likelihood of comorbid conditions being referred. DSM on the other hand employs a "pattern recognition" approach in which matching the criteria for one diagnosis does not interfere with the possibility of making another diagnosis as well.

- You face several challenges not addressed by DSM/ICD, before you reach the most useful possible understanding of the problem:
  - When there are several possible explanations for the problem, find a way to decide between them (see p.365). Or choose the one that is the most specific (e.g. either anxiety or language disability can cause some of the problems of ASD and both are more specifically treatable). Or perhaps the one that is most useful for mother, your colleagues, and the local education department.
  - Working out which symptoms are impairing is not just an academic question (see also impairment with *single* problems, p.17). Most referred children have multiple "symptoms", so one might argue that the main task of assessment is to work out which symptom(s) are most impairing, in order to treat them first. In some cases this is easy because the impairment and symptoms started at about the same time. In complex cases, though, even when a full formulation involving multiple predisposing, precipitating, perpetuating, protective and feedback causes is available, assignment of impairment is impractical and treatment planning may be organised differently, i.e. on the basis of the treatability and dangerousness of symptoms; the availability and acceptability of treatments; and the principle of treating as close to the "root" of the problems as possible.

    You will often meet a child with multiple problems, that act together to impair him, yet he has obtained no help, because one problem prevents him using standard treatments for the other; or on the grounds that none of the individual problems is severe enough to justify treatment, or to have been the basis of a randomised controlled trial.
  - You need to look for other features that are not in DSM/ICD:
    - psychological processes (e.g. perception, learning, memory, adaptation, thinking, motivation and emotion)
    - cognitive distortions or biases (p.534)
    - interactional patterns in the family (p.211)
    - any other factors that can guide treatment (p.393).
  - Make a formulation (p.468), and also attempt to make a diagnosis[1598]. Formulations are more useful than diagnosis when (a) the child needs to achieve trust; (b) the child needs to deal with an inner conflict/cognitive dissonance (p.355); (c) the child's identity (or lifestyle, etc.) is at risk [1598], (d) when the problem is a learned behaviour such as excess use of imaginary friends (p.231); (e) when a teenager will rebel against a label more than against an idea; (f) when the label misleadingly pathologises the child, as in Conduct Disorder (☝ p.249) and Attachment Disorders (☝ p.195); (g) when the DSM is clearly wrong, e.g. in omitting the "not better explained by another disorder" in the definitions of PDDs or prohibiting diagnosis of ADHD in the presence of autism (which is widely viewed as a mistake and is ignored). DSM/ICD are weak in these areas (a–g), though many cases of a,b,c could be broadly described as anxiety.

- Ways of thinking
  - ○ Brainstorm to find the simplest formulation able to account for all of the abnormal items. The lists of "causes to consider" in this book help broaden one's thinking. Background knowledge of clinical features, age, sequence, comorbidities, etc., help to eliminate impossible explanations.
  - ○ Colour-matching/pattern-recognition, labels. This happens automatically after you have seen a few hundred cases, and it would require a lot of very methodical thinking (about DSM, comorbidity, research, etc.) to achieve it much sooner. It is also useful to recognise that x is different from what you expected.
  - ○ Intuitive, like a GP: what is the salient feature today: what do they want today?
  - ○ Use a scientist's or detective's approach, making and testing hypotheses during history taking. Ideally, try always to have a list of alternatives in mind, and be exploring evidence for branches of a "tree" of possible explanations. With increasing experience, you can recognise sooner which branches are less likely to be productive. This kind of "exploratory assessment" necessarily takes longer than the pattern-recognition approach.

> A quick route to formulation: Complete a P,P,P,P table (p.394) for an individual child, then isolate the unusual aspects in the table and weave a story around them, that can explain the presenting problems and all other unusual findings. Think mainly about findings that are clear, undisputed, and have high predictive value.

4.   Checking

  - ○ Ideally, work out which parts of your formulation are least certain, what are the alternatives in those places, and what further information will help you decide. This is particularly important when some of the possible causes are easily overlooked (marked by ☞ in this book) or urgent/potentially emergency (marked with ‼).
  - ○ *Discuss, debate, go back to the family and ask more questions.* Institutionalise staff time for discussion and debate: this is most effective if staff feel comfortable enough to think broadly and express their ideas freely.
  - ○ *Use the family* to check your conclusions: they know more about the child than you do, and your conclusions need to be both understood and believed by them (in almost all cases).
  - ○ If you are not sure, consider *reassessing* in a day or month; using investigations or treatments to clarify the situation (pp.365,371); getting a second opinion; or a trial of stopping stressors (e.g. see *overwork*, p.521).

Cognition

Causelist 1: Poor results in school or testing☼

This has first place in the book because it needs to be considered in every child, even when it is not the presenting complaint. Knowing a child's developmental level is a prerequisite for understanding his or her behaviour. Children referred with behavioural problems are far more likely to have cognitive problems than the children who are not referred.

Comprehensive school reports, including examples of recent written and drawing work, are indispensable to reliable assessment (see p.371). The teacher's assessment of mood is also useful: severe emotional problems can prevent learning for years, and conversely cognitive problems can severely damage confidence.

It is crucial to distinguish between not having skills, not having the ability to acquire them, and not demonstrating them. Children with normal performance on an IQ test may function in the ID range on tests of attainment (e.g. National Curriculum or WIAT) for many reasons listed in the accompanying table.

Problems are not often confined to just a single area (as in dyslexia, p.51; callosal agenesis, p.445), but a single area can be spared (e.g. children with severe ID often have excellent gross motor skills, presumably because this is subcortically controlled).

Of the three umbrella concepts of developmental psychiatry (ADHD, autism, and ID – pages 83, 183 and 498 respectively), ID is where functional subdivisions are least recognised. Currently a CAMHS worker is doing well to reliably recognise the following *functional* areas: levels of ID, verbal and non-verbal learning disability, and some so-called "specific" problems that can be usefully remedied or bypassed (e.g. poor speech, poor reading, p.149).

Nomenclature is a sensitive issue, discussed on p.498. Regression means loss of skills (p.41).

Contributory factors in poor performance	Notes
Not actually poor performance	
Not living up to parents' expectations	High-achieving family
Inappropriate test	e.g. the Flynn effect, p.59
Can't learn well	
👁 Intellectual disability (low intelligence)	Isolated areas of (relatively) high performance can be caused by assiduous parental teaching. Often causes school refusal (p.217), and multiple cognitive problems wrongly described as "specific". Commonly overlooked in immigrant families (p.488)
Uncomplicated delay Specific learning disability	Family history of delay; no physical problems (p.551)
Verbal-performance (VP) discrepancy	A *substantial* difference between verbal and performance scores on IQ testing. 6% of the population have a verbal IQ 20 points lower than their performance IQ, and 6% have the reverse[148]. The latter group is one of the definitions of NVLD (see below)
Non-verbal learning disability (NVLD)	There is no consensus on the best way to define or detect this, e.g. performance IQ 20 points below verbal IQ; or 20% below; or 10 points below verbal IQ with other criteria used as well[429]. For test interpretation, see p.33 and[429]; and for the distinction from Asperger's see[414]. The term *learning disability* within *NVLD* uses the DSM/American sense (see p.498), so does not imply anything about the full scale IQ.
	Though not in DSM, NVLD is crucial for teachers, EPs, and parents to know about. The child is articulate, possibly enjoying English but hating maths, science, and geography, often misbehaving in school, or not paying attention (p.82), or anxious about attending. If the NVLD is accompanied by good verbal intelligence, the result is fluent speech lacking in ideas or structure – there can be denials, disengagement, or rude practiced excuses. People with NVLD are sometimes labelled as argumentative because they repetitively produce illogical arguments. They also cannot understand normal reasons, so are very difficult to persuade. For example, a highly articulate boy with NVLD and needle phobia rebuffed every attempt at reasoning about the blood tests, with practised and superficially logical excuses, but was completely unable to weigh the pros and cons of having the test (in the end he was persuaded in an essentially non-cognitive way, by a staff member who spent enough time with him to build up trust).

continued ▶

Questions useful in screening depend on age, e.g. can he tell time, estimate distances, tell whether a bird or plane is faster; or a bike or loaf is bigger, work out change (or even that there should be change).

It may be that NVLD can be caused by any condition in which the neocortex's connectivity (p.444) is sufficiently disrupted[1385,1483,1683]. Hence a large number of physical conditions have been implicated: Fragile X, p.468; Turner syndrome, p.570; Williams syndrome, p.177; VCFS, p.572; callosal agenesis, p.445; Cornelia de Lange syndrome, p.445; hydrocephalus, p.482; chemotherapy; leukodystrophy, p.498; foetal alcohol syndrome, p.467; multiple sclerosis, p.510; traumatic brain injury, p.477; Sotos syndrome, p.551; congenital hypothyroidism, p.485; septo-optic dysplasia, p.547; and chemotherapy/toxic encephalopathy.

Poor vision or hearing	(Screening tests in clinic: see vision, p.133; deafness, p.130)
Disorganisation	Sometimes seen with dyspraxia (see clumsiness, p.89)
Memory problems	(p.37)
Cerebral palsy	(p.437)
☞ Physical problems	When major these can reduce opportunities for learning
☞ Medical /genetic	The most important to detect are the treatable causes, p.32
Learns usually but not recently	
☞ Regression	(p.41)
Avoidance (p.429)	• Caught in dilemmas – may avoid discussion of difficult subjects, e.g. marriage in general or her parents' marriage. • Shyness, p.181; other anxiety, e.g. selective mutism, p.153. • (see also *Learned avoidance* below).
Wrong attitude (p.425) to homework or schooling	
OCD	(p.65), with repeated checking or crossing out. On IQ testing, often has a low "processing speed" score, p.36
Sleepy	(p.321)
Rebellion	Against swot label or parental pressure
Relationships	e.g. Bad relationship with teacher, such as threats and sarcasm
Lack of confidence	Well engaged with simple questions. Often due to unrecognised educational difficulty. May be due to problems with parents, teacher, or peers.
Boredom	Child may have outpaced class, or lessons are repetitive
Preoccupied / interested in something else	Autism (p.183), books, family problems, bullying (p.219), abuse (pp.273-275), obsessions (p.517), tics (p.101), ruminations (p.543)
☞ Depression	(p.309)

Drugs	Anticonvulsants, antihistamines, sedatives, solvents in lunch hour
Medical	• ☞ Epilepsy (subclinical, esp. petit mal) (p.73)
	• Head injury previously dismissed as trivial (p.477)
	• ☞ See treatable causes of ID, p.32

Can learn but hardly ever did

Autism ☂	(p.183)
Learned avoidance (p.429)	Suspect this if general milestones are slightly delayed, but test results are behind them, and are falling further behind peers. Child doesn't engage even with the simplest questions (IQ testing always starts with these). This is most common as a partial picture, with the child opting out of just those subtests he thinks might prove difficult, producing some isolated low subtest scores. The same occurs in conversation, so it is helpful to start with simple questions (p.405). It is a rare child who doesn't want to do work if he can (see p.527).
Language different at home	Especially if mother doesn't speak English. Usually only a problem in the first year or two of school. Consider selective mutism (p.153).

Can learn but not taught

Lack of learning opportunities	E.g. few toys, prolonged or repeated absences from school, or no suitable place for homework
Unusual verbal environment at home	Dual language delays language by a few months. Poor interactions (e.g.maternal depression, p.174) have broader effects.
Schooling problem	e.g. school for ID; incompatible teaching assistant
He has been treated as a little child	i.e. not stretched or given responsibilities. Rewarded with cuddles for acting immature.

Can learn, but doesn't use the learning well

Hyperactivity, impulsivity, inattention	Often familial (p.79). Inattention can also be caused by *any* of the other causes of delay in this table.
Malingering	(p.503)

Investigations to find the cause of ID in a child

Some have claimed that it is possible to find the underlying cause of ID in 80% of children with IQ below 50, and 40% of children with IQ from 50 to 70[563]. Other published results have much lower figures. In any case, using a hierarchical approach to diagnosis, as shown below, improves efficiency. Details vary depending on local resources, but the overview (broad arrows) needs to be completed before any deeper investigations (narrow arrows) are considered. For more details see p.32 and[559].

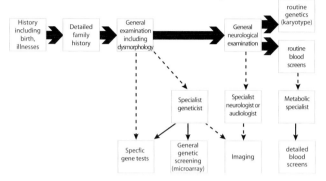

Figure 4. Sequence of investigations for ID.

Pros and cons
The amount of investigation that is justified depends on the situation. Children who suffer through their disability deserve the most detailed possible assessment of *treatability*. Carers can obtain support, information, and *practical help* more easily with precise diagnoses. Parents and siblings of a disabled child who want further children justify the most detailed possible assessments of *risk*. (This last category is often worth deferring a few years, as genetics is advancing so fast[124].)

Some of the more precise diagnoses can actually make life more difficult for some parents, by confirming a degenerative course, or by making them feel there are no other parents nearby who have similar problems; or by confusing them into thinking that *all* the child's difficulties are due to the disorder and are untreatable. The rarer diagnoses can also disempower clinicians, making them wonder whether they know enough to help this family (they always do, because most principles of behavioural and social management are universal).

Knowing the past
In general, if one finds a factor known to be *associated* with ID, one cannot be certain that it *caused* the ID, or the extent to which it did so. For several examples of this, see p.553 and *birth*, p.432.

Genetic causes
You are most likely to succeed in finding a *genetic* cause if there are multiple objective physical signs (especially if they are in multiple bodily systems); if there is a positive family history including similar symptoms or unexplained deaths in infancy; if there is an objectively demonstrable true regression; or if there is a history of metabolic crises (p.381). If you have found any of these it is invaluable to consult a geneticist (p.379), even by phone. If you are looking for a *genetic* cause of ID in a child who has none of these factors, then the search is likely to fail, as there are hundreds of known genetic causes, which when combined account for only a minority of cases of ID[818].

Investigation Planner 1: Treatable causes of ID

Some of the most treatable causes are already screened at birth using the "heelprick test". Hence it is very important to test children who missed this test, though parental preference or place of birth. The heelprick test used in the UK in 2009 includes phenylketonuria, p.529; hypothyroidism, p.485; sickle, p.549; cystic fibrosis, p.450; MCADD, p.418.

Many other treatable causes exist, especially in developing countries[1705]. The most common are listed below. In *developed* countries the treatable causes add up to only a few percent of ID.There are many partial forms of disorders (p.384), some of which are treatable. See also the *general approach to medical investigations*, p.373.

	Signs	Test	Excluded clinically or to Order?	Date ordered	Result
Basic tests		Heelprick, chromosomes (p.439), Fragile X			
Thyroid	Hypothyroid: p.485 hyperthyroid: p.484	T3,T4, TSH			
Petit mal status, subclinical epilepsy	p.73	EEG			
Environmental / infective (see general discussion, p.490)					
HIV	p.479	p.479			
Schistosomiasis	p.543	FBC,IgG			
Tuberculosis	p.569	p.569			
Malnutrition	p.504	FBC,LFT			
Genetic (see pp.379,203)					
PKU	p.529	Amino acids			
Homocystinuria	p.481	Amino acids			
Late-onset urea cycle	p.571	Ammonia			
Occipital Horn syndrome	Connective tissue problems: skin & joint laxity, tortuous blood vessels, hernias, dysautonomia, mild or no ID[422]. This is a partial version of Menkes, p.330.	Copper, caerulo-plasmin			
Hartnup disease	p.477	Amino acids			
Cerebro-tendinous xanthomatosis	Chronic diarrhoea with juvenile cataracts (p.436). In school years, seizures & ID. After age 10, xanthomas in tendons esp. Achilles, and in brain[147]. There are many distinct mutations.	Family history, examination, plasma chole-stanol, cheno-deoxycholate, hyperintense dentate on MRI			
Coenzyme Q10 deficiency	p.508	p.508			
Hydrocephalus (early or late onset)	Easily missed after skull fusion, see p.482	MRI			
Mucopoly-saccharidoses	p.501	p. 501			
Some leuko-dystrophy	p.498	MRI			
Biotin (vitamin B₇) deficiency or biotin-related metabolic error	Perioral dermatitis, alopecia, ataxia, seizures, ID[821]; white matter disease, p.574	"Carboxylase activation index" or urinary biotin (see[821])			
Glutaric acid-uria type 1[867] (GA1, GCDH deficiency)	Develops dystonia after metabolic crises (p.381). Macrocephaly (p.502) appears earlier. Rare.	Glutaryl-carnitine in dried blood spots			
Combination					
Cumulation of individually small effects	(e.g.ADHD, anaemia, p.421; severely deficient stimulation, interrupted sleep, chronic infections, p.490; others above)	Thorough history and examination, tests above			

Causelist 2: Inconsistent performance in testing

When two results seem to contradict each other, the first question is whether this reflects an enduring discrepancy within the child, real variability, maturation, or mere artefact. Sometimes this can be clarified by comparing multiple test results, or by doing the optional subtests that weren't used the first time, or repeating the test with subtests in a different order, after a reasonable delay (often six months to minimise the practice effect, but numerical tests are forgotten faster so they can be repeated sooner).

The second question is **how to summarise** the inconsistent performance. This is worth some thought, especially if allocation of community resources will be based on a single number (the full scale IQ) or on a category of ID (as in the table on p.60). Even in such cases, the most useful part of your report may be your suggestions regarding any contributory difficulties that can be alleviated.   Several factors influence the way you describe the child's performance: whether the discrepancy is fixed or variable; whether it is consistent with your clinical observations of the child; and who needs to be convinced by the report. Options, none of which are fully satisfactory, include: (a) exclude the outliers and give a good explanation for why they are unrepresentative. For example, if you think a child has a specific learning disability, give the score in that area as well as a baseline score, which should be calculated by omitting the low score. For example if the verbal score is 60 and the others are 80, 90, and 100, this can be summarised as a baseline ability level of 90, with a specific deficit in the verbal area at 60; (b) give a simple average of all the subscores (this is reasonable only if you have excluded the causes of inconsistency listed on these pages). This can be given in verbal form as "[name] is functioning as a child with [mild, moderate, severe] level of ID but the precise level will need to be clarified on further testing in a year or so"; (c) emphasise the highest scores, making clear that your aim is to emphasise the child's *strengths* (see also discussion on p.568); (d) emphasise the lowest scores; the accompanying prose report should give reasons why these are a fair indicator of a child's *needs*. (e) simply report that the full scale IQ cannot be calculated due to the discrepant subscores; this often does not help a psychologically unsophisticated audience.

Artefactual discrepancies

- Retesting within a few months often increases scores, though this increase is smaller in subtests involving numbers (see discussion above).
- If the child actively dislikes the test administrator, he will avoid eye contact and certainly not ask her about holidays, so even a superb test such as ADOS (p.183) can then give a very misleading assessment of his social interest. This is called *hostile non-compliance*.
- If the subtests are repeated in the same order, the child may consistently grow bored or discouraged at the same point in testing.

Change in ability between test episodes

- Many test results improve in autism[521] and in late developers (p.496).
- Consider the many causes of inattention (p.79) and regression (p.41).
- Many medicines affect test performance (p.568).

Real-world changeability in the child

- Worsening during a test is often due to boredom (p.322), tiredness, or hunger. Hand pain can impair writing tasks. Improvement during a test can be due to figuring out a strategy for the task. Variability over time can be due to anxiety; performing mental rituals (e.g. compulsions) when she is by herself; variable concentration (p.79), behavioural regression (p.41), ruminations (p.543), unrecognised triggers (such as arguments at home, lack of sleep, or who's next to her in the classroom); or if the child is trying to hear what his mother is saying. Many of these causes of poor effort can be detected above a mental age of about 8 by the child's getting exceptionally easy questions wrong [183]. Note that these characteristics can also indicate malingered cognitive deficits (p.503), though this is rare at such an early age. Many of the causes of intermittent problems (pp.61,63,77,69) can also cause fluctuations in performance. Don't forget delirium (p.451).

- Social anxiety (p.298) can make a child perform much less well on verbal tests than on written ones, or better with testers she is comfortable with.

- Factors in the session: sleepiness, p.321; boredom, p.322; medication, p.568; time of day (especially if medicine wears out during testing); expectation (of needles etc).

- Mums often fear that "He hides it in public so you won't see how bad it gets" but other explanations for good behaviour in clinic are more likely, e.g. not respecting the parent's rules, or being more relaxed at home. There are many ways to maximise the chances of seeing the problem behaviour: long sessions (or several in one day), observation in a corridor or waiting room, bringing the siblings along too and letting them play together in a large room with toys while pretending to ignore them, and occasionally observation from behind a one-way mirror, or watching home videos.

- Look for provocations/barbs from parents, or innocuous comments that an adolescent may interpret as barbs.

continued ▶

Enduring, repeatable discrepancies in the child

A child's difficulties with tests
- If the child performs worse in test situations than in real life, consider performance anxiety, p.298.
- There are many reasons for performance being worse in formal written exams than in coursework. The coursework can be elevated by help from parents, or by massive investment of time. Alternatively the exam performance can be lowered by anxiety, p.298; poor essay organisation or handwriting, p.53; tics, p.101; or being rigidly unable to skip questions he doesn't know, p.234.

Isolated low scores (For widespread low ability or attainment see p.27)
- Specific Learning Disabilities (p.551) such as dyslexia and dyscalculia (pp.51,457) are defined based on the performance in a specific area being substantially behind that expected from overall intelligence. Poor performance in timed subtests can be due to dyspraxia or anxiety.
- Because of the content of the questions in the "comprehension" subtest, a low score here can indicate lack of *social* understanding.
- If he performs worse on easy questions than hard ones, consider boredom, p.322; or malingering, p.503. Somewhat similarly, because self-care builds on eye-hand coordination, self-care being years behind coordination (e.g. using the subtests of the Griffiths) sometimes indicates that mother is helping the child too much.
- Occasionally it is possible to be even more precise about a child's problems. In the WAIS-III, "a much reduced Digit Span backwards, compared to forwards, indicates an executive difficulty and if this is accompanied by a selective difficulty in Similarities and/or Picture Arrangement, the evidence for a Dysexecutive syndrome is even greater. A disproportionate difficulty with Picture Completion can indicate a semantic processing deficit implicating the left temporal lobe, even though Picture Completion is a subtest within the Performance Scale. Selective difficulty with Arithmetic and Digit Span may highlight a left parietal dysfunction… The subtest Digit Symbol Coding is a Performance subtest but is directly influenced by a left parietal lesion resulting in acquired dyslexia."[1050]

Isolated high scores
- Highly involved parents often have the child practise standard memorisable tasks such as counting fingers, the letters of the alphabet, reading short words, and writing his name. Furthermore, for children under 10, such memorised information can produce relatively good school marks. School marks, and marks in these specially memorised tasks, are therefore not a reliable indicator of cognitive ability.
- In autism (p.183), isolated areas of (absolute or relative) high performance can be caused by special interests.

Patterns of discrepancies affecting multiple scores
- Reasons for outlying scores in IQ testing are listed in the table at the right, which is based on the WISC-IV but is applicable to most IQ tests. The narrow columns at the right of the table indicate the main functional loads imposed by the test, so you can test hypotheses that all his lowest subtest scores were caused by one underlying problem. For example, if the child's lowest scores are all in written subtests, there are several possible causes of this (p.53). However, note that discrepancies of less than 10−15% are within the noise of the testing and are generally not relevant (for more discussion of this see p.28).

(For general information on IQ tests see p.59.)

Table 3. Components of IQ tests

Subscores / Indices in IQ tests	Subtests	visuo-motor	con-centr-ation	attain-ment	lang-guage
There are many reasons for the **verbal** scores to be lower. It is very important to consider these (p.151) before assuming that the child has an innate language disability. If the verbal scores are *higher*, see the comment below regarding outlying subtest scores.	**Vocabulary** – define a word (tests receptive and expressive vocabulary)			*	*
	Similarities – say how two words are alike/similar. Differences and similarities appear in many cognitive tests. Many children do better in differences, though this does not apply to the easiest similarities (e.g. what is the same about a bird and a plane), because these have a single word answer and have been practised many times in school			*	*
	Comprehension, many of then involving social situations			*	*
	Information (general knowledge)			*	*
	Word reasoning (serial clues eventually permit an answer to be chosen)				*
If the **perceptual** IQ scores are considerably lower than the verbal ones, this usually indicates non-verbal learning disability (p.28). *However* if a single language subtest (such as vocabulary or spelling) is far above the other language subtests, this indicates the child has had a great deal of practice in this area. In such cases the single subtest artificially inflates the language composite score, so dropping it gives a truer indication of ability.	**Block Design** – put together plastic blocks to match a displayed model. Autistic children characteristically do well on Block Design subtests because they are not distracted by the whole picture (see p.163). Extensive play with Lego can also selectively inflate the Block Design score.	*			
	Picture concepts – work out which pictures go together				
	Matrix reasoning – fill in the missing square in an array		*		
	Picture completion – say what is missing in a picture				
An isolated problem in **working memory** subtests is commonly accompanied by inattentiveness in class, with difficulty in reading and maths, and in about half with low self-esteem[28]. It is occasionally due to fits occurring during presentation, or between presentation and response[147]. This applies mainly to children with known epilepsy.	**Digit span** (p.452). Poor performance here is often associated with poor attention at school (p.79).		*		
	Letter-number sequencing – from jumbled up letters and numbers, the child has to say the numbers in order then the letters in order.		*		
	Arithmetic - If a child has isolated difficulty here, consider dyscalculia (p.457) or aversion to arithmetic.		*	*	
An isolated problem in **processing speed** found on testing can be due to slow handwriting (p.53), depression (p.309), obsessive slowness (p.95), hypothyroidism (which has non-cognitive physical signs as well, p.485); or checking (note hesitations, correcting self, saying "hang on let me check") which can indicate obsessionality.	**Coding** – Translate some symbols into others, with bonuses for speed. Uses short term memory (p.555)	*	*		
	Symbol search – find the target symbol in a row of symbols	*			
	Cancellation – in a large set of pictures, draw a line through each animal	*			

Causelist 3: Making mistakes/poor memory☼

This means producing a wrong answer after getting practically the same question right before. This can be very frustrating to a teacher or parent, and can lead to accusations that the child isn't trying or is pretending not to know. This rapidly loses the child's engagement in the task. Obviously everyone makes mistakes, but if they are frequent, upsetting, severe, or odd, then assessment can be useful. The causes should be worked out painstakingly for several specific mistakes.

Actions such as playing the piano, hitting a ball, or speaking can be inaccurate in space or time, and beyond some permitted limit of inaccuracy they are called mistakes (for a similar classification in animals see [1352]). Such inaccuracy gradually becomes smaller as a skill is acquired. Language creates far more options, so more categories of error have been identified (see language and speech problems, pp.145–149; approximate answers, p.357). Other kinds of mistakes are seen in social behaviour, p.169; in monitoring safety, p.539; in disinhibition, p.261; or in degree of focus (e.g. ignoring issues that would be obviously relevant to most people).

It is helpful to think of a child's behaviour as resulting from multiple decisions to act, taken separately by separate nuclei each with responsibility for a category of learning. These major categories are summarised in the following tree[1083]. Each memory system has unique properties[1179,1528], but they can compete, cooperate, or compensate for deficits in each other[659].

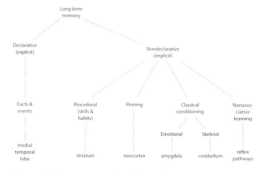

Figure 5. Some categories of learning.

Declarative information, i.e. what people can recall or recognise, is often divided into semantic knowledge (facts) and episodic knowledge (events, see *hippocampus*, p.478). Declarative information goes through the stages: registration → storage as short-term memory[791] → consolidation into long-term memory[1361] → recall → reconsolidation (p.540).

People also acquire much *non-declarative* information that affects their behaviour without being recallable. Examples include preferences; beliefs; the automatic assessment of stimuli as positive or negative[103] (see attitudes, p.425); cognitive biases (p.534); perceptual mechanisms; conditioned emotions (see the General Learning Model[552]); face recognition; and the gradual simplification of motor patterns into habits.

There are many more subtypes of learning than shown in this diagram. About 30 distinct memory mechanisms have been identified, of which a few are habituation and sensitisation, operant and classical conditioning, extinction, punishment; imitation; navigation and language acquisition[1107].

See also *forgetting*, p.468; *extinction*, p.463; *extinction bursts*, p.120; *amnesia*, p.421; *confabulation*, p.443; *perverse effects of training*, p.528; *punishment*, p.538; *superstitiously learned behaviours*, p.558; *working memory*, p.575.

Clinical testing of memory

Declarative memory is the most obvious area to test, and here the key is to check that the child has *registered* the information before passing a time with many distractions, and then testing whether she still recalls the information.

Everyday memory: Testing can immediately reveal practical problems that the youngster faces in everyday life. As well as declarative *facts*, this includes facial recognition, visuospatial information and unprompted recall. For teenagers, the original Rivermead Behavioural Memory Test (RBMT) can be used[1109], but from age 5−10, variants of it tailored to children are used. Because memory is part of everyday life, it can be assessed either objectively or using parental report, and it happens that the two methods give similar results (see[1777] for details).

Table 4. Everyday tests of memory

"Everyday memory": items in a parental questionnaire include:	Related items that can be tested easily in clinic
1. How often does she forget the names of people she has met before?	Name of her teacher. Also ask her to remember "Catherine Taylor".
2. How often does she forget details of her daily routine?	Ask what her class are doing right now.
3. How often does she forget where things are normally kept?	Does she remember the way from the waiting room to the office?
4. How often does she forget things she would normally do?	Ask her to tell her mother the time, when her mother comes back.
5. How often does she forget she has to do something at a particular time?	Show her where you hide some gold stars and tell her she can have one if she reminds you when she's leaving. Set an alarm clock to ring in 20 minutes, and tell her to ask "What time is it" when the alarm rings (5-year-olds need some practice first).
6. How often does she forget what day of the week it is?	Ask her.
7. How often does she fail to recognise the faces of people she has seen before (a) at school; (b) anywhere away from school?	Test using a photo of someone on a TV programme she watches, against an unknown person.
8. How often does she leave things behind?	Make sure she brings a toy and coat to the testing, and see whether she takes them away unprompted.
9. How often does she forget what has been told to her?	Name of her school. Ask her to learn a new name, or to recount a short story (5-year-olds should be given picture prompts for this). Test her recall both immediately and after delay.
10. How often are words on the tip of her tongue, so she knows the word but cannot quite find it?	Observe

Visuospatial memory: This and drawing ability can be tested using a complex *Rey-Osterrieth* figure. The child copies it immediately and tries to reproduce it after half an hour. This is fun and requires minimal input from the examiner. Various suitable figures ▶ and scoring schemes are available online. Some children focus excessively on local details or on higher-level "configural" information, and these styles of thinking are often seen in their normal lives as well[1074].

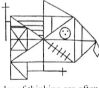

Many other formal tests are available including the *Children's Memory Scale (CMS)* and the *Wechsler Memory Scale (WMS)* (note this does not assess long-term memory). See also *digit span*, p.452. Note that currently available methods test very few of the subtypes of memory (the tests on this page and p.376 and p.400 do not test all the subtypes described on p.37).

Causes of a complaint of poor memory
Things the child has not learned

Inattention	during learning, p.79. See also deafness, p.130; receptive language problems, p.145.
Never learned	• Missed lessons because of teacher change/school change
	• Snowballing effect of child missing one stage (e.g. times tables) so increasingly falling behind on learning based on this (e.g. long multiplication and division)
	• Lack of background knowledge from impoverished home environment; language or reading deficit
	• ID, reading, or memory problems. Some learning about the environment occurs automatically in most children; a dramatic example showing a lack of such learning is a teenager with profound ID who reaches from a 2nd floor window for his fallen ball.
Insufficient consolidation	• Being taught something beyond his abilities (common in ID). In this case the child tries to memorise the answer.
	• Inadequate repetition in class; or no appropriate homework; or parents feel that repetitions are a waste of time
	• Disconnection/lack of synergy between learning at home and school.
	• Hippocampal damage (p.478)
Specific ID	Children differ. Some children generalise very well; some need more repetitions, perhaps just in abstract / motor / language learning. Following neonatal trauma or pneumonia, there are often significant deficits in memory and other cognitive functions[751]. See NVLD, p.28.
No checking	not trained to check answers properly

Inappropriate things the child has learned

Environment	Child taught wrong things (e.g. a mischievous dad teaching the child the wrong name for something)
Idiosyncrasy	Unusual child extracts the wrong core info from teaching (e.g. ASD child focusing on the colours of clothes in a story)

Events between learning and performance

Time	After infrequent use, e.g. over the summer, p.45.
Conflicting learning	Closely related information experienced since then; reconsolidation, p.540

Superior skills reducing performance

Dead end learning	Exceptional mental arithmetic skills may prevent attention to the simple examples used by teachers to introduce procedures for multiplication etc; then the child is lost when mental methods cannot cope with very large numbers.

Performance problems during testing

Impulsivity	Look for rapid wrong answers and rapid self-correction, p.79
Inattention	Focused or sustained attention, interest, preoccupation, p.79
Language	Look for answers that relate to just one of the words in your question; or ignoring of prepositions and secondary clauses.

Emotional / motivational	• They panic when the answer doesn't come fast – improves when there is no time pressure and no one is watching
	• What's the point in talking to you? The question may be so easy that it feels demeaning, or the answer is too boring and getting it right will just lead to another question.
	• The Yerkes–Dodson law states that there is an optimal level of arousal or stimulus strength[1808]. Performance reduces when we are too relaxed (see *inadequate anxiety*, p.423) or too aroused/anxious. Anxiety may draw us to non-task issues (such as threat), or may increase self-monitoring; in either case less cognitive capacity is available for a task[1778].
	• The performance decrement seen in aroused states, as described in the Yerkes–Dodson law, may be an artefact of artificial experimental situations in which the level of anxiety was not matched to the task. Arousal (a) increases automatic responding[1319]; (b) restricts our attention to the most salient objects; and (c) prepares the body for rapid action. This is not a failure but is evolutionarily useful. When the task is searching for threats, fearful subjects perform fastest (see[647]). Anxiety causes most difficulty on tasks requiring methodical or lateral thinking; or when the anxiety biases memory function toward threats that are not relevant to the task[309], e.g. in PTSD and OCD.
	• Repression (p.421)
	• A sensitive teen, especially, may respond not to the actual question, but to what he thinks is the implication of the question. He may not be aware that he is doing this, especially if the implication makes him defensive or cross.
	• Focusing on details; pedantry, p.163; showing off, p.548
Speed issues	• Slow thinking can prevent subsequent checking.
	• Habit of answering fast favoured by teacher responses?
	• Competing with siblings to be fast.
Memory distortions (see also standard cognitive errors, p.534; false memories, p.465)	• E.g. "hindsight bias" – thinking something must have / couldn't have happened.
	• Priming, in which recent thoughts affect current answer
	• Environment during recall different from environment in which learning took place. This is not simply state-dependent learning: a person's judgment of what is right, or what he would do in a situation, depends on his current state of mind[Chapter 5 of 57].
Immaturity	A normal 4-year-old cannot say what she did at nursery today. Her organisational skills are too immature to organise recall of the information.
Minor confabulation	E.g. remembering the right sentence being said, but attributing it to the wrong person (see *confabulations*, p.443)
Errors of the test	
Cultural	Test may be out-of-date or culturally biased. The teacher's model answer can be wrong. The child produces content or format which is reasonable to him, but incorrect according to teacher's preconceptions / knowledge.
Environment	suggestibility or distraction, in the test or the environment.
Pseudo-acquisition	The assumption that the child previously knew how to answer this question may be mistaken (p.44)
Structure	Forced choice of "the most similar" is inherently subjective.

Causelist 4: Regression

True regression is the loss of skills, not due to disinclination or to loss of the *physical* ability. The change, to behaviour characteristic of a younger child, can be in: [1056]

- Language (words, pronunciation, grammar, communicative intent)
- Motor skills (gripping objects; posture, p.93; gait, p.471; self-help skills; constructive or imaginary play, p.221).

Several related behavioural changes are considered in other sections of the book. Rapid severe losses, over a week or less, are considered with *hardly doing anything*, p.97. Isolated reduction in *social* interest or skills (such as interest in people, social smiles, waving goodbye, looking at people, and orienting to name call) usually has emotional causes, p.181. Reappearance of wetting has many causes and is considered separately, pp.339–340, as are cosleeping, p.198; soiling, p.341; school refusal, p.217; and crying, p.315.

Loss of skills is one of the more urgent presenting complaints in child mental health, because of the possibility of a treatable physical illness, though this is fairly rare. If in doubt, involve a paediatric neurologist.

Ways to work out whether a child is regressing.

Unproductive avenues
If you ask "is he losing skills?" the parents and teachers will often say "yes, every day we teach him skills and the next day he has lost them and we have to teach him again." – which means he is not really learning them (p.468), not that he is going backward. Word-finding difficulty has many reasons other than regression (p.149). Not using words when you know he can, e.g. common words such as yes/no – also has many reasons (p.151).

Indicators of real regression
- The most convincing sign of regression is loss of simple activities that he likes to do, has done daily, and still tries to do but does less well than he used to, e.g. does he make new mistakes while dressing?
- Loss of skills he used every day for more than a year is important, as he won't have simply "forgotten" the skill (most children lose academic skills over the summer holidays, p.45).
- He is more likely to be having real difficulty (rather than *choosing* not to do something) if he becomes frustrated or tries to hide the disability, or uses a more primitive form of the behaviour without drawing attention to it (e.g. using a multifinger pencil grip instead of a tripod grip – still consider the possibility of a physical explanation such as his finger hurting).
- If he plays with toys, is he stacking them less high than he used to?
- Is his handwriting becoming less clear (examples obtained from school are invaluable, or the teacher's opinion from Christmas onward when she knows him well).
- Has his handedness changed?
- For speech, don't look for speaking less, but for worsening pronunciation.
- The presence of any hard neurological signs (p.58).

Indicators that he is not regressing
- Acquisition of new skills simultaneous with the apparent loss, is reassuring to some extent, as it means the regression is not global. However, it does not exclude physical illness or local CNS lesion.
If there has been a brain insult (e.g. head injury, p.477; encephalitis, p.461; or even severe chickenpox, p.490) the regression that took place then is effectively accounted for. In such cases loss of skills is only worrying if it takes place between two timepoints *after* the brain insult.

continued ▶

Regressive-like changes	Diagnostic notes
Voluntary behaviours	
Self-comforting	During illness, and for up two weeks afterwards, bed wetting and thumb-sucking are common. Similarly, when a new baby arrives, a child may take comfort in the familiar, going back to previously abandoned toys. The child may choose childish clothes or a previously discarded comfort object (e.g. thumb-sucking).
For social effect (seconds to minutes)	Many children do this several times a day, until age 10 or so. Behaviours are explicitly shown to parents (especially mother) and disappear when parents are absent. If persistent, it is reasonable to call this pseudo-regression of behaviour (see p.363). In such cases, mother is often inadvertently rewarding the behaviour, e.g. by smiling or cuddling or paying attention.

Other behaviours that a child may incorporate include:
• clinginess
• "baby talk", i.e. clear meaning with word substitutions (e.g. me for I); immature pronunciation (e.g. intermittent lisp); protruding/pouting the lower lip only while talking; tipping the head down so they have to look up at the other person.
• "baby noises", i.e. intermittent little squeaks when he can talk
• "baby walk", i.e. taking short awkward steps, or on all fours when he can walk
• making himself smaller, pulling elbows or wrists together
• scribbling when he can draw
• flapping (p.106)
• an unusual sign is feigning (or exaggerating) stranger anxiety. Demonstrating this requires a major show of anxiety on meeting, then the child happily accompany the stranger within minutes, e.g. to fetch some super pencils for drawing.
• trying to breastfeed, or insisting on a feeding bottle.

Who the behaviour is modelled on:
• the child himself, after physical illness in which the benefits of regression were experienced.
• infant sibling: occurs most when that sibling is given attention.
• peers in special school: can produce dramatic behaviour. |
| Habitual (months to years) | If the child is habitually over-dependent on mother, the child may be still an infant cognitively (ID may have been missed); or the child is abnormally anxious; or the mother is not sufficiently encouraging maturation (p.189), or a combination of factors (e.g. attachment in autism, p.196).
If a child or teen permanently adopts an immature manner of interacting with others, see p.237. If the immaturity extends to lack of initiative, consider Dependent Personality, p.242. For an immature voice tone, see p.147. |
| ☞Super-added psychiatric disorder | As well as symptoms, consider which disorders have this characteristic age of onset. For example, loss of complex activities at age 10 in a learning disabled boy could be caused by the onset of tics or anxiety disorders. Familial disorders also sometimes have a familial age of onset. Examples include:
• Depression often starts around puberty, especially in girls (p.313) |

- In autism, stereotypies (p.553) are usually maximal at age 4 to 6.
- Obsessive compulsive *behaviours* are maximal from age 4 to 8 (p.63), but OCD usually starts from age 10 to 16 (p.65).
- Schizophrenia is very rare before puberty (see p.543).
- Tics (p.101) are maximal from age 7 to 10.
- Characteristic anxieties depend on age (p.295) but in general anxiety often worsens at puberty. Panics rarely start before late adolescence, but they can be so severe that a very small number lead the person to change his life to avoid them, causing major impairment (p.301).
- Migraines, p.141

Some substances tend to be abused (p.257) at specific ages, e.g. solvents (p.258) in pre-pubertal children, and stimulants (p.555) before exams.

Environ-mental change	E.g. new stepfather, breakdown of foster placement, change of school, or a change to a new less compatible teacher (see p.215)

Pseudo-acquisition of a skill

Random behaviour: accidental achievements	An infant may accidentally babble "mama" and "dada" while having no clue what they mean, leading to suspicion of regression when these "skills" are lost. Similarly, a child may upend a bucket on the beach and accidentally make a "castle".
Memory	E.g. a child may learn all the sentences in a story book by heart, giving the impression that he knows how to read. Change of interest, or time away from the book, lose these memorised "chants" but can also give the impression of loss of ability to read.
Partial skills	E.g. hyperlexia (p.483)

Artefacts

Plateauing	Skills that develop to a certain level and then stop will yield decreasing scores over time when compared to age-related norms.
Regression to the mean	If he had an exceptionally good day, or testing session, his next is likely to be worse.

continued ▶

Factors in true regression	Diagnostic notes (Note that the causes often coexist.)
Isolated regression of speech	
Normal	• Brief mild *regression* of speech is common between age 1-2, sometimes with an infective or emotional cause (when it will be accompanied by behavioural regression).
	• Transient mild regression confined to speech is also common. This is most common when a sibling is born.
	• Very occasionally there is a reduction in the use of pat phrases (not vocabulary) as the child makes the transition to full phrase speech (perhaps because the use of the same word in different contexts is a challenge).
Landau–Kleffner syndrome	("Acquired epileptic aphasia", AEA) should be considered in speech regression, over days to months (p.73). In contrast with autistic regression, non-verbal intelligence and non-verbal communication are preserved and the onset is later (see [1539] for a dimensional view). Often it causes no convulsions so an EEG is essential to confirm. It often remits in early adolescence. Other circumscribed losses due to epilepsies at other foci are possible
Other cerebral	Lesion of Broca's area or supplementary motor area; bilateral thalamic lesion; pseudobulbar palsy (p.537)
Isolated regression other than speech (of behaviour, skills or motivation)	
"Summer learning loss"	Especially when children are unsupervised, knowledge and skills are lost during long school holidays: up to two months in maths and reading level[315]. Hence, if developmental milestones have only recently been passed, they can be lost dramatically over holidays. For example, a boy with ID who had only just learned to speak before the Christmas holiday lost all speech by the time he returned to school after the holiday. The reason was revealed by his new preoccupation with computers, which had filled most of his waking hours during the holiday.
Motor / muscle disorder	See deterioration of gait, p.471; weakness, p.87; Guillain–Barré over weeks, p.87; muscular dystrophies over months to years, p.510. Long term following brief illness: see GA1, p.32.
Schizophrenia	or schizophrenic prodrome (p.544)
General regression (of skills and speech, lasting at least weeks). Often circumscribed problems start first or are noticed first.	
"Autistic" regression (p.183)	• Seen in at least a third of children with autism, between 18-36 months[1538]. Social or motor regression is more common than language loss, *even if parents have not noticed*[1739].
	• The history of 1–30 words largely disappearing over weeks to months around age 2, rather than leading to phrase speech, supports a diagnosis of autism, but about 10% of such regressions have other causes. Regression *after* phrase speech has been acquired carries a worse prognosis.
	• The *impression* of loss of speaking ability is sometimes created by acquisition of stereotyped interests (p.553), in which case the child can sometimes be tempted to speak better if asked quietly about his interests when well relaxed, and without eye contact.
Epilepsy (p.73)	• there are many subtypes of epileptic encephalopathies that cause visible fits.
	• Stopping in mid-sentence can indicate absences (p.75).

- In epilepsy with continuous spike and wave during slow sleep (CSWS), severe regression can be caused by epileptiform activity (p.73) rather than by discrete fits.
- Fits can cause cognitive impairment even if the fits are not externally visible [160].

Other medical combined	(see investigation planner, p.47) Medical problems are often exaggerated or perpetuated by children, particularly if there is secondary gain (p.471) such as time off school or time with mother. Confrontation can exacerbate this.
Pervasive refusal	(p.527)
Rett syndrome	(p.541)
Childhood Disintegrative Disorder	This is a behavioural description for deterioration often found in neurological disorders (see[298,318]). It can be similar to autism but with a regression that is more severe, late, or atypical.
Specific regressions	Some conditions previously identified in a child can increase the risk of future regressions. Some of these are listed under *medical causes of regression*, p.47. Others include:

- Down's greatly increases the risk of Alzheimer's, but this is very rare before age 30 and has not been reported in children or adolescents. Deterioration in teenagers with Down's has several causes, such as hypothyroidism, p.485; coeliac disease, p.441; deafness, p.130; depression, p.313 or vitamin deficiency[1648].
- HAND, p.479
- tuberous sclerosis, p.569

continued ▶

Investigation Planner 2: Medical causes of regression

Conditions that cause ID or autism can, if they are somewhat milder or late in onset, cause regression or psychosis. Hence this list overlaps lists for ID and psychosis (pp.32 and 349), which should also be consulted. Treatments are generally more effective at the "psychiatric stage" than after irreversible neurological damage has occurred[1448]. A careful developmental assessment sometimes reveals stepwise losses previously wrongly thought to be one-off events. Periodic neurological reassessment is useful[1349].

See also the *general approach to medical investigations*, p.373, and[512,703].

	Signs	Initial tests	Excluded clinically or to Order?	Date ordered	Result
		Physical examination, thyroid, renal, FBC, UECr, LFT,ESR/CRP, B6, ammonia, lead, mercury (p.330), serum amino acids and urinary organic acids, white cell enzymes (p.572). Consider MRI, EEG.			
Infections					
Meningitis, encephalitis	hours to days. See p.42	FBC, CSF, blood culture			
HIV	p.479	p.479			
Whipworm, etc.	see [1168]	stool microscopy			
Sequelae of infections					
Guillain-Barré	p.87	history, CSF, nerve conduction			
Chronic fatigue	p.323	(see initial tests on p.325)			
Intracranial lesions					
Head injury	p.477	MRI			
Occult hydrocephalus	p.482	MRI			
Multiple sclerosis	p.510	MRI			
Progression of neuro-fibromatosis	p.514	history, examination, MRI			
Progression of tuberous sclerosis	p.569	history, examination, MRI			

Metabolic

Storage disorders (p.556)	various	Look for cherry-red macula (p.501).
	mucopoly-saccharidoses	p.501
Urea cycle disorders	p.571 (often with intestinal complaints or protein refusal)	ammonia MRI **
Wilson's disease	p.575	p.575
Phenyl-ketonuria	relaxation of diet in some PKU[616], p.529	phenylalanine MRI **

Toxicological

CO	carbon monoxide from car or boiler	carboxyhaemoglobin
Drug abuse Medication	p.257 side-effects of medication especially sedatives, antiepileptics antipsychotics, p.422	urine drug screening blood levels

Endocrine

Addison's	p.419	BP drop on standing, low Na

Other

Epilepsy, whether mild or severe (e.g. Rasmussen syndrome, p.539)	p.73	careful history and EEG
Xeroderma pigmentosum	p.454	history and examination
Leuko-dystrophies	p.498	MRI
Juvenile Huntington's disease	p.482	p.482
Autoimmune	p.427	for SLE: p.560

** if plasma amino acids are normal, this condition is excluded

Causelist 5: Deviance

This word is used in several different ways to describe behaviours:

- Patterns of behaviour that would not appear on a normal developmental trajectory[612,1402]. An example showing the normal trajectory and a deviation from it is shown on p.169. This is not as straightforward as it may seem. For example, simple delay can lead to unusual patterns of behaviour which are then misleadingly called "deviant", e.g. the child with ID or very low verbal ability, who becomes excluded from games at school, and then starts talking to himself (p.560). In addition most clinicians are "deviant" in the sense of being unrepresentative of the population, typically in the top 10% intellectually, and having behaviours not shared by others.

- "Qualitatively different from normal". This can mean "severely different" or "so obvious that you don't need to use quantitative measures to see it" or "not just attributable to delay" or "not seen at any age in normal people." DSM-IV confusingly specifies that *impairments, lacks, and failures* are "qualitative".

- Deviance is sometimes used by professionals as a shorthand for "characteristic of development in autism." Certainly, abnormal behaviours are common in autism (**A** in table at right). However, there are other causes of these behaviours (many can be found by following the cross-references from the DSM symptoms listed on p.388). Also, autistic children often become deviant in idiosyncratic ways, rather than ways characteristic of the disorder[1661]. Furthermore, DSM-IV explicitly allows the diagnosis of autism based on delays, rather than insisting on abnormality.

- An obsolete sense is immoral, persistently naughty, or psychopathic (p.280).

The word also has several related usages in the social sphere:

- Some, probably a minority, feel that the notion of deviance is merely a convenience for the rest of society. "The belief that such persons are crazy and do not know what is in their best interests makes it seem legitimate to incarcerate them. This is a socially useful arrangement: it allows some people to dispose of some other people who annoy or upset them."[1577]

- The usual meanings for parents are evil/worrying/inappropriately sexual/needing to see a psychiatrist.

- The term "deviant peers" is often used to refer to peers who are not adequately driven by society's norms or by the need for approval from parents or teachers (see *gangs*, p.472; *conduct disorder*, p.249).

One approach to apparently deviant behaviour is to consider the following groupings:

Contributory factors in deviance	Examples in language	Examples in social behaviour	Examples in drawing	Examples in spelling
not actually deviant but often thought to be, i.e. much more common than people realise, and not usually indicating pathology	Most pronoun reversal difficulties indicate simple immaturity. Most stilted speech is a pattern learned from respected adults (p.163). A	Preferring solitary tasks cross-dressing (p.267) Different patterns of eye contact in some cultures (p.175)	Drawing violence seen in computer games or TV	Immature: has learned regular plurals but not irregular plurals. Most letter reversals in writing indicate simple immaturity.
Unable to follow the usual path	Deafness causing problems with pronunciation and cognition (p.130). Using holophrastic phrases (p.480) in areas of cognitive deficit (example on p.158).	Many autistic children find social contact overwhelming so avoid eye contact, and move parts of others' body as instruments (figure, p.169). Masturbating in public A (p.115)	Unable to face difficult facts, or dissociating (p.453), so cannot draw family.	Letter reversal in some dyslexia (p.51).
	Unusual voice (p.147) or accent (p.417) or word order (e.g. Susan, be naughty her). A	Gang membership, p.472	Finds people stressful so draws them much simpler than other things A	Finds it too boring to spell normally, so spells backwards (can also be to show off)
Drawn toward an unusual path	Unusual verbal environment (e.g. 2nd language). Very idiosyncratic language can result from combination of this with cognitive deficits.	adopting an unusual persona (p.238)	Drawing violence within the family, or pustulent genitalia for the sake of peer approval	Elements of a previously learned language intrude.
	Accents learned from nannies. Private slang used in gangs, p.472.		Repeatedly drawing something from his autistic special interest A	Autistic people may learn only spellings associated with their special interest. A

In the table above A indicates behaviours suggestive of autism (not diagnostic)

Causelist 6: Difficulty reading

Difficulty with reading cannot sensibly be considered separately from the child's general developmental level (including IQ), his educational history, and other related developmental areas such as language and speech[1240]; vision, p.52; attention, p.79; and clumsiness, p.89. Difficulty with reading is usually accompanied by other cognitive problems[669].

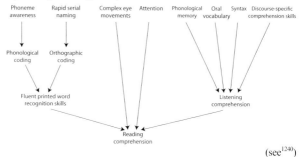

(see[1240])

Figure 6. Skills involved in reading.

Some languages are more difficult to read than others (Chinese is very difficult; English is quite difficult). Because reading develops late, it is unrealistic to identify a specific reading problem before age 8.

WIAT-2 (the updated version of W.O.R.D.) and CELF can be helpful. The Neale Analysis of Reading is well standardised up to age 12 ¾. For remediation, it is sometimes useful to try to be more precise, e.g. finding out the child's level in all the skills underlying reading, as follows:

Measures	Description	Examples
Single-word reading	Read aloud some unrelated words of increasing difficulty.	cat chair
Spelling	Spell some words of increasing difficulty.	mushroom television dictionary laboratory
Phonological decoding	Read pseudowords to show the use of phonetic rules.	siglop dorkit pamdin
Orthographic coding	Recognise words that cannot be decoded by phonetic rules alone	yacht salmon
	Choose which is the real word (a forced choice)	rain or rane? fight or fite?
Homonym choice	Choose between two real words that sound the same(forced choice)	Seven days are a: week or weak?
Phonological awareness	Move phonemes around within words	Combine the first sound of "spoon" with all but the first sound of "dog". (spog)
Rapid automatic naming	Rapidly name numbers, colours, objects	▲2♥

Table Some simple tests to describe a child's reading difficulty [1216]

Common errors in diagnosis

• Diagnosing dyslexia, or any "specific" cognitive problem (p.551), without obtaining a wide ranging Developmental Quotient or IQ (p.59).

• Ignoring developmental comorbidity: Children with dyslexia *usually* have attention problems and *often* have visuospatial or language deficits[1504]. Some dyslexia is caused or exacerbated by attentional problems[1676]; and dyslexia produces many more reading errors in children if they have ADHD too[1599].

• Ignoring the impact on mood and behaviour of being multiple years behind peers, even if this is in an apparently isolated area.

Contributory factors in reading difficulty	Notes * = mainly superficial dyslexia ** = mainly deep dyslexia
Problems not specific to reading	Recognise these by deficits on non-reading tasks[1300,1301]
Hyperactivity, inattention	(p.79) */** Most children with dyslexia meet criteria for attention deficit as well[1504].
Cognitive problems Language impairment*,**	See diagram and table at left for examples. (p.145)
👁 ID	e.g. overfocused testing, familial delay. Consider mild, borderline, or patchy abilities, which are often unrecognised.
👁 Vision* (p.133)	In *most* children with reading difficulty, this is only a small factor. Aspects include: • poor acuity • pattern-related visual stress (Meares-Irlen syndrome), exacerbated by high contrast stripe effects of text, often improveable with filters[27]. • eye movement problems*. There are six eye movement systems working simultaneously (saccade, p.543; fixation; vestibular; optokinetic; smooth pursuit; vergence). They have all been implicated in some cases of reading difficulty (see e.g.[812]).
Auditory problems*	Deafness, p.130; CAPD, p.121 (see[1635])
Poor short-term memory**	Check whether the problem is specific to reading by using digit span (p.37) or melodies. Reading comprehension will be worse for longer (not necessarily nested) sentences.
Obsessionality**	Uncertain he read correctly so he repeats. High neuroticism scores are also associated[708].
Movement	Imprecise or extraneous movements[1630].
Poor processing of rapid information	This is a major "theory of dyslexia" but affects also oral language and motor coordination.
Brain damage	Many brain areas can rarely cause distinct dyslexias[1350], e.g. alexia without agraphia[780].
Reading epilepsy	Most often language-induced jaw myoclonus[876].
Epileptiform activity (p.73)	This can impair reading even in the absence of overt fits[655].
More specific problems than reading	
Suboptimal teaching of reading	E.g. embedded phonics ("whole language" reading) emphasising reading whole words. Use of adult Ay, Bee, See. Letter–sound relationships not emphasised enough for the child.
Social learning, p.550	E.g. parents do not model reading at home
Reading phobia	If he has been repeatedly shouted at for misreading.
Pseudo-dyslexia	More likely in older teens[658].

Dyslexia

Many methods are used to argue for this as it can produce useful extra time, a reader, and a scribe for examinations. In order of decreasing rigour, these are:

• The clearest demonstration that a child has a fairly circumscribed reading deficit is that his performance on tests is much higher when they are read to him. However the 1:1 attention usually overcomes attentional problems too.

• DSM-IV *suggests*, though it is not part of the definition of "Reading Disorder", that *substantially below* means "usually" 2 s.d. below expected based on age, IQ, past education, and any sensory deficits.

• Most schools cannot offer special help to children whose reading is in the population average range, even if this is far below what would be expected from their very high IQ. So in practice IQ is rarely considered, and a child whose reading is two years below his peers usually gets help in school.

• Some colleges employ a "Dyslexia Assessor". A typical assessment includes several standardised tests, but "Specific Learning Difficulty (Dyslexia)" is sometimes diagnosed so loosely as to be misleading, e.g. even in cases where reading comprehension and accuracy are the person's best skills.

Causelist 7: Difficulty writing

Writing has several components: imagination, knowing what to write, making ideas flow, forming sentences and paragraphs, conjugation, following appropriate lines and spacing; writing the alphabet; spelling; joined-up writing; punctuation and capitalisation.

Obtaining a sample is easy. You need to watch the child doing some written work, as previous work supplied by school or parents may have been practised, copied, or prompted. Above age 8, "write for 5 minutes about anything you like or how to make a ham sandwich" tests many of the skills in the preceding list (for other methods see MMSE, p.400).

The child's written work must be compared with that of children with the same sex, mental age and educational experience. For most children with average IQ, this means comparing their handwriting with other children of the same sex in their class at school. There are various ways to decide whether a child's writing is poor enough to be impairing, but this does seem to be the case with around 8% of boys and 3% of girls[816].

The causes of writing difficulty (dysgraphia) ♠ are numerous and the diagnostic difficulties have much in common with those of dyslexia ♠, p.51. Isolated problems affecting single aspects of writing are rare. The conditions shown in the table at right usually interfere with several aspects.

For secondary effects of handwriting difficulty, see effects on mood, p.89; on arithmetic, p.457; on posture, p.93; and on cheating, p.439.

See also: changes of handwriting indicating regression, p.42; handedness, p.475; proto-writing, p.56; belief that a child's difficulty is just in writing, p.237.

Contributory factors in writing difficulty	Notes
Problems not specific to writing	Recognise these by deficits on non-writing tasks such as drawing or use of cutlery.
Hyperactivity,inattention	(p.79)
ID (p.491)	e.g. overfocused testing, familial delay. Consider mild, borderline, or patchy abilities, which are often unrecognised.
Dyspraxia (p.89)	See testing of dysdiadochokinesis on p.457.
Low processing speed	(This has many causes listed on p.36)
Language problems	p.145
Medical conditions	Many medical conditions cause movement problems (see lists on pp.89-92 and p.86).
Problems specific to writing	
Writer's cramp / dystonia	p.458 (much less commonly, this affects other tasks such as piano practice)
Insufficient training	Lack of training or practice (especially for children who manage to avoid work)
Aversive training experiences	E.g. severe criticism from parents or teachers – who often see untidy writing as morally reprehensible.
More specific problems than writing	
Problems affecting written *tests*	Special factors influencing written *testing* include the long duration (in comparison with verbal questions), complex scoring schemes, and the need to organise one's time.
Being watched while writing	p.298. This can be analogous to selective mutism, p.153. As with selective mutism, anxiety needs to be fully considered.

Special Topic 1: Is this child developing normally?

Few behavioural symptoms can be properly understood without knowledge of the child's developmental stage. This can be obtained with a broad developmental inventory (e.g. Griffiths, p.451), a simple checklist (e.g. Denver Developmental Screening Test), or a more cognitively focused test (IQ tests, p.59). A good holistic alternative is to check the height and weight (see below), plus motor milestones (p.91), language milestones (p.143), social milestones (p.55) and the drawing age (p.56).

If a child develops a skill sooner than 99% of his peers, this has little importance clinically. However if he is later than 99% of his peers, this is often important clinically. The most difficult question is *when to do further investigations*. This depends hardly at all on the developmental level, and much more on the likely degree of treatability (see e.g. p.32) and the benefit to be expected from extra support.

Milestones

Physical development: For growth charts see www.cdc.gov/growthcharts/ and[1795]. See also *puberty*, p.411; physical examination, p.409.

Motor skills: Note that *gross* motor skills are well dissociated from cognitive development, e.g. children with severe ID often run and climb well. See *motor milestones*, p.91; neuro examination, p.409.

Sensory: See *face−hand test*, p.464.
Feeding: p.331
Toilet training: pp.339-340
Dressing: pp.441, 91
Memory/digit span: p.452
Language milestones: p.143
Other behaviours: Play, p.221; jokes, p.495; sexual behaviours, p.267; age norms for sleep are on p.321. Various kinds of naughtiness increase or decrease with age (pp.511,249).

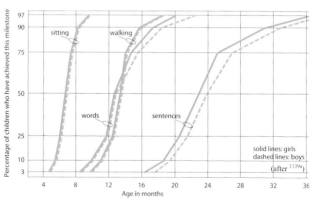

Figure 7. Age distributions of acquisition of early skills.

Social milestones: Social interactions with strangers are greatest before 5 m and after 3 y, because attachment behaviours (p.195) are maximal in this gap, and stranger anxiety starts at about 5−10 m. Smiles: p.549. Interest in other babies: 2−6 m; smiling and babbling at other babies: 6−9 m. Joint attention (p.494) should start by 15 m. Social behaviour by age 2−3 should include interest in people, pointing, imitation or pretend play, and response to praise (these items are especially useful as they are not confounded by language delay). Turn-taking is acquired between age 3−6 (p.570). Egocentricity (p.180) is common until a year or two after school entry. See also social play milestones, p.222.

Academic achievements: These depend greatly on exposure and practice, so have less predictive value than untrained cognitive tasks. However the *cognitive* level of children's drawings can be assessed in useful ways (semantic and emotional interpretations are speculative). Several proprietary tests are well validated against IQ[1] so it makes sense to use the simplest[1133] or most readily available. More crudely, ask him to draw a person as well as he can with no prompting; calculate $3+(P/4)$ with P being the number of parts in the drawing (doubled body parts such as eyes are counted as just one); this gives a reasonable mental age from about 3 to 7. Preschoolers' scribbles, drawings, and proto-writing can be compared with examples in[938]. Drawings can be assessed using this table[331]:

	% of children who draw this feature, at age...									
	6	7	8	9	10	11	12	13	14	15
Head										
hair	25	32	40	52	65	68	70	...		
eyebrows	10	12	15	18	22	25	30	33	35	...
ears	5	7	10	15	22	28	34	40	45	48
chin	2	6	12	22	32	36	40	44	46	50
Figure										
neck	42	45	49	55	68	75	77	80	84	90
shoulders	2	2	4	8	12	18	22	28	35	40
waist	2	2	3	10	15	20	22	24	...	
shoes/toes	2	2	3	10	15	20	22	24	...	

Ages by which immature behaviours should disappear (or only be done for effect): When seen in interview, these behaviours establish the likely mental age more reliably than individual achievements, which may be specially trained or misdescribed or unseen.

Infantile behaviours:

- Hand-regard, i.e. delight in looking at the hand, often while turning it or wiggling the fingers, is normal at a mental age of 6−7 months. Rarely, gazing at a non-moving hand persists for many years as a learned way of limiting over-excitement.
- Casting (p.103) is normal at a mental age up to 18 months.
- Tactile exploration of a room (p.132) is common until a mental age of 18 months, as is prowling around and climbing over furniture without regard for its normal use.
- Many children mouth objects (other than dummies and digits) for over half an hour each day under 18 months, but then it rapidly reduces[795]. (If extreme consider *Klüver-Bucy*, p.496.)
- Flapping usually disappears by a mental age of 3 (p.105)
- Echolalia usually disappears by a mental age of 3½ (p.459).
- Upgoing big toe on stroking the sole (called upgoing plantar reflex, or Babinski sign), usually disappears by age 2. After age 3 it is a clear sign of organic disease or developmental delay[1791]. For other primitive reflexes, see[1441].

Other immature behaviours: Dummy-sucking usually finishes by nursery, and thumb-sucking by age 10. By age 7, most children have found more entertaining ways of spending their time than imaginary friends (p.231). Daytime wetting usually stops by 24 months, but night-time wetting lasts much longer (p.339). Most children lose interest in Duplo (big Lego) by age 6, small Lego by about puberty, and Techno in their teens.

Familial milestones should be considered, e.g. age of reading or being dry at night.

continued ▶

Prediction based on early milestones

Occasionally this information can be retrospectively obtained from parental or professional records.

Even though *most* preschoolers' future academic ability cannot be reliably predicted[319], there are obvious exceptions in many genetic syndromes. There are also a few early behavioural signs that, when positive, are highly predictive of substantial ID [1004]. Having any one of these signs makes such an outcome many times more likely (the same reference also gives predictors for younger ages):

Table 5. Symptoms increasing the likelihood of special schooling

Age (months)	*If the child cannot perform these tasks*	Odds Ratio of later ID (moderate or severe)*
12	Walks (with aid)	9.5
	Plays give-and-take	7.5
18	Builds tower with 2–3 pieces	6.8
24	Runs	9.2
	Kicks big ball without falling	10.7
	Names familiar objects in a picture	27.2
36	Jumps with both legs	13.9
	Talks in sentences	15.6
	Differentiates sizes	20.1
48	Can walk on a straight line for a few steps	40.1
	Able to copy a cross	43.5
	Knows 3 primary colours	16

* This column shows how many times more likely is the outcome in this child, compared to children who *can* perform the task. The outcome measured was eventual "Level 3" Special Educational Placement in Finland.

General neurological maturation
The reliability of neurological signs ranges from fair to substantial (i.e. from 0.2 to 0.7[975]).

Hard neurological signs indicate definite abnormality in brain or nerve, i.e. in general they cannot be attributed to mental processes. The most reliable ("hardest") signs of upper motor neuron lesions are increased tone, clonus, and upgoing plantar over age 3[907] (p.56). Nearly as reliable are unilateral movement abnormality, and loss of function in spinal or cranial nerves.

Soft neurological signs can be assessed using NES (Neurological Evaluation Scale), which has the advantage of a fairly detailed description of signs[232]. An alternative is NESS (Neurological Examination for Subtle Signs[392]) in which three or more signs are taken to indicate developmental immaturity. This is *occasionally* correlated with the development of schizophrenia, or with frontal dysfunction[347] (see *frontal signs*, p.469). (The following is from [919]; unfortunately the precise tests and thresholds used are not recorded):

Table 6. Symptoms of general neurological immaturity

Soft sign	No affected in UK sample of 12 000 at age 11 (%)
Left eyed (p.497)	4068 (32%)
Left kicker (p.475)	1444 (11%)
Left handed (p.475)	1414 (10%)
Left thrower (p.475)	1218 (10%)
Unsteady heel-toe	1090 (9%)
Tics (p.101)	923 (7%)
Speech defect (p.147)	651 (5%)
Clumsy (p.89)	605 (12%)
Unsteady on left foot	443 (4%)
Unsteady on right foot	426 (3%)
Coordination (p.89)	351 (3%)
Bowel control (p.341)	332 (2%)
Twitches (p.101)	280 (2%)
Convulsions (p.73)	265 (2%)
Coordination/balance (p.122)	193 (2%)
Hand control (p.476)	158 (1%)
Speech difficulties (p.147)	158 (1%)
Dysarthria (p.89)	83 (0.7%)
Neurological problem	60 (0.5%)
Enuresis (p.339)	52 (0.4%)
Incontinence (p.340)	43 (0.3%)

(see also ambidextrous, p.475)

continued ▶

IQ tests are the best way to test thinking ability. The importance of this is discussed on p.27. The overall (or *Full Scale*) score is most important, but the differences between subscales are also important (see NVLD, p.28) and sometimes individual subtests (p.36).

In many children there are practical challenges such as boredom (p.322), anxiety (p.298), differences in educational background (see pp.27–33) and whether they speak (see *testing non-verbal children*, p.516). IQ tests are administered 1:1 which often overcomes attention deficits, but stimulants still often improve test scores (p.568).

The WPPSI can be used from age 3 to7; the WISC from 6 to 16, and the WAIS from age 16 upward. The WASI is a shortened form, valid from age 6 upward.

It is important to realise that IQ tests do not test all abilities, as developmental tests try to do (p.451). Furthermore, IQ tests do not cover even all cognitive skills. For example, a child with normal overall IQ (and even normal scores on all the subscales) can be quite unable to learn to read (p.51) or to talk, or to find her way (p.512). Another shortcoming of IQ tests, that occasionally causes practical difficulty, is that the tests are less well calibrated and the results somewhat less repeatable in the very high and low regions[1484].

IQ testing methods usable in infants (and in children with mental age under 5) utilise preference, habituation, and violation of expectancy[68], but usually observation and history of skill acquisition are much more practical (see *developmental quotient*, p.451; *object permanence*, p.517; *P-levels*, p.522).

IQ tests are recalibrated within developed countries every few years, to keep the mean at about 100. This is necessary because of the Flynn effect[702,1756]. This is the steady increase in IQ scores produced as societies develop, and is thought to have many causes including improvements in nutrition, health care, urbanisation, a trend to smaller families, improvements in education (especially special education), test-specific skills, increasing use of abstract concepts, and greater environmental complexity. Using an old test produces a misleadingly high score, and conversely using a test calibrated for more developed societies produces misleadingly low scores. Hence using an up-to-date IQ test in Britain produces a population mean of about 100; using the same test in Britain in 1948, or in Nigeria in 1992, produces a population mean of about 80[1756]. The Flynn effect may have plateaued in the most developed countries by about 2000[1594].

Children who are physically ill produce lower IQ scores[1484]. Medication can improve or worsen IQ scores (p.568). See also *intellectual disability*, p.491; *gifted children*, p.473; memory testing, p.38; *components of IQ tests*, p.36; inconsistent performance in testing, p.33.

Table 7. Terminology for IQ levels

Medical term	IQ	Description of ability used in education & psychology	Closest term in UK Education (for more details see p.497)
	130+	very superior	
	120–129	superior	
	110–119	high average	
	90–109	average	
	85–89	low average	
	80–84		
Borderline intellectual functioning, p.434	70–79	borderline	Mild Learning Difficulty
Mild ID	55–69		Moderate Learning Difficulty
Moderate ID	40–54	extremely low (see *intellectual disability*, p.491)	Severe Learning Difficulty
Severe ID	25–39		
Profound ID	below 25		Profound Learning Difficulty

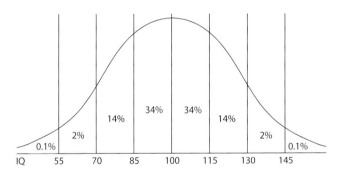

Figure 8. Population distribution of IQ.

General temporal patterns

Causelist 8: Periodic or rhythmic behaviours

The idea here is that the timing of behaviours may give a clue as to what is fundamentally going on.

When trying to find the cause of a problem that comes and goes, the first thing to work out is the trigger. A diary of symptoms can help work out whether the behaviour is rhythmic, which often makes the cause clear (as in the list below). The diary can also include A, B, C (antecedents, behaviours, consequences) to reveal situational triggers (p.365).

Sometimes, intermittent problems can give the impression that they are steady. For example, the child may only come to appointments when he is at his best (or worst). Or a parent may give the impression that the problem is incessant, especially if they are desperate for help (pp.80,205).

Timescale	Types of periodic behaviours	Notes
Periodicity in the child		
	Tremor	All people have slight tremors, which are increased by sympathetic activity (p.428). *Resting tremor* almost disappears with active movement whereas *intention tremor* increases when the finger nears a target. For intention tremor consider cerebellar disease, p.437. Resting tremor can be increased by hypocalcaemia, steroids, lithium, or heavy metals, p.330; if it is accompanied by akinesia see *parkinsonism*, p.525. Consider Wilson's disease, p.575. Contrast *asterixis*, p.105.
Several per second	Myokymia	Involuntary activation of groups of motor units, insufficient to move a joint. The commonest is twitching within an eyelid. Cannot be reproduced voluntarily so are not tics (p.101). Increased by caffeine, tiredness, severe exercise, thyrotoxicosis.
	Normal rhythmic behaviours	E.g. pencil tapping, finger tapping, foot tapping, humming tunes, flapping (p.105), walking, laughing (p.111), masturbating (p.115), and rubbing oneself to warm up. Like normal non-rhythmic habits (p.63), many increase during stress, and only deserve attention if physically or socially impairing.
Each second	Self-soothing: thumb-sucking (p.564), chewing movements when settling at night, head rolling, some headbanging (p.119)	• *Rhythmic* self-soothing activities may replicate mother's heartbeat or the parental rocking of babies. Used when tired or anxious or bored (p.322) – or in emotional or physical anguish. (compare self-entertainment, p.545; gratification phenomena, and specific sensation-seeking, p.123). • *Non-repetitive* self-soothing is often achieved by holding a treasured toy, a transition object (p.567), someone's hand, onself[786] or (mainly in ID) one's penis.
	Body rocking[1420]	If cultural, persists to adulthood. Otherwise disappears as head rolling (above).

	Palilalia	Etymologically means simply repeating oneself. Sometimes this is subdivided based on the length of the repeated chunk,so that a stutter repeats one sound (see p.157), palilalia repeats a word, and palilogia repeats phrases[907]. Occasionally heard in Tourette's.
Each second	Tachyphemia	Decrescendo accelerando repeat of the last syllable of an utterance, in parkinsonism, p.525.
	Tardive dyskinesia	Usually consists of rhythmic tongue or jaw movements. Many other movements are associated but it is difficult to know whether they are due to t.d. or to other underlying causes[1486]. Very rare in children but worrying because disfiguring and difficult to treat. Occurs in about 1% of those on atypical antipsychotics for ten years, most in ID. (for other tardive movements see p.561)
	Music	Sometimes the body is rocked to help keep the rhythm (e.g. in singing and religious recitation). May not be recognised if a child is singing to himself.
	☞ Depression	(p.309)
	Hypoglycaemia	(e.g. after school or before breakfast)
	Inflammation	often worst in the morning (e.g. p.93)
	Intracranial hypertension	(p.493) Persistent vomiting, particularly in the morning.
Time of day	Medication	e.g. rebound (of overactivity or tremor) when stimulants (including caffeine) are wearing off.
	Parasomnias	(p.200)
	Segawa syndrome	Leg function (e.g. walking) worsens as the day progresses, p.458.
	Juvenile parkinsonism	(p.525)
	Premenstrual	can occur even before menarche: p.506.
Monthly	Other	Rarely, urea cycle disorders[189], p.571; Kleine-Levin syndrome, p.496; juvenile parkinsonism, p.525; or, in the second half of the menstrual cycle, porphyria[336], p.532.

	School	• The morning rush to prepare for school creates many opportunities for conflict.
Time of day and time of week		• In school – bullying (p.219) or teasing can affect mood outside school too.
		• Getting out of school: enjoying physical activity, hunger after school, releasing tics (p.101).
Time of term		Children get tired toward the end of term, especially if they are being pushed. Also, exams are approaching. Occasionally the child's mood may be affected by a tired teacher's mood.
	Seasonal affective disorder	(p.314)
Time of year	Anniversaries	Specific months or dates can be associated with bereavements (p.430).
	Heat	Heat can increase irritability (p.494).
	Holidays	e.g. stress, antimalarials, time with relatives
Various	☞ Presence of abusers	Usually via anxiety, violence: see frozen watchfulness (p.470). See also Fabricated/ Induced illness (p.359)

Causelist 9: Invariant non-rhythmic behaviours ☼

In other words, behaviours with a highly consistent form that is repeated
often, making the behaviours inappropriate. The list here is of *causes*, but
some of the specific *movements* are described in more detail starting on
p.99. See the glossary for terms used to describe behaviour.

Even more than with rhythmic problems, the key is working out the
triggers for each episode, and the maintaining factors for the pattern. A
diary often helps. Many triggers are not known to the child (see
unconscious, p.570). For repetitive *speech*, see p.156. For overwhelming
states, see p.69. For dominating interests see p.229. For behaviours that
are odd even when they occur singly, see pp.99, 347, 353.

The three categories below that most often concern psychiatrists are classic
OCD (not enjoyed, and usually driven by fears); autistic stereotypies
(enjoyed); and forced touching (most common in people who tic).

Types of repeated actions	Notes (NB multiple factors are often present)
Normal non-rhythmic habits and motor patterns	These only deserve attention if physically or socially impairing. Some are particularly associated with anxiety (see below). • Everyone yawns, stretches, scratches (p.110), blinks (p.108), clears their throats (p.109). • More variable patterns include hair pulling (p.117), cheek chewing, tissue tearing, nail-biting (p.511), leg jiggling, and knuckle cracking.
Sleepiness, and pre-sleep	(p.200)
Developmental / Learning-related	
Limited self-entertainment skills (p.545)	Particularly in ID when accustomed toys are not available and fantasy/imagination is poor. Use of muscle groups is less constant than in tics (p.101). Examples include clicking a pen or tapping a radiator. Unlike autistic interests, these increase when the child is bored, such as late in a session with no one interacting with him.
Play	Normal play often seems repetitive, but usually has some challenge or variation (p.221)
Normal repetitive behaviours /OCB	E.g. "Step on a crack, break your mother's back.": avoiding cracks in the pavement; bedtime rituals; counting rituals, unlucky numbers, favourite colours (p.247), wanting things in their right places. They are common from age 2−8. They are often called obsessive compulsive *behaviours*, childhood rituals, or normative repetitive routines,to distinguish them from Obsessive Compulsive *Disorder*. Like OCD they are sometimes enacted to ward off harm, and often include a demand for sameness or symmetry; but unlike OCD, OCBs are not distressing and do not impair the child[473]. They may help the child learn about rules v flexibility, individuality, and perhaps anxiety management. OCBs are a very weak predictor of later OCD[191].
Overvalued lesson	I.e. the over-rigid application of a learned rule (p.521).
Addiction	both drug and "behavioural addiction" (p.259)

Stereotypies	For definition see p.553.
Forced touching or forced completing or forced balancing	Forced touching is most often seen in Tourette (p.101). The child touches something, usually himself, in order to balance a feeling or get it just right. It is a common feature even though it is not one of the diagnostic criteria. For example: if he knocks one shoulder on the door he has to then do the same for the other shoulder; if you tap one knee he has to tap the other (or he may feel even better matching is achieved if *you* do the second tap); a tiqueur who drove the left wheel of his car over the curb had to then drive the right wheel over the other curb; he may need to straighten everything on every table; he can be preoccupied with the discrepancy between clocks Many tiqueurs *go back* to make things *just right*, (e.g. going back to balance a tap, or in one case retracing steps to check he didn't walk past a nest of snakes) whereas motor tics go with them (as do stereotypies or obsessions in those with autism or OCD). Forced touching is also different from these other conditions in that it is generally inactive until triggered by something in the environment. *Contrast with OCD* Forced touching is hardly seen in OCD. Tiqueurs do not have an underlying fear: they just feel uncomfortable until they have performed the action. Treatments are distinct
Autism ☂ (p.183)	"Stimming" is a jargon word for stereotypies, used mainly by carers of autistic people. Many repetitive *behaviours* exist to serve an underlying abnormal autistic *interest* (p.229): • To directly create a desired sensation (e.g. the sight of fingers wiggling). In autism-related disorders the repetitions are usually simple (p.229) or sterile (p.554); not directed at an underlying fear (p.307), and not resisted. Unlike the other causes of stereotypies, autistic ones seem to be desired, and often hold the child rapt with attention for several minutes (e.g. a boy who pushes a car back and forth in the same line until it grinds its way through the table; or a teenager who will find a leaf and focus on it indefinitely). • To indirectly contribute (e.g. tearing strips of paper that can then be dropped to create a desired sensation; or throwing flowerpots because of fascination with the distribution of earth made on the carpet) Some repetitive *behaviours* associated with autism do not result from *abnormal interests*, but from:neurological immaturity (e.g. flapping, p.105; utilisation behaviours, p.572); developmentally appropriate interests (e.g. casting, p.103); sensory intolerance and intolerance of change (p.126); behavioural spandrels: rigid sequences or styles (mannerisms, p.505) in the way that an interest is pursued; lack of social constraints (e.g. public nose-picking, masturbation, p.115). See posturing (p.93) and [1631] for more discussion.
Midline stereotypies / hand movements	These usually involve both hands acting together. They are sometimes associated with minor developmental problems, especially autism-related disorders; or the precipitants may indicate that they are variants of flaps (p.105). Hand-wringing with regression may indicate the rare Rett syndrome (p.541).

continued ▶

Anxiety related	
Anxious movements	Hand-wringing, lip-sucking, foot turning, writhing, deep breathing, pursing , etc. There can be lots simultaneously; they are slower and more variable than tics (p.101). They usually reduce with time in the session, and increase with social or performance demands. Consider panic (p.301).
Depression (p.309)	Can cause rumination, self-harm, obsessive behaviours. Consider bipolar affective disorder (p.264).
Phobias	Keeping one's distance from the feared object helps in phobias, but not in OCD**
Obsessive Compulsive Disorder (OCD)[1023]	Obsessions are unwanted repetitive thoughts; compulsions are repetitive behaviours used to ward away fear. Traditionally it has been assumed that obsessions must have arrived before the corresponding compulsions; but the compulsions often start first in children (i.e. in at least some cases the obsession is a post-hoc explanation for the compulsion). In adults diagnosis requires obsessions and compulsions to be time consuming and distressing but this is often not the case in children. 80% of the general population have had obsessional thoughts at some time[1293]. The diagnostic difficulty is that most people are embarrassed about the underlying obsession and don't disclose it (p.452), so the only clues are the behaviour (i.e. the compulsion, which may be an invisible ritual), what can be learned in direct sympathetic questioning in private, and self-completed questionaires[1636]. Characteristic categories of underlying fears (**obsessions**): contamination, disaster, asymmetry, religious, sexual, risk of becoming violent, unlucky numbers; categories of **compulsions**: cleaning, checking, repeating, counting, ordering, hoarding (p.480). These can be combined on 5 main dimensions: symmetry/ordering, hoarding, contamination /cleaning, aggression/checking, sexual/religious. Content is culturally determined so fears/obsessions about the internet, and compulsions of recycling, are increasing. Below age 9, the commonest obsessions are dirt and catastrophe, and the commonest compulsions are washing and checking[538]. The resulting behaviours are generally not stereotyped, but variable within the demands of the fear. Onset is usually age 10−16, but can be as early as toddlerhood, in which cases a family member often has OCD [1574]. OCD often leads to depression, or symptoms can appear during depression[912]. See also *intrusions*, p.493; *rage*, p.71; *obsessive slowness*, p.95; OCB (above); distinction from tics, p.101; obsessive compulsive personality, p.242; other anxieties, p.297; attractor, p.397.
Prospective memory impairment[351]	Can necessitate checking actions have been done or that objects are really there. Can be confined to visual check
Other psychiatric	
substance abuse	(p.267)
Anorexia nervosa (p.334)	Anorexia is often very similar to OCD, and there is considerable comorbidity. Pervasive repetition of exercises "to get them perfect" would be viewed as OCD, but compulsive exercising to lose weight, or as a result of weight loss, is usefully described as an eating disorder. Similar inflexibility is seen with other causes of starvation (see p.553).
☞ Psychosis (p.537)	Ask the patient why he does it. In adults, resistance, i.e. trying not to comply with the urge, is more characteristic of OCD (above) than of psychosis**. See *catatonia*, p.98; *cycloid psychosis*, p.449.

Deprivation related	
"Deafisms"	• E.g. rhythmic vocal noises, or hitting one's ear.
	• For people who are deaf in just one ear, head turning can allow them to work out the source of a sound. In children, such oft-repeated behaviours can form the basis of repeated experimentation, producing a whole family of turning-related self-entertainments and habits.
	• The word also refers to variations in the written and spoken English used by Deaf people.
	Note this word can be experienced as pejorative.
Behaviours in visual impairment (sometimes called "blindisms"[588])	• Light gazing lasting longer than 15 seconds almost always indicates cortical visual impairment rather than ocular impairment[763]. An extension of light gazing is wiggling the fingers in the visual field, sometimes between the eyes and a light source; or repetitive blinking (compare p.108).
	• Eye pressing, or even hitting, is *sometimes* to obtain visual stimulation. This only happens with severe bilateral ocular visual loss[763].
	• Central dazzle is painless intolerance of light, usually caused by thalamic damage
	• Bilateral anterior visual path disease sometimes causes complex compensatory behaviours. For example, nystagmus can be partially overcome by repetitively turning or shaking the head[587].
	• People often try to look around scotomas, e.g. by "overlooking" the object of fixation. This can give the impression of poor eye contact as in autism.
	• Expect to see perimeter hugging and touching everything. The opposite, a nearly complete disuse of the hands for exploration, is seen in some blind people with cerebral palsy. It is important to recognise as it is remediable[1411].
	• Rocking is more common in the blind – often due to comorbidities such as ID; such movements are better called self-soothing (p.61), self-entertainment or stereotypies, depending on other features (p.553).
☞Severe deprivation	as after 3rd world orphanage care.

Neurological & other medical	
☞PANDAS	(p.522)
Motor symptoms	(p.85)
Head injury	(p.477)
Perseveration	(p.527)
Mouthing (p.56); excess persistence with a toy	Klüver-Bucy syndrome (p.496)
☞Migraine	(p.141)
Cluster headache	(p.140)
Medical	• reflux (GORD, p.472), cardiac arrhythmia, syncope (p.74), absences (p.75), reflex anoxic seizures
	• Some metabolic disorders are periodic, e.g. ketotic/nonketotic hypoglycaemia (cf p.82), and disorders of the urea cycle (p.571) or of fatty acid metabolism (p.418).
	• Infection (especially UTI, URTI)

** These apparently simple rules are often impossible to use in young children, and in any case may arbitrarily separate things that are on a continuum or whose underlying cause is identical.

Conundrum 1: OCD within autism

When an autistic teenager starts a new stereotypy that is more complex than any he has had previously, it is reasonable to wonder whether he has developed OCD (p.65), other anxiety disorders, tics, or depression. All these problems are somewhat more common in ASD [193]; for examples see[557,1317]. Repetitions, intermittent exacerbations by stress, and inaccessibility of thought are characteristics of both disorders, hence many parents imprecisely use the word *obsession* to describe the stimming of autism (p.64). If symptoms occur only in specific places or in the presence of a particular person, both ASD and OCD are unlikely[e.g. p.20 of 1574] but not impossible as either can be worsened by anxiety.

Assigning a symptom to OCD or autism
- ➢ Mounting anxiety while repeating a behaviour is highly likely to be OCD; but mounting excitement (autistic **rapture**) is often seen while repeating a stereotypy.
- ➢ In OCD there is often sadness or frustration (p.291) and fears even if the fears are **hypothetical** or vague (e.g. "I scared"). In autism the fears are usually concrete, e.g. sensory intolerances, p.125.
- ➢ Obsessions of OCD are usually omnipresent, but its behavioural out-bursts are often confined to **home**. ASD can go unremarked at home if parents are very accommodating (see p.207).
- ➢ Behaviours in autism are highly **stereotyped**. Compulsions of OCD are more variable or complex. Even though OCD is often associated with Tourette's, the tics from Tourette's can usually be distinguished from autistic stereotypies by their greater speed (also, contrast common stimming patterns, p.64 with common tics, p.101).
- ➢ Thought content is not a reliable marker of OCD as there are other causes of thoughts or behaviours related to sex (p.267), and cleaning (p.112); for others see above. However, **somatic** obsessions, and **counting** compulsions, make OCD more likely than ASD[1395], as do hundreds of crossings out, and fear of losing one's temper.

Usually OCD starts in **adolescence**, whereas autistic ritualism starts much earlier. In the rare cases of OCD with onset in toddlerhood, there is often a family history of OCD (p.65).

Causelist 10: Sudden changes in emotion

Only a few emotions (of the list on p. 395) are subject to troublesome
sudden change, typically producing episodes lasting a few minutes. There
are many terms for the tendency of a person's emotions to vary more than
most people's: *Emotional instability*, *dyscontrol, episodic dyscontrol,
emotion dysregulation* all usually refer to disruptive or dangerous
behaviours. *Lability*, *emotionalism*, and *emotional incontinence* most
often refer to excess or sudden crying. See also impulsivity, pp.79,489;
autonomic instability, p.428; distinction from epilepsy, p.71.

Some variability of emotion is of course highly desirable in life, but in the
clinic high emotional variability is associated with mood related
diagnoses[889]. Aspects worth enquiring about clinically include the
frequency and speed of emotional shifts, the triggers for them (e.g.
threshold, episodicity and spontaneity: see p.63 and functional analysis,
p.365), the intensity (see rage, p.71) and duration of any states achieved.

Linking categories to mechanisms

The categories described below overlap, as do their names, which are often
used imprecisely. The terms generally refer either to excessive impulses
(and their presumed causes) or to the inadequate control of them.
However in practice such distinctions are difficult.

Excessive impulses: e.g. testosterone is often suspected as the cause of
excess aggressive impulses in adolescent boys (but see p.554).

Emotional dyscontrol (i.e. *dysregulation*) is an exceptionally complex
concept, as regulation itself is so complex.   A rigorous analysis[622] suggests
that people's primary aim is to regulate their internal emotional state (their
affect), and to do this they use diverse means including coping
mechanisms (p.445), defense mechanisms (p.303), external emotion
regulation[307], and (longer term) mood regulation.

Causes of sudden emotional change	
Any kind of episode	.
Learned, acted (p.418)	Children will learn to use any kind of emotional display to get what they want. Crying and aggression are the most common.
True instability of emotion	*True (pandirectional or directionless)* instability can cause episodes of any of the types listed at the right. It is often seen in mild form in ADHD (p.83). • A mild sign is overt emotional change that tracks the changing subjects in a conversation. • In unusual cases instability can be far more extreme than the child's hyperactivity. Note that even one or two outlandish *non-aggressive* episodes (e.g. jumping backwards over a chair or lifting her mother's shirt briefly with a grin) show that the problem is not aggression but true instability.
"mood dysregulation"	In future a "severe mood dysregulation" category may be used, combining irritability (p.494) and hyperarousal (e.g. insomnia, physical restlessness, and pressured speech) as well as, in some cases, persistent sadness[222,1217]. The construct is so far little used, perhaps because it conflates developmental with emotional issues, emotion with mood (p.461), and high with low mood, all in a counterintuitive way. Other problems with the concept parallel those of Intermittent Explosive Disorder, below.
hallucination	(p.343)
flashback	in PTSD, p.532.

Aggressive episodes	Aggressive outbursts may appear to clinicians to be more common than elated ones, simply because many children are referred after someone is hurt, or if they are unhappy as well. Such outbursts when extreme are called *rage*, p.71. Physical aggression is normal in frustrated toddlers (see pp.286,289), though it does not usually cause damage. Nearly half of children and adolescents referred to clinic (for any reason) have aggressive episodes lasting over 30 minutes[98], but this is unusual in unreferred youngsters. For causes of aggression see p.289.
Irritability	(p.494)
Bipolar Affective Disorder	There is a recent trend, currently mainly in America, to classify children with emotional instability as having Bipolar Affective Disorder (for diagnostic issues see p.264).
Intermittent Explosive Disorder	DSM-IV uses this term for aggression too great for the provocation, when it occurs in adults (*Intermittent Explosive Disorder*). Unfortunately the definition would include most infants. In one study, 7% of the adult population received the diagnosis, having typically 1-10 episodes per year; 4% of assaults required medical attention and the average property damage in an outburst was $40. In such adults, serious anger problems are typically recalled as having started between age 10 and 18[15], no doubt in part because of the teenager's increasing capacity to cause physical damage. Episodes in diagnosed adults typically last seconds to minutes and are followed by remorse. It is not yet clear how much of this disorder results from specific causes (see p.291) and how much is a separate condition in its own right.
Other episodes with a specific emotion	
Elated	Such episodes are often called *overexcited* (p.520). Occasionally, hypomania or hyperthymia is the cause (p.264).
Depressed	Surprisingly, depressed people show greater "emotional inertia" from moment to moment, both for positive and negative emotions[889].
Anxious	See *panics*, p.301; *startle syndromes*, p.552.
Emotionally unstable or borderline personality (p.242)	Characteristically the behaviours in these conditions are highly emotionally and socially laden (e.g. self-harm, p.318; threats of harming self or others).
Crying (or less commonly, laughing or smiling)	Emotional lability or emotionalism or emotional incontinence is uninhibited laughing or crying, sometimes lasting for minutes, that can be triggered by mild stimuli. This is common in numerous diencephalic conditions, such as a stroke affecting the globus pallidus[841] or the subthalamic nucleus. In contrast, emotional episodes caused by a hypothalamic hamartoma (p.76) occur out of the blue and are typically affectless. Neurological assessment is essential. When lability is combined with dysarthria and dysphagia it forms the clinical syndrome of pseudobulbar palsy, p.537. See also other causes of laughing, p.111; and crying, p.315. Hormonal causes of emotional lability (pp. 506,315-316)

Causelist 11: Brief overwhelming states

Deliberate self-harm (p.317) and aggression (p.289) often occur when a
person's normal self-monitoring is overwhelmed, but his ability to direct
actions is not.

Overwhelming states	Notes
Obviously fully alert	
‖ Tantrums	(p.286)
Rage	A rage is an extreme, explosive, uncontained (i.e. completely out of control) outburst of anger or aggression. It is not always sudden, and it can last as long as two hours. Rages are similar to tantrums in age trends, causal associations, and temporal organisation, so are probably severe versions of tantrums[1272]. Rages are more common in ADHD, ID,and language disorder[1272]; indeed in many physical and mental conditions (p.289). Concealed OCD (p.65) is an important cause, because of the cognitive rigidity (p.234), and disliking their rituals being interrupted, and not being able to explain why. Less dramatic rage-like feelings often contribute to impulsive violence, rudeness (p.161), and tantrums (p.286). Schools are often more sympathetic to children described as having the internal state "rage" than the external-sounding "aggression". Distinguish between moral rage (strong sense of values, not accepting that adults have more rights, etc.) and spoiled rage (frustration, p.291). For a more general discussion of aggression see p.289. For the relationship between rages and epilepsy, see p.75.
Breath-holding spells	(p.434)
Hyperventilation	(p.484)
Panics	(p.301)
Shuddering attacks	These occur in older infants and young children, with sudden flexion of the neck and trunk and movement inwards (adduction) of the arms. The child shivers and the body stiffens. This lasts 5–15 seconds, and needs no treatment[137].
Orgasm (see also masturbation, p.115)	• There may occasionally also be orgasm-like states when there is intense focus on a desired sensation, such as in scratching a severe itch (p.110). • The "rush" following use of heroin (see opiates, p.519) has been described as orgasm-like • orgasm-like auras can precede epileptic fits (rare).
Autism ☂ (p.183)	Intense focus on something simple (e.g. a line, or bumps in paint) can be pleasant or can be a learned way of avoiding being overwhelmed by information from the world (p.125).
Apnoea	(central or obstructive, p.518)
Dropping to floor	See *drop attacks*, p.75

TIAs	Transient ischaemic attacks. These cause negative symptoms (neurological deficits) that are maximal at onset, and typically improve over minutes. Consider moyamoya disease in children[529].
Phaeochromocytoma	Sudden onset of headache and pallor/sweating : p.529
Impaired alertness	
Catatonia	(p.98)
Syncope	(p.74)
☞ Epilepsy	(p.73) Can be very infrequent.
Dropping to floor	See *drop attacks*, p.75
Sleep-related	
☞ Microsleeps	Look like absences (p.75); poor sleep may be the cause.
Narcolepsy	Attacks of irrepressible sleep in the daytime, mainly during monotonous activity. Usually has continuous background sleepiness. May also have cataplexy (p.436), dreams immediately on sleep onset, sleep paralysis (partial waking), and sleep shouting[1561]. The usual molecular cause is autoimmune[369], lowering hypocretin and somehow allowing REM phenomena to intrude into other states of consciousness[343]. *Investigations* Low CSF hypocretin (p.485) is found in over 90% of cases with full narcolepsy (including cataplexy). Some of this association may be due to obesity. Rapid REM onset can be confirmed by the Multiple Sleep Latency Test (MSLT). Cases not reaching standard diagnostic criteria are sometimes clinically impaired.
Parasomnias	(p.200)
Simulation	
Pseudoseizure	(p.74) Other fabricated conditions: p.359.

For common fit types consult a textbook of neurology. This section addresses some common causes of diagnostic confusion.

It is often thought that an EEG (p.459) will show whether a child has epilepsy, and if so it can be treated with antiepileptic medicines. The reality is more complicated: Three issues need to be considered somewhat separately, not in this order but in this eventual order of importance:

Does any **treatment** help? In the end this will only be certain after a trial of treatment. However treatment benefit does not prove that the child has epilepsy, because anti-epileptic medications also help conditions other than epilepsy.

The old adage "treat the patient not the EEG" (discussed in[1524]) is widely cited. Often this adage is interpreted as limiting treatment to observable fits; however a more useful and modern interpretation is that the measured outcome of any individualised treatment trial needs to be clinically relevant. Such outcomes can be observable fits, attention, cognitive level[168,1089] or reading ability[655].

Is there a *tendency* to repeated unprovoked* seizures, with observable externally recognisable **fits** ? After exclusion of other causes (p.69) this tendency is called epilepsy.

> **EPILEPSY IS**: In epilepsy there is *usually* no trigger; there is *usually* a sudden change in level of consciousness, and a fairly sudden end to the episode; during the episode there are *usually* simple repetitive movements; the person *may* be incontinent or bite his tongue; and he is *usually* very sleepy afterward (except after absences).

> **EPILEPSY ISN'T**: If the action is (a) motivationally directed, (b) *fully* aware (i.e. full vigilance, reactivity and orientation), and (c) clearly recalled without suggestion, then it is *not* epileptic. If the awareness and recall (b and c) are present, it could be dissociative (p.453), part of a complex partial seizure, or very rarely, nonconvulsive status epilepticus. The vigilance named in (b) is considered to be present if the episode can be terminated by a light touch.

Physical investigations do not usually make or break the diagnosis of epilepsy. This reliance on an externally observable syndrome is analogous to the observable syndromes of psychiatry (e.g. ADHD, p.387). However, the diagnosis is strongly supported if there are epileptiform EEG changes that are synchronised with observed seizures, or if there is a characteristic pattern such as the 3-Hz spike-and-wave of absences.

Are there **epileptiform EEG abnormalities**? This is not a straightforward question as the limits of normality are not clear. Subtypes are spikes, sharp waves, benign epileptiform discharges of childhood, spike-wave complexes, polyspikes, hypsarrhythmia, seizure, and status pattern[1166].
- In some cases there are epileptiform EEG changes synchronised with brief cognitive lapses. This can be detected by computerised testing[168], most simply responding to a click[1166].
- A substantial number of complex partial seizures have a normal routine EEG – special electrode positions may be needed.

Medical emergency if:
!!   Tonic−clonic fit lasts longer than 5 minutes
!!   Series of fits lasts longer than 30 minutes
!!   This is the first fit, or is much longer than previous ones.

* unavoidable provocations, such as flashing lights, are allowed.

Causes of fits and fit-like episodes

Careful observation (ideally with video recording) and knowledge of standard patterns are invaluable. These include phenomena in up to four spheres: sensory, motor, consciousness, and autonomic (see[1165]).

A. *Epileptic fits*

Epilepsy cannot be diagnosed simply by observing *fits*: there are many non-epileptic causes of fits (see B below). Prolactin (p.536) is raised following both epileptic and syncopal fits. Tongue-biting can occur in epilepsy and in pseudo-fits. Following tonic–clonic fits, post-ictal EEG slowing and raised CK are good indicators of grand mal. Transient focal neurological deficits can indicate focal epilepsy or migraine.

B. *Non-epileptic fits* (or secondary /physiological seizures)

These are true fits, with loss of consciousness, and abnormal brain electrical activity during the fit, but they differ from epilepsy in not having an enduring brain abnormality that can produce fits. Non-epileptic fits are often multifactorial, with causes including fever; syncope; head injury, p.477; medication or illicit drugs and their withdrawal; sleep deprivation; encephalitis, p.461; tumours, p.569; hypocalcaemia, p.485; hyponatraemia,p.338; hypoglycaemia[388], or other causes of extreme bradycardia such as reflex anoxic seizures. These factors also exacerbate pre-existing epilepsy.

Syncope is fainting. There are usually clear precipitants such as dehydration, prolonged standing, severe coughing, blood loss or venepuncture (i.e. vasovagal fits) or a severe startle (p.552). Signs include lightheadedness or vertigo, pallor, feeling odd or nauseous, followed by a visual backout or "whiteout" and/or visual hallucinations; falling; and rapid recovery. Especially if the person does not lie down, syncope can trigger a fit (epileptic or not). Sometimes in ID, an intentional Valsalva manoeuvre can cause pallor and a vacant look, or full syncope.

C. *Psychogenic*, i.e. pseudoseizure: (the term non-epileptic seizure by rights includes both B and C, but is often taken to mean only C) This is not either/or: many children have both A and C. Upgoing plantar reflex (p.56), absent corneal reflex, or elevated prolactin soon afterward, make seizure likely, but are difficult to obtain. Tongue-biting, incontinence, and good response to antiepileptics all tip the balance toward seizures. There are many clinical signs that favour pseudo-fits over actual fits: Non-response to medication, "fashionable" diagnoses, psychiatric diagnoses[137], pelvic thrusting, stop/start (especially pausing to see who is around or who has just come in the door); non-rhythmical activity, side-to-side (no/no) movements, weeping, eyes closed. A complete absence of post-attack confusion/sleepiness makes pseudoseizures more likely, but is also found in some epilepsies. Pseudoseizures are more likely to be provokable by suggestion or hypnosis[1192]. Pseudoseizures occur mainly when people are around – but if only one individual carer has witnessed frequent daytime episodes, the veracity of the reports needs to be considered [see 1551]. None of these signs is perfectly reliable and video-EEG is the gold standard. Pseudoseizures lasting over 30 minutes are always grand mal-like, and have been called "pseudoseizure status"[1318]. See pseudo-behaviours, p.363.

Behaviours that often make parents wonder about epilepsy

Rages (and other overwhelming states, p.69)
Epilepsy can usually be distinguished from rage or breath holding (p.434), by the absence of precipitants (even very slight) or of directedness during the attack. Fits prevent organised behaviour so are very unlikely to be the explanation for destruction of property, with the exception of property falling and breaking during a fit. Rages can (rarely) be due to pre-ictal fear, restraint during post-ictal confusion[1359] (see also bewilderment, p.431), or 'hyperkinetic seizures' with fairly random hitting of anything nearby[1566] which can confuse by appearing purposeful[1003]

- Epilepsy (e.g. TLE) can cause sudden mood change without precipitant.
- Epileptic automatism (p.427) can cause sudden irrational acts.
- Some rare epilepsies can cause brief fear which causes violence (p.76)
- In young children, an *akinetic seizure* (which often includes falling backwards) may be blamed by the child on someone pushing them, so they then attack that person.

Drop attacks
The commonest cause is dropping to avoid moving (which happens with full alertness, when he is tired, a change of activity has been suggested, and he expects to be pulled). Syncope is also quite common (p.74). Much rarer causes include atonic seizures (following which loss of consciousness is limited to seconds[137]); vertebrobasilar ischaemia; and cataplexy in narcolepsy (p.72).

Absences or zoning out (staring spells)
Absences, or petit mal seizures, happen many times per day, and interrupt behaviour suddenly, even in the middle of a sentence. There are many variants of absences, e.g. with or without 3 Hz eyelid movement; with or without eye opening part-way through the absence; with or without awareness[1415]; and with or without minor automatisms (p.427). The combination of stilling with upgaze (showing sclera only) is highly suggestive of an absence attack – but some children learn to do this voluntarily to shock (usually distinguishable by other movements of the face) or to zone out. Counting to 100 can sometimes make absences obvious, and hyperventilation (p.484) can be used to precipitate an absence. EEG-confirmed absences are often preceded by subjective negative affect or feeling "blocked"[980]. Each child has a characteristic range of seizure durations (e.g. 1−2 seconds or 10−30 seconds)[1415]. After the attack, the child usually resumes what he was doing (he may resume speaking where he left off or more often loses the thread of conversation Fig.6 of 1166,1241) – without any sleepiness, in contrast to the sleepiness that both precedes and follows *microsleeps*, p.72. **Zoning out**, meaning letting the mind wander or letting it go blank, happens when the child is bored, and is ended by a touch. If the child can describe something fun he was doing during the episodes (ask if he was being in a movie) this is an *imaginary world*, p.231.

Panics
The features of these are listed on p.301. People with panics usually have other symptoms of anxiety too. However, fear can also be an aura in mesiotemporal epilepsy[137].

Twitches.
Almost all of these are tics (p.101). However if they are not temporarily suppressible and not identically reproducible at will, consider myoclonic jerks or epilepsia partialis continua (p.461).

Symptoms that should raise the question of epilepsy

Regression : Epileptiform changes (p.73) can cause general or circumscribed regression[1089,1524], see p.41.

Night-time fits (nocturnal seizures): These can remain unwitnessed for years. Signs are noise, sweatiness, and secondary enuresis. They should not be ignored as they reduce learning. They usually happen several times a night, as opposed to night terrors (p.200) that happen only once a night.

Personality change: Sudden changes in mood/behaviour/ personality may be temporal-lobe fits [or other sites: 9]. Frontal epilepsy can change personality, or induce automatisms (p.427), or be seen as misbehaving.

Behavioural fluctuations: (a) Monthly "premenstrual" symptoms are common in peripubertal girls (p.506). These include migraines, mood changes, and occasionally epilepsy.   (b) Some children (boys and girls) show a gradual deterioration in their behaviour over 4−8 weeks, that is then relieved by a few days of odd behaviour that can only be proved epileptic by EEG.

Other rare manifestations of epilepsy
- Epilepsy causing hyperactivity or inattention: p.82.
- Repeated bewilderment or alerting, p.431.
- Epileptic hallucinations: p.351.
- Gelastic (laughing) seizures (p.111) are rare but serious, and usually start by age 2. The laughing is characteristically mirthless, and the person may not remember having laughed or cried. The seizure usually arises within a hypothalamic hamartoma (a noncancerous lump of cells), and the location and size of this affect symptoms to some extent[834]. The focal seizures tend to become more complex within months, so that the child might develop diverse other fits, or have a laugh followed by a generalised fit.
- Hypothalamic hamartomas can also cause other intrusive experiences (p.493), such as visual or auditory hallucinations, delusional experiences ("Mummy she's pulling my skin off!") and brief emotional changes, such as dacrystic (crying) seizures, fearfulness, or brief aggression[991]. They are often missed on routine EEG. The episodes are characteristically brief (15−120 seconds) with a sudden onset and offset, and no trigger. Half of cases experience precocious puberty[834].
- Autonomic/vomiting fits (Panayiotopoulos syndrome, childhood autonomic epilepsy)[1215]
- Out-of-the-blue fear or anger or threat, suddenly intruding while doing an enjoyed activity, usually strange in some way and usually undirected. Diagnose by video EEG. See *intrusions*, p.493.
- Odd subjective experiences occurring truly out of the blue should raise the suspicion of epilepsy. The most obvious are visual hallucinations (p.344).   Less obviously, a sudden strong feeling of depersonalisation turned out to be an aura; in another case a sudden odd feeling in the throat was due to frontal epilepsy.
- Cycloid psychosis (p.449)

Causelist 12: Crescendo of activity

Timecourse
Crescendos can be sudden, step-wise, or gradual over various timecourses. One type is the commonplace escalation of aggressive behaviour over tens of seconds to win an argument, often culminating in a full temper tantrum. An habitually violent child may be somewhat cautious in using this on a stranger (e.g. clinic staff or a new teacher) so starts with a stare or gentle tap to gauge its effect, growing to larger blows in subsequent confrontations. A *sudden* increase in excited, out-of-control behaviour can be called emotional dyscontrol (p.69). Out-of-control behaviour that is started by an interaction, lasts just a minute or two then disappears is anger (p.287).

The duration of the calm is important for management in school. If the child stays calm for half an hour or more, it is usually practicable for the school to manage him (regardless of what he does after that time) by changing his task before he erupts.

Nature of activity

The list below refers to an increase in activity level, during a clinical session or a half-day at school. Intrigue and anxiety can both suppress hyperactivity for the first 5–30 minutes of a clinic appointment. If the new behaviours that then appear are social, relaxed, or appropriately exploratory, they were being suppressed by anxiety. If they are chaotic, it was hyperactivity or impulsivity (pp.79,84). If both appear, it was both.

Factors contributing to crescendo during a session or lesson	Notes
Of repetitive behaviour	(compare self-soothing, p.61)
increasing anxiety	E.g. results of anger frighten an autistic child, increasing the repetitive behaviours, often ending in headbanging. These behaviours will be well known to the carers.
sensitisation to noises or smells	(p.546)
exploratory success	Child has found something fun and repetitive to do, e.g. a blind to whizz up and down.
needing to use toilet	
attempts to achieve just-right sensations	Crescendos over seconds to many minutes occur during masturbation, p.115; and in some headbanging, p.119 (see also tics, love of exactness: p.163).
Of non-repetitive behaviour	
increasing boredom (p.322)	Signs are increasing chaos, agitation, and protests (p.84; or the opposite: see p.322. Can result from any cause of hyperactivity / impulsivity (p.79)
relief of exhaustion	E.g. after a frantic run to the clinic (unlikely unless mother is very fit).
lifting of rules	Gradual testing and extending boundaries in this situation. The child may suddenly realise that in the clinic adults don't tell him off (perhaps mum wants to show staff how loud he gets).
Of either sort of behaviour	
reducing anxiety	Look for signs of anxiety (p.296) early in the session, and then reduction in these accompanied by increasing interaction with people present.
increasing hunger temperature	
approaching the time when he wants to be somewhere else.	
getting a reaction	When children are trying to elicit a reaction, there is both repetition and variability. They select an activity that is known to get a reaction (e.g. throwing keys, climbing up shelves) and repeat it with escalations until they give up and try something else. During this they are not actually excited, but intermittently monitoring adults' reactions. They are partly out of the parents' control but not out of control of themselves.
Winding up	This means that the child's purpose is actually the upset in the parent, rather than the parent's physical reactions. This is rare before puberty, but common afterwards. Many other behaviours are often interpreted as winding up (e.g. casting, p.103; getting a reaction, above) but this incorrect interpretation should be avoided as it can damage the parent–child relationship and prevent effective management.

Causelist 13: Hyperactivity, Impulsivity, Inattention ☼

The reason to consider these three characteristics together is that they are often associated and difficult for referrers to distinguish from one another. They all affect behaviour and performance in school; in most children they are highly variable; they are all improved by stimulants (p.555); and taken together they form the criteria for a diagnosis of Attention Deficit Hyperactivity Disorder (ADHD ⬆, pp. 387,83).

There are many apparent paradoxes in this area (see *paradoxes of ADHD*, p.523), one of which is that stimulant medication helps almost regardless of the underlying cause. This may be an artefact of (a) the ways in which we conventionally test performance – requiring speed, focus, predictability, and precision, all of which are part of an evolved response to stress, and (b) the rather similar ways in which children's classroom behaviour is judged.

Detailed assessment is necessary to avoid missing social and cognitive problems and substance misuse (p.267). This is important because some of the underlying causes have treatments that are specific, effective, and long lasting. Others, such as ID or NVLD (p.28) require major changes in the way the child is taught.

The first question is duration. For changes from minute to minute see *emotional instability* on p.69; for escalation within a session see p.77; and for longer-term difficulty (which can act via these short timecourses) see the table below. The hyperactivity of hypomania typically lasts weeks (p.264); in TLE no more than a few hours after a sudden start; in Prader-Willi up to a week (p.533).

It has been commonly thought that ADHD is a discrete disease entity with a distinct pathology. According to this view, the other entries in this list are "medical mimics" of ADHD [252,1236]. This would imply that all the problems in the list need to be excluded before ADHD is diagnosed. A more modern view is that ADHD is merely the combination of all the other causes in this list, when they are either unrecognised, or too small to attract individual diagnoses [1080,1770].

Basic screening should include school report, developmental or cognitive testing (p.59), detailed sleep history, FBC, thyroid, lead, ferritin. Further tests to consider are described on p.82.

Factors contributing to hyperactivity, impulsivity, or inattention	Diagnostic notes (Note that many of the differential diagnoses commonly coexist.)
👁 Immaturity and ID	The entire triad appears in normal babies and toddlers, so disorder should not ordinarily be diagnosed under 4, or indeed in children whose mental age is under about 4. Assessment should therefore include the establishment of at least an approximate mental age. Children with a chronological age below about four are not as a rule observed next to their peers in a controlled academic environment, making assessment less reliable. Children with mild or borderline ID children are somewhat more active[1485], and this escalates dramatically when given work they find difficult. Many children with profound ID explore or climb almost continually.
Boredom	Bright children (see *gifted*, p.473) who are bored as well as hyperactive sometimes do 2−3 things at the same time (see p.322). Children brighter than their peers can be bored in a special school.
👁 Sleep problems	Both night-time sleep and (more importantly) daytime sleepiness are abnormal in hyperactive or inattentive children [1202]. Young children can become hyperactive when they are very tired. People at any age concentrate less well when tired. Consider narcolepsy including mild forms of it, p.72; obstructive sleep apnoea, p.518.
Letting off steam, or burning off energy (See also *exercise*, p.462)	• Children, especially boys under 10, who have not been able to run around for several hours, often tear around or roughhouse for 10−20 minutes in the playground, or at home. The noise and movement can be repetitive. However, unlike autistic repetitions they welcome other people bumping into them or getting excited with them. (There is scant information on this effect in children, but a similar effect is seen in rats, in whom it also reduces with ageing[697].) • More directly boredom-alleviating behaviours: cleaning, rocking, drumming but different from self-soothing, p.61 • Over-control by parents increases the likelihood of severe outbursts or rebellion. • (The term also refers to talking about pent-up frustrations, or the idea that children should "release their aggression" by punching a pillow…; or a role of demonstrations in a democracy.) It is often interpreted as *sublimation*, p.305 – but there is usually no underlying meaning or conflict.
👁 Parental difficulties	Parental difficulty coping is a possibility if referral is initiated by parents or comes before the child has entered nursery. A much more reliable indicator of problems at home is the presence of great difference between the parents' and the teachers' rating scale scores, with behaviour reported as much worse at home than at school. Complaints of *hyperactivity* may indicate nothing more than overburdened, overworked, unresponsive, or depressed parents, particularly when preceding children were very easy to manage. Related, but less common causes of inattentive restless behaviour include disturbed attachment (p.195), witnessing interparental violence, and physical or sexual abuse (pp.273−275).

continued ▶

Learned behaviour	• Hyperactivity is sometimes used for attention-seeking, but in such cases it tends to be specific behaviours selected to get attention (e.g. climbing high on furniture within the parent's field of vision.) • Occasionally, children learn that hyperactivity stops mother talking, or distracts them from painful discussions, or their parents from marital rows. Hallmarks are the sudden starting and stopping of behaviours (especially noise, leaning from windows, etc.) that selectively disrupt conversation, triggered by specific topics or combinations of people.
Impulses	
Oppositionality (p.253)	This can exist either as a comorbid complication of ADHD, or as a separate entity.
Tic disorders (p.101): "Fidgetty Tickiness"	Attention difficulty and impulsivity are often seen in children who have tic disorders. Conversely, tics themselves occasionally give the impression of hyperactivity and impulsivity. This can be difficult to spot if the presence of many different tics conceals their repetitive nature. Additionally, tics, attempts to prevent them, and premonitory sensations, all distract the child so can create "secondary inattention". Head tics are particularly likely to cause visual inattention.
Deficient suppression of behaviours	Causes include inadequate anxiety, p.423; frontal deficits, p.512; and monoamine dysfunction[236,1351].
Ineffective punishment	(p.538)
Mood	
Mood or preoccupation	**Conundrum 2: Mood causing inattention or vice versa** Anxiety and agitated depression can cause inattention, hyperactivity, and impulsivity, but the reverse is also true. These possibilities can be distinguished by asking which came first. Inattention occurring only at school may be caused by worry about forthcoming playtime bullying. It is usually straightforward to distinguish hypomania and hyperthymia (p.264) from other causes of hyperactivity and impulsivity. PTSD (p.532) or anything else that preoccupies the child (e.g. obsessions, p.517; psychosis, p.537; being in love, p.501; anger, p.287; frustration, p.291) will give the impression of inattention.
Emotional instability	In most hyperactive children the behaviours are chaotic and flitting (p.84), and the emotional state is boredom (p.322). However more overtly emotional problems can also occur: see emotional instability, p.69.
Schizophrenia or prodrome	(p.544)
Cognitive	
Deafness, auditory processing difficulties	These can usually be distinguished by not being a problem when the other senses are used. Screening for deafness should be routine (p.130). Behaviour problems in deaf children don't increase with level of deafness, but with degree of expressive speech difficulty[1545]. See also CAPD, p.121.
Visual impairment	(p.133)

👁️ Non-verbal learning disability (p.28)	"Attention is usually reported to be impaired and testing supports this, but the affect is desultory as opposed to distractingly impulsive, as in ADHD. It is as if people with NVLD do not know what to attend to, but once focused, can sustain attention to detail. The distinction between figure and ground is disturbed, resulting in attention errors" [414].
Autistic Spectrum Disorder	Hyperkinesis here may be of stereotyped movements (p.553), or of situationally inappropriate behaviour. ASD (p.183) has several characteristics not shared with ADHD ☂. It can look as though they have poor concentration because
	• they don't understand what is said to them but they don't want to admit it,
	• they prefer thinking about a special interest. Sometimes you (or parents / teachers) glimpse what's going on through off-the-cuff remarks when he had looked bored.
	• they don't see the point,
	• or even don't know how to say "Can you say that again" – they don't have that skill in "repairing" the conversation.
Poor memory	Screening for digit span (p.452) should be routine, because this can reveal working memory deficits which appear as inattention[28] (and which benefit from stimulants).

Physical

Hypoglycaemia	This responds rapidly to food. It is most common after school when stimulants are wearing off; for other causes see p.331. The child is irritable (p.494), hungry, weak and often anxious. Even mild hypoglycaemia reduces the energy spent on thinking [1022]. Severe hypoglycemia causes tremor, nausea, pallor, sweating, repetitiveness, inflexibility; and rarely, hallucinations[736], p.349; or myoclonus, p.511. Extreme hypoglycaemia can cause coma or death.
Allergy or hypersensitivity	There is a common small effect of food colours and preservative[1032]. In a very few children the effect is large, but this is very unlikely unless an association with a specific food has already been noticed by the parents.
Itch (p.110) and pain	Especially when the child cannot reduce them. Consider pinworms.
👁️ Neurological	• Suspect epilepsy (p.73) if hyperactivity is episodic without precipitants
	• In inattention: overt or "subclinical" epilepsy [73,819] including absences[168] (pp.73−75)
	• Consider neurological causes of regression (p.41)
	• Frontal lobe deficits (p.512), particularly post-head injury (p.477), can cause inattention and hyperactivity, as can chorea (p.439), and ataxic cerebral palsy (p.437)
	• PANDAS (p.522)
Other physical causes [see 1588]	Caffeine, sympathomimetics (p.428), SSRIs causing "behavioural activation" (p.552); paradoxical effects of benzodiazepines (p.430) and antiepileptics; other licit & illicit drugs (e.g. sedatives and cannabis (p.258); solvents (even normal use of some glues) poor concentration and disinhibition; cocaine (p.258); anaemia (p.421), malnutrition (p.504), kernicterus (p.495), lead poisoning (p.330), hyperthyroidism (p.484), neurocutaneous syndromes, Fœtal Alcohol syndrome (p.467). Low iron is unusual but possibly useful to correct [870].

Special Topic 3: Is ADHD a useful diagnosis for this child?

ADHD (Attention deficit Hyperactivity Disorder) does not appear in the causelists in this book because it is an umbrella concept embracing many causes (figure on p.385, table on p.79) rather than a cause in its own right.

ADHD is defined to include all of the causes for hyperactivity, impulsivity, and inattention for which there is not a better category in DSM (see p.387 for the full DSM definition of ADHD.) The diagnosis of ADHD has been beneficial for millions of children, because it has reduced the likelihood of their being labelled as naughty (or worse), it leads to useful interventions in classrooms, and medications often help. Unfortunately the high frequency of diagnosis can lead to the overlooking of important remediable reasons such as abuse or poor sleep (other causes are listed on p.79).

Many people have strong views on whether the diagnosis of ADHD is useful, ethical, or scientifically sound. Because hyperactivity, impulsivity, and inattention follow a normal distribution in the population, a real practical difficulty is working out what level of symptoms justify diagnosis or intervention (see figure). Another issue for practicing clinicians is that all causes of these behaviours need to be carefully considered (p.79) because some of them require quite specific interventions rather than general ADHD interventions.

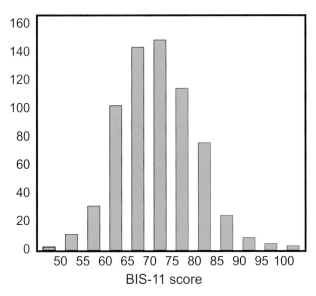

Figure 9. Population distribution of impulsivity.

Distribution of scores on the Barratt Impulsivity Scale for an unselected sample of 662 teenagers aged 15−17 [after 950]

It is important to realise that the diagnosis of ADHD ☂ cannot be ruled out solely on the basis of observations in clinic, because children with ADHD are often less active in novel environments. However if the session lasts at least an hour, most children with hyperactivity in class will be showing a crescendo of chaotic activity in the second half (see p.77). The diagnosis cannot be ascertained or ruled out simply on the reports of the parents, because they may have personal reasons for perceiving (or missing) problems; they generally don't ask the child to engage for long periods in unwanted tasks, and they do not have several peers to compare. Teachers are the most useful observers: If they have no concerns about inattention or hyperactivity, that almost completely rules out ADHD. There are two exceptions: (1) where the teacher is strongly influenced by the belief that misbehavior is a moral issue rather than a biologically based long-term condition (2) where ADHD is suppressed by anxiety in school (p.207).

Try to observe the duration of focus; then what pulls the child away; how he searches for something to take his attention, and then how strongly he is drawn in. The following are not in the DSM criteria but seem to be useful indicators that the child is impaired by inattention and/or impulsivity (conversely, the first three greatly reduce the likelihood of ☂ autism):

- *chaos*: randomness, constantly trying new little activities
- *flitting*: starting an activity and almost immediately moving to something else. The duration on tasks can be measured. See *distractibility*, p.453.
- *simultaneous non-habit behaviours*: e.g. drawing and looking around while talking to you.
- *crescendo*: increase in activity level during the session (p.77)

From the point of view of statutory educational support (statementing), ADHD ☂ is given much less weight than Autism ☂ or even Autistic Spectrum Disorder ☂. Parents often believe that a diagnosis of ADHD (or indeed, any other diagnosis) explains every conceivable difficulty their child has, especially misbehaviour, so it can be worthwhile stating clearly at the time of diagnosis that even though the child meets diagnostic criteria for ADHD, this is a relatively minor problem in him, compared to his ID or the lack of consistent management, for example.

Common errors in diagnosis
- Diagnosing ADHD without discovering that the child can't understand what is happening in class (e.g. due to ID, p.491 or specific learning disability, p.551; or language problems, p.145)
- Not considering the multiple remediable contributors to hyperactivity (table on preceding pages).
- Paying much attention to the subtypes as children frequently move back *and forth* between subtypes, and the subtypes have little prognostic or therapeutic significance[896].

Motor (General) ☼

For movements as for all behaviours, the frequency and triggers (p.61) need to be worked out, as do broader contributors such as emotion and learning (p.63). Most repetitive movements are more common in autism than in global delay or in normal development[1112]. Some very unusual movements are listed in[924].

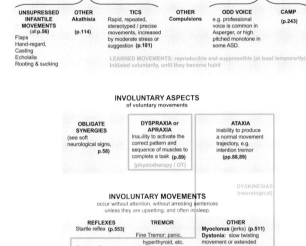

Figure 10. Standard categories of movements.

Investigation Planner 3: Treatable medical causes of movement disorders

(after[924])   See also the *general approach to medical investigations*, p.373, and[703]. For a much broader list see p.92.

	Signs	Test	Excluded clinically or to Order?	Date ordered	Result
Hyponatraemia	(p.338)	UECr			
Streptococcus	See PANDAS, p.522	(p.522)			
AIDS / HIV	(p.479)	p.479			
Epilepsies	(pp.73-76)	EEG			
Wilson's disease	(p.575)	(p.575)			
Leukodystrophy	(p.498)	(p.498)			
Segawa's disease	(p.458)	(dopa response)			
Coeliac disease	(p.441)	(p.441)			
Whipple's disease	rashes, diarrhoea, fever, joint pain, myoclonus (p.511), oculomasticatory myorhythmia, supranuclear gaze palsy	intestinal biopsy			
Myoclonic hereditary dystonia	Jerky head and arm movements	Striking improve-ment with alcohol or clonazepam			
Wernicke's encephalitis	(p.574)	vitamin B$_1$, MRI[1826]			
Thyrotoxicosis	(p.484)	TFT			
Renal failure	myoclonus (p.511), asterixis (p.105), restless legs	UECr			
Liver failure	myoclonus (p.511), asterixis (p.105), tremor, chorea (p.439)	LFT			
Non-ketotic hyperglycaemia	chorea (p.439), myoclonus (p.511)	fasting glucose			
hypoglycaemia	(p.82)	glucose			
Polycythaemia	chorea (p.439)	FBC			
SLE, antiphospho-lipid syndrome	(p.560)	(p.560)			
paraneoplasia-opsoclonus	myoclonus (p.511), chorea (p.439), dystonia	(complex auto-immunity)			
CoQ10 deficiency	(p.508) diverse; commonest is ataxia[460]	p.508			
Hypopara-thyroidism	(p.525) dystonia, chorea (p.439)	Ca++, phosphate			
PDH deficiency	episodic dyspraxia[105]	lactate & pyruvate			
Lesch-Nyhan and variants	may have dystonia with no other signs[778]	(p.318)			
Nonketotic hyperglycinaemia	(p.350)	(p.350)			
anti-NMDA	(p.422)[507]	anti-NMDA			
Autosomal recessive / metabolic ataxias[460]					
abetalipo-proteinaemia	(p.417)	(p.417)			
Refsum	(p.499)	(p.499)			
cerebrotendinous xanthomatosis	(p.32)	(p.32)			
Ataxia with inh-erited vitamin E deficiency[866]	progressive ataxia starting at any age. Babinski sign.	Serum α-tocopherol (vitamin E)			
GA1	(p.32)	(p.32)			

Neurological review is essential. Demonstrating a strong stretch reflex, or non-conformity to known distribution of motor nerves, is not sufficient to exclude a physical problem. Weakness (paresis) can become exaggerated to full functional paralysis if the sufferer feels she is not believed[850]. Fatiguability of muscles can be demonstrated by repeated foot tapping or repeated finger–thumb touching. See also chronic fatigue, p.323.

Causes of weakness & paralysis Part of body	Notes
Disuse	e.g. following plaster cast.
Guillain-Barré	Ascending paralysis starting 2 weeks after a severe fever, lasting months then disappearing downwards. There is a broad group of related acute and chronic inflammatory demyelinating polyneuropathies (AIDP/CIDP). About a third of patients with severe GBS have psychotic symptoms, especially in the first few weeks[302]. There are numerous variants and underlying causes that must be considered urgently in order to guide treatment[939].
Pseudo-paralysis (see pseudo-behaviours, p.363).	• Arms: e.g. disuse of arm when awake, but not when asleep. Try the face-hand test (p.464). • In unilateral leg pseudo-paralysis, attempts to lift the good leg off the bed force the heel of the affected leg deeper into the bed (Hoover's sign[907]). Conversely, attempts to lift the affected leg force the good heel down in organic weakness, but not in pseudo-paralysis.
Rare	• Monomelic motor neurone disease (Hirayama disease) • Multifocal motor neuropathy with conduction block
Widespread mild weakness	
Self-limiting illness	
Exhaustion	
Lack of exercise	
Ataxia	This takes so much energy that it reduces stamina
Malnutrition, anaemia	pp.504,421
Widespread severe weakness [1787]	
Proximal weakness	• Spinal muscular atrophy (p.551), muscular dystrophies (p.510), myopathies, Congenital / structural, Metabolic, p.379; Inflammatory, motor neurone disease • Neuromuscular junction disorders (myasthenia, p.510) • Myotonic dystrophy type 2 (p.568)
Distal weakness	Neuropathies • Hereditary: Charcot-Marie-Tooth disease, the most common inherited neuromuscular disorder, is actually a group of disorders involving peripheral axons and their myelin sheaths, initially affecting just the longest nerves to the feet[1219]. • Acquired: Guillain-Barré (see above)

Causelist 15: Ataxia

For life-long or long-term (chronic) ataxia see the discussion of terminology, p.89; and *metabolic ataxias*, p.86.

Causes of acute ataxia	Notes
Medication side-effects	Especially anticonvulsants and sedatives.
Post-injury	
Basilar type migraine	(p.142)
☞ Varying or increasing	
Maple syrup urine disease	(p.505)
Episodic ataxias	There are several rare genetic causes: Hartnup disease 477; channelopathies, pp.438 and 142.
Pseudo-ataxia	acute onset in highly emotional situations. See pseudo-behaviours, p.363.
☞ Medical /genetic	The most important to detect are the treatable biological causes, p.86. Examples: • Urea cycle disorder, p.571 • Segawa disease: worsens as the day progresses, p.458 • Pyridoxine toxicity, p.329 • Labyrinthitis • PANDAS, p.522 • Hartnup disease: episodic ataxia, p.477 • ☞ Cerebral tumour, p.569 • ☞ Encephalitis, p.461

Causelist 16: Clumsiness

There is no clear divide between dyspraxia, apraxia, chronic ataxia, and clumsiness, so they are grouped together here[559,743]. *Dyspraxia* ("wrong actions") and *clumsiness* are terms describing difficulties with organising or coordinating complex or fine movements. *Apraxia* usually refers to high-level organisational difficulties: "disorder of skilled movement not caused by weakness, akinesia, deafferentation, abnormal tone or posture, movement disorders such as tremor (p.61) or chorea (p.439), intellectual deterioration, poor comprehension, or uncooperativeness."[679]. *Ataxia* is generally reserved for much more severe difficulty affecting all movements ("no actions", see p.88).

None of these terms is a diagnosis in the sense of describing the origin of the problem, except that *dyspraxia* is often used as a shorthand for *developmental coordination disorder*. This affects about 6% of children mildly, and 2% severely[559]. It is important to look for underlying causes as in the list below, plus sequelae such as low mood; being told off for messy writing; or teased for poor performance in sports[461].

Occasionally, *dyspraxia* is used in a very broad sense ☂ as an "explanation" for numerous difficulties including not only gross and fine motor dyscontrol but also restlessness, poor organisation, and poor high-level reading skills. This does achieve a single name for all the child's problems (as does ☂ DAMP, p.450) and it has a theoretical basis (embodied or grounded cognition ([51,1285] but see [1271])). However such a broad use of the term fails to engage useful services – in education, social services, and health. Identification of smaller categories of problems amenable to targeted help is more useful: these can include ADHD, p.83; NVLD, p.28; DCD, above; hypermobility, p.483; sensory intolerances, p.125; and others.

Some categories of apraxia/ dyspraxia	notes (see[1251] for others and for details)	ways to assess
Ideomotor or executive a/d	Fluency and speed of movements (including timing, sequencing, and spatial organisation).	Movement ABC or DCDQ or BNS (age 6-7)[566]
Constructional apraxia a/d	Unable to build with blocks, or to copy complex drawings.	Griffiths (p.451), blocks, Rey-Osterrieth (p.38)
Visuomotor or oculomotor a/d	Disruptions to actions requiring visual support (catching; fine motor skills with cutlery & writing).	TVPS VMI (Visual–Motor Integration). rapid alternating movements (dysdiadochokinesis, p.457)
Oromotor a/d	Unclear speech, choking, dribbling (p.456). Oromotor dyspraxia causes unclear speech and problems with feeding, latching, chewing, and choking on lumps. Occasionally this is associated with a more widespread cerebral palsy including abnormal jaw reflex, in which case it is called Worster-Drought syndrome.	Test for oromotor dyspraxia by repeating "p-t-k" (because unpractised) or "buttercup" or "power rangers" repeatedly – Sainsbury's, clucking, tstststs, peter piper (try several).
Gait apraxia, p.471	Clumsy gait (gross motor)	Difficulty on stairs, history of falls
Dressing apraxia	Difficulty with dressing	From parent
Orienting apraxia	Difficulty orienting one's body to other objects.	Bumps into doors or tables.
Ideational or planning apraxia	Planning or the conceptual organisation of movements.	A severely affected child (without other deficits) could name a toothbrush and comb, and explain their use, but would eat with the toothbrush and brush his teeth with the comb.

Rareties in children		
Mirror apraxia	Difficulty reaching to objects that can be seen in a mirror.	
Gaze apraxia	Difficulty in directing gaze	
Conduction apraxias	Able to name someone's movements but not to copy them.	

continued ▶

Motor milestones

Where a range of ages is given below, the first is the age at which about 10% of children will have acquired a skill, and the second the age at which about 90% have. Delay in several skills beyond this 90% age merits further assessment (see p.55).

(After [640,1470,1522]. See also language acquisition, p.55; clothing, p.441.)

Age	Gross motor	Fine motor, eye-hand coordination	Self-care
0–1	Holds hands together from 2–4 months. Sits unsupported at 5–8 mos. Stands unaided at 9–14 mos	Follows person with eyes from 6–12 weeks. Looks at own hands and reaches for toy from 10–20 wks. Passes toy from hand to hand from 22–24 wks.	Finger-feeds self starting from 4–8 mos. Chewing starts 5–7 mos. Drinks from cup starting at 6–16 mos. Pincer grip starts at 10–12 mos.
1–2	Walks well at 10–16 mos, pushes ball with foot, crouches to pick up object at 10–16 mos	Scribbles round and round at 12–24 mos. Stacks 4x1-inch cubes at 18–24 mos.	Takes off clothes from 14–20 mos. Starts using spoon or fork.
2–3	Broad jump over small object, rides tricycle	Draws straight line at 17–36 mos, copies circle at 24–36 mos; stack 8x1-inch cubes at 24–39 mos, simple jigsaws	Dry during day starts 18–38 mos
3–4	Hopping	Pencil grip is mature tripod grasp, copies cross at 32–58 mos, starts drawing a person at 32–58 mos (see p.56). Builds a bridge from 3x1-inch cubes at 27–45 mos:	Fastens row of buttons, brushes teeth without help, puts on socks.
4–5	Alternating feet on stairs. Balances on one foot for 5 sec, from age 4 to 5 ½.	Cuts paper along a line, ties and unties simple knots, complex jigsaws	Fastens zip and all fasteners, independent toileting (including paper, washing hands, clothing), uses knife and fork separately
5–6	rides cycle without training wheels. Heel-toe walking	Cuts complex shapes from paper, ties shoelaces, catches small ball from 3 metres	Dresses independently, takes bath or shower without help
6–8	skips		Uses knife and fork together, can make his bed

Causes of clumsiness [559,743]	Notes
The most important to detect are the treatable causes, p.86 and below.	

Steady, or gradually improving with maturation

Normal variation or immaturity	
Delayed motor maturation	(often familial)
Developmental coordination disorder[1262]	Also called developmental dyspraxia (p.89)
Joint hypermobility	(p.483)
ADHD ♣	Careless when doing several things at once, or in a great hurry. *Also* inaccurate, i.e. handwriting is poor.
ID and small-for-dates	Particularly clumsy with the hands. Often whole-body movements remain very agile.
Minimal cerebral palsy	(p.437)
Mirror movements	(p.507)
Metabolic ataxias	(p.86)

Varying or increasing

Medication	Especially sedatives. Check the dose.
Emotional	Can be related to insecurity
Visual / Visuospatial defects	
Migraine	(p.141)
Head injury	(p.477)
Epilepsy	(p.73)
Precursor or prodrome of schizophrenia	Worth considering if there is family history [see 1747]. For signs of prodrome see p.544.
Heavy metals poisoning	(p.330)
Substance abuse	(p.257)
Hypothyroidism	(p.485)
Brain tumour slowly growing	(p.569)
Muscular dystrophy	(p.510)
Multiple sclerosis	(p.510)

Rare syndromes (for a fuller list see [1276])

Peripheral

Hereditary sensory & motor neuropathies, congenital myotonia, myasthenia, p.510

CNS

Lipidoses[1573], chorea, p.439; Wilson's, p.575; basilar type migraine, p.142; Rett, p.541; von Hippel-Lindau, p.514; ataxia telangiectasia, p.454; spina bifida, p.551; cerebral gigantism, pyruvate carboxylase deficiency[59,1710] (episodic acidosis and ID); cerebellar lesion, p.437.

Mixed central & peripheral

Hereditary ataxias such as Friedreich's ataxia (iron buildup in cells by age 20, causes stumbling and problems with vision, hearing, and speech), leukodystrophies, p.498; abetalipoproteinaemia, p.417; xeroderma pigmentosum, p.454.
Marinesco-Sjogren syndrome[1062] (cataract, p.436; ataxia; ID)

Miscellaneous

Ehlers-Danlos, p.460; GM1 gangliosidosis, p.501; inherited vit.E deficiency, p.86

Visual

Ataxia-telangiectasia[915] (p.454); Cogan's syndrome (p.442)

Causelist 17: Posture

This is the way the body is held upright. *Posturing* means adopting an unusual position of all or part of the body. (See also *gait*, p.471).

Tummyache, diarrhoea, idiopathic scoliosis (see below), back pain, a pressing urge to micturate, and dysmenorrhoea are the commonest causes of unusual posture. Unusual postures can be adopted by children for secondary reasons, e.g. in order to write better (for left-handed writing or to stabilise an unstable shoulder girdle), to masturbate (p.115), to look around a visual field defect, or to prevent them falling (see W-posture, p.483). Holding one or both hands fixed for a few seconds or more is common in autism, usually but not always looking at them (p.64). For disinhibited body postures, see p.261. For odd postures with unresponsiveness, see *catatonia*, p.98.

Back arching: Eye-gaze turns upward in oculogyric crises, a common side-effect of some antipsychotic medication. This often progresses to dystonic retrocollis (extension of the neck). Opisthotonus (arched back) is the most severe form of this, seen in syncope, pseudoseizures, kernicterus (p.495), meningitis, hydrocephalus (p.482), tetanus (p.490), posterior fossa lesions, and anti-NMDA encephalitis (p.422). Tonic convulsions arch the back, but if children sink slowly to the floor while arching their back, there is a good chance that it is a pseudoseizure (p.74). Other reasons for back-arching include masturbation, yawning (children stretch more), breast display, airway obstruction, some cerebral palsy (p.437), and after epidural injections or midbrain lesion.

Back pain and stiffness: Children who have had chronic back pain often avoid cuddles, which can give the impression of social aloofness. However they are likely to develop other behaviours that demonstrate social involvement, such as joint handholding or saying "please don't touch my back" . Keeping the back rigid while sitting and standing may be due to paramilitary training, copying role models, or back pain. If other joints and muscles are affected consider overexercise (which athletic parents may consider normal). If there is a general paucity of movement consider depression, p.309; sleepiness, p.321; fatigue, p.323; and physical illness. Ankylosing spondylitis affects up to 1% of the population, and usually has its onset in adolescence: look for family history, large joint stiffness worse in the morning, and eye inflammation[237].

Scoliosis is curvature of the spine from side to side. It can be mobile or fixed. Mobile scoliosis can be due to pain (e.g. backache, sciatica) or to difference in leg lengths; but most often is a transient developmental stage seen mainly in teenage girls, in which case it disappears on bending forwards. Consider central neurological causes (spina bifida, p.551; cerebral palsy, p.437; spinal muscular atrophy, p.551, Friedreich's ataxia, p.92; dystonia e.g. Segawa disease, p.458; syringomyelia); physical trauma; connective tissue diseases (Ehlers−Danlos, p.460; Marfan, p.505; asymmetrical arthritis); peripheral nerves (Charcot−Marie−Tooth, p.87); Prader-Willi, p.533; muscular dystrophy, p.510; neurofibromatosis, p.514.

Other causes: Side-to-side asymmetry of the body or of body parts is not rare, and sufferers often adopt unusual postures to compensate or to conceal this. In Sandifer syndrome, reflux oesophagitis (GORD, p.472) causes torticollis for several minutes at a time. Posturing the whole body or a limb, sometimes for hours at a time, is seen in catatonia (p.98); in dystonias (scoliosis in Segawa disease, p.458) and with a wide range of rare intracranial and intraspinal pathologies. People with Stiff Person syndrome (p.555) have a sore stiff back and walk with their arms held out to the sides because of fear of falling.

Causelist 18: Passivity/Slowness

Passivity
In common usage, passivity means a lack of initiative, and a willingness to be led. The psychiatric term *somatic passivity*, in contrast, denotes the subjective *feeling* that this is so, in other words the experience that one's actions, thoughts and/or speech are created by others. This is often a symptom of psychosis (see Schneiderian symptoms, p.544). Compare *passive–aggressive*, p.525; *pseudo-passivity*, p.354; *automatic obedience*, p.98.

Slowness
The rest of this section addresses objective, observable slowness. This includes two distinct problems that often come together: slow individual movements and paucity of decisions to act. The paucity of decisions to act can give the impression of passivity, above. Speech makes more aspects obvious, including time-to-reply, word rate, volume, size of lip movements, floridity of accompanying gestures, and flattening (p.467).

Distinct aspects of slowness are separated in the list at the right. However several of the aspects are often found together, particularly in depression (pp.309, 313), hypothyroidism (p.485), parkinsonism (p.525), and catalepsy (p.435). The combination seen in depression (marked with *) can be called "psychomotor slowing" (see p.537).

Obsessive slowness (OS) 🦅

This term has two main uses:

a) The term is often used to refer to people who take a long time to complete a task (e.g. hours for a bath) but such usage is inaccurate because there are usually many repeated activities within that time[47].

b) The term better describes people whose movements are slow as in a slow motion film[1292]. Usually the movements are precisely monitored and lack spontaneity. It is useful to work out which movements are slowed as this may indicate what is being compensated for. For example:
   - Mild slowness just while writing can usefully compensate for lack of practice, but if it also occurs during eating consider dyspraxia (p.89).
   - If it affects all movements, but only when non-family are present, consider social anxiety (p.298).
   - If it only happens in situations that have to be endured (such as class or assessment, without social pleasure), consider situational low mood. If the child is bored, tasks can be intentionally stretched out, e.g. drying each finger separately.
   - When anxiety is combined with autistic inflexibility, arm movements when moving objects across a table become linear with a uniform speed, quite unlike the spontaneous accelerations and redirections seen in most people. Perhaps this is due to a focus on the movements, of near dissociative intensity. When severe, complex movements can be broken down into component parts, giving a robotic impression. The most automatic behaviours (e.g. walking, and perhaps talking) can be relatively spared.

Despite its name, and the observable fact that it is more common in obsessive people, OS 🦅 is not simply part of OCD. OS seems to most often start in toddlerhood [1581] whereas OCD usually starts at age 10−16. OS may be another term for the bradykinesia which is very common in those people who have both OCD and cognitive deficits[1224].

Causes of slowness, passivity	Notes
Perception	
Sensory problems	(acute or chronic)
Slow thinking	
ID	Gross motor skills are usually age-equivalent or nearly so.
☞Depression *(p.309)	For consideration of the timecourse see p.564.
Performance anxiety	Social anxiety (p.298) can prevent normal lateral thinking on an open-ended question such as "tell me about your family's car", so he cannot find an answer, or if he finds a word or two he may get stuck and unable to find more, occasionally repeating the first ideas he found. His thinking is not slow and his words or sentences are not slow, but his production of ideas is. Confirm this by much better written performance.
Thinking of something else	
Allocation of resources	Some people automatically drive more slowly when they think of something interesting.
Stress	Some people become slower when stressed: they may be partly disengaged, or preoccupied, or needing to check more because their attention keeps switching between tasks.
OCD (p.65)	OCD has characteristic obsessions and compulsions: checking and being over-exact can cause slowness (p.95). Other sufferers learn that slowness helps them to avoid activating other obsessions (such as tidiness or exactness).
Obsessive slowness	(p.95)
☞Rumination*	(p.543), e.g. in depression, p.309.
☞intrusive thoughts	Pychosis, bereavement, p.430; PTSD, p.532.
Reluctance	
various situations	See inflexibility (p.234)
Disinterest*	E.g. saying nothing, looking around in a meeting
Oppositionality	(p.253) Becoming slower when pushed
Initiation	
Sleepiness	(p.321)
Learned helplessness (can be part of depression)*	Learning that there is no way to avoid pain or unpleasant stimuli. A minor form of this can be seen in children who are continually told to obey. Eldest girls constantly enlisted to help a bossy and critical mother may lose any initiative.
☞Fears	Learned immobility (on guard) in frozen watchfulness (p.470). A much stronger response is the total passivity which is an evolved response to extreme fear, p.307
Motor neglect	Some lesions to frontal, parietal, and thalamic areas (p.512) cause an underutilisation of the contralateral side, without defects of sensation, strength, or reflexes[906]. Normal strength and dexterity can be demonstrated only by prompting an extraordinary effort. The deficit may also affect the ipsilateral arm when in contralateral space.
Execution	("True bradykinesia")
Weakness	Physical illness or fatigue (p.323). Spasticity
Self-consciousness	Excess control/checking: obsessive slowness, p.95.
Muscle/joint pain*	(p.135)
Catatonia (p.98).	May be manneristic (p.505).

Causelist 19: Hardly doing anything

There is a "conflict of paradigms" here, between neurology and psychiatry, and medical causes must not be neglected. There is obviously a need to work out whether information is getting in to him, whether he is thinking anything, and whether he can express himself. The GCS does this:

Glasgow Coma Scale[1593] (from Wikipedia, calculated instantly on www.sfar.org/scores2/saps2.html#glasgow)

	1	2	3	4	5	6
Eyes	Does not open eyes	Opens eyes in response to painful stimuli	Opens eyes in response to voice	Opens eyes spontaneously	N/A	N/A
Verbal	Makes no sounds	Incomprehensible sounds	Utters inappropriate words	Confused, disorientated	Oriented, converses normally	N/A
Motor	Makes no movements	Extension to painful stimuli	Abnormal flexion to painful stimuli	Flexion / Withdrawal to painful stimuli	Localizes painful stimuli	Obeys commands

Terms for acute levels of consciousness

Conscious	Oriented in time, place, and person
Confused	(Or clouded) difficulty following instructions
Delirium	(p.451)
Somnolence	Incoherent mumbles or disorganised movements. Very sleepy
Obtunded	Little interest in surroundings, slow responses, cannot be fully roused
Stupor	Only rouseable by intense or painful stimuli. The only responses are grimacing or pulling away from pain. (The psychiatric sense is different, meaning a severe reduction in action and speech, whether organic or psychogenic[158,1487].)
Coma	Not rouseable. In 500 "comatose" cases referred to a neurologist, the following diagnoses were reached[1270]:

Supratentorial lesions	101	Hepatic encephalopathy	17
Subtentorial lesions	65	Uraemia/dialysis	8
Encephalitis	14	Endocrine disorders	12
Subarachnoid hemorrhage	13	Drug poisons	149
Concussion, non-convulsive fits, post-ictal	9	Temperature	9
		Dissociation	4
Anoxia	10	**Depression**	2
Hypoglycaemia	16	**Catatonia**	2
Nutritional	1		

Terms for chronic levels of consciousness[1270]

Abulia	Appears fully awake but doesn't initiate activity and responds slowly if at all to speech. Suspect a frontal lesion.
Akinetic mutism	E.g. with damage to the midbrain, medial thalamus, or anterior cingulate cortex.

Other severe causes of not moving

- Locked-in syndrome / persistent vegetative state (does not indicate coma). Can communicate with blinking or eye movements[228].
- Decerebrate rigidity, with limb extension
- Frozen: see frozen watchfulness, p.470. Amygdalar lesions can produce "catatonic-like frozen states"[1270] (compare p.296).
- pervasive refusal, p.527.

Less profoundly disabling

- See languor, pp.321−323; non-behaviours, p.515; brief zoning out / absences, p.75; passivity/slowness, p.95; rigidity, p.234; muscle weakness or paralysis, p.87; Stiff person syndrome, p.555.
- Occupational: human statues, commandos, guardsmen, microscopists
- Motor neglect (e.g. underutilising an arm, p.96).

Catatonia

This is very odd, *largely unresponsive* behaviour with abnormalities of movement, lasting hours or days. It is a "behavioural syndrome" like delirium, i.e. there are many underlying causes. It is most often seen at the start of psychotic episodes, especially in non-whites.

Catatonia is not well understood. However, grimacing, posturing, and stereotypies suggest catatonia rather than metabolic delirium[1270]. Rapid relief by lorazepam (1−2 mg each 3 hours for 9 hours) is felt by some to confirm the condition as being catatonia[497], but it may be more useful to regard this as a large and important subgroup of catatonia[1375]. In patients with catatonia caused by affective conditions, 80% are relieved by lorazepam, but if the catatonia is long term or the underlying condition is schizophrenia, the success rate is much lower[1375,1638].

Although descriptions of some of the symptoms of catatonia can *sound* somewhat similar to those of autism (e.g.[804]) conventional usage reserves the term *catatonia* for states persisting continuously without a break for days and preventing any aspect of the child's normal interactions – which is quite distinct from autism, which is a lifelong condition in which the regression, if any, occurs gradually over weeks to months.

A few cases actually have obsessional slowness (p.95) or psychotic depression, but this distinction can only be made if the patient's preoccupations or mood are accessible.

Symptoms include:
- Stupor (see p.97)
- Ambitendency (repeatedly starts then stops a behaviour)
- Automatic obedience
- Aversion (turning away from the interviewer)
- Forced grasping
- Gegenhalten or counterpull. With lesions to the supplementary motor area, the patient is aware but cannot decrease the resistance[793].
- Waxy flexibility (can be moved to uncomfortable positions, then stays still). This is very similar to gegenhalten (above) except that the resistance starts after the movement finishes.
- Mitgehen (body can be moved with the slightest touch, then returns to the original position)
- Negativism (resists attempts to be moved; more complex than gegenhalten)
- Obstruction (stops in the middle of a movement, like thought block)
- Rigidity or posturing (p.93), including psychological pillow (lying as if one had a pillow: compare stiff person syndrome, p.555). These can also result from frontal lobe lesions[793] (p.512).

Less specific symptoms
- Mannerisms, stereotypies, perseveration, staring or grimacing, echolalia and echopraxia
- Excitement (distinguish from mania or delirium)
- Logorrhoea (incessant incoherent speech)
- Catalepsy (p.435)
- Partial immobility, e.g. stiff jaw preventing eating or talking

Do not forget medical causes (p.99), nor the complications of immobility, such as dehydration, hypoglycaemia, hypothermia, and DVT.

continued ▶

Investigation Planner 4: Medical causes of catatonia/stupor

Investigations for decreased conscious level are complex, and comprehensive guidelines are available[1210]. Even if a diagnosis of catatonia has been made, a wide range of causes need to be urgently considered (pp.97, 451 and [1270,1297]). Start with a detailed neurological examination including the points listed on p.100.

Useful investigations include: FBC, UECr, LFT, TFT, glucose, CPK, CRP/ESR, B6, ammonia, lactate, urine dipstick; urine drug screen, heavy metals (p.330), calcium, phosphate, magnesium, autoantibodies, urine and blood culture and microscopy, white cell enzymes (p.572), organic acids, urinary amino acids. Consider also the medical causes of hallucinations and delusions (p.349) and these further tests: MRI, EEG, LP.

See also the *general approach to medical investigations*, p.373, and[703].

	Signs	Initial tests	Excluded clinically or to Order?	Date ordered	Result
Infections, p.490					
encephalitis	p.461				
malaria	p.503				
tuberculosis	p.569	p.569			
HIV	p.479	p.479			
mononucleosis					
viral hepatitis					
Drugs & intoxicants, p.257					
alcohol	p.258	blood alcohol,ketones			
stimulants	p.555	--			
antipsychotics	p.422	--			
neuroleptic malignant syndrome	p.514	p.514			
abrupt neuroleptic withdrawal	history	--			
cocaine	p.258				
ecstasy					
serotonin syndrome	p.548				
steroids	p.554				
antiepileptics	p.422				
disulfiram					
aspirin (Reye syndrome)	severe vomiting, fever, lethargy, aggression, confusion	!! history of viral illness & aspirin use, glucose, LFT, ammonia			
Metabolic (p.379) and endocrine					
hypoglycaemia	p.82	glucose (fingerprick)			
Addison's	p.419	sodium, potassium, cortisol			
Cushing's	p.449	p.449			
ketoacidosis	p.338	urinary ketones			
hypercalcaemia	p.483	(Ca++ and phosphate)			
porphyria	p.532	p.532			
Wilson's disease	p.575	p.575			
Neurological					
supratentorial lesions, e.g. head injury	p.477	MRI			

Conundrum 3: Psychiatric or paediatric brain disorder

Collecting information
Paediatricians and inpatient staff are often needed to monitor level of consciousness, fluid intake and output, and put up drips. Paediatricians have an important role in looking for localising neurological signs, and arranging special investigations. Psychiatrists should assess carefully for secondary gain (p.471), for changes when family members are around, for previous social and academic functioning, and for signs in recent months that could indicate psychological deterioration (e.g. schizophrenic prodrome, p.544).

Formulating
Psychiatrists and paediatricians should discuss this together, avoiding the temptation for each to say "It's not any condition that I know of, so it must be one of yours." *Psychiatric* and *paediatric* are not diagnoses of exclusion.

- Suggestive of organic brain states: variable or partial behaviours; abnormal neurological examination (including fundi and frontal signs such as perseveration, p.527, utilisation behaviours, p.572; other hard neurological signs, p.58; other frontal signs, p.469); abnormal EEG or other investigations; severe sleep variability; good recent social functioning; visual hallucinations; true loss of skills (p.42).

- Suggestive of psychiatric conditions: psychosocial trigger; family history; markers of specific pseudo-behaviours (p.363); good response to lorazepam[497]; behaviours that depend on who is present; behaviours that are important symbols for the patient (e.g. the patient explains that she is making swimming movements because she is in the sea – which was the last time she was with her father); all-or-none behaviours (but see p.361); secondary gain (but see p.361); auditory hallucinations with highly emotional content.

- There are many mixed conditions. For example, the following conditions characteristically start from an overt physical illness such as infection, yet have major psychological components: Guillain-Barré, p.87; chronic fatigue, p.323; pervasive refusal, p.527.

Treatment
This depends on the underlying causes that have been found or suspected.

Motor (Specific Behaviours)
Causelist 20: Twitching

Twitches are rapid movements. They include myokymia, p.61; myoclonus, p.511; sleep starts, p.200; and tics, which are addressed here.

Tics

Tics are sudden, rapid, recurrent, non-rhythmic movements which recur isomorphically (i.e. are stereotyped/invariant over weeks) and can be reproduced voluntarily. They can be increased by suggestion, and suppressed temporarily at the expense of mounting discomfort. Several can occur simultaneously, especially in severe cases. Tics can occur in the middle of a sentence without interrupting it, though they will if they are upsetting or are being demonstrated or exaggerated. Some standard tics are easily recognised, such as hard blinking, head jerks and shoulder jerks, but for less common movements one needs to work through each word of the definition above.

Tics look or sound purposeful and can sometimes be supressed. This often leads to parents or teachers telling the child off.

Some clinicians use the word *tic* more broadly than the above definition, to include sensory tics (p.231), tonic tics, dystonic tics, mental tics[765] and even echolalic tics[766] – perhaps most appropriate when preceded by a premonitory urge.

Conundrum 4: Tics or a limited repertoire

Children with autism ☝ (p.183) and/or severe ID ☝ often have such a small repertoire of behaviours that the "recur isomorphically" criterion doesn't help to identify tics, unless you can find a different sitting/standing position that re-forms the movement, thereby disqualifying it from being a tic. Similarly, "can be reproduced voluntarily" is less useful in these children, but tics are usually fast and start at a later age (7–10). If you are lucky enough to see a longish purposive action interrupted by one or more tics, especially several near-simultaneous tics, this clearly shows the movements to be non-purposive, so they cannot be self-entertainment.

Conundrum 5: Tics or compulsions

There is much comorbidity, and many cases are transitional between the two[1574]. When the movement is performed to neutralise an underlying fear, the diagnosis is OCD rather than tics (see ** note with Causelist 9); but if underlying fears are unclear or absent, other means are sometimes needed to distinguish them.

Generally tics are much simpler than compulsions, but compulsions can sometimes be difficult to distinguish from complex tics. The traditional inclusion of resistance in the definition of obsessions is unreliable, particularly in children. A feeling that something bad will happen (often with no more details) is more likely in OCD than with tics. The age of onset is generally later with OCD (10–16) than with Tourette's (7–10). Family history can also help.

Observation
Parental history is crucial because many children can suppress tics through a class or an hour-long interview. This does not mean that the tics are unimpairing in real life as efforts to suppress them can prevent the child concentrating in school, and the unsuppressed tics at home can cause friction with parents. Covert observation in the waiting room, or after the session (from behind, in the corridor) can reveal the tics.

Causes of tic-like movements	Notes (see[84])
Not actually tics	
Normal fast blinking	Confusingly, this fits all the criteria for tics. However, it is a hard-wired reflex, and is much faster than other tics. Normal blinking has many non-tic causes (p.108).
Throat clearing (p.109)	can be tics; more often due to prolonged mucus production or other local irritation lasting months after infection.
ID, autism	The repetitive movements made by children with autism, and some with severe ID, are sometimes confused with tics, but are usually easily distinguished as they are more variable and less rapid.
Pseudotics	These are copies (often partly intentional) of the real thing, but imperfectly acted. The "real thing" can be learned from friends, TV, or the child's own tics. Typical imperfections are making them too slow, or too variable, or too suggestible (like echopraxia), being focused on each individual tic, using them communicatively, or only doing them while looking for a response. (See pseudo-behaviours, p.363.)
Describing the behaviour	
Transient childhood tics	Occur in 25% of children; disappear within a few weeks and do not interfere with normal life.
Tic disorders	Standard criteria require tics be present for most of 12 months; some definitions require impairment. Extra-hard blinking, often prolonged to achieve a particular feeling, is often the first "clinical" tic to appear, about age 6−8.
Tourette's syndrome	This is defined as chronic motor plus vocal tics. The subdivision of tics into motor and vocal interprets vocal broadly, to include swearing (p.161), laughing (p.111), throat clearing (p.109), clucking and even sniffing (p.109). Swearing is not a very common vocal tic, but characteristically after swearing he will often apologise. Swearing is sometimes triggered by frustration, but more often appears without distracting his train of thought. Occasionally a child says he's doing his movements intentionally to annoy people, and this turns out to be his explanation of his tics. For an intriguing description of the internal experiences of an adult with Tourette's, see[1412] (though note that adult tiqueurs are a tiny and atypical group).
Underlying causes	
Drugs reported to induce tics or worsen pre-existing tics	Stimulant drugs (dose-dependent) e.g. methylphenidate, antipsychotics, p.422; antidepressants, antiepileptics, p.422; levodopa, antihistamines, anticholinergics, lithium, opiates and opiate withdrawal (pp.519,258)
Primary neurologic disorders manifesting tics Most of these are rare [887].	• **Acquired** head trauma, encephalitis (p.461), stroke (p.556) trigeminal neuralgia (pain can cause "tic douloureux") ☞PANDAS (p.522), carbon monoxide poisoning, hypoglycemia (p.82), Creutzfeldt−Jakob disease, neurosyphilis, schizophrenia (p.543); see also myoclonus and epilepsy partialis continua (p.75)
The most important to detect are the treatable biological causes, p.86.	• **Genetic** Huntington's disease (p.482), Neuroacanthocytosis (p.514) Hallervorden−Spatz disease, Idiopathic dystonia Duchenne's disease, Tuberous sclerosis (p.569) Chromosomal disorders (p.439), Fragile X (p.468) Down's syndrome (p.455) Sex chromosome abnormalities (p.548)

Causelist 21: Throwing

When a child throws something, watch his eyes to learn his motivation.
Several of the following kinds of throwing can be seen in a single
consultation. See also *gender differences*, p.473.

Causes of throwing things	Notes
Anger	If he throws or kicks several objects in quick succession, unconcerned with outcome, the cause is usually anger.
	Parents and teachers sometimes say "he throws chairs". They are usually trying to emphasise the degree of aggression. You need to find out whether the chair follows an arched trajectory across the room (which is rare and dangerous), is knocked over, or picked up and dropped in order to make an annoying bang, or scooted across the floor.
Winding up	If he looks immediately at an adult, he is monitoring the reaction, a far more sophisticated process than casting, which may indicate that he finds the usual parental response rewarding (even being shouted at can be more pleasant than being ignored).
	Objects can be thrown in the toilet for this reason, or due to anger.
Fun	Throwing in fun is accompanied by laughter and looking at the person who is supposed to be amused.
Discarding	In autism and in completely untrained (near feral) children, toys can be discarded with a gentle toss, or just pushed off the table. The gaze is already on some new activity.
Casting	If he gazes at the object while it flies, lands, and perhaps bounces, this is "casting", a primitive sort of play characteristic of age 12−18 months. Like mouthing, when seen in children over 5 it points to a diagnosis of Profound ID. Such children will throw anything they can get their hands on, and throw them much further than a 15-month-old, so there is some risk.
Pseudo-casting	This can be seen in more able children who are envious of a disabled sibling who gets more attention. This can be recognised by being inconsistent with their developmental stage, by the objects being carefully directed (e.g. at people they are angry at), and by their not following the object as it flies. (See pseudo-behaviours, p.363.)
Trying to get sibling in trouble	If he quickly looks away from the thrown object, he is trying to pretend he didn't throw it.
Rare	In Lesch-Nyhan syndrome (p.318) children sometimes throw things in an apparently well-controlled way across the room, then apologise (see unwanted actions, p.353). Consider also hallucinations (p.343).

Causelist 22: Spinning

Spinning is fast turning (akin to running being faster than walking). A
related behaviour is circling, which autistic children and people with
schizophrenia do somewhat more to the left[1097]. Spinning is also similar to
dogs' tail-chasing, which has been used as a model of OCD (p.65).

The most important issue in the table below is whether the spinning is an
abnormal stereotyped interest that would contribute to a diagnosis of autism.
This depends on several aspects of the interest (pp.227–229). Key aspects of
spinning are whether it is variable and evolves (p.227); and duration factors,
as follows.
- A. *Duration of each episode*. Many children could cycle in a circle for
  more than 20 minutes, if there was added interest such as varying the
  circle, or someone talking to them, or having just learned to cycle. If
  the child needed no such variety for 5 minutes, that is abnormal.
- B. *Duration of the interest*. If a child continues such a habit daily over a
  month without changes, that would increase the likelihood of autism.

Watching washing machines turn has similar causes (whatever the cause, this
can evolve into a useful interest in loading and unloading them): watching
them turn (would also watch ceiling fans, and moving rather than stationary
cars); watching clothes falling; feeling the vibration or heat; copying mum.

Causes of spinning	Notes

Whole spins of self	Spinning oneself produces many unusual sensations:
	• Visual:
	   o Looking up to see the ceiling spin
	   o Looking sideways, either to see the world rushing by or (turning slowly) to enjoy the changing perspective
	   o Reorienting when they open their eyes again
	• Tactile: feeling the wind; falling down
	• Vestibular

Intrigue	Normal children spin, but only briefly, and usually with laughter. Experimenting with the unusual feelings.
Roleplay	E.g. making noises while flying Thunderbirds.
Other play	Chasing in circles, fairground rides, dancing, etc
Excitement	Spinning as the result of extreme excitement is self-limiting.
Autism (p.183)	A very energetic autistic boy leapt at the start of any activity, making a half-turn in the air (see also above).
Partial spins or turns of self	
Experimental	Spinning the head back and forth is tried by many children, and is more fun with pigtails.
Excitement	Spinning back and forth
Tics	(p.101)
Deafism (p.66)	Children with unilateral deafness turn their head usefully to locate the source of sounds. This can be done in a uniform, habitised way, but can also lead to an inventive child finding many variations.
Spinning other things	There are several motivations for spinning, e.g. toy car wheels: • Enjoying watching them turn • Copying dad who is a mechanic (or who plays with cars) • Interest in the numeric codes on tyres (some children with Asperger's (p.424) recognise the family car in this way) • The challenge of getting something to spin – or a competition • Proud he has a car with such excellent wheels • Enjoys the noise (would only turn noisy wheels) • Likes the feeling on his finger.
Normal play	e.g. spinning tops, or spinning a chair with something on it.
Autism ☝ (p.183)	Evidence of an excessive, stereotyped interest (see also above): • Spinning even things that don't spin well • Spinning in odd contexts, e.g. every time he puts something down • Has learned ways of making things that spin, in order to be able to supply this need in any environment.

Causelist 23: Flapping

This means repeated movements of the arms or hands.

Causes of flapping	Notes
Bilateral	
Normal until age 3 (after this age, more common in autism, hence dubiously called "autistic flap")	This is (a) moving the hands rapidly up and down, (b) when aroused. The flap is bilateral, with elbows bent, and palms forward.
	Flapping is useful clinically as a sign of immaturity (for other signs see pp.55 and 58), and also as a sign of what excites the child. The arousal can be due to frustration (p.291) or pleasure.
	Most flaps are easily recognised and clinically unworrying. When the movements are very atypical, recognising the trigger to be the same as conventional flaps allows them to be identified.
	Variants include: • Wiggling the hands at the end of arms hanging straight down • Pushing the hands together or pushing one hand back • Unilateral flapping in hemiplegia • A more advanced variant sometimes seen in older children during excitement is running in place while moving arms alternately as if drumming. • In extreme emotion, it can spread, e.g. to legs, causing leg-straightening synchronised with the arm-flaps (which suggests subcortical control) or running in place (whether sitting or standing). This may be the origin of the term "jumping for joy" . It may be related to the bouncing that gives springboks their name, and which lambs do when excited or trying to negotiate a novel obstacle.
Poor mime	E.g. during the song "head and shoulders, knees and toes" in a mute boy with ID.
Asterixis	Flapping of the wrists at about 1–3Hz caused by repeated brief loss of tone when the person tries to hold his wrists dorsiflexed, said to look like a bird's wings flapping. It usually indicates encephalopathy due to toxins, e.g. in kidney or liver failure.
Unilateral	
Dismissal	Single hand, toward someone
Artistic pointing	Ulnar deviation of hand, fingers straight and separated, to indicate an area of a painting or landscape
Unilateral or bilateral	
"Bye bye"	Very odd movements make autism more likely (p.183).
Camp gesture (p.243)	Only one movement rather than a repeated flap. Wrist mainly in flexion, often combined with other communication such as pointing finger or limp wrist.
Learned body language	• Learned from an influential adult with idiosyncratic behaviour. Here the movement is used when people are around, to communicate frustration. It may be atypical, e.g. with hands in fists or accompanied by "Grrrr!" • Culturally or subculturally determined, usually as an expression of frustration.

During mental tasks	Multihertz bilateral movements, to communicate the level of effort, or indicating frustration at the difficulty of recall, or perhaps occasionally to aid recall (as a Valsalva-like or semi-dissociative act or for state-dependent learning)
Pseudo-regressive flaps	E.g. copying a younger brother or children in special school. Detect this by late age of onset timed with exposure to other flappers (see p.363).
Normal gesture for attention	Unilateral or bilateral, palms backward or to midline, directed to other person
"Complex flaps"	Some autistic children incorporate flaps into more complex rituals, e.g.:

- unilateral flap while posturing with the other hand
- Flapping when approaching anything (looks as if trying to frighten a fly; unclear whether this is copied, superstitious, or an aid to concentration).

Causelist 24: Flinching

Flinching is a natural rapid self-protective response to sudden, unpredictable, or painful events. It includes blinking, squinting, withdrawing, and protective arm movements. This useful sign can be picked up during the introductory handshake, physical examination, and naturalistic observation of the child (a game of catch reveals the level of flinch to minor threats such as a foam ball approaching the face).

Flinching can be directional in two ways: either to protect a part of the body, or to avoid a risky individual, e.g. a child flinches away from a punitive parent after dropping a pencil. When the stimulus is *non-directional* (e.g. thunder & lightning), or localised but severe, a generalised startle response is seen (e.g. withdrawal; panic, p.301; anger).

There are two phases: an initial fast reflex, and a slower more prolonged one with varying degrees of muscle tensioning, facial grimacing, and subjective discomfort. The rapid phase of flinching is a true reflection of surprise; it is a brainstem response (exaggerated in hyperekplexia, p.483). The slower phase is under higher control and can be shaped, e.g. being louder or more expressive (related to the neuropsychiatric *startle syndromes*, p.552). Spatial avoidance (e.g. keeping space or objects between another person and oneself) is a related sign (p.429)

Wariness by a parent, especially flinching on approach by spouse or child, usually indicates major difficulty coping, and needs urgent attention.

Causes of flinching	Notes
Elevated	
Specific trigger	Judging whether this is normal depends on its severity and what caused the hypersensitivity, as well as current triggers. *Example 1* A child flinched from anyone touching her wrists. This was more than a reaction to physical pain because she could not talk to people while they were holding their own wrists. • Recent physical injury must be carefully assessed. • If the child or a relative had severe wrist injuries (e.g. fracture), such strong reactions could last a year or more. • If the child says this is just because the aesthetics of wrists disturb her, this is a specific sensory intolerance (p.125) *Example 2* A teenager flinched only from men approaching his face with their face or hands. The possibility of physical or sexual abuse with PTSD-like sequelae needs to be carefully considered using a much wider array of evidence (p.275). Innocent injury can cause similar flinching, and could also be restricted to men. *Example 3* Flinching from shouting is due to noise and fear of violence.
Non-specific	Anxiety. Compare general sensory intolerance (p.125)
No trigger apparent	Can indicate intrusive perceptions or thoughts of danger. The fear can be quite appropriate yet invisible to others, e.g. a girl with allodynia (p.136) affecting one shoulder, who flinched when anyone passed near that shoulder.
Reduced	
Fatigue	(p.323)
Weakness	(p.87). Famine victims ignoring flies on their eyes.
Prolonged exposure	Learned helplessness, p.96 (consider depression p.309; physical abuse, p.273).
Secondary gain (p.471)	Father of autistic teenager trying to believe that the teen's hitting him isn't worsening, because father wants to believe things are manageable so the teen can continue to live at home.

Causelist 25: Blinking

The main physical causes that need to be excluded are vision problems, allergy, and dry eyes. Blinking can be transiently altered for a few *seconds* when orienting or trying to concentrate; or for *hours* if the person has been awake for a long time, particularly in an unaccustomed dry environment. Extra-hard blinking is often a tic (p.101), whereas most *rapid* blinking is normal. Blinking can also be caused by tearfulness or crying (p.315). Myokimia is more rapid and not voluntarily reproducible (p.61).

Most people blink 18 times a minute during conversation.

Reduced blinking is seen in depression, exhaustion, Möbius syndrome (p.178), parkinsonism. Individual blinks are slower in hypothyroidism, p.485.

Unilateral blinking, i.e. winking, occasionally occurs as a tic (bilateral blinking is the most common tic). This can be socially crippling, particularly to girls. Some in religious families have been subject to exorcism. A rare cause is TLE[1165].

Causes of complaint of excess blinking [after 300]	Relative Frequency if unilateral	Relative Frequency if bilateral
"habit tic" (i.e. common tics. can last weeks to months after physical problem resolved)	2	21
Tourette (i.e. phonic plus vocal tics, p.101)	1	1
"Psychogenic" (simple habit, sometimes increased by anxiety)		10 *
Marcus–Gunn jaw winking	2	
Orbicularis myokymia (p.61)	2	
Nasolacrimal duct obstruction	1	
Uveitis	1	
☞Conjunctivitis		14
Keratitis		5
Dry eyes		5
Intermittent extropia	1	10
☞Uncorrected refractive error		14
CNS disease		4 **
Lid abnormalities		3

*   Some of these have photophobia (p.529) or a blinking blindism (p.66).

**   Some of these have Jeavons syndrome, which is the combination of eyelid myoclonia and absences. The absences can be so brief as to be hardly observable[328].

Causelist 26: Sniffing

Throat clearing shares many of the same causes as sniffing, and in addition is exacerbated by anticipation of speaking.

Causes of sniffing	Notes
Common	
Respiratory tract infection	Runny nose, cough, sore throat, malaise
allergy	Hayfever is seasonal with itchy eyes, worse outdoors.
Habit	
As the first stage of eating	To prevent a surprise (like feeling water before diving in)
As part of crying	After blinking has sent tears through the nasolacrimal duct.
Tic (p.101)	Characteristically identical, brief sniffs, without signs of other causes such as a runny nose or itchy eyes. Reverse sniffs have fewer causes, i.e. they are much more likely to be tics than normal sniffs.
"Sensory tic" (p.231)	E.g. smelling fingers when they're *not* likely to have unusual smells such as the flower just touched
Investigating (smells lots of different things)	E.g. food (fussiness or gourmets), fingers when they *are* likely to have special smells, recently read about smells.
Enjoying particular smells	If he always smells the same few things, e.g. roses (common), books or fingers (uncommon) – that is a stereotyped interest (p.553).
Invoking memories	(e.g. invokes childhood memories or visual imagery when smelling cut grass).
Contagion	See *mirror system*, p.507.
Uncommon	
To get a high	Solvents, cocaine (p.258).
"Being sniffy"	Non-verbal expression of disapproval (now rare).
Stereotypy	(p.553) E.g. an "in-out-in" pattern of sniffs and reverse sniffs.
Anxiety or distrust	(checking that the food is OK)
To stick the nostrils together at very low temperatures	Can be experimental, or a "sensory tic" (p.231) or habit

Causelist 27: Scratching

For scratching in a specific spot, see also *skin picking*, p.549. Relieving an
itch may take unusual forms (see *Prader-Willi*, p.533).

Causes of scratching	Notes
For itch	Itch gradually grows in a single location (as does pain). Relief by scratching may be by the same mechanism by which pain terminates itch[175]. Itch is not uniform over the whole body, but can arise from the local bodily function (e.g. anal itch, itchy eyes). Unfortunately, the precise quality of itch or its daily timing do not assist in finding the cause[1533]. 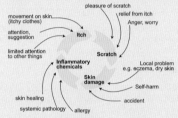 **Figure 11. Contributors to the itch−scratch cycle.** (After[1029,1669]; for physical causes see also [1111,1533].)
Localised itch	Dry skin, eczema, repeated washing, infestation, insect bites, herpes, poor hygiene (p.483), healing, nerve injury (e.g. trench foot), peripheral nerve lesions.
Generalised itch	(Requires thorough investigation as 10−50% have systemic causes): low weight as in anorexia (p.334), impaired renal/hepatic/thyroid function, zinc or iron deficiency, malabsorption (p.502), pregnancy, multiple sclerosis (p.510), common side effect of opiates (p.519), lymphoma *Neuropathic itch* is often accompanied by burning or stinging, and can arise from disorders of the central nervous system, or from peripheral nerve injury or herpes[742].
Epilepsy	E.g. an automatism (p.427)
For pleasure	
	The relief of itch can be exquisitely pleasurable [742]. In scratching a severe itch the immediate tactile sensation (which can be painful) is sometimes followed by a more diffuse, very pleasurable sensation lasting seconds. This contributes to the itch−scratch cycle.
Psychogenic	
Preoccupation	E.g. after touching a person with nits.
Contagion	See *mass psychogenic behaviour*, p.505; *mirror system*,p.507
To harm self	
	Signs are scratching particularly painful or obvious areas such as the face; use of sharp objects; and scratching in public. See p.317.
To hurt others	See p.289.

Causelist 28: Laughing

This is a hard-wired response to incongruity and, below a mental age of about 3, to tickling. During maturation its suppressibility, intensity, duration, trajectory, sound (initial syllable and the repeated vowel) and associated facial expressions come under conscious control, allowing several distinct normal types of laughter (see list below). Culturally inappropriate features in any of these should make one consider impulse-control (p.79) and developmental social problems (pp.175, 183). Humour and tickles are both expressed through laughter, or when milder a smile (see 526, but also see 603). Laughing has anti-anxiety and analgesic effects. It occasionally causes giggle incontinence (p.340) and rarely syncope (p.74) or cataplexy (p.436).

Giggliness is sometimes inherited, as is smiliness (some families keep grinning even when discussing difficult things), and both can be used to disguise social awkwardness. It is also determined by mood, and over a shorter timescale of minutes has some inertia in both directions, i.e. a hysteresis. See 657.

Laughing has a detection phase and an expression phase. Reduced laughing can be due to not getting jokes (p.495) or not feeling like showing it. Trying *not* to laugh has obvious causes such as trying not to annoy people; but some teens do it to look cool, to be unobtrusive, or to avoid interaction – occasionally in selective mutism (p.153) or social anxiety (p.298).

Because it is difficult for a listener to work out whether he is being laughed *at* or laughed *with*, a listener's interpretation of laughter can be a useful indicator of paranoia (p.524).

Causes of laughing	Notes
Not really laughing	
Sex	Masturbation or sex, overheard at night sometimes with a crescendo, can be interpreted by parents as laughter. Eskimos describe sex as "laughing together".
Social	
normal	Defusing a previous communication, self-deprecating. Nervous/embarrassed, not knowing what to do or say. Coquettish; enacting a girlish persona. Creating a relaxed atmosphere; sardonic/mocking.
Fits of the giggles	
Suppressed laughter	Giggles about private jokes. Japanese ladies cover their mouths.
Infectious	(Hence laughing sounds in comedy TV). See *mirror system*, p.507.
Copying someone	Laughing to join in or to be like the others.
Courtship	(See [1108])
Semisocial	(I.e. strengthened, but not appearing out of the blue)
Tickling	Laughter is a direct effect of tickling that reduces after a mental age of 3. *On self-report*, ticklishness is correlated with tendency to crying; and perhaps to propensity to smiling, goosebumps, and blushing; but not with noise-intolerance, anxiety, or sexuality [325].
Hypomania	Giggles are loud and prolonged, highly social, and with a low threshold.
Substance abuse	Solvent/aerosol, cannabis, nitrous oxide (p.267)
Autism, psychosis	(p.538)
Non-social	(Laughing out of the blue, without social cause)
Gelastic epilepsy	(Usually from hypothalamic hamartomas, p.76; but see[1214]). Can occur with or without subjective feeling of mirth ("sham mirth"). Other subtle behavioural/mood changes due to epilepsy: p.76
tics	(Laughing tics are rare)
Other neurological	Multiple sclerosis, p.510; motor neurone disease, brain tumours, pseudobulbar palsy, p.537; emotionally incontinent laughter, p.70.

Causelist 29: Cleaning

The causes are usually revealed by a careful history. This includes date and rapidity of onset, triggers, methods, family norms (which can be unusual) and geographical extent.

Reasons for *not* cleaning include: immaturity, depression (p.309), schizophrenia (p.543), rebelliousness, hating water, fear of soap in eyes (esp pre-school), male role-models.

Causes of cleaning	Notes
Normal	
Hot weather	Teenage girls can shower 3 times a day.
Hobby/role-related	E.g. a boy cleaning and adjusting his bike for an hour or two a week.
Not really cleaning	
Water-play	Common until puberty, but from age 5–6 needs extra complications to maintain interest, e.g. competition, swimming, ball games. Simple water-play can occupy hours per day under a mental age of 3, especially with autism.
Hand-washing and hand-wringing movements	(p.477)
Specific benefits of cleaning	(See also non-specific causes of any dominating interest – p.229)
Care: practising a maternal or caring role	
Loves the repetitiveness / sensations/water & soap	Autistic (if highly repetitive, has a favourite place/motion)
Keeps mother happy	(Would do more when mother around). May be because of rewards or because frightened of the consequences if she doesn't (e.g. fear of mother's depression, or fear of being hit).
Territorial / self-image	(if she only cleans her room or only her house)
Compulsion in OCD (p.65)	There will be other signs of the fear, e.g. avoidance of dirt – or older children may be able to describe a vague or specific fear. Measuring the duration or amount of soap used reveals timecourse & treatment effect.
calming	
Tourette (p.101)	This can cause two special kinds of cleaning: • Demands for exactness, and cleaning when no dirt is visible, until it feels "just right". • Forced balancing (p.64). This happens just after his parent has washed him: he then needs to wipe in the same or opposite place to achieve the "just right feeling".
Learned / reinforced	(p.540)
Overlearned lesson	She has learned that cleaning is good, but not how much is good.
Habit	(p.475)
Can't think of anything else to do	Does she often clean in the same way, quite unimaginatively or repetitively? (see p.185).
Symbolic	(p.14)
☞Feeling impure, unclean	E.g. following sexual abuse (p.275) or rape, pre- or intra-menstrually.
Maturation and independence	Makes her feel clever (if ID), grown up. There is a story of an unemployed adult with ID who, during hypomanic phases, was sure he would get a job cleaning public toilets.

Causelist 30: Self-biting

Typical places are the side of wrist, back of the wrist, and the knuckles. Some children bite their knees or arms, but these areas are less accessible and tend to be used by the children who bite less frequently.

Self-biting is particularly common in autism ☂ (p.183), when it appears to be used to self-soothe (see *stimming*, p.64). However children (whether autistic or not) can also self-bite to avoid demands or to make their mother remove them from a situation.

The key to working out the causes is careful observation of antecedents and consequences (p.365). Hand-biting shares many of the same causes as headbanging, but the biting is easier to manage because it is less worrying to carers. For causes of self-harm in general, see p.317. For biting other people, see p.289.

Causes of hand-biting	Notes
Common	
Self-distraction	Under a mental age of about 3. Sometimes a useful sign of physical pain (examples are on p.119) or sensory intolerance (p.125). Most common in autism, presumably because of the lack of social and linguistic outlets.
Task avoidance	Because hand-biting hurts the child less than headbanging, it is more often used to avoid demands from carers. In such cases:
	• biting may be concentrated on the less painful areas such as knuckles
	• the act or the marks will be shown to the carer
	• biting will terminate when the demand does
	• after the carers have learned to back off quickly, the child will not need to do it hard or often – so a detailed history will be available, but skin will not be thickened.
Lesch-Nyhan (p.318)	Includes biting lips and fingers, with tissue loss.
Klüver-Bucy (p.496)	The child's focus in this syndrome is on continual mouth stimulation (by fingers or other objects). Note that constantly putting fingers in the mouth shows the motivation to be quite different from most mouthing, which is investigative and exploratory. Self-biting may be absent or only fill a small proportion of the time.
Endogenous opioid addiction (see p.317)	That this is not a common cause is shown by the fact that most hand biters only do it sporadically, not continually.

Causelist 31: Pacing

Causes of pacing	Notes
Anxiety	
Relieving pain / urge to micturate	
Helps thinking	
(Restless legs syndrome) (p.200)	Worst at night.
(Leg jiggling)	
Akathisia	Side-effect of antipsychotics. Can be highly distressing to patient or carers.
Pacing around the perimeter of room	Ritual (if room isn't shut) or if it is, like a caged animal
Pacing with special meaning	Depression, psychosis (p.537)
Walks to door because wants to leave	
Counting something	
Can't sit down	
Excited, excess energy	
Mania	(p.261)
OCD	Afraid of dirt on chair; afraid he will have to do rituals when he stands up, which will be embarrassing until he gets the "just right" feeling.

Causelist 32: Masturbating

This has several components, typically acquired at very different ages:
- Genital rubbing
- Interest in opposite sex
- Orgasm (p.71)
- Knowledge of sex.

Genital rubbing has little relation to sexuality when it occurs in children without sexual knowledge or interest or orgasms; and in small children the terms *gratification behaviour* (p.474) or *self-comforting*, implying an analogy to thumb-sucking and rocking, are more acceptable to many parents and teachers. Removing clothes, or threatening to do so, is not part of masturbation and can be analysed like rudeness (p.161). For other sexual and sexual-like behaviours see p.269.

In *infant girls*, masturbation can be difficult to recognise because there is usually no genital handling. Each child has a standard (stereotyped, p.553) posture, usually with thigh adduction and hip flexion, but other positions also occur, such as sitting on a foot, leaning over a table, or straddling objects; there is usually rhythmic movement of pelvis or stimulating hand accompanied by quiet grunting and sometimes flushing or sweating; and the episodes *always cease with distraction* and the child then appears annoyed [412,1807]. There may be grimacing, pouting, or back-arching. Orgasm is often inconspicuous or absent pre-pubertally, but some episodes end with a sigh and drowsiness.

Some of the causes in the list below increase the interest in masturbation, often by reducing the repertoire of alternatives; others reduce the inhibition against masturbating in public; a few do both (e.g. ID, autism, mania, and sexual abuse). This distinction is difficult to use in practice as it is rarely known how much masturbation occurs in private. Also, when the masturbation is mainly done in a public place (e.g. the inpatient staff office or the doorway of a restaurant) it cannot simply be attributed to disinhibition because there may be quite separate factors acting simultaneously (e.g. loneliness, p.500; or wanting to monitor who is coming or going; or suddenly being unable to cope).

Anal masturbation can be done with fingers, with foreign objects (p.118), by pressing against a hard object, or by voluntarily pushing stool "in-and-out" of the rectum[62]. The trigger for the "in-and-out" is often excited affectionate play, with parents, therapists, or other children [62]. There are often social or emotional factors, but it is also conceivable that these children have greater anal sensitivity than most people[62].

Causes of masturbation	Notes
Normal	30% of boys masturbate before puberty, and nearly as many girls, with no harmful (or beneficial) sequelae [928]. At least double this number masturbate in adolescence. Masturbation with objects is less common (p.267).
ID ☂, autism ☂	In ID this is less hidden and can be much more frequent, because of a limited self-entertainment repertoire (p.545). Some children with severe ID and autism (p.183) masturbate almost constantly against furniture or stairs, or with their hand. It is increased by inadequate toys or space.
Mild anxiety	I.e. masturbating as a comfort / coping mechanism (p.445)
Hypomania	Or other causes of disinhibition (p.264)
Sleepiness	Sleep-onset is accompanied by many repetitive behaviours, p.200.
Manipulative (p.504)	Listen for "If you don't… then I'll do it, I'll pull down my knickers".
Attention-seeking	This is unconvincing if the masturbation is silent and involves only tiny movements. See what happens when people leave.
Desire to offend	This is not the reason if the masturbation is silent and involves only tiny movements. Happens when angry.
☞ Tactile deprivation	When parents *reduce* their cuddling or hugging (rather than never having done it), masturbation sometimes increases, and then it can be rapidly stopped by reinstating the cuddles [1036]. The reduction in cuddling may be caused by separation, weaning, puberty, or arrival of a new baby. Other types of sensation-seeking are listed on p.123.
Sexual abuse	Rarely causes sexualised behaviour (p.270).
Perineal irritation	Vulvovaginitis (can be cause or effect); urinary tract infection.
Clothing	Wearing thin clothes or no underwear can increase masturbation; a thick unopenable coat can reduce it.
Premenstrual tension	Can occur even before menarche: p.506.
Pornography on internet	Can act as *superstimuli* (p.558) which some teenagers cannot stop looking at, even to the extent of watching/masturbating all night and being exhausted the next day.

Causelist 33: Pulling own hair

NB Trichotillomania is defined as pulling hairs "to the point of alopecia", i.e. bald patches 2 cm or more across. Exclamation-mark hairs (growing thinner toward their base) are seen in both conditions, though it may be more useful to inspect the distal end, which is usually frayed in alopecia but not in trichotillomania[741].

The relief of mounting tension is akin to that in discharging tics (p.101) or compulsions (p.65), but hair pullers have fewer neuropsychological impairments than people with OCD[279]. If razors or other methods are used interchangeably, the aim is appearance rather than the pulling itself. Compare playing with hair (p.225).

Causes of pulling own hair	Notes
One-by-one	
Habit	Attention is not focused on it, i.e. no tools or mirror. Precipitant can be any other other causes. Perpetuated by any working position that keeps hands near face.
Local irritation	Attempts to remove irritating ingrowing hairs, especially in beard area and with very curly hair.
Around zits	Possibly a learned way to relieve pressure in comedones
Grooming	Eyebrows, nose hair. Only important if pursued to an impairing or disfiguring degree. More frequent in hairy girls with unhairy friends. Increased by boredom (p.322) and lack of better occupations.
Anxiety	Anxiety about something else can focus attention on that, leaving a hair-pulling habit to act unchecked.
Rare	Excessive pursuit of symmetry; intrusive tic-like need for the pulled or "just right" feeling (as with cracking joints). Copying role model; Body dysmorphic disorder (p.433). To inflict pain (but pain reduces with repeated hair-pulling); Lesch-Nyhan (p.318).
	OCD (p.65) is increased in people with trichotillomania, but still not common, and the hair-pulling need not be a response to an obsession. Ask why they do it: true obsession is an exaggerated fear with normal content. One study suggests inflexibility (p.234) and obsessionality are *not* associated with hair pulling[280]. Impaired inhibition of motor tasks is associated with both OCD and hair pulling[280] but this seems to be just a theoretical consideration.
Pulling clumps of hair	
Unintentional	Byproduct of grooming, as by a tight ponytail
self-punishment	Pulling large clumps (see historical references to pulling hair)
Rage (p.71)	Pulling handfuls of hair, but not usually pulling much out.
Headache in ID	May be screaming while pulling hair (see pp.139,142)
Cultural	Or religious
Either / Other	
☞Psychosis	(p.537) rare. Ask why they do it: hallmark is bizarre reason.
Not hair pulling at all	Alopecia, like other causes, often follows stress. Girls often twiddle their hair. Some hairstyles pull hair so tight that alopecia can result.
Waxing	Normal in girls, but in boys it is worth exploring to find causes (which may be benign or worrying).
Symbolic	A boy who was confused about whether he wanted to be like his father plucked *or shaved* his eyebrows. This was intermittent depending on his mood and on when people told him his eyebrows were just like his father's.

Causelist 34: Inserting things in body

This is very common, particularly in small children (for numerous examples with X-rays see [734]).

Small children often insert objects into the **ears** and **nose**, where they can cause chronic pain and persistent unilateral discharge with an offensive odour. In the ear, a common cause is the child's copying a parent's use of a cotton bud.

Laryngeal foreign bodies are usually mis-swallowed food or small objects (pills, fishbones, peanuts, hard sweets, or blowpipe projectiles). When the objects are thin or flat they can remain stuck for weeks without causing acute airway obstruction[959]. Usually they are freed by coughing; however if the airway becomes obstructed an emergency Heimlich manoeuvre is required.

Vaginal foreign bodies necessitate consideration of sexual abuse[691]. **Rectal** foreign bodies can result from anal self-stimulation, sometimes called anal masturbation[62]. Sometimes this is done with stool (compare faecal misplacement, p.341; masturbation, p.115).

The example used below, inserting things in the **penis**, is obviously unusual, but included here to illustrate the search for potential explanations, even for rare or highly circumscribed behaviours. There are several components in the development of such an unusual and unpleasant behaviour: First, having a reason to do it (unless it is accidental); second, overcoming the pain or fear of pain; and third, learning which kinds of tools work. It may be useful to look for causes of each of these components separately; to look at related causelists in this book (e.g. p.342); or to work through a classification of causes (p.393).

Causes of inserting things in penis	Notes
Exploration	May explore other orifices too
Itch (p.110)	E.g. post-operative healing can cause itch, and the attempts to scratch this can cause further injury and itch.
Copying	Re-creation of catheterisation (remembered or reported)
Exploration or habit	Nothing else to do (especially if confined to bed without many toys)
Ignorance of how to masturbate (p.474)	Very unlikely as a cause.
Paraphilia / fetish	Requires that the penis be erect.
Self-punishment	E.g. punishment for sexual thoughts
Self-harm	If isolated to penis, must find out why. See sections on deliberate self-harm (p.317) and headbanging (p.119)
Self-distraction	Increased at times of stress, comparable to some cases of wrist cutting done with the purpose of self-distraction
Related to skin picking?	Reduced pain-sensitivity and skin picking are found in Prader-Willi (p.533, with rectal digging) and in Smith-Magenis (p.550).
To get attention/help	He ensures that he is seen or that the blood is found.

Causelist 35: Headbanging

This means repetitively banging the head on something. Hitting the head with things is more common and usually quite different (p.317), but in children who headbang, objects can also be used to bang the head for the same reasons as are listed below. Infrequent headbanging occurs in 10−15% of normal children aged 9−36 months (especially at sleep onset), and at least as often in ID at any age.

There is usually no immediate danger, unless it is done on glass, or if the child runs forcibly into hard corners or surfaces, or there is loss of consciousness. There is substantial longer-term risk of brain or retinal damage if he enjoys it (look for banging on very hard objects, and self-absorption with a contented face), or if he is seriously damaging himself in other ways too (p.317). Protracted bursts in children with autism or ID can be dangerous (it can be used to self-stimulate endorphin release, akin to eye-poking blindisms, p.66). Worrying signs are bruising, cuts, and particularly skin thickening as they indicate forcefulness, frequency and chronicity. Children can bother neighbours in the night with fairly gentle bangs on something that resonates.

It is worth taking a detailed history to discover triggers. Some children headbang in different ways at different times of day, each needing different management. If a child headbangs severely but not on all days, it is worth looking hard for what makes those days different (see intermittent problems, pp.63 and 365). Settling into a rhythm suggests he's happy with the feeling, and this is often a sign of sleepiness. When headbanging seems to be out of the blue (without obvious antecedent) consider especially pain and attention-seeking in the following list. Epilepsy is very unlikely.

The first question parents *pose* is whether the headbanging is dangerous (see above). However their *puzzlement* is usually about whether the headbanging is manipulative, anger, or self-soothing (the hidden question is: is it the child's fault, the child's immaturity, or the parent's fault). The answer is often a combination of these, and in any case most causes respond fairly well to assiduous behavioural management.

Types of headbanging	Notes
Fairly normal	
Accidental	Is not repetitive
Exploratory	• A child tries a bang to see what it feels like, and gets upset if the surface is harder than expected. • Headbanging on the TV can be due to wanting to get to something just shown.
Rage (p.71)	In this the child is out of control, and the headbanging is accompanied by rapid movements, flailing of the arms, an angry expression, and sometimes screams or growls.
Repetitive parasomnia	(p.200) and see left.
Caused by other pain	
Distraction from pain	☞ **Facial pain**, especially from ears and teeth[see 1542] ☞ **Other head pain,** p.139 especially cluster headache, p.140 ☞ **Non-head pain**: reflux (GORD, p.472), constipation (p.444), hernia, phimosis, urinary infection, dysmenorrhoea
Autism related ☂ (p.183)	Treatments can aim for protection (cushions or helmets), distraction, or extinction (by preventing any of the rewards; there will be a temporary increase called an extinction burst which shows that the loss of rewards has been noticed).
Communication	Children with communication difficulties may bang their head in frustration on the person (or even the hand or MP3 player) that they wish would do something. A mild version of this is banging the head on the side of mother's knee, presumably to make the leg move (this only happened when the child was bored or wanted to leave). This can give the impression of using their head as a weapon to hurt the other person, but that is not usually the case.
Distraction from external stimuli	The most common cause in autism, to escape from pain, fatigue, unpredictability, rapid change (e.g. the speed of people's approach), fear, crowding, noise, heat, fluorescent lights.
To achieve a particular feeling	Signs are looking for the right surface hardness, hitting carefully and gradually harder, and relaxation at the end. The aim can be noise, touch, or rhythmicity – or pain in general, in which case there would probably be other kinds of self-harm too (see[1749]).
Effects on other people	The child doesn't do it when alone. He either checks that people are looking, or chooses noisy surfaces.
To stop something	E.g. to stop people talking, to terminate washing, or to go home.

Sensory ☼

Many kinds of abnormal perceptions have been described, and they are initially subdivided into illusions and hallucinations, depending on whether a real external object actually triggered the perception or not. (For hallucinations see p.343.) There are many subtypes of illusion, e.g. the Alice in Wonderland-like size-distortions sometimes experienced in migraine; *synaesthesia* (p.559); *allochiria* meaning mislocation of sensory stimuli to the other side of the body; *allachaesthesia* meaning other displacements of stimuli[1055].

Apart from pains (p.135), feigned or exaggerated sensory problems are rare (see p.359). For suspected pseudo-anaesthesia, a wide range of tests are available[904], of which the simplest are worse-than-random performance on a two-choice sensory discrimination task, and functional brain imaging. For other pseudo-experiences, see p.364.

Using any sense well has a motor component. For example, some children learn to overcome ocular motor apraxia with head-thrusting movements or by blinking before voluntary saccades[588]. Children with hemianopia develop extra head-turning[588]. See also *deafisms*, p.66.

Sensory integration problems are mentioned on p.125. Many pursuits, preferences, and actions also have a sensory element, described in their respective chapters.

Categories of sensory deficits

Sensory problems can be categorised by modality, and anatomically subdivided into problems of end-organs, nerves, sensory nuclei, and cortical processing (see table). In general, cortical processing problems are less obvious, less well understood, more flexible, and more likely to have multiple associated deficits – so testing can be very difficult. Sensory-evoked potentials (p.462) and EEG are useful for checking how far the sensory signal reaches.

	End-organ effects	Nerves, brainstem	Cortical processing
Auditory	(p.130)	(p.130)	**Mild**
			"Central auditory processing deficit" (CAPD ☝) should be suspected if the child is not deaf, but is much impaired following verbal instructions, compared with his peers, even though his written performance is normal. According to the broadest conceptions of this construct, one of the subgroups would simply have poor auditory short-term memory (e.g. they cannot follow multi-part verbal instructions). The concept of CAPD is reasonable, but unfortunately it has been defined to require the *absence* of closely related problems, which aids research but is impractical for clinical work (given the high degree of comorbidity).
			Severe
			"Central deafness" includes "pure word deafness" and "auditory agnosia", i.e. not recognising what the sound of a telephone ringing is.
			Functions preserved despite cortical damage There is preservation of startle reaction to a clap.
Visual (p.133)	Visual impairment (*blindness* implies that	damage to optic nerves, optic chiasm (e.g. pituitary	**Mild** See reading difficulty, p.51. **Severe** "Cortical visual impairment"[588]

	this is complete) Cataracts, p.436, trauma, retinal degeneration	neoplasm), optic radiation or lateral geniculate nucleus.	Functional blindness but with a normal pupillary light reflex. There can be damage to all or part of the visual cortex, or to the temporal "what" pathway (visual agnosia or prosopagnosia: inability to recognise faces) or the parietal "where" pathway (simultanagnosia: inability to perceive more than one object at a time)[1350]. **Functions preserved despite cortical damage** Blindsight (can avoid bumping into things).
Temper-ature		In distal poly-neuropathies (as in diabetes) affecting the smallest axons, the feet can feel as though they are burning; and this can be accompanied by *reduced* temperature-sensitivity.	Cold can be painful following central or peripheral lesions[108] (see *neuropathic pain*, p.136); and can be experienced as hot in uraemia. (See also temperature of body, p.562).
Pain		See Fabry crises, p.464.	(p.135)
Other somato-sensory		Impaired touch or proprioceptive sense.	**Mild** Contributes to dyspraxia, p.89; synaesthesia, p.559. General developmental difficulties, such as low birth weight (p.432), are associated with impaired somatosensory processing[389]. **Severe** Astereoagnosia (inability to identify object by touch) **Functions preserved despite cortical damage** See spinal cord, p.551; brainstem, p.434.
Taste and Smell	Nasal infection, rhinitis, and cigarettes can dull these sensations or cause bad tastes. Very many medications can alter percep-tion[425]. Mercury excess, p.330		Seizures can have a specific olfactory aura, e.g. of burning rubber. Migraines can also have such an aura, or can cause osmophobia (p.126). Tastes and smells can form part of a flashback in PTSD. Olfactory hallucinations can arise in schizophrenia (p.543); in amygdala lesions; and in depression (p.313), in which case they are unpleasant and perceived as emanating from the patient[1373]. For variation in taste preference by age and metabolic needs, see p.124; genetic variation, p.128. For taste training in childhood see p.331. For cognitive effects on enjoyment of tastes see p.534. See also sniffing, p.109. For more details see[219].
Balance		Vestibular neuronitis / labyrinthitis	Vestibular symptoms and anxiety are mutually enhancing[757]. Many people with vestibular dysfunction develop panics and agoraphobia, p.297. Conversely, hyperventilation can cause dizziness. Vestibular dysfunction also occasionally contributes to reading difficulty, p.52; secondary hypermobility, p.483; and apraxia / dyspraxia, pp.88-89. See also predictive relevance of falling, p.57; vestibular intolerance, p.127.

Causelist 36: Sensation-seeking ☼

This term is ambiguous, as seeking *to be stimulated* or *aroused* is very different from seeking a specific sensation, or seeking the general feeling of relaxation. These are listed separately in the accompanying table.

People also have social drives (p.168) and many other separate needs [1024] of which some take clear precedence over others (figure, p.505).

Every activity can also be used as a distraction from other things (identify this by whether the activities only happen when those other things are present). Every sensation in this table can also be avoided (see defensiveness, p.125). To some extent people get used to the long-term level of stimulation of each of their drives (e.g. [1036]) but such adaptation is limited in practice.

Often a single stimulus has several aspects – for example joking (p.495) often satisfies many of the drives in the following table. This means that the aspects that this particular child values can only be worked out by looking at *several* desired stimuli (p.307) or the triggers and relieving factors.

Types of sensation-seeking	Means of gratification
Exciting/Ennervating/Arousing (see play, p.221; self-entertainment, p.545; relief of boredom, p.322).	
General visual stimulation	Eyes open, looking around *Indirect*: pressing on eyeballs (blindism, p.66)
General tactile stimulation	Mainly in autism (p.183), ID, and sensory impairment/ deprivation. Mouthing objects (p.56). An extreme and rare example is seeking a footscratch.
General auditory stimulation	Listening to music (iPod), tapping, singing, shouting.
Energy, enthusiasm	Stimulation, hyperactivity (p.79) *Indirect*: stimulants (p.555)
Novelty	Exploration, e.g. seeking *new* sensations/situations, or seeking *specific unusual* sensations, p.104. Simple experimentation is often called self-entertainment (p.545). Children with high *behavioural inhibition* (p.296) reduce their activity when exposed to novelty (see also p.322).
Complexity	"We systematically underestimate the human need of intellectual activity, in one form or another, when we overlook the intellectual component in art and in games. Similarly with riddles, puzzles, and the puzzle-like games of strategy such as bridge, chess, and *go*; the frequency with which man has devised such problems for his own solution is a most significant fact concerning human motivation." [677]. Learning (and advancement to the next Piagettian stage, p.530) may be encouraged by this.
Incongruity or surprise	The drive to novelty might more accurately be called a drive to surprise or to incongruity: "A side-show in a fairground will attract more patrons if it exhibits a two-headed but otherwise normal man or a bearded but otherwise undistinguished lady than if it offers a collection of beetles or birds' eggs, all of which may be completely new to those who inspect them." [152]. Similarly we pay attention to non-sequiturs in sentences.
Challenge / anxiety/fear (p.307)	As in risk taking / thrill-seeking (love of controlled fear in horror films, roller-coasters). Gambling has complex motivations (p.259).
Specific sensations	
Gratification phenomena	Implies hard-wired, strong, simple, and perhaps relaxing (p.474).
To get a particular feeling	Repetitive phrases or squeals, echolalia (p.459), gazing at something, spinning (p.104). See sensory tics, p.231; autism, p.183; tidiness/just-right/exactness, p.163.
To stretch and get exercise	Physical play: p.221
Tastes	Regulated by metabolic needs, e.g. salt. Sweet taste is enjoyed more in childhood.
Social approval Feeling of mastery	E.g. obtained by joking or engaging in scary activities (can also relieve a feeling of inadequacy)
Self-soothing (see p.61)	
Calmness / rest / sameness	Often labelled as oppositionality, p.253, sometimes as Pathological Demand Avoidance, p.527.

Causelist 37: Sensory and other intolerances ☼

Enjoyment of sensation has an inverted-U distribution in the population, from sensation loving (p.123) to the opposite, sensory intolerance (or in milder form, over-awareness). The term "sensory defensiveness" refers to the intolerant end, somewhat inappropriately as defence, like avoidance, is a learned strategy rather than the initial problem. *Sensitive* sometimes means *intolerant*, but it has other meanings too (p.546; see also Chapter 8 of [890]).

Additivity: Sensory intolerance is much more common, and more obvious, in children who are anxious, ill, in pain, tired, angry and/or who have neurodevelopmental problems (compare the additivity of rigidity, p.233). Sensations are also additive, e.g. he is more sensitive to noise when he is in a small room or if people are very near; or he is usually sociable but hates being comforted when he's hurt himself. The overwhelmed state is often called "flooded" or "meltdown."

Timecourses of causes: Startle syndromes (p.552) and trait anxiety are lifelong, overaroused hence the opposite of psychopathic (p.280). Autistic children have a massively raised cortisol response to new situations, lasting 1−2 hours[317]. More common short-term contributors include exhaustion and hypoglycaemia (p.82) after school, and sleepiness.

Sensory intolerance (like sensation-seeking) is not an observable behaviour, but an interpretation of that behaviour. If you think a child is intolerant of X, you have to check (a) whether he is really intolerant of just a small part of X (using the reasoning as for phobias on p.307), (b) whether he is intolerant of a larger group of things than just X, and (c) whether his intolerance of X is usually insignificant but grows to an impairing level when he overwhelmed by other things (e.g. information overload, depression, anxiety, intolerance of Y).

Anxiety and low mood are the most common associations of sensory intolerance [582]. Sensory intolerance causes instantaneous responses, and it can also lead to phobias which cause longer-lasting arousal, that characteristically disappears when the child is sure the stimuli won't reoccur. Such intolerance can cause school refusal (p.217) and party refusal, giving the impression of social anxiety (p.298).

Other sensory processing problems
Some clinicians believe that autism, or at least its intolerances, result from sensory processing problems, rather than the more cognitive deficits usually cited. The logic is flawed because these sensory processing problems are not specific to autism[1364]. This does not reduce their clinical importance.

Occupational Therapists talk of children being hyper- versus hypo-sensitive in various sensory modalities (in present terms, intolerant versus having reduced acuity) and use the concept of Sensory Integration / Processing Disorder. Of patients whom carers believe to be intolerant of noise, functional analysis can demonstrate this objectively in fewer than half, probably for reasons such as situation dependence, additivity of stressors, and incorrect observation[1035]. There is good evidence that the early environment guides the development of multisensory integration[1706], and while this adds to the face validity of environmental adjustments to help children who have difficulty integrating information from multiple senses, there is little evidence that this contributes to any recognised impairment, or to its treatment. Some parts of brainstem auditory evoked responses are magnified in anxious states[81]. The effects of expected versus unexpected uncertainty are also under scrutiny[1813].

General strategies invoked by intolerance (normal & abnormal examples)

General strategy	Intolerant of what	Observable behaviour
Avoidance (p.429)	Physical discomfort	Relieving hunger, thirst, hypoglycaemia (p.82), nasal drip (p.109), itch (p.110)
	Danger	The fast phase of flinching (p.107)
	Something we enjoy in smaller amounts (p.123)	E.g. regulating body temperature; avoiding exercise (and enjoying rest) by lying down; covering ears (p.131)
	Psychic discomfort (e.g. fears, p.307)	Avoiding tasks he is likely to fail (usually by inattention; refusal, p.540; tantrums, p.286; rarely with frozen watchfulness, p.470; or even dissociation, p.453). Some self-harm (p.317), compulsions (p.65). Resolving cognitive dissonance (p.355) is sometimes observable.
	(Not always clear)	Avoiding physical contact or eye contact or people
	Forgetting, not knowing	Organising life to avoid not knowing what's going on.
	Boredom, p.322	Do more as boredom increases
	Tension, horror, nausea	School refusal, p.217; the slow phase of flinching, p.107; dissociation, p.453. Tidying to avoid messiness.
Self-distraction / redirection / masking	Anything	Headbanging (p.119) can produce pain or be addictive (hence the effectiveness of naltrexone [1749]).
	Tiredness, anxiety loneliness, p.500	self-soothing behaviour, p.61. imaginary friends & worlds, p.231
	Over-excitement	Averting gaze, walking, spinning, hand-regard (p.56)
Some problems cannot be successfully avoided /distracted, i.e. there is still anxiety (p.295) or violence (p.289).	(Various)	E.g. OCD, p.65; also pp.295,307. frozen watchfulness, p.470. use of sedatives, p.267.
	Change itself	Anger or violence when the routine changes (see rigidity, p.234)
	Not understanding	Anxiety or violence in unfamiliar situations (contrast intolerance of change itself, see above).

Conundrum 6: Autism with anxiety and intolerance

Intolerance in autism

Intolerance is common in autism ☂ (p.183), causing avoidance or signs of frustration (p.291). See stimming, p.64.
Only a minority of intolerant children are autistic[582]. However, intolerance of unpredictability, noise, or social contact would in practice increase the likelihood that a clinician would diagnose autism. Avoidance of feeling overwhelmed sometimes causes poor eye contact and, in autistic people, may be the reason for gazing at or holding objects.

Anxiety in autism

Anxiety is very common in ASDs [317,1746]. It often increases intolerance and in practice contributes to ruling the diagnosis of autism in or out. If an anxious child seeks his mother for reassurance *in a normal way*, or seeks siblings for interactive play at home, he is unlikely to be autistic; whereas if anxiety makes him engage in sterile stereotyped behaviours (p.554) this is likely to be an autistic trait.

continued ▶

Working out what the child is intolerant of	Notes
Specific sensation intolerance	
Aversions	Some common sensations cause discomfort or are disliked by many people, e.g. the feel of cotton wool, the sound of a baby crying or fingernails on a blackboard, the line by the toes of socks, ugliness. Complex dislikes can be learned (akin to fears, p.307). Rarely, aversions can be impairing[1010].
Complex	This most often comes to attention as context-specific anxiety (p.307).
Pain sensitisation	Physical injury can cause hypersensitivity that persists long after healing is complete (p.107). This involves both central & peripheral mechanisms[777].
Conditioned arousal, or sensory amplification	(a) Some children have aversive cumulative (i.e. sensitising, p.546) arousal responses to repeated minor aversive stimuli, such as pans dropping or school fire alarms, that are unusually resistant to *extinction*, p.463. Many diagnosed cases of PTSD (p.532) have this problem[1741]. (b) Sexual and physical abuse can cause intolerance of touch or even proximity lasting years. (c) Innocuous sensations can become aversive if one pays too much attention to them. Reasons for this include: • worry (as in idiopathic environmental intolerance[1489] or hypochondriasis, p.362) • if one believes that offense is intended, p.188 • failure of habituation, e.g. to tinnitus, p.565; an itchy shirt, p.110; a ticking clock; or someone tapping in the library (contrast failure of pre-pulse inhibition of startle, p.462). • discomfort, in people prone to pains such as fibromyalgia (see p.466)
Modality-wide intolerance	
Auditory (p.131)	Auditory perception sensitises easily, causes startle responses, and can carry more deeply unpleasant social content than most senses. Hearing is also the most difficult sense to block, due to the difficulty of avoiding noise and the ineffectiveness of shielding the ears (p.131). Hence auditory intolerance is a fairly common complaint. This has peripheral causes (e.g. paralysis of stapedius; ear infection; exposure to loud noises) and central causes (e.g. sleep deprivation; migraine; autism). Central causes are more likely to be affected by mood. The term *hyperacusis* is sometimes used to mean both central and peripheral groups; sometimes just the peripheral ones; and sometimes all non-stapedial causes. Deafness often causes both auditory intolerance and tinnitus (p.565). For other aspects of loudness detection, see[85]. Another special characteristic of hearing is that it is the last sense to go during anaesthesia or sleep.
Visual	*Intolerance of specific visual information* Shutting or shielding or averting eyes, to avoid unpleasant sights, rollercoasters, scary parts of films. *Intolerance of illumination* Anxious people prefer lower levels of illumination, although they are not actually fearful of light (see data in[828]). See also *photophobia*, p.529.

Tactile	(To fabrics, labels, gloves, touch, toothbrushing, getting hands dirty). Physical and sexual abuse (pp.273−275) contribute, though rarely. Dry hands also contribute. Both feet having to feel the same (consider whether related to tics, p.101). Especially if the intolerance is limited to specific parts of the body or follows injury, consider *allodynia*, p.136.
Vestibular	Consider joint laxity, BPPV (p.454) with avoidance, gross motor dyspraxia (p.89).
Olfactory	(See migraines, below). Children with autism are often more idiosyncratic, e.g. one breathed out hard whenever he came near people, because he couldn't tolerate their smell.
Taste	70% of humans have a genetic predisposition (PROP) to dislike and avoid bitter and strong-tasting foods and juice[1597].
General (or cognitive or meta-sensory) intolerance	Senses share many properties that can be aversive, while being distinct from the modality itself. Suspect such general intolerance if the aversion can be elicited by more than one modality, or if it is seen only with meaningful stimuli, or with stimuli from some people but not others, or when a mistake is detected (caused by self, others, or no one). General intolerance is worse when sleepy, and is cumulative between modalities, e.g. the child is more intolerant of touch when there are loud noises going on. **Assessment***:* This can be tricky as you need stimuli with each of these characteristics. Apart from *distraction*, causes need to be assessed when the child isn't trying to concentrate. Lorries skidding to a halt a few feet away should surprise anyone. Fire alarms, thunder, and loud airbrakes on lorries are surprising but not novel; they usually cause a few seconds' arousal. Pencil drops, cat miaows, and hoovering in another room are not novel and should not be arousing. A doctor looking in your ear and saying Boo is both novel and surprising.
Arousal / surprise	Unpredictability and painfulness increase each other's anxiogenicity [620].
Being distracted from what he is doing	Any sensory input can be annoying to a child enjoying his homework, imaginary world (p.231), or autistic preoccupation (p.183). Contrast *distractibility*, p.453.
Multisensory	Migraines (p.141) bring not only headache and assorted neurological symptoms, but also avoidance of light, sound, touch, and smells (osmophobia).
Interpersonal	Getting annoyed by the way someone sounds, or the way they walk, or previously inoccuous habits.
Change	May refuse to change clothes, and repeatedly wipe off kisses, p.234
Social contact (p.181)	Common examples are walking away and avoiding eye contact. Extreme versions are much less common. They include being unwilling to pass an object to someone else, or trying to avoid doing anything that can be seen (by anyone, or only by strangers).
Novelty	(i.e. you haven't experienced this before)
Symbolic (p.14)	reminders of a difficult period, or an abusive parent
Aesthetic	Petulant intolerance is a learned signal of aesthetic sophistication and of the camp role (p.243).
Pseudo-intolerance	Learned exaggeration should be suspected if responses depend on whether parents are present; and if there is secondary gain (p.471).

Causelist 38: Not listening

This causes enormous annoyance to parents and teachers.

Causes of not listening	Notes
Not concentrating	
Normal	Increased when ill, tired, or in love, or just in difficult classes. Also happens if parents say a lot more unwelcome than welcome things, and even more if parents don't follow through with what they say.
Sleepy/sleeping	E.g. non-response during night terrors (p.200)
Hyperactive	Bright hyperactive children often do several things at the same time, and can seem not to be listening when they are. A hypomanic child can ask a question then fly onto another idea.
Difficulty responding	If you can't get the child to respond to anything else auditory, try his name! See disobedience (p.253)
Hypoglycaemia	(p.82)
Insufficient cardiac output	Child complains of feeling strange and may pass out completely (and fall over). Clammy (cold damp hands)
Absences	(p.75), also rarely other seizure types.
Pays attention to you	
Oppositional (p.253)	Hears and understands but chooses to do something different.
Poor comprehension	You need first to check the hearing (see above). • To detect receptive language problems, ask the parents what the child can understand and try a few instructions like "touch your nose" (with no non-verbal cues). Spread toys out and say something age-appropriate e.g. "give dolly to mum". • In NVLD (p.28), it is bewilderingly impossible to reason with the highly verbal child.
☞ Deafness	This can be transient or permanent, see right.
Pseudo-deafness	Estimates of prevalence are as high as 7% of children referred with hearing problems[960,1113], e.g. because of academic difficulties or not wanting to hear instructions. Signs include exaggerating their deafness; using information suppplied verbally when out of sight; and blinking to noise. Skilled testing is required: e.g. the false positive rate on audiometry is suppressed[960]. See p.359.
CAPD	Central Auditory Processing Deficit (p.121).
Concentrating on something else	
Depression	Ruminations (p.543)
Imagination	E.g. imaginary friends, p.231; other dissociation, p.453
Autism ⬆ (p.183)	E.g. concentrating on his special interest. These children sometimes hum to mask external sounds, especially speech.
Reverie	E.g. gratification phenomena (p.474)
☞ Hallucination	(p.351)

Deafness

Checking for this should be a routine part of examination.

- Parental report is an important indicator, but not sensitive; nursery reports are excellent but don't generally distinguish between hearing and comprehension problems. From age 3 you can train a child to do something when you say "go", and then say "go" very quietly. Even though this is called the "go test" it is a test of hearing rather than comprehension, as tiny noises such as taps can be used instead of "go" .
- Or test by holding child at arm's length and saying a number (or a toy) as quietly as you can, with some "voice" rather than just a whisper, and asking the child to repeat it.
- Isolated high frequency loss can delay speech acquisition (and cause unclear speech with no consonants): the sounds pssssss , f-th-f-th-f, 66 and crumpling paper can be used to screen for this.

Causes of deafness

These can be classified as conductive (most common), sensorineural, and central (rare; see p.121). Conductive hearing loss is generally no more than 60 dB, so profound deafness is either sensorineural or central.

Prenatal causes include infections (especially rubella in unimmunised mothers; cytomegalovirus); Rhesus incompatibility; and many genetic syndromes (such as Klippel-Fiel, p.507; Waardenburg, p.475; Wolfram, p.575; Treacher-Collins; cleft palate, p.440; Down's, p.455; Turner's, p.570; CHARGE syndrome, p.439.) For syndromes of deafness with psychosis see p.350.

Perinatal causes: preterm delivery; neonatal asphyxia; *stroke*, p.556; kernicterus, p.495.

Postnatal causes: This is generally conductive, caused by OME (otitis media with effusion) or head injury (even a slap on the ear: consider physical abuse, p.273). Causes of sensorineural deafness include meningitis, measles, noise exposure, head injury, p.477; and late-onset genetic syndromes.

Effects of deafness

Effects of deafness are worse if the family can't adapt to communicate well and involve the child in what they are doing. A child with uncorrected high-frequency deafness until age 6 is likely to have permanent reduction in auditory monitoring and comprehension speed. In deaf children, ID is more common, but in addition ID, autism and psychosis can be wrongly diagnosed (or missed) by clinicians unfamiliar with the behaviour of deaf children[699]. Monaural deafness reduces directional sense, filtering of irrelevant noises, and (to some degree) acuity.

Assessment

The local statutory "Teacher for the Deaf", or an audiologist or audiological physician, can be very helpful in assessment. If the child uses sign language, a signing interpreter is invaluable. See[700] for further information. See also *non-verbal children*, p.516.

Sign language

There are many sign languages. American Sign Language and British Sign Language are mutually unintelligible. "Home signs" are signs invented in a home to use there. Contrast *Makaton*, p.502.

For related topics see *ears*, p.458.

Causelist 39: Covering the ears

This is rare as a presenting complaint, but a useful clinical observation as it
often has a big emotional component. The challenge is to work out the
triggers, hence the underlying cause. Relieving this often helps the child's
general mood and behaviour.

Causes of covering the ears	Notes
With eyes open	
Normal	Intolerance of very loud noises
Intolerance of… (p.125)	• most noises (see hyperacusis, p.483) • a specific sound (e.g. high-pitched noises or a particular person's voice) can be *aversive* (p.127). This may be temporary. • complex undecipherable noises, e.g. many voices together (a problem in class or assembly)
Avoiding specific information	E.g. avoiding being told off; avoiding being asked to do something; rarely auditory hallucinations (p.343)
Likes the sound of covered ears	
Modelled behaviour	BeeGees
Fear of losing hearing	May have incorrect or over-valued beliefs about noise-induced deafness
Social communication	• communicating lack of interest • communicating how loud something is (with eye contact)
Stereotypy (p.553)	Puts hands near ears or covers just one, sometimes as part of a multi-step ritual. Not related to noise.
With eyes shut	
Trying to sleep	
Trying to avoid situation	
With eyes open or shut	
Trying to stay in an imaginary world (p.231)	
General or sensory defensiveness	(p.125).
Ear infection	Especially if he is cringing, appears in pain, and is only covering one ear.
Headache	Consider migraine, p.141; and ice pick headaches, p.140

Causelist 40: Touching

Excess touching is in the table below (see also *touching staff*, p.173).

Inadequate touching can be due to fear of dirt (or avoidance of the rituals that the child knows will be necessary after the touching), sensory intolerance (e.g. with very dry or injured hands), or autistic rituals. Avoidance of handshakes is usually due to shyness or culture or autism (in which case it is usually done without eye contact, either limply or as a tap). Many people won't touch the floor, because of dirt. Some inflexible autistic children have only eaten from plates or bags, so cannot eat directly off tables (even crisps).

Causes of touching	Notes
Touching inanimate objects	
Exploration	Handles of doors and cupboards; and other moveable objects. Such tactile exploration is characteristic of mental age under 18 months.
Boredom (p.322)	Touches things he knows he shouldn't, which are visible to someone else he is monitoring for a reaction.
Obsession (p.517)	He has to get the touch "just right", even things up, or do it a certain number of times. Does he wash hands afterwards?
Autism ☝	Drawn to a very small class of objects, particularly simple ones ("sterile", p.554). Sniffing or licking hands afterwards may support this.
Touching self	
Self-soothing	(p.61)
Masturbation	(p.474)
Self-harm	E.g. poking self. See sections on deliberate self-harm (p.317), headbanging (p.119), blindisms (p.66).
Concealment	Concealing a rash, cut, or tremor.
Tic-related	See forced touching, p.64
Touching other people. Types of touch include: caressing, accidental brushing, holding, prolonged holding, feeling, pressing, spot touching, handshake, pat, squeeze, punch, and pinch. Descriptions of the physical movement and the part touched are not sufficient to work out the meaning of touch. Rather, meanings are conveyed in "'packages' of behavioural and situational factors."[789] Between adults there are "12 rather distinct and unambiguous meanings or messages" [789,790]. *Hybrid* touches convey more than one message (e.g. greeting plus affection). *Ambiguous* touches include touching a body part or item of clothing and commenting on it, conveying possible liking or flirtation (see also touching staff, p.173). Disinhibition, p.261 can (a) amplify any of these; and (b) overcome prohibitions.	
Communication[789]	support appreciation sexual interest (see p.269) , affection, playful affection, playful aggression, compliance with requested action, attention-getting announcing a response, requesting sharing of emotion, greetings, departures
Accidental	
Task based	E.g. demonstrating, helping, doing makeup
Provocative wind-up	Bored? Lack of attention otherwise? Looks at person.
Sensory	Autistic interest in hair,earlobes,cheek,feet p.229).
Deprivation	In maternal depression, p.174; exhaustion; or when reunited after separation, p.173

Causelist 41: Visual problems

Functional vision
Vision is not an isolated function; its use is closely integrated with the task at hand, even to the extent of only seeking specific information from visual scenes[673].

Blindness and cognitive development
Children born blind have no visual imagery. Children who lose their sight before age 5 rapidly lose all their visual memories. If sight is lost after age 7, some degree of imagery is likely to last the lifetime (see[851]).

Blindness itself slows children's learning about the environment, but in addition blindness is often complicated by more widespread problems (such as prematurity, birth asphyxia, or various syndromes)[1334]. When it is, the child is much more likely to have cognitive, sensory, movement, or social difficulties, and it is debateable whether such complicated cases can usefully be grouped together with children who have purely optic problems[270]. However, in general blind children lag developmentally behind sighted children from about one year of age. In toddlers the greatest lag is in their exploration of the environment, but by age 5 blind children tend to be a year or two behind their peers in most other areas as well: social adaptation, sensorimotor understanding, verbal comprehension, and expressive language[1334]. By adulthood, blind people *without* other substantial impairments have not developed superior compensatory cognitive abilities but they have developed superior auditory acuity and speech perception[1367].

See also blinking, p.108; eye movements, pp.52,543; eye contact, p.175; blindism, p.66; light intolerance, p.125; covering the eyes, p.176; visual sensation-seeking, pp.123 and104; visual hallucinations, p.343; visual auras, p.141; dyslexia, p.51; screening in clinic, p.409; self-harm involving eyes, p.317; night blindness, p.328. Visuospatial deficits: see *Non-verbal Learning Disability*, p.28. Eye-signs of fits include conjugate eye movements (vertically or horizontally); see also *absences* on p.75.

External appearance of the eye

See eye signs in Down's, p.455; Bitot's spots, p.328; Heterochromia, p.475.

☞ !! Setting sun sign, p.482 (needs emergency paediatric assessment). A "reverse setting-sun sign" with much sclera visible but only *below* the pupil, is normal when people are keeping their head down while looking out at you.

Exophthalmos means literally the eyeball partly out of its socket, but is sometimes defined as protrusion greater than 18 mm from the lateral orbital rim (it can be measured with an exophthalmometer/proptometer). Proptosis is simply less extreme. There are very many medical causes of both, including scleritis and hyperthyroidism, p.484.

Retraction of the eyelids is also worth noticing. It has very many causes[114]. In children, the most common causes of bilateral or unilateral retraction are hyperthyroidism, nerve anomalies, levator fibrosis, haemangioma, craniosynostosis, and Down's syndrome[1553].

Visual problems and social interaction

Blindness (and partial sight) can give the initial impression of autism. Confusion can be avoided by using the non-visual signs of autism (p.183). Blind children sometimes look down, possibly to orient their ears (and in one very unusual case barked successfully for echolocation). To get an idea of whether visual impairment would have impaired social development, consider the age from which vision was corrected, the range of distances over which smiles, frowns, and individuals can be distinguished without glasses, and the use of non-visual communication (language, touch).

Comparison of attachment behaviours in blind and sighted infants[270]:

	Sighted baby	**Blind baby**
Smiling	By 6−11 months: regular and somewhat exclusive smiles to familiar faces	At this age, does not smile regularly or exclusively to familiar voices
Discriminating tactile behaviours	n/a	By 5-8 months: differential and more frequent manual exploration of parents' faces than strangers' faces.
Stranger-avoidance	By 7−15 months, both groups of babies are unhappy about being held by a stranger.	
Concept of mother as an object	At 5 months, extends hand to mother (needs hand−eye coordination only)	Does not extend hand to mother until 11 months (additionally needs object permanence and sound localisation)

Looking at things from an odd angle is related to the DSM autism criterion of part-object preoccupation (p.388). However there are several causes that are normal (subject to duration factors, p.104), such as copying a TV character, sighting along a gunsight, comparing colours, working out which of two things is taller, and learning about foreshortening. Squint and scotomata need to be considered. It would be unusual for a non-autistic child to be frequently preoccupied with achieving particular visual experiences, such as the sensation of a triangle or a particular shade of green or matching objects.

Severe dietary restriction in autism can lead to visual problems (p.529).

Causelist 42: Pain

If a child says he has a pain, he should be believed unless there is strong evidence otherwise. Pain is present 10–20% of the time in children, and about 50% of the time in teenage girls [1245]. However overt distress behaviours during invasive medical procedures tend to reduce at a mental age of about 7[1048]. Normal individuals' pain thresholds differ by a factor of 3[284]. Migraines and fractures cause the most severe common pains. Pain often interferes with school attendance, hobbies, socialising, appetite and sleep. In order to avoid missing physical causes, a paediatrician or GP should be involved if pain persists over more than a week, or is unusual.

It is important to consider psychosocial contributors to the pain, including sports, posture, food intake, exams, mood, family conditions, and surprisingly often the weather[1381], plus the parents' and the child's ideas, concerns, and expectations (p.13). Perception of pain is increased by mental fatigue (p.323) or anxiety[284], and decreased by feelings of control or predictability. If the causation is unclear a functional analysis (p.365) usually helps. Great exaggeration is so common that it should be considered normal, particularly when maternal cuddles follow.

Pain tolerance varies greatly between normal individuals[284]. Some are prone to suffer with pain in multiple areas of their body, with multiple contributory mechanisms (see discussion of *fibromyalgia*, p.466). Most children can hide pain from peers when they are trying to look cool or grown up. Children who are very hyperactive, or who don't like cuddles, or who have ID, often do not seek carers when they get minor scratches and bruises. In mild ID, pain is generally experienced somewhat slowly and expressed imprecisely (e.g.[685]). Some with ID have not learned to get upset by threats to their physical integrity such as bleeding, nor that blood shocks others and can be used to obtain care. Autistic children certainly feel pain (as shown by their heart rate increase during venepuncture, and the fact that they have no more injuries than other children, apart from the self-inflicted ones) but they often do not seek attention when they are in pain[1614]. This seems to be due to their not wanting to interrupt their preoccupations; and their apprehension that any response from carers would be overwhelming.

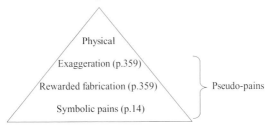

Figure 12. Diagnostic hierarchy for pains.

Explanations higher in the pyramid are much more common.

Psychogenic pain
This is less likely than physical disease to wake children in the night; but careful history is needed on this point as some children and parents will say the child was woken by pain, when actually he was prevented from going back to sleep by it, or he exaggerated it in order to gain attention. Compared to patients with predominantly psychogenic pain, those with predominantly organic pain "significantly more often described a clear localization of the pain symptom, used more sensory words for the description of pain quality, more often described discrete changes of pain intensity and periodicity, more often showed pain-intensifying factors dependent on movement and pain-decreasing factors, more often believed

pain to be a symptom versus as a disease itself, and tended to have fewer difficulties in their interpersonal relationships."[13]

Congenital analgesia
Pain-sensitivity is objectively impaired in Prader-Willi (p.533) and the same may be true in those non-verbal individuals with ID who chronically self-harm[1576]. Some people with impaired sensation on one side (e.g. due to cerebral palsy, p.437) pick the skin on that side only (p.549) or bang objects with that arm when angry. A very few children have little or no pain sensation (usually combined with other nerve deficits, in the rare hereditary sensory and autonomic neuropathies), leading to numerous bruises, fractures, and self-injuries[1169,1183]. In pain asymbolia (p.444) pain can be felt but is not aversive.

Referred pain
This is pain felt distant from its source. Most of the localisation of pain in internal organs is referred. For example heart pain is often felt in the left arm or back, and diaphragmatic pain in the shoulder. *Ice cream headache* is referred from the pharynx to the skull.

Most musculoskeletal pain is correctly localised, but some is referred. Examples include hip damage (for example in Perthes' disease) being experienced in the knee.

Unrecognised pain
In more severe ID, and in autism, non-specific signs such as screaming, self-biting and headbanging (p.119) may indicate unrecognised local or distant pain[1542]; carers may be the only ones who recognise unusual signs of pain[509].

Neuropathic pain.
This is pain caused by disease affecting the somatosensory nervous system, either peripherally or centrally[108,324]. Patients characteristically report strange sensations that they have not experienced before: skin crawling or tingling, electrical pain, burning or shooting feelings. Pains can be induced by trivial stimuli (see *allodynia*, below) or can be spontaneous. The areas of pain can be adjacent to or combined with areas of hyposensitivity. Causes include localised neuropathies, polyneuropathies, and central pain syndromes. Central pain syndromes occur especially with lesions in the brainstem, thalamus, and spinal cord, which can be vascular, inflammatory, or epileptic (for details see[108]). Complex Regional Pain Syndrome Type 1[764,799] (previously called Reflex Sympathetic Dystrophy) is a combination of continuing pain disproportionate to any injury, with localised changes in several of: hypersensitivity, trophic changes (hair, nail or skin), vasomotor function (detectable by skin color or temperature differences), sweating, and motor function.

Allodynia
This is the perception of pain elicited by normally innocuous stimuli. The term should be reserved for actual localised pain rather than more wide-spread intolerances (p.127). It can result from sensitisation (p.546) or can be neuropathic (see above). It is common in herpes neuralgia and is also seen in cerebral palsy and following brain injury. Migraines often cause both sensory intolerances (e.g. photophobia, p.529) and scalp allodynia.

Unusual patterns of pain
Chronic intermittent polyneuropathy can follow glue sniffing[1629] (p.258). Following damage to the supplementary motor area, being touched lightly can be painful even though voluntary actions remain pain free[443]. Also, brain injury can impair the affective or the discriminative aspects of pain, separately[443], presumably because they are processed separately (e.g. in the anterior and posterior insula, respectively[1239]). See also central sensitisation, p.436; Fabry's disease, p.464; temperature-sensitivity, p.562.

continued ▶

Common patterns of pain	Notes (See also *comorbidity*, p.442.)
Tummyache	Only about 10% of children with recurrent abdominal pain have an identifiable physical cause, and conversely the vast majority of them have substantial anxiety or depression [537]. Consider overeating, appendicitis, diarrhoea, peritonitis, torsion of the testis, and *many other conditions*[743] of which a few are inflammatory bowel disease, p.490; irritable bowel, p.494; sickle, p.549; and coeliac disease, p.441.

Colicky pain is pain that gradually builds over several seconds then is relieved quite suddenly, suggesting intermittent blockage of a tube. *Colic* consists of paroxysms of such pain in the abdomen, frequently accompanied by flatulence and drawing up the legs. Colic is a graded phenomenon, and in 10–30% of infants under 3 months, the crying lasts over three hours, on at least three days a week. The causes are diet, immaturity of gut enzymes, infection, gut abnormality, and temperament, in various proportions[1429]. |
| Pelvic pain | Chronic pelvic pain in young women indicates childhood sexual abuse in more than half, and psychiatric disorder in more than half, as opposed to roughly a fifth on both measures in women with other gynaecological problems [1701]. See also menses / premenstrual symptoms, p.506. |
| Musculoskeletal | • Unsurprisingly, one third of those with widespread musculoskeletal pain are depressed [1073]. Musculoskeletal pain is a major factor in chronic fatigue, p.323.
• Growing pains: deep pains in the long bones of the arms and legs, experienced by a quarter of children[1640]. They occur only at night (or occasionally late in the day). Most cases result from high levels of physical activity in children with low pain thresholds. They peak at 6 years and are more likely in children with hypermobility (p.483). If the pains are more related to exercise than to nighttime, consider metabolic muscle disease. Also consider restless leg syndrome, p.200 and fibromyalgia, p.466. In atypical cases consider bone scan.
• Consider joint hypermobility[602], p.483
• Pain in the knee or hip can indicate serious pathology, e.g. slipped epiphysis, polymyositis
• Myotonic dystrophy type 2, p.568 |

Headache	(p.139)
	(Some children will be unable to localise the pain)
Facial pain	Toothache, head injury, p.477; herpes zoster, trigeminal neuralgia

> *Ears*: Sinusitis, nasal foreign body, otitis media, impacted earwax. LOOK IN THE EARS!
>
> *Eyes*: corneal abrasion. *Rarely* glaucoma (p.474) or cavernous sinus syndrome or Tolosa-Hunt syndrome (extraocular palsies and periorbital pain)[391]
>
> *Nose*: severe allergic rhinitis

Sinus: antral infection; frontal sinusitis

Causelist 43: Headache

Headaches are common. Most are minor and soon pass. If they are unusual or disabling it is worth considering general features of pain, pseudo-pain, and psychogenic pain (p.135). However, there are also several aspects that are unique to headaches, as described in this section.

The most important challenge is to recognise headaches with an underlying, potentially dangerous cause. If the headache is sudden, extreme or unusual, "first or worst" or accompanied by neurological signs, neurological examination is needed and sometimes emergency imaging[382].

Questions to ask about headache[1382]:

Questions	Some possible answers
Do you have one or two types of headache?	
How often does it come?	
How & when did it begin?	(E.g. with puberty or head injury?)
How long does it last?	
What kind of pain is it? (severe, burning, throbbing, sharp, dull)	The most severe of the recurrent headaches is the cluster headache.
Is the headache steady, intermittent, or progressive?	(This limits the possible causes, see figure and table)
Is there a specific trigger? time of day? food? medicine? activity?	Most answers suggest a treatment. In intracranial hypertension (p.493), persistent morning vomiting is common
What do you do during the headache?	Sleeping in dark room in daytime suggests migraine
What makes it better? or worse?	
Are there warning symptoms?	Consider auras, p.141.
Where is the pain?	On top or forehead or bandlike usually indicate a tension headache. One-sided suggests migraine or cluster. Face or ears suggests local causes (p.138). Back-of-head is the most worrying[312].
Are there associated symptoms with the headache?	Nausea with flashing lights suggests migraine. Downcast eyes or early morning waking suggest depression (see p.313). Vomitting suggests systemic infection, dehydration, or intracranial hypertension (p.493). For loss of skills see p.41.
Do symptoms continue between the headaches?	(This limits the possible causes, see figure and table)
Do you have any other illnesses, or use any medicines or illegal drugs?	This can suggest a cause (see table)
Does anyone else in your family have headaches?	Migraines are highly familial.
What are your ideas, concerns, and expectations?	(p.13)

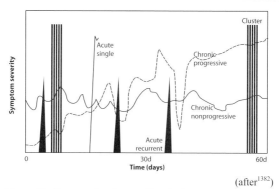

(after[1382])

Figure 13. Temporal patterns of headaches.

Types of headaches...	
Acute single headaches	(NB. See also the list below for *acute recurrent* headaches, as the current episode may be the first of many)
‖ Well-localised pain	Consider head injury, or facial pain (p.138)
Non-localised	*Common causes*:
	• viral infection (p.490)
	• tension headache. Causes include current stress, anxiety or depression (p.313), irregular sleep, overuse of analgesics such as nonsteroidals, school-avoidance (p.217), and ♠ chronic fatigue (p.323).
	• exaggeration or fabrication (pp.133, 364)
	• ice cream headaches
	• head injury and post-concussive syndrome, p.477
	• dehydration (p.450) or electrolyte imbalance, e.g. hyponatraemia, p.338
	‖ • exertional
	Rarer causes:
	• ‼ encephalitis or meningitis, p.461; Lyme disease, p.501
	• ‼ severe hypertension
	• ‼ thrombosis, embolism or haemorrhage
	• hypoglycaemia
	• post-lumbar puncture
Acute recurrent headaches	
‖ Migraine	(p.141)
‖ Tension headaches	For causes see tension headache, above.
Hypertension	E.g. phaeochromocytoma, p.529; autonomic hyperreflexia, p.299.
Medications	
Toxins	lead (p.330), cocaine (p.258), ☞ carbon monoxide, p.330
Post-ictal	(see also p.532)
Autoimmune	(p.427)
Cluster headaches [1391]	Clusters of many unilateral headaches over a few weeks with no clear trigger; rare below age 10. They are so severe that the sufferer may thrash around in bed, or headbang (p.119). There are 1−2 clusters per year. May be difficult to recognise in ID.and to distinguish from other trigeminal autonomic headaches
Ice pick headache	(primary stabbing headache). This only lasts 2−30 seconds.
Chronic non-progressive headaches	
Chronic tension headaches	(sometimes called chronic migraine). For causes see tension headache, above.
Chronic progressive headaches	(progression may be of severity or of accompanying features)
Tumours and other intracranial lesions, p.569	Consider this especially if the headache changes, becomes dramatically more severe, wakens the child from sleep, or is accompanied by neurological signs.
☞ Hydrocephalus	(p.482) or intracranial hypertension, p.493.

Special Topic 4: Is it migraine?

Migraine is probably underdiagnosed as a cause of behavioural disturbance (such as headbanging, p.119; responding to visual hallucinations, p.343). Some people just get on with life if the migraine is mild enough; but severely affected children may have several days in bed, once every few weeks.

Key diagnostic signs:

90+%: headache (50% are unilateral), often pulsatile, aggravated by normal physical activity.

50%: nausea and/or vomiting (children often get abdominal pain). Younger children are more likely to vomit.

60%: sensory intolerances causing avoidance of light, sound, touch, and smells (pp.127–126).

20%: aura with neurological symptoms developing over 5–20 minutes and lasting up to an hour, then being followed within an hour by the other key symptoms. Visual auras such as zigzags or tunnel vision are most characteristic, but are often absent before puberty. "Auras are simple partial non-motor seizures" [665,666] but the auras of migraine last 5–50 minutes whereas epileptic auras evolve over seconds[137,343]. If the auras are dim they may only be noticed in the dark.

Supportive features (for more diagnostic pointers see [743]).

- Triggered by flashing lights, menses, extreme sleeplessness; by many foods, including cheese, chocolate, alcohol, ice cream, food preservatives, caffeine (and caffeine withdrawal)[1081], and even insufficient fluid or getting up late. Note that the triggers are not the same as the intolerances (pp.127–126).

- Migrainous auras spread slowly and often last about 20 minutes, unlike epileptic fits that spread faster and are usually briefer.

- Migraines are always episodic. A useful rule is that migraines cause no symptoms, not even mild headaches, between attacks. This is true even for the atypical migraines such as some cyclical vomiting syndrome (but see p.449), and abdominal migraines.

- Relief by sleep; or partially relieved by isolation in a dark room

- Fatigue usually lasts until the next day, but can be briefer or longer.

- Most cases have a family history, which is very useful as the symptoms are often not classical before age 10.

Developmental changes

Onset at age 3–4, of vomiting without headache, may progress to classical migraine. Benign Recurrent Vertigo (or migrainous vertigo), causing screaming lasting a few minutes at age 4–5 is a variety of migraine and usually progresses to classical migraine[932].

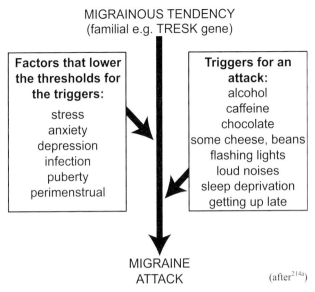

MIGRAINOUS TENDENCY
(familial e.g. TRESK gene)

Factors that lower the thresholds for the triggers:

stress
anxiety
depression
infection
puberty
perimenstrual

Triggers for an attack:
alcohol
caffeine
chocolate
some cheese, beans
flashing lights
loud noises
sleep deprivation
getting up late

MIGRAINE
ATTACK

(after[214a])

Figure 14. Contributory factors in migraine.

Unusual migraines
- In ID, migraine can cause aggression or self-harm, with no obvious classical signs if the child cannot talk. Signs include pulling her own hair while in a rage, screaming, irritability, and photophobia. The only sign of nausea may be temporary loss of appetite. See also *supportive features* (at left).
- Migraine without headache ("acephalgic migraine") is obviously easy to miss unless there are characteristic visual auras.
- Basilar type migraine includes vertigo, ataxia, diplopia, and/or tinnitus (p.565). Occasionally also bilateral tingling, confusion.
- Odd symptoms such as Alice in Wonderland (pp.41, 45).
- Some cyclical vomiting syndrome (p.449).
- Abdominal migraine: dull abdominal pain lasting hours, with a family history of migraines.
- Hemiplegic migraine[465], which can have sensory as well as motor symptoms, can start with tingling, weakness or paralysis in one part of the body (e.g. a hand) and can spread to the other side. Some episodes are accompanied by confusion or psychosis[489] or ataxia[873]. Subtypes are caused by mutations of the Ca channel[1195] and a sodium channel[545].
- Status migrainosus means a migraine attack lasting longer than 72 hours.

Communication ☼

Fundamental rules of communication

The *Gricean Maxims* describe how to logically *convey facts*, rather than the broader question of what is normal in humans:

Table 8. Gricean maxims of communication

Gricean maxims	Related problems
Maxim of quality:	
Do not say what you believe to be false.	Lying, p.255.
Do not say that for which you lack adequate evidence.	**
Maxim of quantity:	
Make your contribution as informative as is required for the current purposes of the exchange.	Pedantry, p.163; not speaking much, p.151; word-finding difficulty, p.149; speaking but not being open, p.166; difficulty talking about feelings, p.152.
Do not make your contribution more informative than is required.	Pedantry, p.163.
Maxim of relation:	
Be relevant.	for circumlocution, i.e. tangentiality and circumstantiality, see [1487]. See also *not listening*, p.129).
Maxim of manner:	
Avoid obscurity of expression.	Pedantry (p.163)
Avoid ambiguity.	**
Be brief.	Pedantry, p.163; repetitiveness, p.156.
Be orderly.	** For extremes, see Thought Disorder in [1487] & p.563

** These rules challenge even bright adult speakers, so children's failure to satisfy them is not usually seen as a problem.

Normal language milestones

In most children, *spontaneity* is seen at all ages, rather than being a developmental stage. For severe or mild speech regression, see p.41. For other worrying signs at various ages, see p.55. For more details see[255,937].

	Expressive	Receptive
0−6 m	In the first month he makes soft, gutteral noises when talked to. In his first 6 months a baby is crying and cooing to a voice.	A newborn blinks or becomes quiet in response to sound. 3 m he turns to sounds at ear level
6−12 m	*Babble* (or "canonical babble") means vocal play before meaningful words have developed (e.g. "lalala dada" to anyone).	By 7 m he turns to a voice
8−15 m	*Jargon* means babbling, i.e. words and part-words assembled into sentences with adult-like stress and intonation, but without meaning.	
15−18 m	Single words with meaning are heard in 90% by 15 months. The content is initially limited to "mama", "dada" and favourite toys; soon it extends to indicating needs and saying "no". Content of first word not significant unless it indicates a unusual interest, or something the family talk about.	At 15 m, he understands in context "give me". At 18 m he can point to 2−3 body parts
2 ½ yr	Phrase speech develops in 90% by 2½. Echolalia should be reducing now, and speech applied to more than indicating needs, i.e. social speech (p.144); naming animals.	Understands prepositions
4 yr	Most children use pronouns, *but*, *and*.	Follows 2 instructions in a single sentence
5 yr	Able to give complex explanations.	

Back-and-forth conversation

This means at least two utterances by each party, with ability to follow changes in the subject imposed by the other person. It is the most advanced common linguistic skill, not mastered by all employed adults. Just as continuing a friendship is more demanding than making a friend, having back-and-forth conversations requires much more than just the ability to convey information, or to ask a barrage of questions. Most of these skills are grouped as *pragmatics*, i.e. social aspects of language (See semantic pragmatic disorder, p.546; criteria for autism, p.388; connectivity syndromes, p.444.)

To elicit whether a child is interested in you (or people in general) and is able to follow a conversational lead, wait until he is relaxed or bored, and say: *I went on a really good holiday* / *I know a really good joke* / *I have a favourite colour. I've got a cat* works better than *I have two children* because they could have a cat too.

Basics
Listen (p.129) and understand reasonably quickly (p.27).
The compulsion to answer questions (even with a "don't know"). This is remarkably powerful – save in anger, severe depression, autism and catatonia.
Desire to make relevant and interesting comments (pp.151,166,152, 149). This requires being interested in the subject and/or person, and not being too tired / preoccupied / low in mood / fearful.
Wait for a reply without interrupting (pp.492, 79). After an appropriate amount of time, amplify appropriately.

Advanced or optional
Using non-verbal communication well (and understanding other's) including eye contact (p.175), smiles (p.549); anticipating, noticing, and responding to listener's boredom.
Maintaining the theme not only in the reply but in the conversation.
Be interested (p.229).
Be interesting (p.163) and use a personal communicative style (p.162).
Being *suitably* polite in interrupting, speaking and changing topic.
Code switching, i.e. fluently moving between the spoken and non-verbal aspects of Japanese, black American, gay voice, etc[905].
See also *thinking together*, p.170.

Semantics

This is the *meaning* of language. The ability to understand words and construct sentences is usually considered separately (see pp.27,149). Deeper aspects of meaning include:

- Knowing what is the main point of a sentence (failure can cause apparent jumps to other subjects during conversation).
- Understanding abstract words, e.g. about feelings or the word "vague".
- Understanding jokes and metaphors.
- Using context to distinguish homonyms such as "hear", "here".

Classification of speech and language difficulties

Aspect of communication	Related problems
• Receptive	
○ Hearing	Deafness (p.130)
○ Discrimination	Permanently impaired if deafness persists uncorrected until age 6.
○ Receptive language	(p.145)
• Expressive	
○ Speech	(p.147)
▪ Voice	(p.147)
▪ Articulation	(p.147)
▪ Fluency	(p.147)
▪ Prosody	(p.147)
○ Expressive language	(p.145)

Causelist 44: Language problems

These are difficulties in the translation between ideas and words. The term does not include deafness, p.130; dyslexia, p.51; thought disorder, p.563; speech (sound) problems, p.147; or word choice such as swearing, p.161.

Of children with language problems at age 5, 73% will still be impaired at age 19[781].

Classification of language problems		
	Receptive	**Expressive**
Phonology	The ability to discriminate sounds in speech is distinct from the ability to discriminate nonspeech sounds. Speech sound discrimination ability differs between people; and is related to their skill in acquiring either 1st or 2nd languages[407]. *Language* abilities can be permanently damaged by severe high-frequency hearing impairment that is not corrected by age 6 (although *sound discrimination* retains plasticity[356]).	
Lexicon	Verbal agnosia Damage to Wernicke's area.	Poor vocabulary Word-finding problem (p.149) Dysnomia Private symbols (neologisms) may be used, in autism or schizophrenia.
Syntax (includes conjugation, word order)	This can be measured with the Test for Reception of Grammar (TROG-2). Some of the children with familial Specific Language Impairment have greater difficulty with syntax than vocabulary[1649].	Mean Length of Utterance (MLU) is easy to measure[1336]. The Developmental Sentence Scoring system is more complex and has published percentiles by age[730,863].
Semantics	A. Disconnection in language disorders: see p.444 B. Categories of plant, animal, or inanimate artefact may be separately affected by discrete cortical lesions[253]. A previous concensus that nouns were represented in temporal lobes and verbs in frontal and parietal cortex may have been confounded by the lower imagability and greater complexity of verb tasks[151]. C. Categorisation problems can be tested with a list of objects, asking the child to match ones in the same category. **Causes:** Brain lesions are more studied than developmental conditions. Rarely, metabolic syndromes can cause this[1347]. The child's personal experience with specific domains of knowledge is crucial.	See *thought disorder*, p.563.
Pragmatics	(p.144)	(p.144)

Just as learning to move around often reduces a baby's crying, learning to communicate often reduces an older infant's frustration and violent outbursts.

Some genetic syndromes include language abilities being worse than non-verbal abilities (e.g. Down's, p.455). Rarely, genes can be identified underlying language disorders. About a hundred chromosome locations have been linked to specific language problems or to autism, and many of the locations influence *both* diagnoses[1503] (e.g. FOXP2 below).

In children with ID, failure to speak is often the first sign that the family notices. Many children are described by professionals as having "specific" language problems when in fact they have broader problems such as ID (in which case the non-verbal / performance IQ will be similarly low) or Autism (p.183). In less severe cases, isolated language problems (i.e. without other cognitive deficits) are often associated with articulation problems that lead to teasing (p.219), selective mutism (p.153), and other social difficulties (p.181). Delayed speech can often be unusual too ("deviant", p.49).

Language problems are associated with many diagnoses:

	Receptive	**Expressive**
Autism ☂	Deficit in recognising ungrammatical speech, especially in verb conjugations, and in sentences longer than 9 words[449]; and in understanding how prosody affects meaning[1242].	Sentences are less complex, and have more repetition. Highly idiosyncratic prosody (from monotone to camp, p.243; singsong, stilted or pedantic, p.163). Association with selective mutism, p.153.
Hyper-activity ☂	Becoming distracted in the middle of a sentence: seems not to understand longer sentences.	Becoming distracted in the middle of a sentence; looking off.
NVLD ☂ (p.28)	Good concrete understanding but difficulty with, e.g., similarities, differences, which of two things is bigger	Verbal/fantasy play (p.222)
ID ☂	Reduced vocabulary and complexity	Reduced vocabulary and complexity
Psychosis ☂		Thought disorder, p.563

See also: Word-finding difficulty, p.149; Pragmatics, p.144; NVLD affecting language, p.28. See also alexithymia, p.152 For *testing* of non-verbal children see p.516.

Language disorders caused by specific genes [619]
FOXP2: Causes impaired performance in most aspects of *speech* (it can be part of autism or of a more specific language disorder[1673]). The most specific deficits are in non-word repetitions (when unpractised sequences of oral movements have to be produced) and in orofacial dyspraxia[1664]. Test the first by saying a non-word, perhaps a few times, and asking the child to repeat it. Test the second by asking him to copy your facial expression, or to show how a named expression looks.

Speech is the effective use of meaningful *sounds* to form words and sentences. Of children with speech problems at age 5, 63% will still have some speech abnormality at age 19[781]. See also speech development and delay: p.143; speech regression, p.45; accents, p.417; selective mutism, p.153.

Speech problems and language problems can obviously coexist: Much light can be shed on the causes by having a written conversation, as well as a verbal conversation, with the child, and comparing the two.

Speech problems are categorised as follows:

A.   Voice impairments (dysphonia): 10% of all speech problems[781].
   - **Pitch**: There are organic and non-organic causes. Abnormally low pitch can be caused by laryngitis, or by poor technique in amateur singers.
        Puberphonia: Mutational falsetto is the psychogenic failure of a boy's voice to drop at puberty[994,1204] but lack of testosterone can cause a similar effect[18]. In girls, a "little girl voice" persists in Juvenile Resonance Disorder, also called juvenile voice. It is often overlooked but sometimes indicates anxiety, adjustment difficulties, or a tendency to histrionics.
   - **Nasal tone** (rhinolalia) is usually caused by a blocked nose, or occasionally by cleft palate, p.440.
   - **Hoarseness** can result from smoking, voice strain / vocal nodules, hypothyroidism, gastro-oesophageal reflux (GORD, p.472), vocal cord paralysis or disease, Parkinson's, myasthenia and other causes[139].
   - **Overall volume**. Being consistently loud is seen in hypomania and late-onset deafness. Consistent quiet is seen in depression. Situation-specific quiet is seen in shyness and fear and in partial selective mutism (p.153).

B.   Articulation impairments: 75% of all speech problems[781]. Lisps affect single sounds (such as *s* being replaced by *th*) and are common until age 5 (and in the "gay voice", p.243). Oromotor dyspraxia typically impairs rapid transitions from one sound to the next. There are many causes e.g. imprecision in deafness, p.130; perinatal cerebellar hemorrhage.

C.   Dysfluency (flow): See *stuttering*, p.157; *cluttering*, p.441. Together these account for 4% of all speech problems.

D.   Dysprosody:

Prosody is the melodic aspect of speech[1103], which is produced by a combination of personal behaviour and local language structure.

Aspects of prosody include:
- Variation in volume
- Variation in pitch. Lack of variation = monotone
- Variation in rhythm / tempo. Lack of variation = e.g. staccato voice, which has a sharp start to each word.

Prosody is used to communicate a lot of information, including (a) grammar, to denote questions and distinguish words (e.g. "**con**vict" or "con**vict**" to indicate noun or verb); (b) emphasis; and (c) feeling and relationships[1231].

Aspects of prosody often are affected together, being reduced (over-controlled voice, p.165; flattened voice, p.467) or exaggerated (hypomania, p.264; camp, p.243). Unusual prosody can can sometimes sound foreign (called pseudo-foreign language) [340]. Unusual prosody is common in autism[1231] and related conditions (see *accents*, p.417). Rare causes in children are dementia and lesions of cerebellum or neocortex.

Causelist 46: Word-finding difficulty

This is over-diagnosed, because it is easy and obvious; broader cognitive and emotional causes are less obvious and less acceptable to parents; full IQ tests are expensive; and occasionally because parents can be offered extra tuition for this "isolated difficulty which is holding your child back." In fact there are several underlying causes worth considering:

Causes of word-finding difficulty	Notes
Normal	Less-used words produce more word-finding errors, in all people, e.g. words about farmyards in city children; English words in Japanese-speaking children.
Broader cognitive problems	E.g. just a small part of ID, or a specific language deficit (p.145), or generally slow information processing.
With checking, i.e. slowed or self-detected errors	I.e. at least partially detected. Detection relies on the number of rules known, and the number of rules broken by a particular word.
Inattention, impulsivity (p.79)	People say "thingy" or "doobry" or the wrong word, usually with a similar sound or in the correct semantic category. Alternatively a word or phrase is dropped from a sentence just because the next part of the sentence is ready a little sooner. Increased when tired.
Finding the wrong word	Words found may be primed e.g. by a preoccupation.
	If the child is reciting the calendar months but gets some wrong, the specific rules broken indicate the severity (and perhaps the cause) of the problem. So if the word mispronounced that is a minor error; if it is something quite different from a month (e.g. a day of week) that's a big error; if a month is repeated that could be an STM difficulty (p.555) or failing to visualise the calendar; if several months are skipped it suggests she doesn't categorise them into seasons.
	A purer test would be an unpracticed sequence such as a list of animals, or family members.
Lack of speaking practice	If children are off school and parents don't interact, performance can temporarily worsen.
Avoidance (p.429)	E.g. reluctance to think about an unliked subject (test this by repeatedly moving between this subject and other ones).
A complete blank	
Not able to put a time limit on the search and say "don't know"	Performance anxiety (p.298) especially when confronted with questions. Obsessionality, or executive function problem
Hasn't learned special strategies for word-finding	E.g. to think about words that sound or look similar, or that would often be spoken together.
Without checking	
Epilepsy (p.73)	
Immaturity / ID	E.g. regular conjugations still overrule special cases.

Causelist 47: Not speaking much

This includes quantitative deficits such as few utterances, low volume, short sentences, and low spontaneity. For speaking much less in certain situations, see p.153.

Causes of not speaking	Diagnostic notes
Long-term problems coming to attention in preschool or primary school, usually broader than just communication	
☞ Deaf	The commonest cause (p.130)
☞ ID	Children, particularly girls, may say very little in order to avoid revealing their lack of understanding of the conversation. ID is also often associated with speech impediments that lead to teasing and hence selective mutism (p.153) [see 937].
Motor function	Cerebral palsy (p.437)
Abnormal language acquisition (p.49)	Poor eye contact and repetitive behaviours suggest autism or related disorder (p.183). Consider also pedantry (p.163), regression (p.41)
Delay of speech	E.g. familial speaking delay, bilingualism.
"Selective mutism grown up"	After fully selective mutism (p.153) has passed, more subtle underlying problems of language, cognition, socialisation and emotion become clearer.
☞ Damaged	Abuse of any kind (p.271)
Social deprivation	Deprived institutional upbringing (as in some orphanages) can produce the appearance of autism (p.183). If severe, this is a form of emotional abuse (p.277). However the tendency is for most such problems to reduce over time after placement with caring parents[1400,1654].
Dysarthria	I.e. orofacial dyspraxia (p.89)
Secondary organic causes after a period of normal speech	If speech returns to normal between episodes, consider migraine, p.141. See also regression, p.45; akinetic mutism, p.97.
Pervasive Refusal	(p.527)
Mute	Aphonia, e.g. from bilateral vocal cord pathology.
Recent onset, usually post-puberty	
Adolescent Truculence	Can look like depression, but distinguishable by how she acts with friends. More often looking sideways rather than downward. No is more common than yes, and sentences, if audible, are delivered sharply.
Depression	(p.309) See also psychomotor retardation, p.537. People lose confidence in speaking their secondary languages first.
Dissociation (p.453) (also called hysterical mutism)	This is a coping mechanism (p.445) that can be conscious to varying degrees. Its hallmarks as a cause of mutism are its pervasiveness (in all settings) and its sudden onset, as in a car crash or on receipt of awful news. Uncommon and usually short lived.
Pseudo-mutism[994]	Sudden onset; patient can cough but doesn't whisper
Obsessional slowness	(p.95)
☞ Psychosis (p.537)	In the early presentation of schizophrenia, catatonia (p.98) is much more common in teenagers than in adults, and can present as mutism. Low mood, distrust, or disinterest can reduce speech. Children are usually happy to discuss unusual experiences; so unwillingness to is sometimes a symptom of paranoia (p.524, though rare). Occasionally delusions can prevent speech, as in the young adult who wrote that "if I start speaking I'll never be able to stop".
Cerebellar cognitive affective syndrome	(p.437)

Causelist 48: Difficulty talking about feelings

Causes of difficulty talking about feelings	Notes
Limited vocabulary or immaturity	Boys' emotional vocabulary matures slower than girls'
Not difficult to name feelings, but unpleasant to think about them	This can also be described as a defence mechanism (p.303) but there are major deficiencies in research in this area[1660].
Embarrassment	Especially with opposite sex and/or strangers
Protecting others	
Boredom	(p.322)
Unengaged	
Disorganised thinking	As in thought disorder (p.563), or even delusional mood (p.544)
Alexithymia	This word has two main senses: a circumscribed inability to access one's own feelings; and difficulty talking about feelings (i.e. everything on this page). Both senses are inappropriate if verbal ability and educational attainment are insufficient for the feeling in question. Comprehensive cognitive testing should be considered to clarify this.
Dyslexithymia	Incorrect recognition or description of feelings. This term is repeatedly reinvented but has never entered common usage. For example, young people often describe themselves as bored, but what they actually mean is often quite different (p.322).
Having an odd (indescribable) feeling	Some feelings are extraordinary, and not everyone is a poet. Consider using wordlists, story stems, other people who feel similarly, or start by considering behaviours rather than feelings.

Causelist 49: Selectively reduced communication

This means communicating less in some situations than in others (for hardly speaking in any situation see p.151). It is a graded phenomenon, so a child may only speak when reading out loud; may always speak in a whisper to teachers; may be completely silent at school; or may become motionless when they feel any attention on them[871].

The following diagram shows that normal drives to communicate can be blocked by anxiety-related phenomena (an innate hypervigilant response to mild fear, p.296; avoidance, p.429; and habit, p.475). Less often, drives to communicate can be blocked by competing behaviours such as very attractive imaginary friends, or stereotypical interests such as trees around the school building. The two blocks can act together, as when a child who has been teased for misunderstanding peers resorts to imaginary friends.

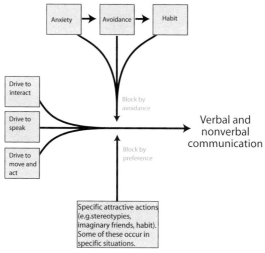

Figure 15. Blockage of drives in selective communication.

Selective mutism (SM): the commonest clinical picture
Among the behaviours that can be affected, selective *mutism* is conventionally singled out because of its obviousness and its social and developmental importance. The commonest forms are not speaking around any non-family adults, and not speaking in school.

The term *selective mutism* is a paradigmatic behavioural description in that it mentions both the trigger (stimuli present in selected situations) and the observable behaviour (mutism, i.e. refraining from speech). Like most behavioural descriptions, this guides therapy well but does not address the underlying causes – which may be much longer-term than the mutism.

Because mutism is common for several weeks in a new school, and rarely bothers peers, and tends to pass, cases often do not come to specialist attention for several terms, or even years. Eight weeks after school entry, 7 in 1000 children are not speaking[524]. By 6 months this has halved. Fewer than 2 in 1000 children remain mute for over a year[871].

SM is usually multifactorial. (a) It is seen characteristically in children with a tendency to anxiety[434], especially social anxiety (p.298); (b) the children often have some difficulty speaking (e.g. dysarthria or non-native speaker). (c) This is often combined with inflexibility[178] (p.234) or intolerance (p.546) or mild learning problems[871] or mild social impairments[871] (p.167). The onset was sometimes when the child was teased for a minor speech impediment or mistake.

The range of behaviours that can be reduced

Many behaviours other than speaking can be similarly affected, whether or not the children are mute. For example, 64% of selectively mute children stop activities when the teacher approaches (compare *behavioural inhibition*, p.296); 46% of them are unlikely to approach the teacher's table, 26% draw less than other children, and 11% of them avoid going to the toilet[224]. A rare few use imaginary worlds (p.231) or approximate answers (p.357).

Among all children (not just the selectively mute), children who know they need help are less likely to ask their teacher for it, under certain conditions. These include: if help-seeking is a rare behaviour in this class; if the teacher's responses are known to be unsupportive; if peers are bickering or insulting (rather than cooperative), and if the child himself is a low achiever[1405].

Children with autism-related conditions have a much wider range of behaviours that can interfere pervasively or selectively with communication (p.156). See also *non-behaviours*, p.515.

The range of selectivity (triggers for the avoidance)

The precise pattern is crucial for intervention planning. It is worth taking a careful history to see whether the mutism occurs just in the presence of non-family adults (the commonest pattern by far); or just men; in school, or in a particular teacher's class, or whether it is more with maths tasks or verbal tasks or just any difficult question. Rarely, a child becomes sensitised to peers' negative reactions so becomes mute with them; this is the opposite of the usual pattern so can wrongly lead to autism being suspected.

If a child's communication is much better or worse on rare occasions (as opposed to being consistently quiet), precise details of those occasions is useful. For example, a child spoke only single-word answers to mum or teachers, but said her first full sentence ("Can I go to the toilet") immediately after another child had said exactly the same thing: The child had severe language impairment and in this situation her speech was scaffolded by the other child.

Investigations

Assessment needs to include all the potential multifactorial causes listed at left, and in the table on the next page.

You should find a way of seeing him talking – this may need a home video, a home visit, or a two-way mirror. You also need to see a situation in which he hardly communicates. A school observation is often needed to see the manner in which he does not communicate at school, and any exceptions to this.

Assessment by a speech specialist, and cognitive assessment, are invaluable to identify any underlying reasons for his anxiety about communication (so they can be specifically remedied). If the pattern of the mutism is at all atypical, autism should be considered (see box on p.156).

continued ▶

Causes of selective communication	notes
Topic-related	
Difficulty in self-description	Poor self-esteem, lack of practice, and conceptual difficulties can all make it more difficult to answer personal questions than impersonal ones in a test.
Hiding a terrible secret	Rare, but perhaps more common if onset is after puberty.
Other	See *Speaking but not being open*, p.166.
Audience-related	
Shyness	(p.181)
Selective mutism	(p.153)
Variants of selective mutism	Many children are better behaved at school than at home. <ul><li>A mild version is a child who talks easily to friends but puts up his hand only in art class, because he's afraid of getting answers wrong in other classes (not of being looked at because that would affect art too).</li><li>An extreme version of this, which is rare, is a child with severe hyperactivity in most situations, who becomes so anxious at school that he is a model pupil there (p.207).</li></ul>
Selective taciturnity	Taciturnity means reduced speech, i.e. it is not as severe as full mutism. It is sometimes called partial mutism. <ul><li>If the child associates an aversive speaking experience with the school or with the presence of non-family, those will become the cues that reduce speech.</li><li>On the other hand, if the child has been teased for getting things wrong or saying "silly" things, he may become generally monosyllabic, or stop speaking in most settings. This can be so severe as to give the impression of depression or even autism (p.183).</li></ul>
Behavioural inhibition (p.296)	This is not just saying the child becomes anxious. One operational definition of behavioural inhibition includes "inhibition of play" in the presence of an unfamiliar adult or robot toy[310].

Conundrum 7: Selective mutism with autism

This combination needs to be considered in every child with SM. Each condition alters the appearance of the other.

Autistic spectrum disorders are defined as pervasive, meaning that they occur in all situations. Thus the truest measure of their severity is obtained in the situation where they are least severe. In children with SM, this is usually at home with no strangers present, which obviously means the assessment of the language and social impairments of ASD – especially in anxious children – often needs to be based largely on parental report or home video.

Selective mutism is, by definition, selective rather than pervasive. A child with ASD finds quite different things stressful from other children. For example, being laughed at for mispronouncing may be irrelevant to him, whereas he is frightened by eye contact with a stranger. Children with ASD therefore develop variants of SM, often with non-standard triggers and/or avoidance mechanisms. Variants of the *trigger* include social interaction in general (e.g. refusing to point or give despite being perfectly cooperative in moving around, putting on a coat, or making a jigsaw.) Variants of the avoidance include not making gestures; complete or partial dissociation (p.453); and obsessive slowness (p.95). Poor eye contact can be due to either condition (the selective trigger or ASD) or to other causes (p.175)

Causelist 50: Repetitive speech

Many of the causes of non-speech repetitions (p.63) affect speech too. But the causes of language repetitions are often more cognitive or social, as shown in this list.

Causes of repeated speech	Notes
Repeating oneself immediately to someone	
Wind-up	Often exaggerated, or sing-song, or with body language copied as well; but crucially monitoring the listener's reaction, usually by looking at his face.
Word-finding difficulty (p.149)	Or similarly, giving oneself time to think.
Stuttering (or stammering; see also p.157 and clutter, p.441)	As this list makes clear, not all repetitions are stutters: the term is only used if the trigger for the repetition is an intermittent difficulty with sound-production. Hesitating and repeating a sound in the middle of a word strongly supports its being a stutter.
	Many stutterers have not just repetitions of a syllable/sound, but also pauses ("blocks" which can be unfilled or filled with empty sounds such as *uh* or *like*) and elongated syllables (especially prolongations of fricative consonants).
	The severity of stuttering ranges from barely noticeable "normal dysfluency" to major communication impairment with increased muscle tension and occasionally whole-body movements. 15 difficulties per 100 words is usually considered a severe stutter. However, underlying factors such as pronunciation or word finding skills, acceptance of imperfection, the subjective feeling of loss of control during speech, and peer responses often have more influence on the level of impairment (see[634]).
	It may be that audible stuttering is a useful behaviour in overcoming (as yet unidentified) neural processing deficits involved in the initiation of syllables[1209]. As a demonstration that it is not primarily a symptom of anxiety, it does not increase in parallel with the post-pubertal increase in anxiety in girls; rather it usually starts in preschoolers, declines therafter, and is more common in boys[1646].
	Stuttering is somewhat more common in people with other speech difficulties. It can be worsened by stress, stimulants (p.476) and other medications. It can disappear during singing, talking to a non-judgmental audience (pets or younger children), or while drunk.
	There are many methods to overcome stuttering, e.g. avoidance, word or sound substitution, circumlocution, and finger snapping. Some of these obviously produce repetitions themselves.
Pseudo-stuttering	Pseudo-stutterers have no struggle behaviours or avoidance behaviours, their stutter is not relieved by singing, and they follow simple rules such as using similar repetitions on every word[994].
Palilalia	(p.62)

Saying the same thing several seconds or minutes apart

Persisting need	If an identifiable drive still exists, e.g. asking for treats, toilet, or reassurance, this is normal (a few times). It can be increased if a child wonders if he was heard, or doesn't have the skills to wait, rephrase, or emphasise, or doesn't understand that the parents' "no" or "I don't know" couldn't realistically have changed.
	On the other hand, if the phrase has no relevance to the listener, is it really being said to them?
Persisting interest (p.229)	E.g. hobby, special interest, preoccupation, rumination (p.543). More likely to annoy if child ignores or can't detect listener's boredom.
Expecting a reply	E.g. a child saying what he thinks might be important information and quite reasonably expecting a response.
Not understanding the conversation	• Misunderstanding parts of a question so using ideas from previous question. This can be voluntary, or based on normal unconscious semantic priming. • Persistence of ideas from one question to the next in a test can be because he doesn't know the rule that the questions are completely independent of each other (he can be thinking of it like a story). • An extreme version of this was seen in a girl with severe language impairment but great drive to participate in conversation. She carefully noted when the speaker came to the end of any sentence, then said sympathetically "He *is* a nasty man."
Weak phrase speech	• If an adult were repeatedly asking for chocolate cake, they would embed this in constantly varying sentences, to avoid seeming rude, and to aid the listener. The child who is only starting to put words together has only one phrase: "chocolate cake". • Losing the train of thought
Perseveration	(p.527)

Saying the same thing on successive days

Pat phrase	This means a standard phrase used with some communicative intent, but less meaningful than it appears. • Normal: "Good to see you", "Have a nice day." • Phrases that fill a wide variety of holes on conversation, usually to avoid revealing a lack of understanding, e.g. "Yes", "You know what I mean", "I know what you mean". • In a child with non-verbal learning disability, everything he remembers from long ago can be described as "in 2006" in otherwise appropriate sentences, with no idea of what the year means or that it is wrong.
Repetitive verbal play	Roleplay ("I am not a number!"); singing/chanting of normal complexity
Stereotyped *reply*	This can have many causes in the same child at different times. E.g. "what?" can be used if any of the elements of conversation have failed (p.144). The reply "what" is reinforced (p.540) by not being told off for ignoring people; bolstering STM (p.555) and attention; and giving time to think of a reply. It then becomes a habit.

continued ▶

Delayed echolalia	Some clinicians use this term if a child uses a phrase learned long ago to answer a current question [e.g. 1283]. It is not the ideal usage because unlike most echoes (described below), it is slow and has some meaning.
Stereotypies (p.553)	Uttered with minimal regard for context, e.g. "bit of a shock" from a teenager with profound ID
Identification/ coping mechanism	Saying something a cool character says, to be like them or to avoid feeling inadequate. (pp.445,487)
Tics	See vocal tics, p.102. If he is trying to make a precise number of repetitions, consider also OCD, p.65.
Obsession (p.517)	Is he afraid of what will happen if he doesn't say it?

Repeating someone else immediately

Habit, mulling over	Especially the ends of questions, to help in thinking about an answer
To aid short-term memory	
Agreeing	"He *does* look funny" with or without the emphasis.
Echolalia	This means repeating other people's sounds without consideration of their meaning, without reversing pronouns, etc., and often with the same intonation (The irrelevance of meaning is also found in babble, p.429, but normal babble is internally driven and more varied.) It can be repeated many times if the person is fascinated by the sound. It is common until age 3 ½, and also in autism (p.183) and ID; also a rare form of catatonia (p.98).
	In practice, if echolalia is significant, it appears without any special effort from the interviewer, because the child becomes interested in particular sounds from the conversation, regardless of whether or not they involve him. "Say hello Tom", "how did you do it?" and "you tripped!" can sometimes elicit the non-reversibility of echolalia, but "Thank you" can't, and "Do you want ice cream?" can't, because "ice cream" is a sensible answer to this. Ask "are you happy?" then if the child replies "happy", ask "are you sad?" to see if he just echoed the last word.
	A child with severe NVLD (p.28) echoed an entire conversation between parents, demonstrating his great interest in the words and the interaction but no understanding of the underlying meaning.
	Phrases repeated more than 30 seconds later are sometimes called delayed echolalia (see above), or just repeated phrases. A variant of this is phrases repeated from a much-loved DVD, which are recreated from memory. If the echo occurs only with accented speech or complex ideas, it is best called not echolalia, but copying, cultural, mulling over, etc. (see *Acting*, p.418). If the child knows he is copying and that this has a special social significance, it should be called mocking or mimicry (p.507).
	Even when a person's only speech is echolalia, you can sometimes work out which words he agrees with more, by his sitting up, making more eye contact, smiling, and repeating the word more times. Pictures aid communication even more (see *Makaton*, p.502).

Mitigated echolalia (also *modified* echolalia)	Phrases with a word changed or added that makes them more communicative. The commonest form is the simplest: echoing a phrase then adding *yes* or *no*.
Fun	Often exaggerated, sing-song. See *Wind-up* above.
To third person	Repeating to emphasise what someone else just said to a third person (e.g. the teacher to the class). Perhaps to identify with, or to try out the same interaction, or to mock.

Causelist 51: Swearing and other rudeness

See also causes of *not doing as he is told*, p.253; *adopting a new persona*, p.237; *anger*, p.287; *aggressive behaviour*, p.289, *argumentativeness*, p.162.

Causes of swearing and other rudeness	Notes
Normal	Normal swearing may be repetitive and done in private, but unlike tics (p.101) there is always a reason.
Subcultural / habit	Swear-words are normal vocabulary in some families and peer groups.
Angry / aggressive (p.289)	He swears *at* people.
Immaturity and attention-seeking	• Repetitive swearing can appear in babble (p.429), i.e. without meaning. Later, swearing can be used in ignorance either of the meaning or the negative impact. • When children, especially boys, are just learning all the aspects of a word's use, excitement may cause clumsy use of the word (e.g. "Hello Butthead!" to a parent to get attention, in either a friendly or aggressive way). Later usage tends to be more precise, even when the intention is merely to obtain attention.
To sound grown-up or tough	May increase when he is asked a question he doesn't know, and reduce when he is not with people he needs to impress.
To reduce pain	Swearing significantly reduces perceived pain[1543].
⬭ Depressed	He swears at himself or at other people.
To shock	
Social communication deficit	He may swear in inappropriate (e.g. happy or non-emotive) contexts, for example waving and smiling while saying "bye bye… ***now Fuck Off!***"
Coprolalia in Tourette (p.101)	Rare. He often mutters it quietly so people don't hear, or says sorry afterwards. Vocal tics (such as swear words) can appear in the middle of a sentence without disrupting the flow of the sentence. When swear tics appear in the middle of a sentence, they are not placed, emphasised, and conjugated as normal swear words would be. Copropraxia is making rude gestures.
⬭ Psychosis (p.537)	Is he swearing at the hallucination (p.351), or being told to swear by the hallucination?
⬭ Obsessionality	Is he swearing the right number of times, or swearing to try to de-activate a compulsion? (p.65)
Hypomania or mania (p.261)	Faster than normal, and sometimes more imaginative. Often directed at other people.
ID	Not having learned politeness, e.g. scratches in public.

Causelist 52: Contradicting and quibbling

Styles of interaction
In groups, a person may adopt a role, such as leader, producer of ideas, encourager, checker, sceptic, spectator, timekeeper, etc. His interactional style will vary with role and mood. Aspects of style include volume, pace, pauses, questions, persistence (and variation of repetitions),acknowledging what people say or feel, letting other people speak, degree of friendliness, enthusiasm and humour, frequency of interrupting (to agree or disagree), interruptibility (see p.144), use of indirectness and assertiveness (below).

A. Argumentativeness
This means a tendency to start or amplify verbal disagreements (arguments). This is often a complaint by parents of teenagers. **Contradictions** are the simplest form of arguing, and usually fairly mild. When arguments are about a personal topic, or when an argument on a public topic becomes personalised, it raises the temperature. The impression of argumentativeness can be obtained if a speaker's style includes lots of interrupting (as is common in teenage girls even with their friends[126]).

B. Assertiveness and considerateness
Young people speak to their parents in an assertive way; both mothers and fathers talk to their daughters more assertively than to their sons [1474].Fathers talk more assertively than mothers, working class parents more than middle class. "High considerateness" speech[1584] is slow, with slow turn taking, longer pauses between turns, avoidance of simultaneous speech.

Causes of contradicting	Notes
Not really contradicting	
Stylistic	(See conversational styles, above)
Not caring what parents think	Included here to point out that it is not plausible: if it were true the child would save their breath.
Contradictions with aggressive feelings	
Verbal expression of aggression	This usually involves milder feelings or better self-control than physical violence (p.289). Irritability (p.494) is a common cause and may indicate mood problems or sleepiness. Signs include ignoring, sneering, scowling, spitting out words, swearing (p.161) or oversimplifying speech, as in: • mocking people's names, origins, odour, etc. • mocking ideas: "I have no *issues, issues* are for dorks."
Confidently picking a fight	In male competition, especially when drunk: "Who you looking at?"
Fear	Argumentativeness is sometimes confined to a single topic of great importance to a child. If long practised it can be very fluent, e.g. in anorexia or needle phobia.
Oppositionality	Would argue on either side (see p.253).
Lack of conver-sational skill	Unable to keep one's own feelings under control, or to de-escalate a conversation.
Querulousness	Escalation of complaints based on belief in rules, being destined for greatness, and wanting retribution[1123].
Contradictions with few aggressive feelings	
Rewarded	Combative repartee (as well as contradiction, wordplay, and pedantry) are rewarded behaviours in some cultures and families. It is then usually accompanied by positive affect.
Lack of politeness	This can be impulsive, ID, autism; or when a person feels so confident in a relationship or group that self-monitoring is reduced. Social warmth distinguishes this from rudeness due to dislike of a particular person.
NVLD	(p.28)
Overexact	In pedantry (p.163) and in people who tic. Valuing precision over conventionality or people's feelings. A degree of showing off is normal (p.548).

Causelist 53: Pedantry

Pedantry has pragmatic, semantic, syntactic, and phonetic aspects.
Pedantry can even be quantified[558] based on:
- Conveying more information than the topic and goals of the conversation demand
- Violating expectations of relevancy and quantity
- Similarity to written language in formal sentence structure and erudite vocabulary
- Conversational turns that resemble rehearsed monologues rather than contributions to a jointly managed dialogue
- Articulation that may be precise and intonation formal.

Many children have not realised that the standard reply is just one or two sentences, and that there are standard cues to exceed this.

Causes of pedantry	Notes
Not actually pedantic	
Simply speaking more	(People who speak little wouldn't be called detailed, & rarely pedantic)
Stretching out the answer	Trying to stay on a topic he knows something about.
Stuttering / cluttering	(pp.157, 441.)
Excess detail or checking: can be increased if the audience or the listener's expected reaction make the speaker anxious.	
Perfectionism	Needing to get sentence just right so repeatedly correcting oneself or improving the sentence. Many children with Tourette syndrome have a great love of exactness that can give the impression of Asperger's (p.424), but their precision when describing their special interest is not matched by prolonged focus on it, nor by depth of specialist knowledge.
Unable to simplify or to see the overall picture	E.g. anxious, language deficits (p.145), or NVLD (p.28). People with autism often focus on details rather than the overview (see also pp.36,442). For a beautiful description of the inability to see the whole picture, in an adult thought to have a brain tumour, see[1413].
Trying to impress	Some children learn a few obscure facts because their friends do; or because they know they're not as bright as peers or siblings and are trying to conceal this. This is different from having a real special interest (p.229) because the child doesn't spend much time studying the topic; the topics are chosen to impress; and the child reveals his most impressive knowledge early in conversation.
Love of detail	The child explores or ruminates on the subject - detailed expositions by savants are rare examples (for description and associated characteristics see[1410]).
Uninterested in simplifying	Self-centred. Not reading others' body language, checking or anticipating.
Thinking the other person will be interested in the detail	E.g. in hypomania (p.261), assuming the topic is so exciting the listener is bound to be interested

Patronising	Explaining slowly or in excess detail. Appropriate if properly matched to listener's ability, otherwise can be calibrated to achieve a particular level of insult.
Over-complicated	Overestimating listener's interest or knowledge
Unusual learned manners	
Reading more than she speaks	…so using the formality characteristic of written language.
Exposed to precise adults	Intellectual parents can teach a child to speak pedantically, giving the impression of social communication difficulties.
Reinforced (p.540)	
Copied	(From society or from hero, e.g. father, teacher, rabbi). Pedantry is only one of the conversational styles that can be learned in this way: see p.162
Academic	Having been praised for pedantry in a particular area (computer game hacks,law, many academics, either just in their area or generally). *"The term, then, is obviously a relative one: my pedantry is your scholarship, his reasonable accuracy, her irreducible minimum of education and someone else's ignorance."* [514] [so pedantry may reflect interest, exposure, or a terrific memory].
Shaggy dog story / wind up	
Monotonous	
Depression	(Other signs of depression are needed; some are listed on p.309)
Autism 🌂	(p.183)
Lack of variety	E.g. of injecting emotion, differing sentence structures, multiple levels of explanation – may reflect immaturity or poor education.
Preoccupied	
Depressed or worried	

Causelist 54: Over-controlled voice

People's voices can be over-controlled voluntarily for up to an hour, or for months during persisting anxiety, or permanently. As with other acts (see pseudo-behaviours, p.363), inconsistencies usually appear, such as a mismatch between the tone and the content.

Among children the most common causes are autism and anxiety. It is also heard in parents, and then is important in understanding them. Voices can be over-controlled in several ways (icy or seductive, clipped, soft, gentle) that are slow with reduced speech modulation but are easily distinguished from the flat slow voice of depression and the idiosyncratic voices of autism.

Causes of over-controlled voice	Notes
Severe anxiety	Sometimes with reduced movement of the mouth during speech.
Hiding anger	• Immediate • Long term: passive-aggressive (p.525)
Theatrical training, voice lessons Copying someone, specific courses, e.g. counselling / psychotherapy. Teaching	
Specific unusual voices	
Autism ☂ (p.183), Asperger's (p.424)	Many variants, e.g. little professor, or sounding camp (p.243) or American.
Psychogenic dysphonia	• Some children become stuck with a childlike-voice after puberty (see *puberphonia*, p.147). • This can also be a sign of pseudo-regression following stress.
Speaking fast	• Afraid people will get bored • Afraid she will forget what she wants to say in the middle of the sentence (occurs more with long sentences) • On stimulants • hyperthymia (p.264)
Detached, or less involved in the emotionality of the situation than the listener expects	Teenagers can be temporarily detached if they are: • bored • annoyed at having to repeat themselves or • are showing their disdain of the listener.

Causelist 55: Speaking but not being open

This problem often arises in talking to a child who does not want to talk to you. If you can pin down the cause and overcome it, this may suggest useful therapeutic strategies. (See also *confidential information*, p.413.)

It is just as important to get to the bottom of this in parents, who may not want to reveal the whole history because they are paranoid (p.524), or because the details of the child's background are very painful to them, or because they think previous professionals have "misinterpreted" something they said – or simply because they don't trust professional confidentiality.

Causes of speaking but not being open	Notes
Just in the session	
Not interested in what you're talking about	If pervasive, consider immaturity or autism (p.183). If in interview, find out from parents what he is interested in.
Dislikes interview	If in psychotherapy→ consider changing to non-verbal interaction (e.g. drawing, play)
Tense	This can often be overcome by talking while walking (stairs can be even better) or in a coffee shop.
Afraid his peers will see	Go somewhere else.
Something about you	If he has difficulty talking to an old person, or a non-Muslim, or an attractive young woman: Can you transfer him to another staff member?
Distrust of interpreter	Rare, but important in small communities or if the interpreter reminds her of someone else. See p.492.
Lack of rapport	E.g. feeling you are uninterested or don't respect him (see p.11)
Fear that parents will find out	Tell him that your conversations are private, and that you will tell no one except colleagues, unless someone's safety is involved.
He thinks the camera is on	Tell him it isn't.
Difficulty hearing or understanding you	This can be hidden, as some children have learned that people get annoyed if they are asked to repeat themselves. Some of their answers may seem irrelevant. You may need to make a special effort to use sentences without subordinate clauses. Consider getting an interpreter (p.492). Consider deafness (p.130) or referral to audiology for possible Central Auditory Processing Deficit (p.121)
General	
Something else on his mind	Try to find out what it is. Try to say something that will sound like what he is thinking, so he feels you are on the same wavelength. He may just be very cross, or angry at the person he's talking to.
Shyness	(p.181)
Slow to warm up	Suspect this if the child becomes more conversational later in the session.
Perseveration (p.527)	Distinguishable from obsessions (p.517) and overriding interests, by the content being short-term, and not anxiety related.
Social communication problems	The cause can be a lack of skill in initiating conversations; a lack of interest in feelings; or lack of experience in talking about them. All these are more common in boys[578].

Social ☼

A child is called *social* if he interacts with others in a non-violent (neutral or helpful) way, or wants to do that. Perhaps the most pure social act is a meeting of minds, but the term is usually used much more broadly than that, to mean anything that two or more people do together.

Social drives (innate or situational) and social skills (often learned) are treated separately below. For social milestones see p.55.

Social drives

There are many social drives (see list on p.168). Some of these are probably independent and have separate anatomical locations. They operate in concert with the non-social drives listed on p.124. For example, the comfort obtained by being near an attachment figure (p.195, a social drive) is balanced against the drive to explore (a non-social drive, p.124).

Pseudo-social behaviours (Social behaviours for selfish reasons)
When assessing a child's sociability (i.e. his social drives and social skills) one should not be misled by non-social drives that force the child to interact with people. Such interactions can be called *pseudo-social* (the *pseudo* does not imply that it is intentional).

The old paradox that no one is social – because people are only social for selfish reasons (see altruism, p.420) – does not generally cause clinical confusion. This is because if children *act* social then they and their classmates obtain the benefits of that.

However the two viewpoints (internal and external) both have to be considered in order to understand unusual children. Some of the reasons for people to be social include:

- A child who *shares* (p.179) may do it to be smiled at immediately, or to earn occasional reinforcers from parents, or to feel more like dad, or to care for others. Or all of these.
- A child may put his arms up to be lifted for reasons defined as *social*, (see list on p.168) such as wanting to talk, or feeling loved there – or for reasons not conventionally thought of as social (see list on p.124), such as wanting to flee a dog, or because he likes being high up. Putting arms up to prevent a sibling from getting attention may seem social, but most people would not call it social in cases where it was done purely to preserve a parent's slave-like readiness to fill a child's demands.
- A child can play catch but be primarily interested in the other person as a ball-throwing machine.
- Eye contact can be made or not made for very many reasons (p.176).
- Pseudo-social behaviours are very common in autism. A child can spread the awareness that he is hungry by banging on the fridge or taking an adult's hand there, without being aware of the other person's social nature at all. Related signs include treating parents the same as other adults, taking a ball from a person just as if taking it from the shelf, and being interested in parts of people (such as earlobes and hair, p.225).

Social drives (i.e. drives conventionally thought of as social)	Examples
Social interaction	Interacting with people (p.173) talking, touching, moving near. This may be stronger in Down's,p.455. *Indirect examples*: imaginary friends (p.231), TV / games
	Loneliness (p.500) is the feeling that this drive is unsatisfied.
Cuddles, warmth (p.574), softness [653]	Touching pets or people (p.173) Masturbation (p.115) Going to bed.
"Being with"	Usually this is used as a loose umbrella term. For example a child who is described as *liking to be with* other people may be so because he is frightened or bored when away from them.
	However it seems likely that most people have a separate desire to be with others. This desire is usually overshadowed by the other drives in this list. It becomes clearer in certain situations, such as the common desire to sleep near other people or animals, and the uncommon situation of an uncommunicative autistic boy who dived in to the sea to be with the tuna swimming next to the boat. By contrast, in illness and depression many people isolate themselves.
Getting attention	Done when other people are around; often looking to check their reaction
Interest in organisms	E.g. visual interest in biological movement[855]. (compare aspects of *object permanence*, p.517.)
Sexual	Sex (p.267), masturbation (p.115) sexual disinhibition, e.g. in intoxication, p.566; sexual orientation, p.481 *Indirect examples*: fetishes, voyeurism (p.267)
Competition (lots of kids, increased by testosterone, p.554)	Sports, fighting *Indirect example*: Writing for publication
To be like someone particular	E.g. spontaneous imitation. Many children do things to feel more like same-sex parent or teacher
To copy or conform	Infectious behaviour (p.490). See also crowd behaviour, p.447
To be liked by people	(or by a specific person). When his work is praised, does he do more, grin, and seek your attention?
Self-esteem (as in the genesis of conduct disorder ☂ p.249)	People usually judge their success relative to other people.
Sharing & altruism	(pp.179,420)
Parenting or caring for	Being a parent; being with your child (see p.189 for duties of parenting) *Indirect examples*: Having a pet; being a teacher/carer
Desire to be looked after	An example is pseudo-regression (p.41). Another aspect of the sick role is the limiting of demands on oneself. *Indirect example*: Munchausen, p.362

continued ▶

Social skills

There are many aspects of social development, and assessing them all in detail is impractical. However, assessing the *areas of current disability* and/or the *presenting problems* is perfectly practicable, and leads naturally to the provision of targeted assistance.

Social skills	Notes
Early skills, first used with mother	
Eye contact	p.175
Facial expressions	See *Facial expressions (using and understanding)*, p.464.
Meeting needs	The following scheme of development is after[154].

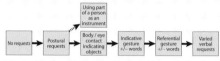

Figure 16. Development of requesting.

	At stage 3 in figure: Children are more likely to use a person as an instrument if communication is difficult (see deviation, p.49.)
Body language	Putting arms up when about to be lifted (p.167); moulding body to the adult who lifted him.
Seeking sympathy	This requires: • ability to detect problem • know who will be interested in it • know how to get help from them. A child may learn that her parents cannot do anything for the pain of severe constipation, so she curls up in a ball; and they will not do anything to soothe her when she has just been told off; whereas for a cut she might go to them immediately. • appreciation of sympathy (or other rewards)
Name	Alerting and responding when one's name is spoken.
Pragmatics	(p.144)
Expressing sympathy (comforting)	This requires: • ability to detect problem • Ability to feel pain oneself, to empathise (p.546), and to bear the feeling without being overwhelmed (autistic, anxious, or closely attached children may not be able to bear it so many turn away.) • interest (or learned rewards) • ability to communicate
Role-play	(p.222)
Security-seeking	Stranger anxiety, and attachment behaviour, p.195
Later skills. Many are developed in play, p.221	
Social rules	There are many (p.261). With maturation, these are learned, given appropriately varying values, and applied to subtlely different situations.
Equal relationships with peers	Requires most of the other elements in this table, plus: • peers who are suitable and available (e.g. arrival in school before cliques formed) • not being too anxious (p.295) • being unstigmatised and physically acceptable (e.g. clean, pp.340–342) and not frightening others, pp.286–289.
Cooperating	The key elements are: • being flexible (p.234); • paying attention and being predictable (p.79). Cooperation on your own task is easier than on others'. This is analogous to conversing on your own chosen topic.
Sharing	(p.179)
Thinking together	• A child can give information to build his self-esteem, or because he likes the topic or the sound of his voice. He can also request information for his own use or to test how much you know. There is no joining of minds.

- A far more social process is to *think about something together*. This requires not just the mechanical capacity for back-and-forth conversation (p.144) but also:

a) interest in what the other person thinks. Without this the child will not stay and pay attention. This is only likely to happen if the conversers have standard interests (p.229) or have somehow found a shared rare interest.

b) interest in the other *person*, with some social warmth and/or diplomacy. Without these, conversation may produce memory-dumps, debate, or intellectual sparring, but only intellectuals will be interested in joining in.

c) the child must have some flexibility (p.234) in what he believes or is willing to think about. Signs of rigidity are conversations repeatedly returning to favoured topics; the conversants never converging to agreement; parallel conversations about personal interests; quoting a favourite idea despite it having been said or refuted before; and using a favourite idea despite the other person having disagreed.

d) ability to monitor the other person's interest. This can be done verbally, but is more fluent if non-verbal. Behavioural signs include showing a found piece of glass to mother, pointing to a helicopter or from a train window, with **gaze monitoring,** i.e. checking that mother looks too, implying an interest in what people are looking at. Does the child follow someone else's pointing (easy) or head movement (harder) or movement of just the eyes (hardest)? Does he initiate *joint attention* himself, using pointing, other gesture, words or other vocalisation, or eye contact?

   - **Gaze referencing** – means working out what a person is talking about by checking what he is looking at (cf. multiple causes of difficulties with this, p.175).
   - Note that pointing on request, or pointing to indicate interest (**protodeclarative pointing**), or to demand something (**protoimperative pointing**) are communications but not sharing (p.179). (*Past pointing* is inaccuracy in pointing, indicating cerebellar disease, p.437.)

e) persistence. Changing the topic rapidly will put off conversational partners.

Responding to other people's feelings	The conventionality of a child's response does not itself indicate the level of his empathy (p.546) or understanding. Other factors need to be considered. *Congruent responses* To some extent, most school-age children are affected by the misery or elation of people around them (e.g. becoming happy or excited or laughing when people around them are, as in a party – see *infectious behaviour*, p.505). This is not always a sign of empathy or of identifying with the other person: some autistic children selectively echo laughter while keeping their back turned. Or a child may become depressed after his mother does, simply because she doesn't feed or entertain him as well as she used to. *Incongruous responses* Some children laugh when others are hurt. This gives the impression they are revelling in the other's pain (psychopathy,p.280) or have no comprehension of it (autism, p.183). Much more often they (a) feel very uncomfortable about not knowing what to do; (b) are trying to cheer up the other child quickly; or (c) are trying to persuade grown-ups that the crying boy is joking, and that the wallop on his head was a joke too.
Showing of achievements	E.g. showing mother his drawing. This is sometimes called sharing (p.179), but it is usually done for self-centred reasons, rather than to make mum feel better!
Back-and-forth conversation	Elements of this are listed on p.144. An early stage is running commentary during parallel play (p.222)
Joking	(p.495)

Peer relationships

This term usually means relationships with children in the same school year, but relationships with children in a slightly older or younger class are similar. Unusual children may have no suitable peers in their school (see pp.489, 181).

Children's peers quickly detect whether a child is behaving normally or not. On the positive side, they will often "mother" a child who clearly depends on them, and ignore odd movements by a child who is otherwise friendly. On the other hand, they mercilessly tease other children as "stupid" or "uncool" (p.219). This means that the number and type of a child's peer relationships is a good indicator of his general development and wellbeing.

The discussion below includes friends, peer status, and pair friction. For other peer issues, see sexual partners, p.548; gangs, p.472; bullying, p.219; effects of home schooling, p.215; sociograms, p.550.

Friends

Friendships are reciprocal enjoyed relationships. They are important in several ways: learning social skills; maintaining one's positive self-image; feeling personally secure; feeling the friend's loyalty will continue; sharing private thoughts safely and learning the friend's viewpoint; being helped and shared with (i.e. it is a *communal* rather than an *exchange* relationship); making play more varied, complex, exploratory, and *fun*.[66]

Friendships can be bidirectional, unidirectional (unrequited), or form part of a small *clique* of friends. Friendships tend to last longer if the friends share many characteristics and are not rivals. Children increase their number of friends during a school year, but larger friendship networks tend to be less stable. Children in primary school keep about half of their close friends for more than a year, and this proportion increases in adolescence. Adolescents make cross-sex friendships that are initially brief and non-sexual, but gradually increase in duration and intensity[1274].

Taking a friendship history has some pitfalls. If the child lists many "best friends", does he know what that means? If he says he has no friends, is this just a reflection of misery or has he recently moved to a new school? If he describes a reasonable number of close friends, are his relationships with them positive and equal, or is he a bully describing his gang, is he mothered by them, or are they just people his mother invites round to the house? Do they ever chat or do they just play video games/football? Does he have the confidence to make social advances? What networking does he do via texts/MSN/Facebook?

There are very many causes of difficulties with friendships, see p.181.

Choice of friends
A child's choice of friends influences his self-identity, and vice versa (for examples, see pp.237–240)

- Liking *younger* friends can result from not making friends in one's own age group (which has many causes, p.181). It can develop into an active preference if the child likes to teach or mother the younger ones.
- Liking *older* friends can result from Asperger's (p.424), bookishness, shared interests (e.g. membership of clubs), or being introduced by older siblings.

Hanging out with the wrong crowd usually indicates an inability to obtain positive feedback from teachers, parents, or conventional peers (p.240). Sometimes less able children are recruited by more able teenagers as assistants (e.g. for drug deliveries).

Status among peers

Status is determined by the value (importance and attractiveness) placed by others on aspects of identity (p.237). Three changeable, inter-related and sought-after aspects of status are described here:

A. Social dominance (sometimes misleadingly called popularity). Often teens who achieve this are seen by their peers as aggressive or stuck up. In order to maintain their status, they often develop skills of social influence (including social bullying, p.219) that result in their being disliked[482].

B. Being liked. This requires being seen as kind and trustworthy.

C. "Cool" means how people wish they were[1360]. In young people's views, confidence is invariably necessary for "cool"; attractiveness and popularity usually are; but other aspects of "cool" are clearly different from society's or parents' views. Examples include age-specific choice of clothing; and children feeling that some types of aggression by their peers are cool (p.219). What is cool also differs between subgroups, with aggressive children finding aggressive peers cool, and non-aggressive children finding non-aggressive peers cool. It varies between ethnic groups, with most black American boys placing very little value on academic achievement[601].

In schools, typically one-third of pupils are seen as "cool", 10% are wannabes on the edge of the cool group, 10% are loners or pariahs, and the remainder form into small cliques (groups) that are not so concerned with coolness[482]. Each of these cliques typically has members with shared characteristics, and a leader who sets the clique boundaries and opinions.

Low mood reduces status, and low status reduces mood, forming a vicious cycle[1608]. Conversely, children who defend a victim of bullying obtain high status through all three mechanisms A, B and C above (see[1421]).

See also: role of status in bullying, p.219; in love of horses, p.248; as a cause of stealing, p.250; or of inter-male aggression, p.291.

Pair friction and antipathy

Friction between two specific peers can be momentary or enduring. It is distinct from bullying, p.219 or from irritability, p.494, or general lack of friends, p.181. When severe it can escalate to anger (p.287) or the longer-term state of hatred (p.187). All these are more likely when there are:

- conflicting goals, e.g. a struggle for status or a particular friend
- simple differences of opinion
- peers spreading rumours
- envy
- extended time together (one reason why sleepovers are usually limited to one night)
- irritating habits or appearance that remind of someone else
- a clash of styles (hyperactive v underactive; intuitive v logical; cautious v adventurous; introvert v extravert; loud v quiet; idea-generators v checkers) – especially when working together against the clock, with role-boundary confusion and lacking skills of negotiation/organisation.

Causelist 56: Oversociability

This means excessive desire to interact with people, or lack of usual limits to social interactions. Do not confuse this with a hyperactive child interrupting or bumping into everyone (p.79); or a severely autistic child interested in the hair of everyone he sees (p.225).

It is essential to find out whether oversociability is life-long, or had a specific onset; and to judge whether his overall drive for sociability is excessive, or whether it is displaced from one place to a place where it is more problematic (e.g. in public or with different people), or whether it is simply expressed in an unusual way. A diary, old family videos, and trial interventions will clarify the reasons for this.

For sexualised behaviour see p.269. For other types of disinhibition see p.261.

Conundrum 8: Touching staff

If a child intentionally touches a staff member during an assessment:

- If running past with attention elsewhere → consider hyperactivity and impulsivity, p.79
- If tapping you to get your attention in a slightly disinhibited way → consider hyperactivity and impulsivity, p.79
- If interrupting and speaking loudly straight to your face → consider hypomania, p.264.
- If violent → likely to be fear, or autistic love of slap-noises, or a child with profound ID who knows no way to get a response other than hitting
- If peripheral, e.g. prolonged interest in socks/hair/part of your clothes → consider the monotropism of autism, p.183
- If leaning on you → see next page
- If sitting on lap → see p.173; or ID who thinks he should treat you like grandma
- If overtly sexual → consider how common is the specific behaviour (table on p.267); consider causes on p.269 including sexual abuse, p.275

For other causes of touching, see p.132.

Causes of oversociability	Notes
With anyone (i.e. indiscriminate)	
Learned	E.g. from behaviour in small villages or army barracks where the concept of family becomes broader
Autism ☂ (p.183)	E.g. a mildly autistic child intrigued by social interactions but repeatedly getting it wrong in characteristic ways such as repetitiveness, awkward or incongruent facial expressions. Contact can be avoided, or conversely the child may lean on others (shoulders, legs, feet) as if they are objects.
Hyperactivity or impulsivity	Look for boredom (p.322), fleeting touches, chaotic behaviour (pp.79, 84)
Hypomania	Look for loud intrusiveness, social non-selectivity, sexual content, and other signs (p.261)
Poor self-entertainment	(p.545)
Mental age under 18 mos	(Attachment behaviours are greatest from age 18 mos to 3 years: p.195).
Lack of anxiety	(pp.423,81)
Smith-Magenis syndrome	(p.550)
Williams syndrome	(p.177)
Mainly mother figures	
Maternal depression	*Causes of this*: Lack of help, several young children, chronic sleep deprivation, behavioural problems in child, poverty (p.533), single parenthood (p.213), parental discord (p.191) or discord with in-laws, lack of a close friend, adverse life events (p.499), family history of depression, chronic illness in child or mother, feelings of guilt (p.475); mother having a history of adversity in childhood or adolescence; and in the post-partum period, delivering a daughter despite wanting a son[223,282,536]. Some of these factors affect the child directly, as well as via maternal depression[330]. Note that having a baby with disabilities does not generally make mothers depressed in the first year of life[900]: the effect tends to start later. *Effects of this*: Perinatal depression delays the infant's maturation a little. Part of this effect is due to worse nutrition[76]. Later onset of severe maternal depression can have a profound effect on the child who will notice the change and may blame himself. Imaginary friends may increase (p.231) and the child seeks not just attention but physical contact with mother figures.
Out-competed by siblings	Mother's parenting style may be adjusted to her depression/fatigue, or simply become primarily responsive rather than proactive due to enormous demands from other children. A child can then be left out if he is less energetic (for physical or emotional reasons, p.323).
Maternal loss	

Causelist 57: Odd eye contact

Normal eye contact is not constant or predictable. Like facial expressions, it reacts quickly to what is seen or heard.

- During a conversation, eye contact is held 30–60% of the time. The lower figure applies to opposite sex strangers less than a metre apart; the higher figure to same-sex strangers 2 metres away[56].
- It often moves from one eye to the other.
- Each time a speaker starts, he usually "checks in" with the listener by locking eye contact for 1–2 seconds.

Eye contact can be absent or very brief in *social referencing* when the child glances at familiar people to work out what his own reaction should be in a new or ambiguous situation (this can be learned with some generalisation[215]). In a group of strangers, eye contact will grow first toward people felt to be unthreatening.

Cultural exceptions: In east Asia, direct eye contact with a senior is rude; and many Muslims limit eye contact with the opposite sex after the first greeting.

Causes of odd eye contact	Notes
Playing	(p.221)
Looking sideways at you	Sign of distrust, torticollis, imperfect glasses.
Divergent squint	When looking through her right eye, the left eye may give the impression of gaze-avoidance.
Visual field defect	Using the preserved portion of retina or visual cortex.[588] (see p.66)
Tipping head	• Backwards, e.g. with droopy lids in myasthenic syndromes (p.510), Cornelia de Lange (p.445). • Tipping the head slightly down (while looking up) is often wary. • Tipping the head far down and avoiding eye contact in depression. • Tipping or turning the head in a consistent direction, with good eye contact can indicate cataracts (p.436) or retinal damage.
Focus on something else	
Preoccupation	(i.e. something in their mind). Turning head while looking the opposite way – perhaps concentrating on the movement or on the edge of the visual field (ID).
Depression (p.309)	Downcast – particularly in children can be briefly overcome by compliments, especially in the third person talking about them (doing this in the third person reduces the problem of shyness, p.181).
Looking at something else	• Some people have learned to focus on other people's nose, mouth, or forehead. This can be a useful taught lesson for people who find eye contact overwhelming (as many autistics and Sir Laurence Olivier did). • (As an executive function, which unlike most executive functions can be seen) trying to force self to focus on what person is saying. • Compensation for shortsightedness • E.g. another person in the room is important or interesting. • Lip reading
avoiding contact in specific situations	
Accessing memories	Eyes upward, or straight ahead and not moving. Avoidance of eye contact while thinking of an answer demonstrably improves accuracy. Somalian culture based on memorising epic poetry – creates habit of looking away to think. Focusing on a taste.

Lying	Perhaps eyes look sideways while preparing an answer, then looking at the listener for longer than usual to check whether they have been detected. Not reliable! For more complex patterns, see http://www.blifaloo.com/info/lies_eyes.php and overoptimistic views such as [954].
Hiding anger	Consider antecedents, speech, body language, autonomic arousal (p.428). *Overt* anger causes intense eye contact.
Expecting criticism	Minutes: worse eye contact with specific parents or teachers. Assess his eye contact before and after a good bit of praise, to see this. Children with low self-esteem can be quite fearful even of rare minor criticism.
	Seconds: A child with ID can "hide" behind his hands, or use his hands as blinkers to avoid a telling off.
Avoiding misery	If mother is depressed it can be painful for the child to look at her face
Concealing reaction, e.g. disappointment	A patient's blank look or non-committal look accompanied by briefly averting the eyes can mean you missed the point and are saying something irrelevant – but she is being polite about it.
Photophobia	(p.529)

Avoiding contact -- prolonged

Imaginary world	(p.231). The child switches into this when lonely (p.500) or bored (p.322).
Shy	(p.181)
Broader categories	See the hierarchy of anxieties on p.295. Within autism: common patterns are avoidance of eye contact, touch, people, or interaction (see p.156). Less often, avoidance of facial expressions and/or heads is sometimes seen in children who happily see/touch other parts of their parents.
Fragile X (p.468)	Aversion and sensitisation to direct eye-gaze [1717]. Characteristically they turn away while shaking hands, or partially cover their eyes (as if the sun is shining in their eyes) while remaining fully socially engaged.
Autism ☂ (p.183)	• Prolonged eye-gaze avoidance is often found in autism, in which it is more often to the side rather than downward. • Some autistic children can talk to a person from behind, or be interested in the eyes but not the person. They may be able to tolerate eye contact from a distance, or by training in the use of "soft focus". • Some autistic children have been trained to look at people in the eyes when talking to them. In this case they usually have a fixed gaze that only appears when required. • In a *few* cases it is limited to covering the eyes rather than turning away, showing that poor eye contact is not always caused by social disinterest or interest in other things. For example, one boy waved to staff while nearly-covering his eyes with the other hand (as if waving at someone with the sun behind them).

continued ▶

Unable to maintain contact

Hyperactivity	Sometimes unable to focus for the duration of a sentence: focus may flit around the speaker's face (visual fidgetiness). The child can look at a face as easily as anything else, but maintaining direct gaze requires intense concentration, to the exclusion of other thinking.
☞Hebephrenia	Acute onset, very rare before teens.
Amblyopia ("lazy eye")	One eye unengaged in task, due to uncorrected visual impairment in a critical period (p.447) in childhood
Hidden epileptic fits	Eye signs & other signs: p.133
Oculogyric crisis	Looking upward, p.93
Myasthenia	(p.510)
Nystagmus	Can make it difficult to focus on one point. The person may give up trying to do so and let the eyes wander – or may adopt extraordinary head movements (p.66).

Excess contact

Aggression	(p.289)
Intrigue	Or anxious monitoring (deer in headlights)
Hypomania	Direct, confident gaze and body posture (p.261).
Learned	• Many gaze-avoidant children are taught by their parents to make eye contact. The result can be a mechanical fixed gaze, perhaps interrupted for breaks. • A child may look mainly at the parent she is usually with, for reassurance, reciprocation, smiles, or to check mother is fine. • ☞Frozen watchfulness (p.470) is sometimes a sign of abuse.
Special interest	Interested in something around your eyes, or the reflection in your eyes. Imagining you can see someone's thoughts, or find an answer in the person by looking into the eyes.
Blank stare	This shares most of the causes of a blank face (p.178) but some interest can be demonstrated by his gaze following someone as they stand up.
Williams syndrome [1018]	Weaknesses: ID (mean IQ is 55, but rare cases have IQ 100), eye-hand coordination, spatial organisation, expressive and receptive vocabulary Strengths: Hypersociability, face recognition, auditory short term memory (see STM, p.555), syntax Special problems: Social disinhibition, indiscriminate relating, anxiety, hyperactivity. They look straight at you but then don't follow your gaze to something else (poor gaze monitoring), supravalvular aortic stenosis.
Psychopathy (p.280)	Psychopaths, and angry or oppositional people (p.253) sometimes return a direct gaze for longer than normal, (whereas people with Asperger's (p.424) generally make very brief eye contact). Overall, however, psychopaths generally make little eye contact, and this may account for some of their deficiencies in fear recognition[353,355]. See also *oxytocin*, p.521.

Causelist 58: Expressionlessness

This can have different social consequences depending on whether the mouth is naturally smiley or frowning. Is he just expressionless in certain situations? Babies look at expressionless faces less than at active or happy faces. See also *faces* (p.464).

Causes of showing a blank face	notes
Not actually blank	
Subtle expressions	E.g. teenage look of disdain has very small movements of jaw, neck, and eyes.
Sullenness	I.e. to show he's not cooperating.
Thinking of what to say, concealing disappointment	A patient's blank or non-commital look accompanied by briefly averting the eyes can mean you missed the point and are saying something irrelevant – but she is being polite about it.
Situational	
Looking at someone	
Uninterested	
Uncomprehending	
Acting tough	Or with less eye contact, trying to act grown-up, knowledgeable, confident
Poker face	Concealing feelings, most often anger (e.g. when looking at a particular person).
Autism, Asperger's (p.424) or other social dysfluency	• Especially in tense social situations, knows that he's likely to get the communication wrong so puts on a blank face. • Relies on formally learned social communication, so when he is concentrating on something else, even something he's doing with people, his facial expression can disappear. • For expressionless violence in autism see p.279
Not looking at someone	
Boredom (p.322)	And sleep.
Social etiquette	E.g. in a lift
High concentration	Many people use habits/stereotypies (p.553) while concentrating – e.g. jiggling leg, rocking, tapping. If during interaction, this can indicate self-absorption.
Social anxiety (p.298)	E.g. can't organise his thoughts when feeling confronted.
Dissociation(p.453)	Recognisable if it appears just in stressful situations
Myasthenia	(p.510)
Sleepy	Lack of sleep, or withdrawal from stimulants
Absences	(p.75)
Poor hearing	(p.130)
Long lasting	
Depression (p.309)	Many other signs such as psychomotor retardation (p.537), downcast (p.175)
Medical	Parkinsonism (p.525). Guillain-Barré (p.87), Melkersson–Rosenthal syndrome (recurrent). Non-dominant hemisphere lesion. Side-effect of some antidepressants (though not usually SSRIs).
Catatonia	(p.98)
Permanent	
Möbius syndrome (hereditary)	Striking mask-like face, with inability to smile and reduced blinking. Though caused by VI and VII nerve lesions, also causes impairment in recognising facial expressions of others, perhaps via "mirror system" (p.507). But he still puts recollections in context so listener will understand; has complex language and shared enjoyment. At risk of bullying.
Emotionlessness	Learned or primed [725], cultural or subcultural. Innate is exceedingly rare.

Causelist 59: Being selfish

Selfish is too pejorative to be used as a technical term, but the word often comes up in discussions with families and needs to be thought about. It generally means to behave as if other people's needs or desires are less important than one's own.

Sharing (of food or toys)
The essence is the willingness to bear a loss for other people, i.e. true unselfishness or altruism (p.420). The degree of unselfishness can be assessed in many ways such as its frequency, spontaneity, flexibility, premeditation, generosity, range of gifts and recipients, and matching to the recipient's desires.

Unavoidable or uncomprehended sharing, and giving away unwanted items, do not count! Giving *information*, from a small child's point of view, is quite different from sharing because he does not lose anything. It usually shows no altruism (except in special circumstances) but it does demonstrate a useful interest in what the other person thinks.

Some children are described as bad at sharing because they don't offer to share with adults or older siblings (who have what they want already) or with younger siblings (who are being looked after and usually getting more attention). However, a willingness to share only with a small minority of other people (e.g. a friend from school, or one particular cousin) shows both that the object was desired, and the motivation was social, i.e. that it was true sharing.

Giving more than other people do, especially of things that one cannot replace, is often called being over-generous. It is easily labelled cynically as trying to buy friends or having low self-esteem, but some people enjoy more than others the feeling of working for or taking care of another, anticipating the smile of appreciation, the subsequent strengthened bond and virtuous feeling of kindness, and following a positive role model. This is an aspect of personality that is very un-autistic.

See also *thinking together*, p.170; *joint attention*, p.494; sharing a bed with parents, p.198.

Causes of complaints of selfishness	Notes
Normal	
Rational selfishness	Everyone is selfish when they feel something crucial for them is at stake, i.e. something fundamental, on their version of Maslow's pyramid of needs (p.505).
Not actually selfish	The complainer may be self-centred or exhausted, or have unreasonable demands, or may not realise the actual need that is driving the behaviour
Cultural / religious	Some cultures mandate sharing, particularly of food. Some religions may make people less selfish, either directly (creating the need to share) or by reducing other needs. Sometimes a person's religion is invoked to explain their unselfishness, even though there could be other factors.
Inadequate maturity to be unselfish	
Preschooler egocentricity (not egotism)	This is normal up to age 7 or so (compare Piagettian stages, p.530). After school entry they start to copy other people's generosity and so become less self-centred between age 7 and 11. Egocentricity is different from autism – they want others to be interested in them. For the distinction from paranoia see p.524.
Delayed social maturation	Egocentricity persists longer in cases of chronic illness, anxiety, overindulgent parenting, ID ☂ (including NVLD, p.28) or indeed autistic spectrum disorder ☂. The component which is genetic can be estimated by looking for other signs of ASD/ID, plus very early development and parental characteristics. The other causes often have an obvious age of onset.
Impulsivity	(see p.79)
Reduced habit of sharing	
Learned self-protection	Learned, e.g. from parents or siblings. Lack of positive role model in parents.
Spoiled	Is the child effectively the head of the household? Is there a over-indulgence, especially by the father?
Only child	(p.518)
Little drive to share	
Psychopathy	(p.280)
Autism ☂ (p.183)	Disinterest in others, and/or inability to know what is wanted.
Unusual needs prevent sharing	
Nothing to share	E.g. very poor or hungry
OCD, other mental illness	Obsessions are often self-centred (p.517). If the obsessions are secret, resulting behaviours may appear very selfish.
Teenage	Usually just that their value are not shared by the complainer (e.g. peer acceptance often overrides punctuality, etc., in teenagers). Sometimes this age sees the onset of anxiety disorders.

Severity of friendship problems can be very roughly put on this continuum: (a) no problems; (b) friendships break down; (c) can't make friends; later aloof; (d) doesn't see need for friends; (e) no interest in others. The *types* of relationship are also important (p.171).

Social problems often lead to a referral mentioning autistic spectrum disorder, because many professionals have a very firm view that ASD ⬆ has a single core, namely a problem in socialising. However, it is now clear that sociability is often inherited separately from the other parts of autism, namely problems of communication and repetitivity. Therefore, for social problems use the list below; and for discussion of the "autism triad" and its other components see p.183.

The difficulty may be due to a lack of interest or *drive*, p.168; or a lack of social *skills*, p.169; or other problems listed in the table below. It is useful to identify the contributory factors because they have quite different prognoses, and several have specific and/or effective treatments.

Causes of social difficulties	Notes
Competing drive	
Mild hyperactivity (p.79)	Difficulty in following the rules (of games, conversations, friendships). Starts a sentence before finishing the last one. Not staying with the subject under discussion, not taking time to judge appropriateness of utterances.
	Different from autism, in that the social errors tend to be overactive and overinvolved, e.g. kissing and hugging peers.
Severe hyperactivity (p.79)	Flitting eye contact. Makes friends but annoys or exhausts them within an hour. Gives impression of disinterest in what other children want, or incomprehension of what they say. Brief but otherwise normal response to brief sentences. Stimulant clarifies.
Anxiety	Unlike autism-related conditions, interactions within the family are fairly normal. • Social anxiety (p.298) causing avoidance (p.429), lack of confidence, awkward speech (e.g. stuttering, p.157; selective mutism, p.153), and more specific signs of anxiety (listed on p.296) • PTSD (p.532) – avoiding social situations that remind him of the trauma (e.g. sexual abuse). • agoraphobia (p.297) – avoiding public places that he cannot escape from. • OCD (p.65) – avoiding social situations that might force him to engage in embarrassing compulsions, e.g. cleaning or counting.
Shyness	• Reduces greatly over 10−60 minutes. • Shyness maximal with adult males • These children are acutely aware of you. • Occasional brief glances particularly when they think you aren't looking – or long stares when their face is hidden, e.g. by a doll. • Interacts well with family or close friends, making good eye contact with them • In class, these children follow people with their eyes but don't put their hand up.
Expectation of rejection or teasing by peers	Can be based on physical, verbal, or mental problems or ability. Typically from age 8 to 10, children with mild ID become increasingly socially isolated in mainstream school, especially if they are anxious by nature.

Paranoia	(p.524)
Sensory intolerance	(p.125)

Lack of skills

Immaturity	This includes • Young age • Young age making recognition of ID harder. Worrying signs for ID are on p.55. • Young age and/or ID making recognition of autism harder. Useful signs at a mental age of 2–3 are limited social interest; absence of pointing; absent imitation or pretend play; and indifference to praise. See also milestones of smiles (p.549)
Inflexibility (p.234)	Difficulty finding solutions, difficulty adapting self to friends' reactions
ID ☂	Difficulty with interaction, attention, speed. Bullying lowers mood and reduces friendships after school entry. Self-esteem worsens as they recognise their impairments, e.g. when rebuffed by the opposite sex in mainstream school.
Poor social skills	Poor understanding of social situations, difficulty reading or expressing emotions (see p.169). This may be due to inadequate interactions in early childhood, e.g. due to social deprivation or epilepsy[161].
Deafness	(p.130) Even if only mild. Especially likely if the child also has ID. If observed in a group, can give the impression of being autistic because unable to follow conversation, find the source of voices, or filter out background noise.
Language difficulties ☂ (p.145)	E.g. SLD (esp. receptive), ID, immigrant (p.488). All these problems reduce self-esteem and social interaction. Use a non-verbal approach to assess social interest and skills.

Lack of interest (see social drives, p.168)

"Socialled out"	I.e. temporarily exhausted by social interactions. More common in males.
Autism, Autistic Spectrum ☂ (p.183)	For a comprehensive overview of social development in autism, see [261]. Unlike anxious children, these have abnormal relationships within the family too. See also early signs, above on this page.
Egocentricity	(see p.180)
Preoccupied	
Depression (p.309)	Not life-long, sociability varies with life events / mood
Enuresis (p.339)	Difficulty with smell, teasing, self-esteem, sleep-overs.
OCD	Rituals or fears preventing mutually acceptable interaction (p.65)
Hallucinations, delusions	Schizophrenia ☂ and schizophrenic prodrome, p.543 .
Physical illness	Consider if a child becomes even less sociable than usual (e.g. in ID or autism or mutism, because he does not communicate the pain).

Social dynamics

Ostracised	Excluded by ingroup, especially in girls' "who said what about whom" .
Lack of suitable peers (p.171)	E.g. the sole child with ID in a mainstream class (see *inclusion*, p.489); or a child who is gifted (p.473) or deaf or linguistically challenged.

Special Topic 5: Would an autism-related diagnosis ☂ help the child?

For the DSM definition of Autism see p.388. In practice, the term Autistic Spectrum Disorder describes milder problems. "High functioning" in this context means IQ over 70. See also Asperger, p.424; "on the spectrum", p.519.

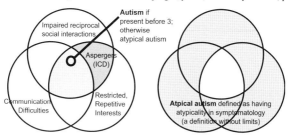

Figure 17. The three aspects of autism-related diagnoses.

Fractionation. It is useful to address components individually: social problems, p.167; communication problems, pp.144–163; stereotyped interests, p.229; and often ID as well (pp.185, 442). Each part of the triad can be further fractionated[855,897] (see also page references on p.388).

Caveat. These are difficult diagnoses to use well. "The use of standardised assessment instruments and the strict application of the DSM and ICD diagnostic criteria need to be employed with caution, as an expert clinical view has been shown to be more accurate"[285]. "Treatment building on an individual's profile of strengths or weaknesses is more important than distinctions between autism, PDD-NOS or Asperger's syndrome"[1684]. If you can produce a comprehensive, useful explanation for the symptoms (e.g. ID with anxiety) there may be no further benefit in using an autism-related term.

Reconciling research with clinical practice

There are several ways to view autism. (a) A traditional research view is that since the definition of autism specifies "a set of purely behavioural syndromes", the multiple underlying causes of it do not replace the diagnosis of autism, but rather are a separate, additional, kind of information[564]. (b) Many people focus on one aspect of autism in the belief that it is the essential core, e.g. monotropism, p.509; deficient Theory of Mind, p.563; lack of social responsiveness, p.519. (c) A more modern view is that autism ☂ is an awkward composite, with separately inherited fractions[1371] that need to be assessed and managed separately, and that in some cases lead to further *emergent* non-familial symptoms[39].

The "gold standard" tests are the ADOS, based on current observation of the child, and ADI/3di, based on long-term history from parents. Both are subject to the problems of checklist diagnoses (p.24). They use phrases such as "cutoff for autism" which reflect their makers' optimism, but disregard the complexities of diagnosis. They are time consuming but can give false positives if the child is ill or anxious or cross, or if the parents have read a lot about autism (which affects their answers). They are best reserved for research, for contentious cases, and for training.

In clinical practice the following system works: For *your* formulation, work out his behaviours sufficiently to fit him into locally available therapies (e.g. language problem plus gaze-avoidance plus anxiety). For the *school*, use what will attract the help he needs (e.g. in some areas Autistic Spectrum Disorder attracts extra 1:1 help but Asperger's doesn't). For the *parents*, try to explain both.

Making the diagnosis

You need an idea of the child's developmental level. The common diagnostic methods are not well validated below a mental age of 3−4 so a "working diagnosis" may be necessary for a year or two (for fairly useful signs at age 2−3 see p.182). Stereotypies and other behaviours characteristic of autism peak at age 4−6, which can clarify difficult (usually mild) cases. Then all aspects improve well into twenties[521]. (If his behaviour is altered by current illness or crossness, that may need sorting out before autism can be rigorously considered.)

In diagnosing, assess the standard diagnostic criteria (p.388) as well as:

- Social problems (p.167): lack of role-play (p.222); lack of empathy; no response to praise; unusual attachment (p.196). In severe cases, playing with earlobes and hair (p.225), or climbing over people as if they are not people. In milder cases:
    - difficulty in understanding why peers are interested in something (such as fashion, hygiene, personal space, football)
    - feeling of injustice caused by not understanding nuances of decisions by peers, teachers, and parents
- Preference for behaviours that are restricted in several ways:
    - interests lacking in complexity, changeability, abstractness, or linguistic content (p.229) and that have minimal human interest (e.g. avoiding eyes, faces, or people's details).
    - Severe inflexibility (p.234), especially insistence on sameness
- Language deficit (pp.143−145). Can seem to be doing back-and-forth conversation, but not interested in the answers coming back (p.143). Often echolalic (p.459) or speaking little, e.g. habitually using gestures or single words despite knowing how to make sentences (p.151).

See also findings on cognitive testing (p.33), "autistic regression" (p.41). Imaging may contribute to diagnosis in the future[442].

Common errors in diagnosis

What is an error? There is a grey area of mild disorder where well-informed experts have different views, not just on the judgment of severity but on the question of whether to take specific DSM criteria at face value or not. Most clinicians are calibrated mainly by published diagnostic criteria, but also to some degree by opinions in the area where they work. Making too many diagnoses of autism dilutes local provision. Making too few creates more difficulty for the child, family and school; some parents will obtain the diagnosis elsewhere. Delaying a diagnosis of ASD/autism until late adolescence can prevent a young person accessing some of the best adult accommodation. Other errors include:

- Misjudging whether a symptom is impairing or abnormal in frequency
- Diagnosing "late onset autism" but ignoring the major physical or emotional events causing it
- Considering language impairment to be a feature of autism without considering whether the child has (global) ID.
- Considering an imaginary world (p.231) or casting (p.103) or balancing/completing efforts (p.64) to be autistic behaviours.
- Diagnosing autism based on ADOS while child was angry or depressed (long term functioning in multiple settings is needed)
- Finding only major socialising problems so concluding simply "Not Autism." However this is "atypical autism" and needs similar care.
- Focusing on the intriguing (an interest in feet) rather than the dangerous (headbanging against windows).

Conundrum 9: Autism with ID

In population studies the two are associated but when assessing an individual child his intellectual ability and his social and exploratory tendencies are separate issues.

Over-broad use of the word "autism"
Some clinicians incorrectly use the term autism as if it implied ID. If you meet a child with severe ID and autism, whose parents have believed for many years that he has "just autism", it is not a trivial matter to tell them that in fact he has ID as well. Consider the likely impact on the parents (especially if single), and whether there are any benefits for his schooling or other provision.

Avoiding overdiagnosing autism in ID
It is crucial to obtain reliable information about the child's relaxed behaviour, as this may be quite different from the behaviour in clinic. Children with ID are especially prone to anxiety, which makes people less social and more focused/repetitive, and can lead to overdiagnosis of autism.
The impression of all three types of "autistic" symptom can result from ID:

➢ *Repetitive behaviours.* Many **non-autistic repetitive** behaviours are more common with ID than without (for examples see p.63). Self-entertaining movements (p.545) sometimes lead to autism being suspected when a child actually has ID. However autistic behaviours (e.g. stimming, p.64) increase under stress while these reduce; and autistic behaviours tend to be invariant and below the child's developmental level whereas most self-entertainment is developmentally appropriate, involves some experimentation, and evolves as fast as the child's learning permits. A child with severe or profound ID causing him to have a very **limited repertoire** of behaviours will generally rotate through these behaviours repeatedly, spending 5–30 seconds on each. In contrast, an autistic child generally shows a marked preference for one or two behaviours, despite having a broader repertoire.

➢ *Social.* A child with **mild ID** or dyspraxia or Asperger's can be quite badly teased or ignored within a mainstream school. This can lead to a child preferentially playing on his own, using imaginary friends more (p.231), or becoming depressed. These socially based problems tend to worsen from age 8 to 12, whereas the more central problems of ID/autism (e.g. not wanting to do what he is told or not understanding his work) arise on school entry. **Profound ID** with a mental age below 18 months can cause indiscriminate sociability (contrast attachment in autism, p.196).

➢ *Language.* Demonstrating that language is behind the other neurodevelopmental areas requires a wide-ranging developmental assessment (p.451). If a child has **no speech**, the diagnosis of autism can be made using mainly the non-verbal criteria and non-verbal testing, p.516. If a child has **limited** expressive language skills, he will often need to use the same words or phrases; but this is different from preferring to restrict his repertoire, as in autism.

Conundrum 10: Autism in high-ability children

High ability sometimes allows a child or young person to work around his social or language difficulties. Social skills improve with age; and a certain formality is useful in some professions.

Introducing this diagnosis, or Asperger's, to a high-functioning teenager can cause her to completely disengage from services if she is quite sure there is a different reason for her problems.

Non-verbal Learning Disability (p.28) can sometimes give the impression of Asperger's, i.e. social difficulty with fluent language (the distinction is considered in detail in[414]).

Investigation Planner 5: Causes of Autistic Spectrum Disorders

Most children with these diagnoses need consideration of causes of ID as well; many treatable ones are listed on p.32. See also the *general approach to medical investigations*, p.373, and[703].

	Signs	Test	Excluded clinically or to Order?	Date ordered	Result
Basic tests		chromosomes (p.439), Fragile X, hearing (p.130)			
Consider the following additional tests as they can be crucial for genetic counselling[966]:					
Rett (p.541)	In girls with ID plus ASD, as when they have Rett syndrome they do not have the other characteristic signs of Rett	MECP2			
Various syndromes	Children with autism and deafness with consanguinous parents	HOXA1			
Macrocephaly-autism syndrome	Extreme macrocephaly	PTEN			

Causelist 61: Hatred

This is more than strong dislike or anger (p.287) or desire to destroy (p.282). True hatred is as out of touch with reality as being head-over-heels in love (p.501): both are prolonged in time and extend to objects associated with the other person. It is arousing and unpleasant even to the hater, and it persists without reduction. It is rarely seen pre-pubertally, except perhaps in abused children. It is almost always counterproductive, but (as a rare example) it can drive a divorced parent to provide superhuman parenting in order to prove the ex-partner inadequate.

Hatred usually includes an accusation that is so severe it prevents the hater from feeling guilty about his hatred. Some suggest it is easier to hate a group than an individual, because we are biased to like individuals; but the extremity of feeling is more easily reached with individuals, who can wind us up in multiple ways at the same time.

Parental alienation

This means beliefs maintained in a child, by one parent against the other, akin to folie imposee. It can amount to emotional abuse of a child (p.277), most often by a separated mother[1730]. The term "Parental Alienation *Syndrome*" is best avoided, as it elicits strong views both for and against.

The effect of interparental hatred changes with age (see [see 785]):
2–3 yr: Anxiety regarding separation from mother is more important than parents' views.
3–6 yr: The child feels allegiance to whichever parent he is with at the time
6–7 yr: Increasing sense of morality, and becoming able to see others' viewpoints. Also trying to avoid hurting parents' feelings.
7–9 yr: Experience the cognitive dissonance (p.355) of their conflicting views.
9–12 yr: Likely to ally themselves to one parent, in an attempt to resolve the confusion.
12+yr: True hatred can develop in the adolescent.

Causes of hatred	Notes
Predisposing	
Rigidity	(p.234)
Splitting	Black-and-white thinking (p.552)
Summation of multiple negative feelings	Many of these are listed as causes of angry feelings (p.287).
Precipitating	
Harm	This can be physical, emotional, or social. It can be real or imagined. An example is parental alienation (see box at left).
Re-creating a previous hatred or fear	E.g. dealing with someone who reminds the child of a prevous abuser. Re-creating primitive feelings. Projective identification (p.535)
Perpetuating	
Persisting harm	(whether real or imagined)
Motivated thinking	Misfortunes can be attributed to the hated person, hence avoiding shame or guilt (p.426). Cognitive dissonance (p.355) can be resolved by making one person wrong and the other right.
Belief that injury was intentional	Persistence similar to that of hatred is seen with the pain of repeated mild physical injury – but only if it is thought to be intentional[605]. This may be exacerbated if the harmer is thought to have gained, or still be gaining, pleasure from the harm.
Lack of other views	Most situations have several interpretations, and the child may have considered only one.
Interpersonal dynamics	The hater can be encouraged by other people who share the same hatred. The hater's unpleasant (even violent) behaviour can produce a reciprocal response in the other person. Or the behaviour can cause exclusion, change of class, or loss of friends and social standing.
Enduring mental status change	Depression, anxiety, and psychotic states can be precipitated by trauma or loss (see *life events*, p.499, and *psychosis*, p.537)

Home ☼

Excellent parenting is practised; warm; prepared for frequent demands
such as hunger; predictable but flexible. Aspects of parenting are
summarised in more detail in the table below. None of the aspects has to
be performed perfectly, and judging what is good enough can be difficult,
as described on the next page.

Table 9. Necessary aspects of parenting

Necessary aspects of parenting[705]	Notes / examples
Physical care	These are the most basic needs (see Maslow's pyramid, p.505)
food, drink, heat	
statutory & medical safety	Prevents accidents, attends appointments sufficiently reliably
Comfort / pleasant feelings	
emotional warmth	(p.574) or love.
physical warmth and contact	Intimates should also be thought of and talked to more than others. Physical closeness has overwhelming importance [653], except for children who can't bear it.
Nurturing/teaching	
dependency	Independence should gradually increase. The balance of control needs to be sensitively regulated.
stimulation	Conversation, attendance at school, reading with child. Teaching by example is especially useful.
boundaries	Parents need to restrict contact with antisocial peers and inappropriate adults. A mother who says her child "insists" or "punishes me" or "won't let me" or "knows how to get at me" needs help in re-establishing her dominance.
Communication	
playful interactions	Look for shared humour, and arranging for interactions with peers. Can the parent enjoy the child, or playing with him?
talking, etc.	Speaking to the child – and listening.
reciprocation	Look for balance of control, shared positive feelings.
Security	
permanence	Changes of school and carers should be minimised (good stable childminders have better emotional outcomes than nurseries which have changes of staff). Child should never be threatened with abandonment.
predictability	E.g. of meals, sleep, parent's mental state, arriving to collect from school. Explanations of family, relationships, duties, etc., should not vary from day-to-day or from carer to carer.
confidence / lack of fear	Relatively minor problems such as being shouted at a lot – or even hearing parents shouting at each other – can have a serious effect on sensitive children. *Learned wariness* is a mild form of hypervigilance, and other responses to fear are sometimes seen (p.296). *Frozen watchfulness* (p.470) indicates substantial fear in the presence of specific carers.
Adaptability	All the above need adaptation for children with special needs.

Good-enough parenting

When it was introduced, this term referred to specific aspects of the mother's interaction with her child, but it has come to be used in a much less theoretical way, as a shorthand for the minimum level of parental care that is acceptable to society. There is no practical working definition of this[1590]. On the contrary, judging what is an acceptable minimum level of each of the aspects of parenting (p.189) depends on local society's specific values, local guidelines on abuse (pp.271-278), personal experience of staff, discussion with colleagues, and the resources available to social services (see p.500).

Donald Winnicott
Winnicott introduced the idea of good-enough care, by which he meant care that allowed a child to progress appropriately. He wrote that a good-enough environment (like a good-enough mother) is "one that enables the infant to reach, at each stage, the appropriate innate satisfactions and anxieties and conflicts" (p.300 of[1783]). As well as being vague, the definition is based on long-term outcomes, so unfortunately cannot be used to work out what forms of parenting are acceptable[1590].

Although it was already obvious that ignoring the child's desires was not good enough (see *neglect*, p.274), Winnicott pointed out the paradox that normal ("good-enough") mothering involves a "carefully graduated failure of adaptation" to the child's desires (p.9 of[1783]). A related idea is that parents don't need to be perfect in order for their children to grow up well[705]. Indeed, if mother is "too good", i.e. if she persists in being totally in tune with her baby, then it may be that the baby's social development can be impaired[713]. Winnicott seems to have viewed this mainly as a fault in the parent, but in practice it is common to find such over-closeness resulting from biologically determined problems based in the child, such as life-threatening illness, ID or extreme inflexibility (these problems are little improved by normalisation of the mother−child relationship, and other children in the family are often unaffected; see p.196).

Good enough for which children?
Population norms and Winnicott's definition offer no guidance in judging what is *good-enough* parenting for a child with special needs. Such children often need unusually resilient, consistent, adaptable, intelligent care – while their parents are often sleep deprived and physically exhausted. Once doubts about the parenting of an individual child have been aired, it is necessary to assess parenting behaviours in detail (usually by comparing them to standard parenting), then to see if the parent can be helped to improve them in any way. It is sometimes difficult to be sure that the parenting is to blame for the child's problems until you have seen the child improve when given substitute parenting and deteriorate again when returned to his family. Occasionally it is possible to be fairly certain, e.g. if the child's behaviour or weight deteriorates during school holidays, or when staying with an uncle, or during admissions to hospital.

Good enough for what purpose?
Winnicott meant for a normal satisfying life, but applicable to more children is the question of whether he is fulfilling his potential. Also relevant in some cases is the question of whether the parenting requires remediation or support or indeed whether the child needs to be taken into care (p.500).

Parents with difficulties

Most parents have difficulties at some time, and most of them manage to be good enough, or even excellent, parents, supplying all the needs listed on p.189.

However, parental burdens can potentially contribute to most of the children's problems in this book. Parental difficulty in coping often makes their children's behaviour objectively more difficult to manage (p.207), and it can also colour parents' reports about their children's behaviour (p.80). The first public problem is often poor school attendance (p.217), or unusual parental behaviour when dropping off or collecting the child. *In extremis*, parental difficulty can lead to the child needing alternative care (p.500).

Parents' social or situational difficulties

See young parents, p.268; single parents, p.213; parental overwork, p.521; parents in prison, p.535; unemployment, p.570; poverty, p.533; refugees, p.540; social isolation, p.212; other patterns of family dynamics, p.211.

Consider lack of information about parenting, or bad experiences of being parented. Too-good parenting, p.190.

Parental physical illness

See parental cancer, p.569; maternal HIV, p.479.

Parental deafness

If the child is deaf: Deaf parents have complex and subtle reactions to discovering their child is deaf, but they are well placed to support the child throughout childhood[245].

Hearing children generally suffer little or no difficulty from having deaf parents, and develop speech well, especially if they have a television and contact with hearing children[339].

Parental discord

This can be a temporary reaction to stressors such as unemployment, cramped housing, alcohol abuse or physical illness. It may also progress over years, usually following this sequence:

- Parents often express their hostility to each other by criticising each other's parenting – or bickering about seeking help, or about what treatments are acceptable. Years of such bickering are more damaging than a quick divorce, and can amount to emotional abuse, p.277. Marital rows are especially upsetting for perfectionist or anxious children, and can make a child antisocial, withdrawn[342] or even more anxious.

- Domestic violence, p.454.

- Separation: the impact on children depends very much on how the parents manage this[474]. Most children will feel some responsibility.

- Divorce. This affects the *majority* of children in some countries and ethnic groups[692].

- Post-divorce. Relationships between parents often worsen after divorce. Parental alienation is an example of this (p.187). A gentler pattern is of each parent trying to outdo the other's gifts.

Parental mental illness

Usually, children's level of disturbance does not fluctuate with their parents' episodes of mental illness; however children of parents with mental illness have double the rate of long-term difficulties[1402]. Reasons include greatly increased parental discord[1402]; genetic inheritance (exacerbated by assortative mating); unemployment, p.570; and poverty, p.533.

When assessing children, parents' difficulties usually receive little attention. This creates a special hazard for the clinician, of unawareness of disorders the parents are unlikely to complain about, such as drug addiction or bipolar disorder[830]. This can usually be overcome by obtaining information from other family members separately, or from the GP, or by prolonged professional involvement.

See maternal depression, p.174; parental drug abuse, p.257; folie imposee, p.347; grandiosity in parent, p.262; parentification, p.214; Munchausen, p.362; Munchausen by Proxy, p.204. For a wideranging view of the psychosocial impact of parental mental illness see[329]; for the heritability of each disorder see[1049].

Common disorders that also affect parents: schizophrenia, p.543; bipolar affective disorder, p.264; anxiety (esp. social phobia), p.298; alcoholism, p.420; eating disorders, p.458.

Parental ID

Assessment of parenting ability should include not only what the parents can do (p.189) but also what services (to the child and the parents) are needed to meet the child's needs. Tasks that often need attention are managing hygiene and diet, travelling independently, timekeeping, managing finances, and disciplining the children[426]. Most mothers with an IQ under 60 cannot provide competent parenting on their own, but with support from the father and extended family some do cope[156].

Parents with mild ID have a high risk of having children who also have mild ID[1154], and who also have increased rates of emotional and behavioural difficulties that tend to require better-than-average parenting. There is higher risk of abuse and neglect by parents with ID, but it may be due not to the ID itself but to associated factors such as childhood deprivation and social isolation[426,1043]. There is conflicting evidence on whether children of parents with ID have better outcomes if they have *more* or *fewer* siblings (see [426,704]).

Causelist 62: Poor relationship with mother ☼

(Mother is used here as a shorthand for the main carer.) The first task is to work out what aspects of the relationship are poor. Constant friction between mother and child typically results from problems in several areas in this table, which can often be remedied. The commonest challenge for parents is to balance sensitive responsiveness against the need to be authoritative and set boundaries – in other words to balance love and rules.

The second task is to consider whether the parenting is *good enough* (p.190).

Causes of odd interactions between carer & child	Notes
Not really poor	Most unusual relationships between mother and child are not pathological. Separations and reunions have less effect in older children, and greater effect in children who have rarely been separated from their mothers (e.g. the Japanese)
Child's short-term feelings	
Cross	E.g. after being told off. Sulking because coming to clinic makes him miss football.
Staying with relatives on holiday, or in hospital	After an absence, children may take a few days to get used to normal continuous interaction with a parent, e.g. getting in the habit of asking them for things.
Child's long-term feelings	Try to assess all the factors on p.189.
A. Closer to mother than to others (but still problems in the relationship)	
Autism, Autistic Spectrum ☛ (p.183)	Can produce very odd stuck relationships (p.196)
Shyness (p.181)	Child seems oddly stuck to mother, but only when strangers present.
"Inhibited attachment"	Extreme fear of strangers, sometimes following very severe maltreatment. Note most abuse does not prevent attachment.
Anxious attachment	
Disorganised attachment	(p.195)
B. Does not discriminate carer from other people (sometimes called non-attachment)	
Lost faith in carers	E.g. lots of changes of carer
Global deprivation	E.g. following poor institutional upbringing
Extreme hyperactivity, impulsivity (p.27)	Can be strikingly similar to "disorganised attachment" (p.195)
General oversociability	(p.174)
Many carers	
C. Less comfortable with this carer than with the public	
Parental alienation (p.187)	
Abuse (p.271)	Learned wariness is a milder form of frozen watchfulness (p.470).
Learned disinterest	E.g. due to long-term lack of affection. Carer can be critical or extremely judgmental, or very depressed.
This carer not as nice as the previous one	
Carer's long-term feelings	
Carer's fear	Particularly in ID, a teenager can overwhelm mother.
Carer's mental problems	• Mother's depression (p.174) or preoccupation or severe cannabis use can lead to child no longer seeking comfort from her • Timidity or ID can lead to the child becoming boss when they overtake mother. • Mother's alcoholism can lead to fear of her being violent; conversely the child is afraid to be away in case mother can't look after herself.
Autistic /Asperger's parent	(p.183)
☞ Carer's reaction to child's OCD (p.65)	Teenager manages to impose his rules on the parents.

continued ▶

Attachment

Much of the research in this area is based on the assumption of the *uniqueness* of the mother–child (or parent–child) relationship, and the *permanence* of its effects. Subjectively there is no question that the relationship with the attachment figure has a numinous, unique quality for the child. However, Romanian adoptees, intercultural differences, and the protective effect of a good relationship with another adult make it likely that relationships with other people in the child's life are quantitatively, not qualitatively, different [see 1446].

"Attachment is but one of several components of the child–parent relationship, and so it is important not to equate parent–child relationships with attachment relationships." [1176]. "Parents usually have an attachment relationship with their children but the relationship also includes caregiver qualities, disciplinary features, playmate characteristics, and other aspects. Each of these may predominate in different contexts…"[1399]. "Similarly, sexual relationships may show strong attachment qualities but they do not necessarily do so. Thus, a person may have a strong sexual longing for someone else in the absence of a committed relationship and without that relationship bringing any sense of security." [1399]. Attachment qualities can also be seen in some relationships between people and pets (p.246).

Normal attachment. Attachment is usually defined as the child's feelings (particularly of **security or comfort**) towards the main carers, whereas bonding is what happens in the carer's mind. Attachment *behaviours* are greatest from age 18 months to 3 years. They include:
- anxiety in moderately stressful situations when the parent is absent
- brief delight and contact-seeking when the parent reappears
- seeking the parent when hurt.

Abnormal attachment. Attachment behaviours are what you may see, in the waiting room or in your clinic on separation; but inferring an impaired attachment relationship is considerably more complex. The conceptual chaos in attachment work (e.g. *Reactive Attachment Disorder* ☝p.390; disorganised attachment in the Strange Situation Test, p.556) means that it is best to avoid disputed labels, and instead describe what is observed (e.g. frozen watchfulness, p.470 or wariness during approach to mother, or flinching when mum moves, p.107); what can be consistently demonstrated; and what is reliably known about the child's treatment.

There is no doubt that attachment difficulties are statistically associated with life-long problems. However, few studies of attachment have carefully assessed autistic spectrum or IQ problems so it is not known how often the association is causal. It is likely that attachment is a function of general processes such as learning and social relatedness[e.g. 749], which allow a child to benefit from aspects of his carers, especially permanence (p.189). Recognition of attachment difficulties should not produce an "aha" moment but a careful search for causes, such as (a) depression in the mother; (b) maltreatment syndromes (p.271); (c) abnormalities in the child (see [1818]).

Practice note. "observing…the *lack* of attachment behaviour where it would be expected, could present a substantial challenge for the clinic setting. [This is because] the lesson from developmental research is that a moderately stressful situation is needed to elicit attachment behaviour from the young child." [1176].

Common errors in assessment

- Focusing on poor attachment when there are bigger or more directly addressable issues, e.g. the child is autistic or profoundly ID, or has been physically or sexually abused, or mother is depressed.
- Considering poor maternal attachment as damaging, when there are excellent protective attachments to father, auntie, grandparents, etc.

Conundrum 11: Attachment in autism

In autistic children (p.183), attachment is usually secure [1366]. However attachment *behaviour* is sometimes odd, such as brightening when mum appears but not seeking proximity or contact. More severely affected children may hit only their parents. Rarely there is attachment to hard uncuddly transition objects (p.567), such as hoovers.

Addressing this question in reverse: when attachment behaviours are fully normal, the likelihood of autism is greatly reduced. This is because normal attachment behaviour requires the desire to explore, and the ability to be comforted by closeness to mother, both of which are reduced in most autistic children.

Attachment in autistic spectrum disorder (ASD)
The situation with ASD, as opposed to full autism, can be subtle and confusing. The returns to mother can be rarer, or conversely oddly repetitive or stereotyped. Language difficulty can increase the exclusivity of interactions, especially if only mother is able to understand the child's signals. Inflexibility and violence can allow a small child to totally dominate his mother.

Assessment
Extreme attachment behaviours can make medical, psychiatric, or developmental assessment very difficult, for example if the child clings to mother continually. In this case, keeping the child strapped in his buggy can allow mother and staff to move around. The effect of mother's standing, giving instructions, moving further away, or leaving the room can then be assessed. Developmental testing equipment can be scattered around the room, or put next to his buggy when he isn't looking to see what he does with it. Availability of his favourite toys from home will help to calm him and also allow his practised play to be assessed (p.221).

Causelist 63: Difficulty separating from carer

Multiple causes often coexist, e.g. the mother and child may both be anxious, avoidant, and mutually protective (compare school refusal, p.217).

Causes	Notes
Normal	It is normal for children to be unable to settle without mother for one week at the start of nursery / primary school.
Problems in parent	
Other rewards from carer	E.g. carer may be the only adult who makes no demands on the child, or may feed him what he wants or give in to his rituals.
Parental perception of anxiety	An anxious mother may see a perfectly happy child as anxious, or try to avoid causing him any anxiety.
Parenting	Parents may be unable to implement a behavioural plan for separation at bedtime, or may not be aware that children need to learn to fall asleep by themselves.
Mother is bored without him.	
Parent can't separate	This is not the whole problem if the mother can happily go out shopping while the child stays at home.
Problems in child	
True separation anxiety	Anxiety for self (feeling unsafe) when separated from main carers. This is a sign of attachment (p.195).
(for DSM criteria see p.391)	Determining whether it is within the bounds of normality demands consideration of age, experience, and simultaneous stressors such as unfamiliar environment, people and noise. It is normal if the child has not often been separated from mother, as is common in some cultures until school entry.
	It should not be diagnosed when the amount of separation has just been substantially increased, as in the first weeks of nursery. Also, it should not be a main diagnosis if the child can stay at home quite comfortably while mother goes out shopping, or can happily pop out to the corner shop for chocolates by himself.
	The majority of children diagnosed with separation anxiety will later suffer from panics and depression[945].
Anxious about what might happen to others especially family	Occurs when, e.g., a sibling walks ahead, or when a lift door is closing with family separated
Anxious about what may happen to carer	Common if another parent has been lost, or this parent has been ill/hospitalised/threatened.
Anxious about planned events for self	E.g. going to school or clinic. Consider fear of abandonment, fear of the dark, fear of being alone, fear of strangers, fear of hunger or of having nothing to do
Resisting change	Sometimes can be distinguished from the above causes, by happening in both directions, e.g. both preparing for school & preparing to come home.
Resisting imposed change	Some mothers report their child can easily leave them, but that if they leave their child, the crying lasts for hours.
Autistic spectrum	Can cause abnormal attachment behaviour (p.196).
Problem in environment	
Insufficient safety signals	E.g. an unfamiliar place, people, toys, and routine. Children should be allowed time to get used to a babysitter before being left alone with them.

Causelist 64: Sharing a bed with parents

Co-sleeping is generally not a problem in itself before puberty. At any age, cases involving sexual contact are serious, rare and usually difficult to detect (p.275). The much more common innocent cases need to be carefully considered for a different reason, which is that there are often causative problems in parent and/or child, especially if co-sleeping persists after school entry. Co-sleeping can perhaps delay achievement of sleep independence in the child, but on the other hand it fosters security and closeness.

Causes of bed sharing	Notes
Infancy	Increased risk of Sudden Infant Death, especially under 6 months, if sleeping between parents, more so if they smoke or have been taking alcohol or other sedatives.
Poverty	(p.533)
Warmth	(p.574)
Cultural	In some cultures, over half of 7-year-olds sleep with their parents, and in Italy 3% of 11-year-olds do so[1203].
Older child	Sleepovers can be a useful incentive. Try gradual change. Partial solutions may be easier to achieve, e.g. cot in parents' room or sleeping on the floor.
Parents unable to impose rules	Not returning the child to own bed if he comes to parents bed in the night.
Habits	E.g. parents staying with child until asleep.
Separation anxiety	(p.197)
Temporary	E.g. thunderstorms or after a bad dream
Postpubertal	Sometimes associated with sexual abuse (p.275) but much more often done just to feel secure.
ID in parent or child	
Medical condition in child	E.g. epilepsy (p.73), vomiting, sleep apnoea. Mum's concerns continue for years afterwards.
Any age	
Preventing parental sex (intentional or not)	Or preventing single parent from acquiring a new partner.
👁 Incest (p.489)	Higher risk if opposite sex and post-pubertal.
Protecting other parent's sleep	
Parental loneliness	(p.500)
Parent still feeling like child	(E.g. if her parents still have dominant role)
Special fears (p.307)	(Exaggerated or mis-handled fears are much more common). Try a dimmable nightlight.
Subcultural	The "family bed" has some vocal proponents.

Causelist 65: Insomnia

For age norms see p.321.

Causes of sleep difficulty	Notes
Parents want him to sleep excessively	(Understandable in, e.g. ID with severe hyperactivity).
Normal variation	Recognise by self-waking in a.m., & no daytime naps.
Circadian rhythm out of sync	e.g. due to staying up on previous nights, sleeping late in the mornings, or jet lag.
Social / Organisational	
Reward for getting up	Hugs may be more readily available when the parents are calm and only one child is up. Food may be available from parents or by raiding fridge. Toys or TV in bedroom; or unsupervised pornography on internet (p.115).
Irregular bedtimes	(Especially after weekends)
☜ Parents' belief that he cannot fall asleep alone.	Remind parents that most people wake several times in the night, and then go back to sleep; parents should almost always leave the child while still awake, so he develops this skill. Parents may be frightened by their infant's *crescendo crying* (p.316).
Daytime naps	
Inadequate exercise	
Overcrowding, heat, cold	Also: music and televisions on at night; excitement of parents returning late, hunger.
Excitement	Remind parents of the need for a wind-down period before bed.
Parents fighting	
Mood	
Worries (p.295)	• about dark, school the next day, dirt, bugs in bed, a recent horror film, etc. • separation anxiety (can be normal or not, see p.197) • worries can be sufficient to trigger rituals
☜ Depression, mania	(p.309)
Physical	
Minor illnesses	Cough, blocked nose, earache, vomiting, diarrhoea, frequency, abdominal pain
Medications	Decongestants, stimulants (though in a similar proportion of cases this improves sleep if given early enough in the day), citalopram, risperidone (rare). If long-acting stimulants wear off after bedtime, child may wake up extra hungry.
Drugs, p.258	Caffeine, nicotine, cocaine. Also heroin withdrawal, p.258
Other medical	Hyperthyroidism, p.484; thiamine deficiency, p.328; obstructive sleep apnoea, p.518
Growing pains	(p.137)
Severe itching	(p.110)
Smith-Magenis syndrome	Poor settling, repeated prolonged waking, early waking, and daytime sleepiness (see p.550).
Sleep structure	
Nightmares	(p.456) Or fear of nightmares
Parasomnias	(p.200)

Causelist 66: Other sleep problems

Sleep problems affect a third of 1-year-olds and gradually reduce with maturation. A sleep diary is invaluable. For each day it should include: waking time, naps (time and duration), time told to go to bed, time in bed, time asleep, wakings (time, duration, and behaviour during them), time of medicines. See also *excess sleepiness*, p.321; and *microsleeps*, p.72.

Behaviours seen mainly during settling and sleep onset

- Settling difficulties (see p.199).
- Repetitive parasomnias: Headbanging (p.119) in the cot is common, as are hypnic jerks (see below). Other common examples are rocking, or rolling from side to side, during waking or settling (jactatio nocturnus). People with ID can become much more repetitive at bedtime, presumably because of tiredness and parasomnias (e.g. partial sleep syndromes), even to the extent of giving the impression of autism.
- Restless Legs (see below) are sometimes seen in children at bedtime.
- Hypnagogic hallucinations, p.345
- Sleep starts (hypnic jerks, which are benign myoclonic jerks without the emotional component of true startles, the reproducibility of tics, or other features of fits[137]). Compare other causes of twitching, p.101.

Behaviours during sleep

- Night-time waking. All people wake intermittently during the night, i.e. when parents complain about night-time waking the real problem is the fact that the waking comes to their attention. This is mainly due to available rewards such as cuddles or drinks or sleeping in the parents' bed (p.198).
- Extreme unrouseability. Especially in the first 90 minutes of sleep, prepubertal children are very difficult to wake[238] – which is very useful to parents carrying the child from the car to bed. Children who wet the bed tend to be much less rouseable than children who are dry[1786].
- *Night terrors* are commonest 1½ hours after sleep onset. Child is terrified, sitting up, and mumbling or shouting. He may hallucinate or speak but rarely listens or understands. The terror is not remembered (unlike nightmares, p.456). Sometimes caused by minor infections or over-heating. The nature of the signs often make parents think they are due to traumas, but this is not the case.
- *Sleep-walking* and sleep-talking.
- *Bruxism*: Grinding or repetitively clenching the teeth. This is very common in sleep. Occasionally it is a daytime sign of stress, and in autism it can be self-soothing or a stereotypy, p.553. In a small minority it leads to substantial tooth damage.
- *Restless Legs syndrome*: This term is used in two ways. (a) a well-defined syndrome of severe unpleasant creeping or crawling sensations deep in the legs that comes on at rest (e.g. in bed or in the cinema) and is rapidly relieved by movement[450]. It is more common in adults and can be caused by iron deficiency, pregnancy, kidney disease, or rheumatic disease. It is quite distinct from akathisia (p.114) in that the paraesthesias of RLS are strictly localised and cause most trouble at night. (b) an ill-defined concept used in some research, that has much overlap with ADHD, but is defined based on night-time behaviour [892] whereas ADHD is based on daytime behaviour.

Behaviours at the end of sleep

- Early waking. This is usually due to the availability of unmonitored television. In teens it occasionally accompanies depression or anxiety.
- Partial waking syndromes (such as sleep paralysis), particularly on mornings when normal waking routine isn't followed.
- Hypnapompic hallucinations, p.345
- Sleep paralysis is sometimes as part of narcolepsy, p.72

Causelist 67: Behaving better with dad than with mum

This needs to be broken down into two questions: whether the child behaves unusually badly with mum, and whether he behaves unusually well with dad. It is very useful to put together information about behaviour at school, and on school trips, and when eating with or staying with friends or relatives. This often allows one to see that the child behaves well or badly in just one situation.

Parents' behaviours
What the parents actually *do* needs to be known as objectively as possible. Reports from a relative or friend are usually biased one way or the other. The parents may be able to recite lessons on child management but put none of it into practice.

Two useful methods are observation in the waiting room, and observation during long sessions. Schoolteachers can often give extremely valuable accounts of how the parents behave, especially if the teachers are approached verbally rather than asked to put anything in writing.

Parents' motivations
It is important to keep the parents' motivations separate from their actual objective behaviour: they may act quite differently from the way they want to (p.353); and children will be far more aware of their parents' actual behaviour than the underlying motives.

Nevertheless, the individual parents' motives are useful to know, especially for organising any treatment. The parents themselves, and relatives, may try to give useful explanations, but the truth of them needs to be independently verified if possible. In some cases, especially when we have access to only one or two family members, we are unable to find out why parents are behaving in an unexpected way.

Behaving worse with mum than with staff / grandma	
Not actually behaving badly with mum	Mum may be self-critical, or unable to cope, or dad may be criticising mum for being too lenient
Mum gives in Feeling most confident with mum	} Evidence is the child giving in to other people.
Poor relationship Copying dad	Mum may be consistently critical or demanding. Is there domestic violence or denigration of mum?
Mother's circumstances	
Mum is around at difficult times	Mum prepares him for school in the morning, and is around when he is exhausted after school
Attention-seeking	If a friend or professional visits the house, mum will direct her attention towards them, and an only child, used to attention, can react violently against this
Mother's motivations	
Self-blame	Mum may blame herself for the marriage breakdown, and so be less confident about her role as a parent
Cultural	In some cultures, mainly Arab ones, some mothers feel their role is to serve, not to discipline, boys
Mother's capacity	
Physical	Mothers are more likely to suffer from physical illness, pain, or exhaustion
Mental	Characteristics of mother such as low intelligence (p.192), or a low mood, or a dependent personality can make it more difficult for her to impose authoritative discipline

Behaving better with dad than with staff / grandma	
Not actually behaving better with dad	• Dad may hardly enforce any rules • Dad minimises problems because in denial (which is more common in males because not exposed to so much information about children)
Dad is intimidating (intentionally or not)	Large body size, louder deeper voice, unpredictability, short temper (even if he has never physically chastised)
☞ Physical abuse	(p.273)
Able to enforce his rules	E.g. due to having great strength or energy.
Cultural / child identifies with dad	The child may be trying to be more like dad (most common with boys).
Rewards	Dad gives more rewards / bribes / fun / novelty / travel / physical play / ballgames.
Good relationship	Dad is a specially supportive person. Or they have something in common – even enjoying each other's humour
Father's circumstances	
Focused	Many fathers have the luxury of concentrating fully on their children when they are with them, undistracted by household duties or other children; the children obviously react well to this.
Not often there	He is less often around so is able to make a more detached overview of infractions and progress.
Father's motivations	
	Dad may be repeating the "script" of his own relationship with his father, making him feel that he should be domineering; alternatively he may have adopted a "corrective script" to try to prevent his difficulties from repeating.

Special Topic 6: How to use a genogram

Drawing a genogram with the family gives you much more than a chart of parentage. Sometimes children's symptoms become clear when they are seen in more florid or mature form in parents, who are more likely to have been diagnosed, and better at introspection and describing their reactions to adversity.

Drawing the genogram together is an ideal opportunity for asking about personalities, life changes, and relationships. Doing this is time consuming but helps the parents feel understood, and demystifies all those family names they keep referring to. Doing it to three generations prevents the parents feeling blamed.

See also *Genetic testing*, p.380; *sociogram*, p.550.

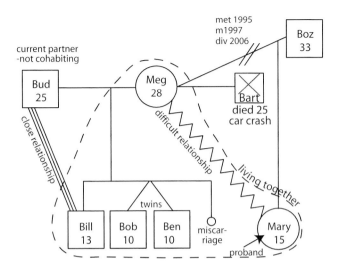

Figure 18. Sample genogram showing standard symbols.

There are many other standard symbols for putting information in genograms but most of them are best avoided as they are known only to specialists.

The best layout depends on what the genogram will be used for. For purely genetic purposes the siblings are best all together (with couples connected by |_____|) but this makes it very fiddly to show who lives with whom. Social relationships are more easily shown if couples are brought closer together (connected as shown in the figure above), which inevitably disrupts the row of siblings they come from.

Sometimes it is helpful to put the following information into a genogram, especially if the family is very complicated:

- family rifts and coalitions (this can be done with simple lines as above, but for more complex examples see[1090])
- child has moved around between branches of the family (can show with dated arrows)
- distribution of various diseases in family
- patterns of deaths, including miscarriages (p.507)
- prison (conviction, date, and expected release date), p.535
- locations such as houses and countries (both of which can have major emotional importance)
- helpers and influential people (related or not).

Timelines spanning decades can also be invaluable in understanding families.

Causelist 68: Parents complaining about normal behaviour

This can lead to a helpful intervention, if the situation is not dismissed as "just another anxious mother". The key point is to realise that the complaint indicates a problem, even if the problem is not at all what they say it is.

Related problems are inappropriate complaints by the child (p.359), and excess parental worries about real but small problems. A variant is parents complaining about a school's inability to teach, when in fact the child has ID.

Causes of complaining of normality	Notes
Normal is difficult	E.g. baby's crying keeping parent awake.
Parents having difficulty coping	Eg. single parents p.213; parents with other problems, p.191. See also p.80.
Tangible goals	Trying to obtain extra benefits or help in school.
Misled	E.g. by friends or the internet or professionals. There may be false positive results (p.373), e.g. an EEG may have been "over-read"[137].
Ignorance	E.g. first born, no extended family to provide experienced advice, environmental differences preventing parent using skills that were useful in home country
Parents sensitised to a particular behaviour, or "over-vigilant"[137]	• Minor change in child's eating or breathing reminds them of a dangerous illness in this or another child • Child stealing biscuits raises fear of escalation of criminality and violence, as in a relative. • Baby won't settle because parents can't manage consistently because father remembers over-strict parenting or abuse • Parents who have been primed by reading symptom lists place excess importance on rare occurrences (p.183)
Looking for information	• In order to see what the doctor knows about unsociability, phobia, etc., when the problem is bigger in parent or spouse • Heard about this symptom on the television, etc • Wondering if the behaviour is an early sign of a serious disorder suffered by another family member.
Excuse for consultation	Checking whether you are sympathetic so she can ask something more sensitive, e.g. risks if she has another baby.
Querulousness	(p.162)

continued ▶

⟨⟩ Parental mental illness and other problems

- Maternal depression is common (p.174).
- Anxious parents can complain vociferously that their child is terrified to visit friends, when he simply doesn't want to or has a different problem such as Asperger's (p.424).
- A parent can be addicted to a child's medicine, e.g. exaggerating the frequency of fits to obtain midazolam.

The following categories are difficult to use well. The words suggest clear distinctions, but in practice there isn't.

- Munchausen by proxy is rare, and describes carers inappropriately seeking help for their child, typically in multiple hospitals, often fabricating or inducing symptoms in the child. The case has been cogently made that the term focuses inappropriately on the carer's motivations, rather than the effect on the child[750]. For practical management the term *medical child abuse* is much more appropriate. Look for other signs of physical or emotional abuse (pp.273, 277). Symptoms deteriorate objectively when mother visits. MBP is fairly often suggested by professionals but in practice is rare; in any case it is still a behavioural pattern necessitating a search for causes (see p.359). Consider tertiary gain (p.471) or personality problems in mother.
- Hypochondriasis (pejorative)
- Wanting reassurance on a specific point (esp. if mother can't say that's what she needs)
- Doctor-shopping (most of which is caused by doctors failing to communicate well)
  Seeking a scan or a top or favourite hospital.

Causelist 69: Behaviour worse at home than school

This is often assumed to imply poor parenting, but there are many other reasons. Look at the time-of-day (p.62), and whether adding a person (e.g. a tutor) or taking people away (e.g. siblings) makes the problem worse or better.

Causes of behaviour being worse at home	Notes
Parental problems	Several are listed on p.80
Mistaken school report	The school report may be based on a period during which the child was medicated; or occasionally the report may be confused, or distorted to avoid diagnosis or medication.
Physiological	
Tired	(Parents and child, at start and end of day)
Lack of medication	E.g. methylphenidate not given at weekends or school holidays, or in the evenings (evening rebound from ADHD medication).
Emotional	
Anger	Home is always emotion laden, and often argumentative. Parents may be nagging or using barbed criticism, making power struggles, having to have the last word – even sometimes without realising it.
Upset	E.g. by anger, noise, lack of space, lack of privacy, siblings. Parents may upset the child by being strict or unpredictable, or disagreeing with one another.
Rush	There is a morning rush to prepare, and also evening homework.
Excess anxiety at school	In most childen, anxiety regarding possible consequences counterbalances their tendency to hyperactivity and impulsivity. Hence: • Social anxiety (p.298) can suppress misbehaviour at school: e.g. fear of being teased, fear of being told off . This can produce simple good behaviour, or in more severe cases selective mutism (p.153), or a variant of it. • If the child is innately hyperactive (p.79), suppression of behaviour at school by anxiety (of normal degree or more) can produce the unusual pattern of ADHD ✦ that is worse at home (see [165]).
Boredom	(p.322) 1:1 attention may be given at school.
Self-control	Energy (and tics, p.101) can be stored up while sitting in class, and later released at home.
Low mood	Misery, e.g. feeling stupid or teased for being fat
Environment	
Lack of toys, space, or exercise	E.g. severely ID children who can't go in the garden or who break everything in the house.
Physical environment	E.g. noisier, crowded, glass not replaced with perspex, doors not secure
Lack of structure	Structure is particularly helpful in PDDs and ADHD.

continued ▶

Social	
Complex relationships	• Chaos or other disturbance in family dynamics (p.212)
	• Confusion (in parents' as well as child's mind) between parent as attachment figure (p.195) and source of discomfort.
Learned	• Consequences intended by parents to be negative can be unreliable or actually enjoyed by the child. For example, timeout in a room with a TV and bed can be very comfortable. More ambivalently, a child being shouted at can simultaneously enjoy parental closeness.
	• Some autistic children learn quite distinct patterns of behaviour at home and school. This can be strikingly demonstrated if a child's level of cooperation, proximity-seeking, or regression suddenly *improves* when a single cue such as mother (or brother or desk) is altered.
Poor examples	Violent videos/games, parents, siblings, peers
Good examples	Wanting to fit in, or to be like admired peers (see mirror system, p.507)
Combination	Child likes (or knows) schooltime structure and predictability. But home is the opposite: less planned, less staff support, siblings compete in many ways; parents are manipulable, home strife can trigger it. These patterns can be perpetuated by habit or rigidity (in child or parents: p.234).

This can last seconds or hours. The running can be just walking, and it may be from a school or playscheme or inpatient unit rather than from parents. It can be terrifying to parents if a child is found miles away, as he may have crossed roads or been abducted.

There are obvious parallels between toddlers' running off, teens' staying out late, and actually becoming a runaway (p.210). In all these cases, as in most other misbehaviour, a full explanation cannot be purely in the child: the carers at the time were participating in the situation during which the child went off; and, at least in preschoolers, they were responsible for monitoring and controlling if needed.

Glancing back shows the child is weighing two things in his mind: where he has been versus where he wants to be; or his desires versus his fears; or his doubts versus his desire to be in control. Looking back usually increases with time and distance, due to fading of anger, increase in fear, and uncertainty about what mum is doing.

Causes of running / wandering off	Notes
Causes in the child	
Try to get somewhere	E.g. trying to get home after deciding to leave school during break time. Walking across a large shopping centre to reach a known toy shop does not imply rejection of parents, though it can be exacerbated by anger at parents for not letting him go there.
For fun	Trying to be chased. Look for eye contact and grins. Does it happen mainly when he feels deprived of attention?
Trained	Assumes that parents will follow as they always have?
Following overriding interests	E.g. in autism. He is preoccupied and there is little emotionality in the act or in the reuniting.
Poor impulse control	• Darting into the road to get a football • Love of running/exploring
Low anxiety (p.423)	Temperamentally anxious children run off much less.
Angry	Rejecting either the carer/carers or something they just said. This is one kind of sulking (p.557)
Unaware of leaving	E.g. in profound ID.
Causes in the care	
Abuse	Momentary fear as in the fight-or-flight response (p.466), as when physically attacked by parents. Can occur with abuse of any sort (p.271).
Poor monitoring	• Parents have not established clear rules and sanctions for staying within sight • Parents tired, chatting, or otherwise engaged.
Difficulty following	E.g. carers looking after multiple children, or parents with impaired mobility.
Strictness or harsh punishments (p.538)	Can be over-strict, or can be simply more abrupt than the child's temperament can tolerate.

Causelist 71: Running away

"Running away" usually means going without parental permission, and establishing a base elsewhere, with food and shelter.

Sleeping rough for a night or two is similar – they have similar causes and a similar prevalence, about 7% of U.S. teenagers[1606]. At the severe extreme, seen in psychotic or badly abused children, sleeping rough carries its own risks: e.g. of frostbite, gangrene, and assault.

Running away overnight is a turning point in the child's life, and over the following year a teenage girl is twice as likely as non-runaways to start having sex: 84% of Malaysian prostitutes have run away from home[982]. Running away to a relative is much less risky.

Occasionally, some of the causes of children's running off (p.209) are relevant to a child's or teenager's running away.

Causes of running away	Notes
Not really running away	Some children learn to pack their bags, take a teddy, and say "right I'm going if you don't…" This is a learned behaviour to get their own way.
Causes in the child	
Following overriding interests	E.g. to be with boyfriend/girlfriend (especially if sexuality is not accepted by parents)
Following an example	E.g. a role model (real or fictional) ran away, or friends are having a party tonight.
Delinquency[1632]	Increases opportunities and contacts, and decreases monitoring.
Causes in the care	
Abuse	(See under Running off, p.209)
Poor monitoring	E.g. parents arguing, on drugs, doing shift work.
Strictness or harsh punishments, p.538	Can be abusive or merely over-strict, e.g. imposing curfew for weeks due to an infraction.
Neighbourhood	Feeling unsafe or victimised around home[1632]
School exclusion	Previous school exclusion increases the likelihood of running away, though there is no evidence that the running away is actually increased during the exclusion[1632].

Special Topic 7: Is this behaviour due to family dynamics?

Because anxiety can worsen almost any symptoms in a child, and because disrupted home life makes it more difficult for the parents to cope, unusual family dynamics often contribute to referral (see diagram, p.295).

Signs that family dynamics are contributory include symptoms being worse at home than at school, having their onset at the same time as the discord, and exacerbations similarly coinciding. Less specific but suggestive signs include parental arguments, mental illness and alcoholism, other children being affected and leaving home at an early age, or any sign of abuse (p.271). History from older siblings, adult relatives, and teachers is often invaluable (as is observation of the whole family, and occasionally the behaviour of parent-copying children).

The best documented situations in which family dynamics affect mental health are:

- relationships with mother, including attachment (pp.193,207,197).
- negative expressed emotion (p.512) which increases the likelihood of a relapse in schizophrenia (p.544).
- Anorexia nervosa (p.334), often worsened by conflicts in the family.

The converse: Family dynamics altered by an individual's problems
Here are a some examples: ADHD is not often worsened by family dynamics, but mothers' hostility to their sons *is* increased by ADHD[956]. Negative attributions (p.426) can make a small personal mistake spiral out of control into arguments or fighting. The same thing can happen if a parent and child doesn't know any way to get what they want apart from threats, shouting, and violence (or are too tired to think of those other ways): the result is a vicious cycle of escalating coercion, usually won by the parent at the cost of a worse relationship and a bad example for the child. Separation anxiety or OCD (p.65) can make an individual feel he has to impose his will on others in the family. Splitting (p.552) can have dramatic, usually disruptive, effects on interpersonal dynamics. Some children with autism or schizophrenia are fine when left alone, but become rapidly overwhelmed by their mother's closeness. Complex family interactions can result from one or more individuals' need to be wanted or to be cared for or to have a particular distance from (or relationship with) other family members – or from one child wanting to have the same privileges as another. Children with non-verbal learning disability (p.28) sometimes say obviously wrong things with a straight face, leading people to think they are being sarcastic or humorous (which can lead to bizarre conversations). Sibling rivalry (p.213) often results from parents' reactions to one child's strengths or weaknesses. ID in children causes a bereavement-like phase while parents recognise it and come to accept it, but also often a long-term sorrow exacerbated each time the child experiences extra difficulty or fails to meet a normal developmental milestone[517]. A child's behavioural problems in general contribute to maternal depression (p.174) which in turn has adverse effects on the whole family.

See also: parenting, p.189; unemployment, p.570; trauma, p.567; immigration, p.488; resilience, p.541

Most of the following can be emotionally abusive if sufficiently severe, though demonstrating the pattern does not by itself prove that the child's development is being damaged. Unfortunately there is no standard system for describing all these patterns or their effects on a child[398].

Table 10. Some patterns of family dynamics

Pattern	Notes
Chaos, or environmental confusion	This is the best environmental predictor of poor cognitive development[242]. It consists of: • noise, disorganisation, inconsistency (e.g. parents having different rules or different sanctions, or not reliably collecting child from school) • parents repeatedly intoxicated or mentally ill
Multiple stories	• Including telling the child lies (e.g. about parentage) that he knows are wrong • Double bind (see cognitive dissonance, p.355) • Family myths
Enmeshed	• Members are over-close, with little independence • Parent-as-sibling. For example, in some families grandparents are really in charge, often because of youth, anxiety, or ID in the child's mother. (see *subsystems*, p.213) • Grown-up sibling constantly disagreeing with parents on the treatment of a younger child
Combined families	• Stepmothers, stepfathers, stepsiblings • Stepchildren are sometimes cared for less well than biological offspring (the Cinderella effect includes an increase in abuse and homicide[364]). • Adoption (p.419) • Conflicts between real mother and whoever has taken over from her (e.g. stepmother, father, powerful aunt or grandmother)
Generation gaps	These are most severe in immigrant families where the values of teenagers often conflict with traditional cultural views (or with Westernised parents).
Abuse (p.271)	Abuse by a parent or sibling (see incest, p.489), carer, or outsider. Mother's attitude to the allegation of abuse can be critical (p.275).
Informal family	Especially in poor rural areas, children often live with relatives or friends, for practical reasons.
Similar or different	E.g. mild ID is often a characteristic of all family members; but severe LD usually affects one individual[1154]. Many common disorders such as anxiety, depression, and especially alcoholism are highly shared between family members.
Relationship to community	
Isolated families	Families that have little contact with the outside world are more likely to have mental illness, ID, and abuse. They are also less likely to obtain help.
Trapped wives	She may fear she will never find another partner; she may blame herself for the difficulties; or she may identify with her mother who also endured domestic violence. In non-mingling ghettos of recent immigrants, it can be almost impossible for a mum to flee to a refuge, where she and her children will be cut off from friends, family, school, religion, language, culture, and familiar food, and may become permanently ostracised.
Multigeneration families	
Grandparent-led	Grandparents can function as main carers, taking over from young or disabled parent. In practice, this prevents many parent-based interventions.
Skip-generation families	occurs when parents are working abroad or have died, e.g. from HIV.

continued ▶

A parent's influence	
Influence of parents' childhood	E.g. parents who were cruelly treated as children may be so frightened of being like their parents that they can impose no rules (and see p.201).
Single parent	Increases the risk of maternal depression, p.174. Children of a single parent are more than twice as likely to have a psychiatric disorder in childhood, and over three times as likely to abuse drugs (even after accounting for parental mental health and socioeconomic status)[1736].
Controlling	E.g. a tyrannical father (sometimes from another culture) tries to impose his will on his wife and children.
Parent in prison	p.535
Dyads	
Healthy	Healthy relationships include open discussions, individual flexibility, and mutual respect (p.191).
Parental discord	
Parental dominance / submission	Traditionally the man has had the greater say in major family decisions, but in practice either parent can. The submissive partner is often less able, or less energetic, or more flexible – or may be following the example of their own same-sex parent.
Stockholm syndrome	Identification with an imprisoner – or, by extension, with an abuser [796].
Sibling rivalry	• To some degree this is inevitable and normal. • The most common cause of significant problems is that parents have focused their care on the youngest, most disabled, or most troublesome child. The other children then escalate their behaviours to get their fair share of attention (e.g. proactive oppositionality, p.253; pseudo-behaviours, p.363) • The opposite happens when parents give all their attention to the wonderful child who is obedient and clever: if her siblings can compete they will, but if they can't they often become depressed or violent.
Mother-daughter	Usually worse during adolescence.
Subgroups within families	
Subsystems	The child subsystem and the parental subsystem need to be kept somewhat separate, and the parents need to have more power[1090,1447]. As well as these obvious groupings there can be more subtle *coalitions*, e.g. between mother and youngest child. These social patterns result directly from the way individuals behave and the way others habitually respond to them[1153]. Disruptive behaviour in a child (e.g. seen with drug taking) can reverse the hierarchy[612].

Roles of children

Adultification	A child having an adult's *role* in the family is a broader issue than his merely having adult *behaviours*.
	Examples of adult *roles* for children include:
	• A parent abdicates the parental role (for reasons of ability, philosophy), treating the child as an equal adult. In most societies, this gradually increases through adolescence.
	• Inappropriate adult demands,e.g.child labour,p.575; parental alienation, p.187; sexual abuse, p.275.
	• Parentification (or parentified *role*). This is common and healthy if the parents oversee the older children, who learn to oversee younger children. A rarer unhealthy pattern is the child not only doing chores, but also reassuring or even commanding the parent. This is most common where mother has mental health problems or the child is treasured (see below).
	Examples of *behaviour* being adult-like:
	• Pedantry, p.163; professorial voice in Asperger, p.424
	• Overconfidence or jocularity in hypomania, p.263
	• Careworn
	• Copying a parent, e.g. dressing like dad, p.441. Copying a parent's mature commands to the siblings is adultified behaviour, but it does not provide evidence for a parentified *role* if the siblings and parents ignore it.
Comparisons between parent and child (mini-me)	This can be driven by parent, the child, or others.
	• A parent may push the child to do what the parent wished he could do, or punish the child extra hard for actions the parent himself feels guilt for.
	• Alternatively the rest of the family can assume boy will be like dad (can be very damaging if dad was violent or committed suicide)
(excessively) treasured child	Children of assisted conception (p.424) or who had/have severe illness or disability can excessively dominate the lives of their parents and siblings. In some cultures, first-born sons have high status that can be reinforced by their mothers' treatment of them, and by their fathers' treatment of women.
Babied / overprotected / persistent infantilising	This can be driven by parent, the child, or others.
	• Contributory factors in the parents include difficulty conceiving; marital problems; mother identifying with the child (so enjoying being looked after) parents not wanting their last child to leave home; and occasionally a mother resenting the child and overcompensating for this feeling
	• Children competing with younger siblings or finding school or home too demanding.
Scapegoat, or other rejection	The child may then become depressed, aggressive, or frantically try to please parents.
Defective	In mild form this is pathologising (e.g. parents wanting a formal diagnosis to obtain help in school); when severe it is fabricated illness (p.359).
Stereotyped unwanted child	Usually with exaggerated contrast between the children. p.571
Child altering the family	To some extent this is inevitable and desirable, but there are specific problematic situations to look out for (p.211)
Others	Pet, peacemaker[1368]

School

Teachers

Teachers in primary school usually have a caring, almost maternal role. In secondary school the children move between classes and the parent-like role is sometimes taken by a school nurse or counsellor.

Underachievement and attention problems can arise when a child and teacher don't get on. This results from factors in both the child and the teacher[614,1007], or if the child resents the change from his previous teacher. Conversely, a teacher may be remarkably flexible, or cherish the child and accommodate many idiosyncrasies. Such differences become obvious when one teacher marks a hyperactive child's behaviour as uniformly excellent (e.g. on a Conner's questionnaire), and another in the same class marks it as troublesome.

Home schooling

This is a complex subject on which involved adults often hold very strong views (for a balanced overview see[345]). Virtual internet schools and home schoolers' clubs provide valuable support for committed parents. With good parental effort, the educational and social outcome for the child can be as good as that attained in mainstream education.

The situation of a child with many siblings or neighbours, being home schooled for philosophical or religious reasons, is obviously more positive than that of a child who cannot get to school due to needing life-support equipment at home, or one who is refusing to go to school (p.217) or one who has been excluded for difficult behaviour.

School leaving

School leavers can be categorised[437] as positive (leaving for a job), opportune (hoping they'll get a job), circumstantial (forced to leave by personal or family circumstances), discouraged (unsuccessful and disinterested in school), and alienated. A few are expelled or kept away by parents (e.g. due to vulnerability). "Reluctant stayers" stay only because they see no alternative.

The legal minimum school-leaving age (called the dropout age in USA) varies around the world. In Britain it is being raised in 2013 from 16 to 18; currently, postcompulsory schooling continues until age 18. For young people with special educational needs (including ID) the usual school-leaving age is 19 but aspects of educational provision continue to age 25.

Young people who leave school *before* the minimum legal age are at increased risk of unemployment, partial employment, and casual employment[1595]. In developed countries, they often continue their family's cycle of poverty, and are at greatly increased risk of criminal conviction (p.446). However if they find good employment, school leaving can be a positive experience for some. The situation is very different in poorer countries, where teenagers often leave school for paid employment (p.575) and the eldest girl may stay off school in order to help mother[463].

See also:

School refusal, p.217 (and *Refusal*, p.540); poor performance in school, p.27; school too easy, p.322; holidays, p.480; school as a cause of periodic problems, p.62; behaviour worse at home than school, p.80 and p.207; bullying, p.219; selective mutism, see below; practical emotions teaching, p.465; school's formulation, p.183; effect of drugs on schooling, p.267; effect of abuse on schooling, pp.274-275; hypoglycaemia after school, p.82; boredom, p.322; tic suppression in class, p.101; using school essays to assess deterioration, p.544; obtaining information from school, p.371; doing school observation, p.372; summer regression, p.45; *homework*, p.481; *inclusion*, p.489.

Causelist 72: School non-attendance

Truancy means being away from home and school without the parents' approval, usually concealing the non-attendance from them and often engaging in delinquent acts with peers. See adopting a new persona, p.237; breaking rules, p.249.

This section discusses only *school refusal*, in which children try to persuade their parents to let them stay home. This deserves attention if it happens more than once or twice a month.   There are often several additive factors (much the same as adults who don't enjoy their jobs are more likely to take time off when ill). An important aspect worth enquiring about is the impact on the family – e.g. does this lead to mother being exhausted or unable to work; does it undermine parents' authority with the other children and lead to their refusing school or other activities. See refusals, p.540. Consider using the School Refusal Assessment Scale (SRAS) [823] and [845].

See also *non-behaviours*, p.515.

Groupings Group by age…	Causes of school refusal
Age 5(peak A) Under 11	Separation anxiety (p.197). Not usually seen in clinics. • Acute onset with separation anxiety (p.197) triggered by life event (p.499) • Unrecognised major or minor learning problems • Not having the right clothes on or clothes not clean enough.
Age 11 (peak B) Over 11	Transfer to secondary school. This is common. Gradual onset, particularly in children with a tendency to withdraw in the face of challenge; poor self-esteem.
Age 14–16 (peak C)	• Acute onset, due to exams, depression (p.309), phobic anxiety, obsessions (p.517, e.g. fear of dirt at school). • Rarely: schizophrenia (p.543)
…or by source…	
☞ Problem in child	*Emotional* • 30% of school refusers have long-term externalising behaviour problems, 20% have anxiety or depression. • Within this anxious group, 40% separation anxiety (p.197), 30% social phobia (p.298), 20% simple phobia (p.307). • Consider OCD, p.65; bereavement, p.430; paranoia, p.524 *Cognitive* • ID; language impairments (p.145); dyslexia; NVLD (p.28): often overlooked. These upset the child who is told off or teased; and are exacerbated when he realises the extent of his problems, often age 10–13. *Other* • physical illness/pain, p.135; drug abuse, p.257; incontinence
Problem in family function (p.211)	• Enmeshed families (p.212) and families in conflict ([see 824]). • Families with no tradition of imposing their will on children. • Parents with anxieties (about self, or child at school) • Parents unable to get out of bed (alcohol, depression) • Some parents and grandparents support the child's devaluation of school, e.g. because they didn't go to school, or successful friends didn't.
or by pull v push	
Avoidance (p.429)	• Of unpleasant situations (presentations, noise, bullying: p.219); • Of travel, assembly, games, teachers (e.g. if told off), pupils (e.g. if bullied) • Of feeling stupid (see *cognitive* above);or depression, p.309 • Of separation anxiety (p.197) or other anxieties (p.307)
Obtaining	• Attention (usually from mother) • TV, computers, video games (p.573) • Couches, favourite food, friendly *au pair*. • Getting his own way

A child is bullied if he is exposed, repeatedly and over time, to intentional injury or discomfort by one or more other children[1193]. Bullying is not a simple operant behaviour involving the bully and victim, but a group behaviour involving relatively permanent social groups and differences in status[1421] (p.172). Bullying spreads if bullying or bullies are considered cool.

In some individual situations, sensitivity to the bullying is more of a problem, and more remediable, than the bullying itself. In other situations the bully or the bystanders are the problem. To work this out requires knowing whether this child is (or has been) affected by the bullying from other children as well, or by other stressors; and whether the bully bullies other children as well.

Prevalence

Being bullied becomes a substantial problem for about 10% of school children[1493], though milder difficulties (such as occasional teasing or throwing a PE bag out of the window) are almost universal. In 1999 in the United States, 80-90% of adolescents reported some kind of victimisation in school. Conversely, 80% of pupils aged 11-15 reported that they had personally engaged in "teasing, name calling, threatening, physical aggression or social ridiculing of peers" (see also *cyberbullying*, p.492).

Bullies and their behaviours

Bullies have problems of their own. Many have low self-esteem or have previously been exposed to bullying at home or at school.

Boys tend to bully physically, whereas girls use more social methods (e.g. spreading rumours, or persuading a victim to arrange a party, to which no one then comes). Female bullies are surprisingly popular, and are accepted as leaders by their peers. Male bullies, on the other hand, are not accepted leaders, even though *provoked* physical aggression does increase social status among boys[1421] (for examples in apes, also of violence achieving social status but not necessarily leadership, see[1427]).

The physical-or-social subtypes are not purely aligned by sex. Learning-disabled children are more likely to bully physically than socially[820]. They are usually unable to do social bullying in a mainstream school, but they can in a special school if they are among the most able.

Results of bullying.

Children's response to being bullied can be assertive, confrontational, help-seeking, self-distracting, or avoidant[1185]. If no such coping mechanisms are available they are likely to feel helpless, and eventually to become withdrawn or depressed.

Bullying by an individual seen as a leader can sometimes escalate into a mob attack on an individual victim, by other children copying the leader[482].

Children who defend the victim have the highest status among their peers[1421].

Causes of being bullied	Notes
Normal	Teasing is bound to happen occasionally. If it leads to tears, low mood, or school-avoidance one must assess not only the bullying itself, but other factors lowering the child's mood (p.311).
Factors in the child	Suggested by being bullied in several classes or schools.
Anything that singles out the child	Awkward movements, learning difficulties (even if not severe enough to be called ID[1753]), deafness, size (especially obesity), rashes or physical unattractiveness, physical disability, smell, clothes, race.
	Even factors that are not obviously teasable, e.g.: cleverness, can unfortunately single out a child (though the associated characteristics of bookishness, poor social skills or shyness are more likely to).
Anxiety, shyness or depression	Children soon learn who is frightened or ineffective in retaliation.
Lack of friends to stick up for him/her	• Newly arrived in school • Autism (p.183) or even mild social awkwardness • Previously offended lots of peers • Just a quiet person, or introverted[1494]
Additional stressors, low self-esteem	A child who could usually laugh off teasing may not be able to when she is worried about schoolwork, or about difficulties at home.
Exaggeration	Because of social difficulty, low self-esteem, liking parents' sympathy, or not having another way to criticise the school.
Genetic difference in response to stress	e.g. 5-HTTLP polymorphisms[140]
Factors outside the child	
Bystander attitudes[1302]	• Not wanting to be involved, or conversely, willing to join in • Admiration for, or fear of, ringleader
Ineffective management by school	• Minimising problems • Lack of effective anti-bullying policy in school • Inadequate supervision
Efforts by socially dominant peers to demonstrate their power	(see *status among peers*, p.172)

Play ☼

Every sort of behaviour can be performed *as play*. Considering all behaviours together, not just play, the simplest behaviours are repetitive (pp.474, 61, 63) or merely random (p.79). *Play* implies more than this, i.e. a degree of "see what happens" from challenge or experimentation. Much play includes exaggeration or surprise, such as a jack-in-a-box, a trampoline, splashing water, or a car that rolls fast. The simplest kinds of solitary play are often grouped as *self-entertainment* (p.545).

Beyond this, play can become more sophisticated along any of the axes of other interests (complexity, abstractness, changeability, social and language: see table on p.227). The following is after[154].

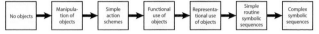

Figure 19. Stages in the development of play.

Generally toys acquire meaning (and a word or name) before they develop personalities, and later, multi-toy interactions reflect the child's social development. Storylines for play are usually made up on the fly, incorporating snippets from elsewhere (e.g. from films or bedtime stories). (See also observation of play, p.372. For milestones of play see[265].)

Types of play

Babble: p.429

Catch/Chasing games: one of the earliest interactional games, initiated by following on the outside of the group during a chase game, or by another child taunting, "You can't catch me!"

Cause-and-effect toys: e.g. press a button and something happens. Interest wanes after mental age 2–3.

Clever play: jigsaw puzzles, crosswords, chess, etc.

Creative play: includes any of the other kinds of play, as long as new goals/challenges are created by the child.

Exercise/physical/locomotor play: most children love running and jumping. One of the main motivations is exercise (see p.462). There can also be a challenge, e.g. to run faster than last time, or jump like Superman.

Exploratory play: discovering the properties of a toy, e.g. can this doll be undressed, does this plane fly. Children with profound ID often move around a room, opening doors, feeling in pockets, climbing over tables.

Free play: letting the child do what he wants. With few toys present this reveals his boredom behaviour (p.322). With many toys present, or free drawing, his interests can be discovered.

Hide-and-seek: can be controlled by an adult, in which case it is simply a *catch/chase* game with an added spatial element; or if controlled by the children it requires counting, keeping the eyes covered, variation in role, and turn taking.

Hobbies: p.480.

Imaginative / pretend play: includes role-play (p.222, e.g. dressing up), miniature worlds (e.g. a toy car representing a big one, as shown by the way it rolls or sounds; a box representing a car or ship; train sets are more complex but less imaginative), domestic play (pretending to hoover or make a tea party). Unlike imaginary friends and worlds (p.231), a child has no difficulty distinguishing *play* from reality. The complexity of this should increase to include more than one character, and a plot, by age 5.

Interactional play: see *social play*.

Parallel play: happy to be next to another child, doing the same thing, but not coordinating activities yet. This helps develop speech and social skills. It is the earliest *social play*, characteristic of 18 to 36 months.

Role-play: this is of individual roles from age 2 to 3, or social role-play from age 3 to 4 (e.g. nurturing play). Enacting an adult role is the main point, not the behaviours themselves – so the use of costumes, which are only available in some homes, is not relevant. Swordplay, etc., is discouraged in some antimilitaristic families. For sexual behaviours see p.269

Stages in the development of role-play
- Copying mother's patting or hugging of a doll.
- Copying mother's hoovering.
- Swearing after dad did
- Enjoying the feel or the complete enclosure of costumes
- Just leaping or roaring, no matter what the costume.
- Using a behaviour or a pat phrase (p.158) appropriate to the character. Since most children will wave a sword if given one, waving a sword when dressed up as a pirate is not necessarily role-play; but miming putting out a fire when dressed as a fireman is.
- Speaking on behalf of toys
- Using the character's accent.
- Being able to do this for more than one character.
- Making up a relevant story
- Being able to do this on the fly, interacting with another actor. Occasionally such roles become continuous (p.237).

Occasionally, an autistic child with normal intelligence plays in a special role-free way: for example, in virtual football, because he always wants Italy to win, he is happy to play "as France" so the game will permit him to make lots of own goals, causing Italy to win.

Rough-and-tumble / muscle play: mainly between boys, and father-son. Actual hitting is rarely used in play.

Social play: at 9–12 months they copy other babies, and from 12 to 24 months do parallel play with occasional comments such as "which is best?", "you do it". Flying aeroplanes are oriented to be seen by the other child, with sound effects, comments or questions. By age 3–4 this progresses to more imaginative, continuously interactive or competitive play. They learn to control aggression, and there are sometimes signals to show that this is play rather than real, such as funny voices, laughing and smiling. Children move fluidly between exploration, parallel play, rule-setting, imaginary play, rule-changing, etc. This builds the skills needed for conversation (p.144) and other interactions. See also non-play social milestones, p.55.

Soft play: describes a type of play equipment rather than a type of play.

Spinning play: p.104.

Structural / mechanical play: e.g. Lego (minimal social or verbal content). Can be done to a pre-set pattern or in a creative way.

Throwing: p.103.

Verbal / fantastic play: a form of imaginative play (see above) with the emphasis on the words. In NVLD (p.28), fantastic stories are sometimes told, their fantastic nature preventing the child from being teased for getting something wrong, and eliciting simple delight from the listener rather than a complicated answer.

Vertigo play: mixture of sensation-seeking (p.123) and experimentation, e.g. spinning (p.104), fairground rides.

"Sigmund Freud was of the opinion that sport, like many other things, existed mainly as a sublimation of the sexual drive, but if it were no more than that, great moments in sport would only be *nearly* as good as sex. What many sportsmen say is that sport can be more fulfilling than sex" [106].

"One thing is clear here and that is that when it is compared to sport, the sex in question is an impersonal matter. No one has suggested that sport is better, or even comparable, to making love with your wife, to the act of procreation. No: sport is compared more to conquest, to the winning of and sexual release within an unnamed partner." [106] In his book with Michael Parkinson, George Best describes becoming sexually aroused before football matches.

(See also non-specific causes of any dominating interest, p.229)

Causes of playing football	Notes
Constant	
Being in a team	Self-identity (p.237)
Enjoyment of the statistics	
Something to talk about with friends	(Useful for small boys, particularly those without great social skills).
While playing	
Physical activity	Enjoying using strength (and feeling good afterwards – see *opiates*, p.519)
Speed	
Following a role model	Usually a famous footballer
Thrill of fear	(E.g. of collisions)
Physical sensations	Trajectory of self, foot, and ball, the sound and feeling of impact
Competition	Power over the ball, inaccuracy, physical constraints, competitors, and audience
Enjoyment of well-honed skills	…and feeling oneself making progress
Group cooperation	Joining of minds, feeling the power of group.
Enjoying how you look, or how you look to others	E.g. wearing the right kit, or scoring a goal.
Love of the equipment	Boys can be very proud of a football. (George Best: "When I was a kid the the only thing I shared my bed with was a football. I know it sounds daft, but I used to love the feel of it. I used to hold it and look at it and think,'One day you'll do everything I tell you'").
Occasional/theoretical targets	
Achieving prowess / goal / winning the game / championship	Geoffrey Boycott: "I wanted to be the best batsman in the world, and I were the best batsman in the world. How can you talk about missing anything?"
Outdoing oneself	Mountain climbing / peak counting. Money, career, escape from ghetto.
Negative aspects	
Minimal social skills needed	Can ignore the other person or treat them as a "ball-returning machine".
Avoiding homework (p.481)	e.g. because not understanding homework
Fear of being worse than peers	

There are many reasons for youngsters to spend a lot of time with computers[553,934,1269]:

Causes of time on computers	Notes
To achieve something else (see also *internet*, p.492)	• social interaction (MSN and email, very common in girls) • virtual enjoyment of activities, e.g. horse-grooming, virtual football, extreme skateboarding, fighting • school projects • to pursue any dominating interest – p.229 • skill acquisition (e.g. typing, foreign languages) • pornography • art • doing something like dad, or like grownups • earning money • computer compensates for his own poor memory or poor handwriting
Something about the computers	• games that are highly exciting or give rapid feedback (that make even hyperactive children sit down) - see *video games*, p.573. • praise for a skill, including "praise" from the computer • gradual manageable increase in difficulty level • computers themselves as a dominating interest– p.229 *Less common:* • time to think • predictability
Inadequate parenting	The computer can be used as a babysitter, or the parent may not be able to control its overuse.
Dislikes	Avoidance of negative social feedback (which the computer doesn't usually give)
Avoidance	Children who are bullied in the playground during breaks can escape to the computer inside the school.
Addiction	(see MMORPGs, p.573)
Default mode	No other toys

Causelist 76: Playing with hair

It is more difficult to control handfuls of hair than just a few strands.
Moving a whole head of hair tidily requires dexterity, visual judgment, and
social confidence.

Playing with someone else's hair generally happens only when both people
are emotionally close, and relaxed. If the child only plays with the hair of
one specific person, the pattern (when, where, how) reveals much about
their relationship.

Causes of playing with hair	Normal examples	Abnormal examples
Likes hair whether or not on a person	Likes the colour, sheen, or texture, but life is not dominated by this.	Autistic: this interest dominates life or surpasses social interaction (p.229). May enjoy the gritty feeling of most hair; or the smooth feeling of eyebrows;or all hanging things, or all long things, or things attached at one end (e.g. arms too).
Own or other's hair		
Experimenting with different styles	Looking at self in mirror, or shared interest with friends.	
Bored; gratification phenomenon (p.474)	Twirling hair	
Deprivation		Stuck behind mother for protection or avoiding her gaze; nothing else to do. Maintains interest in peering over her shoulder. May make imaginary friends (p.231) out of her hair (or child's own long hair)
Someone else's hair		
Grooming	By women, of children or women friends. Varies between cultures.	Child grooming mother (normal only if copied from mother's enjoyment of playing with a daughter's hair, or as part of a bedtime ritual). May calm an anxious or depressed mother, or can be reinforced by mother who likes it.
Adoration, flirtation (emphasised by upward eye contact)	Courtship	Abnormal if done by a child
Copying	Mother is a hairdresser	
Wind-up	Steady pull; flicking	
Something to hold, that tugs back		An autistic girl pulled on people's hair or their collars, her speed incorrectly giving the impression of aggression
Own hair		
Itching (p.110)	nits	Unkempt, eczema, psoriasis
Hairpulling (p.117)		
Habit		

Causelist 77: Collecting stones

Like other sterile hobbies, this immediately raises suspicion of autism, but there are other reasons too.

Causes of collecting stones	Notes
Likes	Appearance, feeling, temperature, sameness/variety (sameness is much more sterile than variety). Copying someone else who collects. Loves mother's reaction when he puts it in his mouth.
Dislikes	Empty hand, having nothing to feel, having nothing to own.
To do something with	• School project, target practice, ☞ self-protection, making a wall, to sell, to give.
	• To focus on to calm self, e.g. in autism (p.183) or when overwhelmed by sensations (p.125)
Default mode	Unable to think of anything else to do

Preferences (General) ☼

Taking the history

Interests are not directly observable, so require more subtle analysis than actions. *Interests* fill the mind. Not all behaviours are due to interests; but those that are are generally accompanied by an interruption of the previous interest; orienting of the body or eyes, some affect, and a continuing reduction in awareness of other inputs. Only one can be pursued at a time (unlike tremors, spasms and habits). It is almost always possible to distract a child from them, though they do occasionally reach trance-like intensity (e.g. in autism or psychotic depression). Key aspects of an interest are *complexity, abstractness* and *changeability. Social* and *linguistic* interests are high on all these measures.

Table 11. Characteristics of constrained and broad interests

	Constrained interests	—Intermediate—	Broad interests
Sensory complexity (p.124)	Single items surfaces, tones	Lists pop rhythms, melody	Hierarchies crowd interaction, orchestra
Motor complexity	Single items tapping	Lists singing, lining up (p.500)	Multiple lines piano with 2 hands
Abstractness	Primary sensations feeling a wall	Patterns,sequences making a goal	Abstract playing chess
Changeability (p.234)	Annoyed if disturbed; even a trance posturing, gripping or gazing at an item	Exploratory, brief intrusions, evolves weekly rugby scores	Creative, rapidly changing conversation
Social (p.167)	Not about people collecting stamps to sort by color and size	*About* people learning about the people & events on the stamps	*Involves* people joins stamp club because best friend is member
Linguistic (p.143)	Non-verbal leaves, hair	Nouns trainspotting	Full language reading stories

Judging normality and severity

What interests are normal depends on the child's abilities and environment; but generally the complexity of interests increases with age and intelligence, and girls' interests are typically more social than those of boys. As long as they are age and sex appropriate, the following special interests can dominate many children's lives, especially in the school holidays, without obviously handicapping them: football, computer games (p.224), horses (p.248), High School Musical, pink (p.247), trainsets, cheerleading, stamp collecting. *Lack* of common interests such as TV or computer games demands an explanation. The same is true of *efforts to constrict* the focus, e.g. doing an activity while facing into the corner of a room.

Most people have both restricted and broad interests, which they move between depending on mood and alertness. An individual's *broadest* interests are generally (a) slightly challenging or novel, (b) not too difficult (see Gricean conversation, p.143), (c) multiple, (d) interesting to other children, (e) somewhat variable and evolving (with enlargement rather than increasing encapsulation). Judgment that special interests are interfering with life requires that he spends an inordinate amount of time on them (p.104) and that his life would be worse without them (especially with severe ID).

Some interests give a rough idea of developmental level (see p.55).

Establishing the cause(s) of a special interest
One diagnostic pitfall is to assume that a child's repetitive activities involve an *interest* at all, as there are many simpler causes (pp.63, 393). Another pitfall is to assume that the aspect of an activity that attracts the child is an obvious one (e.g. a child can like a cigar because his grandma smokes them, or as a penile symbol, or for its smell, or for countless other reasons).

The following may help to identify the multiple factors present in a case:

Table 12. Factors causing special interests

	Factors favouring specific content	Factors that increase repetitiveness in an individual
Predisposing	• The environment can favour certain content (e.g. sexual videos, violence, books) • Models to copy, e.g. families that do something repetitively	• Autistic spectrum ☛ (see monotropism, p.509) • ID • Compensation, e.g. a child with poor language can develop special interest in drawing.
Precipitating	• Experimentation • Whatever was happening when the interest first arose. • Whatever happened straight after the first time (see superstitious learning, p.558).	• Anxiety • Sleepiness
Perpetuating	• Self-image. • Simple sensory appreciation (e.g. stroking hair, sculpture, liking the sound of a phrase). • Enjoys reaction from others	• Can't find better interests • Enforced rules about what can or cannot be done • Lack of rules (e.g. family not correcting bad behaviour).

Sometimes one can account for a special interest in terms of a disorder. In order to do this, one needs to establish that it cannot be adequately be explained as a normal hobby (above), and that it fits known characteristics of the disorder. For example, the ***content*** is characteristically sterile in autism (p.554); depressive in depression; grandiose in mania; food in anorexia nervosa; cleanliness (etc.) in OCD (p.65); paranoid (p.524) or bizarre in schizophrenia (p.543).   ***Timing*** also helps to establish the cause: autistic people use their interests most in novel situations; anxious or dissociating people (p.453) when stressed; imaginary worlds (p.231) are used most when lonely (p.500); and normal hobbies are most used when bored. Some behaviours ***appear*** before the child has any beliefs about them at all (e.g. OCD); they later acquire explanations that make sense to the child. Psychotic beliefs also appear out of the blue (p.348), often as a solution to a conundrum, and also become increasingly complex over time.

However each standard disorder category can be reached via a wide variety of routes (Table 12), which are often more useful in guiding treatment than the broad diagnostic category. Several such causes can work together to create a dominating interest, as in the child with ID who becomes more repetitive when sleepy; a girl who has a mild normal preference to be thin but becomes much more focused on this when her parents are fighting; a rigid boy with an interest in hamsters who uses this as a reason to avoid school; a child who can't excel and so adopts an obscure interest to impress people.

Causelist 78: Dominating interest ☼

Causes of dominating interest	Content	No.of interests	Duration of interests
Normal			
Sensory	Pleasant, varying sensations, e.g. washing and splashing running water	Several	Unlimited duration, but never dominates life unless coexisting with other causes below.
Learned	Same as someone else, esp. father. May be learned too strongly.	(ditto)	(ditto)
Folie imposée	(see odd ideas section: p.347)		
Autism-related	For the relationship between autistic interests and autistic behaviours, see p.64.		
Autism ☛ (p.183)	"Sterile" things that would not fascinate most people (p.554). The autistic person can appear to be in a trance, completely focused on his interest. The interest is definitely not resisted, either because these are the only interests of the child, or (perhaps in a minority) because they are so crucial to his control of anxiety.	One or few	See *duration issues*, p.104. When it does evolve, this is often to a closely related, similarly sterile interest (e.g. wheels → trains → Tube trains → bus numbers). A good sign of useful maturation is interests that become more broad or socially relevant (e.g. wheels → trains → Tube trains → tube systems of the world → Tokyo tubes → Karate) or more like people (e.g. rocks → planets → rockets → Star Wars; or robots → dinosaurs)
Asperger's ☛ (p.424)	These people have good language ability so their interests are much more complex than in autism. Their interests can also have secondary roles such as learning about bookish misfit role-models (Harry Potter or Sherlock Holmes); or learning about people in a safe detached way (law, Guiness Book of Records); impressing peers; or protecting self-esteem.	depends on mental age	
Protected social exploration	Vast social content but one-way (e.g. films, law reports, wedding videos).		(Could evolve to internet research then internet chatrooms and socialising)

Inflexible temperament (pp.234,561)	Normal	(ditto)	May change more slowly than in normal children – i.e. years; or change can be more painful. Perhaps distinguish speed of change of this minute's plans, versus long-term hobbies & goals.
Language impairment (p.145) ↑	Can be somewhat impaired due to lack of social and language input.		Matures and broadens like other children, but slower.
Anxiety related			
Childhood rituals / OCB	(p.63)		Age 2–8.
☞ OCD	Based on worries. Usually but not always resisted. Often characteristic content (p.65).	(ditto)	Many years
Separation anxiety (p.197)	Can appear similar to OCD but not resisted (see caveat on p.65).		
Phobias	Not really a "dominating interest" because it disappears when the feared object is not nearby		
Performance anxiety (p.298)	Can make a child stick to performances that he knows he can do easily.		
	Conundrum 12: Avoidance or autistic preoccupation Distinguish this from a real dominating interest by (a) seeing what he does in free play or drawing; (b) judging his long-term degree of interest by the level of specialist knowledge he has accumulated; (c) asking the child to draw something even simpler, but from outside the putative dominating interest.		
Tics (p.101)	Most tics are not an *interest*, as shown by the fact that several can occur simultaneously (in some children) and that they can occur in the middle of a sentence without interrupting it (even a "shut up" tic can). However, many children with tics develop an *interest* in preventing them, which can severely impair classroom concentration. *Very* rarely, a	Several	

continued ▶

child enjoys the social impact of a tic, so choosing the right time, audience, and performance then becomes an *interest*.

Some experts suggest that the desire to achieve a particular feeling (e.g. cracking knuckles, straightening, matching sides) is a *sensory tic*, though it could also be described as a temporary sensory *interest*. When a person wants to achieve a particular sensation, many muscle groups can be used together. For example, if a child wants to achieve a particular feeling of twisting his neck, he may use both hands to do this, and simultaneously close his eyes to allow him to focus on it; the final movements are quite slow and precise, and when he gets the right feeling all these muscle groups simultaneously resume their previous activities.

To calm mother	Grooming-like activities can calm mother, and make a bedtime routine that both enjoy. A child who is bored with this can make it more interesting by weaving it into an imaginary world (see below).	Few	Indefinite
Imagination, or "overactive imagination"	This term does not imply that great imagination is used: the simplest imaginary worlds are most likely to cause repetitive behaviours and hence to be referred, often with a query about autism. Ruling out autism is not sufficient because the simplicity of the imaginary world is sometimes caused by ID and/or severe social deprivation. The content of the world is usually either extra sociable or extra exciting or extra complimentary, depending on the child's needs. The key to the diagnosis is that a situation or game is invoked at appropriate times of deprivation such as boredom (p.322) or loneliness (p.500), and has content that compensates for the triggers. It is common until age 7 or so. *We must all, in order to make reality more tolerable, keep alive in us a few little follies.* (Marcel Proust, Remembrance of things past).		
Imaginary friends	Always welcome, used to overcome a felt need (e.g. social deprivation, maternal deprivation, p.174; anxiety). Can be human, animal, ghost, robot, etc.	Depends on IQ, age	These can also be described as defence mechanisms (p.305) and/or as dissociation (p.453). They persist until no longer called

	If a doll is available, the child may have a conversation with it; this is not usually called imaginary friends even though cognitively and emotionally it is the same. The content and the timing indicate the underlying motivation, and the frequency indicates severity.		for by the situation; or until superseded by other defenses. They may be revealed in later life when stress overwhelms more recent defenses.
Imaginary ideas	e.g. "I am a robot" to avoid feelings of vulnerability	(ditto)	(ditto)
Imaginary worlds	A forerunner of dissociative states (p.453): an imaginary world which may come from a film/book. To help him/her stay in this state, the child may avert his eyes, cover his ears, or look at picturebooks or magazines of popstars. Compare *daydreaming*, p.450.	(ditto)	(ditto)
Imaginary play (p.221)	Normal. More varied than imaginary friends/worlds. Child knows it is unreal		
Acquired			
☞ Psychosis / schizophrenia (p.543)	Accompanied by deterioration in other areas. Catatonia (p.98) may resemble OCD rituals (p.65). Even if there are no hallucinations or delusions, the reduced self-monitoring allows more bizarre ideas to be used within other frameworks described in this table.		Duration of psychosis (plus time to question then supersede these ideas, which can be very long in rigid or ID people)
Acquired epileptic aphasia	Develop sterile interests (p.554)		Landau-Kleffner syndrome (p.45)
Temporal lobe epilepsy (p.562)	Deficit in social interaction		
Symbolic	(p.14)		
Communica-tion	Even numerous communications do not constitute a dominating interest. Communication may be intentional or not (as in semantic priming). Partial concealment can allow the child to check the listener's views.		
Repressed ideas (p.421)	e.g. interest in aliens because he identifies with them; interest in boxing as a safer version of preoccupation with parents' arguments.	Few because so emotional-ly loaded	

Causelist 79: Difficulty changing what he's doing

Persistence of states is a key aspect of a person. Some people prefer variety and only become inflexible when stressed, but others are attracted to routines. Most of us become more inflexible in stressful states such as exhaustion or starting a new job, when we have few options in our repertoire, and feel we need to stick with the most familiar ones.

Generalised severe rigidity is often found in autism (p.183, with non-engagement), and in NVLD (p.28, with fluent non-comprehension often accompanied by anxiety). In other conditions rigidity is often an underlying temperamental characteristic, but is characteristically *most severe on a topic* which has led to referral. Examples of this include anorexia nervosa, p.334, OCD (p.65), cognitive dissonance (p.355), prejudice and hatred (pp.187, 282).

Even though prolonged focus on most topics is benign (e.g. hobbies and homework), persistence is a characteristic of all conditions that deserve a diagnosis. Inflexibility is often hastily ascribed to oppositionality (p.253) or to Asperger's (p.424). Many other causes are listed on the following pages.

Conundrum 13: Short-, medium- or long-term rigidity

The longevity of rigidity, is often key to understanding a child, and working out how to help him.

a) Life-long (trait) rigidity[1445] tends to very gradually ameliorate. It causes characteristics such as black-and-white thinking, perfectionism, egocentrism, bossiness, unimaginativeness and a tendency to rages (p.71)[696]. A few have a specific learning disability (p.551) or extinction deficit (p.463). Some cases are severe enough to justify a diagnosis of autism or ASD (p.183).

b) Rigidity imposed by enduring stresses or mood. Anxiety or low mood or physical illness can make a child resist doing anything novel or challenging.

c) Rigidity created by the situation: fear (p.307), exhaustion, crossness, and many other factors in the table below. In some cases rigidity may be learned, by long reinforced practice, social learning, punishment, or even abuse. In such cases the rigidity is usually confined to specific social relationships, or societally relevant rules or rituals. It is important to discover these triggers for rigidity, in order to reduce them (see frozen watchfulness, p.470; oppositionality, p.253).

The categories do not neatly separate because the kinds of rigidity are cumulative: a child with innate rigidity is more likely to resist changes in learned lessons, or to have mood-based rigidity; and a child with mood-based rigidity is more likely to be situationally rigid as well (much as anxiety and intolerances add up, p.125)

This is difficult to identify with certainty if the onset of the problem was before school entry, though home videos taken before and after a change can be very helpful. Home videos can also help you to believe the parents' description of the occasional child who behaves very differently at bedtime, or out of the blue.

For broader issues see avoidance, p.429; and fight-flight-freeze (p.296)

Table 13. Types of rigidity / inflexibility

Note there is no standard terminology for this.

Sensory
- Being upset when things around him change (intolerance, p.125).
- Difficulty in unlearning things (p.571).

Behaviours driven by self
- Not spontaneously varying what he chooses to do (testable using a repetitive drawing task). A severe version of this is perseveration (p.527).
- Not adjusting his behaviour according to the situation. This can be due to overriding interests (p.229), rituals and rules (p.353), social disinterest, cognitive limitations (such as the task switching deficits in OCD[626]), or lack of learning experiences[14].
- Adjusting his behaviour to the situation, but in an idiosyncratic way that observers only discover by chance, e.g. able to eat a crisp from a piece of paper but not from a table; another boy was cooperative in situations that reminded him of school but regressed and un-cooperative in situations that remind him of home (with his little brother present competing for attention).
- Dictating what other people do. This quite common in OCD (p.65), when it is often enforced by rages (p.71). It also occurs when a child has difficulty quickly understanding other people's variants of rules for a game.
- Pedantry (p.163).

Behaviours driven by others
- Difficulty in listening to, understanding, or accepting suggestions. The following are increasingly difficult changes that can be tested in clinic:
  - ▶ Accepting help with a choice of where to put something down
  - ▶ Accepting suggestions while playing, e.g. having decided to draw, accepting someone's idea of what to draw
  - ▶ While unoccupied, agreeing to draw
  - ▶ When he wants something, agreeing to do x or y first, with no time limit
  - ▶ When engaged in drawing, being asked to start a different drawing
  - ▶ While doing an enjoyed task, agreeing to write numbers
  - ▶ While doing an enjoyed task, agreeing to do something foolish, or something he dislikes, with no explanation.
- Intolerance of not understanding (p.126).
- Not accepting that there is more than one way of doing things; or not remembering and following these.
- Difficulty separating what he believes from what he does; or difficulty doing something he thinks is wrong just to please someone or as an experiment.
- Refusals, p.540; non-behaviours in general, p.515; contradicting people, p.162; ignoring instructions from particular people.
- Failure to unlearn (p.571).

A child may suffer from several of these problems, each appearing in certain situations, plus long-term (trait) levels of rigidity and anxiety. For planning any remedial measures, the key distinction is between difficulties about the *state*, and difficulties about the *change* (see next table). Usually this distinction is easily worked out by comparing the situations in which he is most and least flexible.

continued ▶

Causes of difficulty changing what he's doing	Notes
Issues about current state	
Likes what he's doing now	A careful assessment of the child's level of unwillingness when switching from activity A→B versus B→A can be useful.
Liking continuity	Equal difficulty leaving either home or school.
Liking doing nothing	Rare in healthy well-rested children and teens.
Issues about the new state	
Not liking what is offered	More difficult going to school than to McDonald's; or frightened that he won't do well in the new situation.
Not understanding what is offered	E.g. in ID
Anxious about what might accompany the change	E.g. social anxiety, p.298 (this fluctuates with the child's overall anxiety) E.g. unable to perform rituals in new place
Issues about the change – a. external	
Disliking something that accompanies the change	E.g. disliking the speed of preparation, or travel
Unreasonable speed of change	E.g. if parent or other child is impatient (e.g. impulsive, p.79) and changing tasks often
Disliking the method of presenting the news, or the bearer of it	Consider parental bossiness or short temper. Child and parent might both be rigid, causing inevitable clashes.
Issues about the change – b. internal	
Trying to assert status	Disappears when request for change comes from respected people.
Not having a reason to change	Insistence on having a reason may indicate a basic inflexible personality, or may be learned from parents' practice of explaining.
Oppositionality	(p.253)
Cognitive limitations	Having a limited repertoire of things to say, i.e. it is a lot simpler to say "no I don't want to" than to compromise, negotiate, or work out an alternative.
An underlying belief that makes the proposed change untenable	• A rigidly held belief such as "If you eat something straight off the table you get germs and die." • He may think that being moved on to a different task means he's failed at this task (often happens in cognitive testing) or be an admission he was wrong. • Not understanding that he can return soon to his preferred task (or that a toy taken from him will soon be returned). • A new idea can have unacceptable cognitive dissonance with existing ideas (p.355).

continued ▶

Unable to change set

Inflexibility imposed by anxiety	• In autistic spectrum conditions ☞ (p.183), special interests serve in many cases to reduce anxiety. • In OCD (p.65), compulsions are experienced as reducing anxiety, and so being thwarted feels extremely dangerous. • Preoccupations (as in depression, or when life feels insecure with parents constantly fighting) can have a similar effect. • Fear of forgeting what he is doing, or not getting it done in time.
Basic rigid inflexible personality	People with tics (p.101) are often inflexible. Schizotypal disorder is associated with rigidity.
Only child (p.518)	Particularly with over-acccommodating or depressed parents, when there are few other children around.
Slow learning	Willing and able to follow an example just shown him, but needs many trials to learn to make this transition automatically, and to perform it without supervision.
Perseveration	(p.527)
Starvation	(p.553)
Stimulants	Occasionally, even a low dose of stimulants will make a child with ID so fixated on tasks (such as colouring in, or searching on the internet) that he may be thought autistic.
Non-cognitive	See causes of repetitive behaviours, pp.61–67.

Causelist 80: Adopting an identity/persona

Self-identity

A person's *self-identity* (or self-concept), consists of ways in which he is similar to other people – or different from them. Most people develop a self-ideity that is an amalgam of *people* (television characters, sports stars, and people they actually know) and *groups* they belong to. People are sometimes said to identify with a *label* that has been applied to them, but most of these involve actual people and groups (see[1800]).

One identifies with groups based on (or understands oneself in terms of) many individual characteristics shown in the table below. All of these characteristics require patterns of behaviour that need to be learned, experimented with, and calibrated to the current society[848].

Self-knowledge is a broader notion than self-identity, including as well an ecological self (relating to the immediate physical environment), an interpersonal self (relationships with other people), the temporally extended self (with memory and anticipation), and the private self[1139].

Aspects of identity	Associated problems
Gender	Gender dysphoria, p.267
Name	(p.239)
Age	(for examples see *Living one's identity*, below)
Family	One's identity can be opposed to the family, or part of it.
Sexuality	(p.239)
Body image	Attractiveness; Body dysmorphic disorder (p.433)
Religion	(p.541)
Intelligence	If a child has mild ID, his self-esteem can be protected to some degree if he and his family maintain an acceptable identity, e.g. believing he only has problems with reading and writing; or believing that he has been let down by the school.
Conformity	Girls tend to value conformity more than boys, and this contributes to depression and anorexia nervosa (p.334). The value placed on fitting in varies between cultures.
Health	Chronic illness can change self-identity in many ways that depend on not only the physical effects but also their own, their friends', and sometimes their religious interpretation of the illness[1388]. (See also sick role, p.487).
Diagnoses	Teenagers do not find diagnoses such as autism simply bad or good or painful, rather they look at practical questions such as what the diagnosis explains in their life, whether it reduces bullying, whether it is better than their previous self-identity (e.g. "alien" as one boy said) and whether it changes their life hopes[737].
Disability	E.g. disliking the way disabilities are described[1825]
Possessions	Teenagers often try to define themselves, and understand others, on the basis of their possessions (e.g. Converse trainers, hat, etc.)[416].
Other	E.g. nationality, ethnicity, class, caste, race, school, gang, club, clique, sportiness, laziness, conformity, fashionableness, interests, strengths and weaknesses, future expectations for self
Status: popularity, "cool" and whether one is *liked*	If stable these can become part of one's identity, but they are discussed separately (p.172) because they are more fluid and more actively sought.
Permanence	Self-identity can switch between learned states in multiple personality conditions (p.510).
Automaticity	Usually one's identity doesn't need to be thought about. If it becomes an object of preoccupation it can be disabling

Identification with a known person
This is an important aspect of maturation, as when children copy their parents' behaviours and beliefs.

Identification with a real person often alters behaviour towards that person. So a mother who identifies with her child can be overprotective (p.214) or excessively demanding (p.214) or damaging (see Munchausen by proxy, p.206). Staff also need to be able to empathise (temporarily identify) with children and patients, in order to understand their behaviours and their difficulties.

Identification with a real person also affects behaviour when that person is not present. Outside observers will see a girl using the same stance and phrases as her mother. A boy who identifies with his mentally ill father will soon be wondering what it feels like to be mentally ill, and will wonder when he will become like dad.

Identical actions do not always indicate identification
If a girl does what person X did, identification with X is just one possible explanation. There are many others:

- to test whether she can do it
- to show she can do it better (or can't)
- because she is similar to, or has similar motivations to X
- just coincidence: she does the action for reasons different from X's, such as experimentation or because it's *right* or because someone else did it.
- because X is popular (or a hero or attractive), and she wants to be too (p.156). People are especially likely to copy a powerful oppressor if they feel weak, as in the Stockholm syndrome, p.213.
- because X was oppressed, and she is too, so she might as well submit to having the same life story (p.212)
- because she likes imagining herself as X (for the above reasons or other ones (see p.237) and doing the action helps the imagination.
- because she feels she *is* X (some call this *total identification*).

The choice of person (or thing, p.232) to identify with is important as it usually indicates the motivation (akin to the motivations for *imaginary friends*, p.231).

The presence of mirror neurons (p.507) suggests that identifying with other people (temporarily and to a limited degree) may be a routine part of observing and understanding them[1187].

Lifestyles (living one's identity)
Self-identity can be remarkably inflexible. This can cause problems, e.g. if a 15-year-old sees himself as an adult and the others in his class as completely childishly incompatible, he will usually stop participating in education (perhaps in an attempt to reduce cognitive dissonance, p.355). As a more common example, if a preteen girl identifies with a teen idol, it can feel insulting or even traumatic not to be allowed to wear makeup, and to spend a lot of time on it.

The range of intensity varies from mere interest, to occasional adaptations of manner or phraseology (see *styles of interaction*, p.162), to party or weekend "role-players", to permanent lifestyle shifts of varying degree including name change, and finally to conviction of beliefs or identity.

Lifestyles are correlated with important health issues. For example, Goth subculture has a 50% prevalence of self-harm (p.317), compared with 25% for Punk and Garage subcultures, 7% for Pop and 0.3% for Indie[1811]. Self-selection and modelling by group members both contribute. Somewhat

continued ▶

similarly, early sex, multiple sexual partners, and same-sex sexual behaviour are correlated with increased suicide attempts [1757]: 75% of lesbian, gay, and bisexual youths are verbally abused, 15% are physically attacked, and 33% lose friends because of their sexual orientation; and 37% make a suicide attempt[352].

Some people live their identity for a conscious reason such as fun or friendship; in others the identity affects their choices in more subtle ways.

One mechanism is the unpleasant feeling of cognitive dissonance (p.355) that a person feels when he acts out of character. He will also not want to do anything that endangers group membership. Self-identity could be described as changing during physical illness, especially if prolonged (p.487). The resulting behaviours often help overcome physical illnesses, but they carry the risk of perpetuating psychological conditions (p.323).

Changing identity
Identities and lifestyles are not fixed. Many examples are in the table at the right.

Changing names
Societies differ in the extent to which name changing is permitted. In some societies transitions in life are marked by name change, and the most common examples of this are at marriage or divorce. Adding "Madame" or "Doctor" is similar. Changes can be made on immigration simply in order to have a more pronounceable name, or can indicate a need to avoid ethnic prejudices[221]. Change of gender usually necessitates name change.

Some parents change their children's names, and may give the child a major say in this. The change can be in law or simply in practice. The child may do so in order to indicate the parent they feel closer to. They may be more sensitive to the name's connotation than their parents; or the parents may not have noticed what the child's initials would spell.

Occasionally, name changing indicates a problem. Reasons given for name changing by long-term psychiatric inpatients include the innocuous (avoiding teasing, disliking the old name, adopting a pet name, choosing a simpler name, thinking it was a "good idea"); common relationship issues (making or breaking family ties, wanting to protect others, or wanting to change to a pre- or post-adoption name) and the more unusual: starting a new life, religious meaning, deceit (e.g. to escape creditors), wanting the power or notoriety of a name (very worrying if satanic), or wanting to change personality[1689].

Repeated name changing or use of multiple names simultaneously is very unusual. It can indicate confused self-identity, preoccupation with names themselves, Munchausen syndrome, or pseudologia fantastica (p.256)[609,1689].

Choice of a bizarre name may indicate psychosis and the reason for the choice should be investigated[1689].

Causes of adopting a new or odd persona	Notes
Pulls: attractors	
Group identity	Adolescence is probably the time when people most need to feel they are members of a group.
	• This need is greater if they have low self-esteem, or if they expect failure. If positive groups are not sufficiently welcoming, negative ones will be joined: see *deviant peers*, p.49; *gangs*, p.472.
	• Lesbians, gays, and bisexuals move from first awareness, typically at age 6–13, to self-labelling about age 12–17, first disclosure (p.452) at 14–19, and first disclosure to a parent at 15–19[352]. The "gay" lifestyle usually has a simple sexual meaning for early adolescents, but as they mature many gay teens adapt their persona, either to fit in with a smaller subgroup or to find a persona that is more individualised[678]
	• Adoption can partly change self-identity.
Copying a role model	• The range of role models is enormous here, including family members, teachers, friends, deceased relatives, cartoon characters, and the most noble – or powerfully evil – characters.
	• Children who are more exposed to computer games than to other people occasionally develop an American accent (not a whole identity).
	• The vampire "scene" offers powerful and seductive role-models wearing elegant clothes, with only a small minority involved in actual "blood play" (see http://vampires.meetup.com/120).
Establishing a strong identity to reduce bullying, or increase self-confidence	E.g. small boy dressing as superhero; children and teens defining themselves by clothing or brands (p.237). Less commonly, an adolescent who feels a failure in school can adopt punk style to show they have made a lifestyle choice rather than failing.
To express maturation	(p.244)…or to emphasise being different from parents
To match self-identity	• E.g. as gay / imaginative / odd / violent / alien
	• One's role in a job or gang can become an identity
	• Within families, trivial differences between children are often noticed, commented on, and inadvertently reinforced.
Pushes: Avoidance / dissatisfaction	
To avoid interaction	Due to teasing, low self-esteem, or poor social skills. Bookish and aggressive personas work for this.
Experimentation	Short timecourse or variable persona
To annoy parents	
Pulls and pushes or neither	
To express immaturity	Baby talk and many other related signs (p.43).
Medical	E.g. changes in health and diagnoses (p.237)
Not constrained by social group	(Due to characteristics of individual or group). See disinhibition, p.261.
No interest in appearance	E.g. in ID, depression (muted colours), Asperger's (p.424)
Drug abuse	(p.257)
Mental illness	• Odd, over-individualised, appearance such as wearing redundant clothes, dark glasses, or odd tattoos can result from odd ideas (p.347) or paranoia (p.524) [251]
	• Depression and borderline personality increase the rate of changing appearance[251].
	• Grandiosity can result from mania (p.264).

Special Topic 8: Does this teen have a personality disorder ♣?

Personality

This comprises the long-term social and emotional characteristics of an individual; sometimes also used to include his values and habits. This shapes the person's life experiences, e.g. his susceptibility to bullying [1494].

Often personality is regarded as a minor or vague characteristic that barely needs to be considered in diagnosing serious behavioural problems. However the personality (or temperament) preceded most post-infancy behavioural problems, and is an important part of understanding why those problems arose. Hence personality is the basis of assessment according to OPD-2 (p.519), though we would argue that consideration of developmental level is even more fundamental (see discussion, p.15).

There are several ways of describing personality, of which the most commonly used is the five-factor model. The five factors are (see [268,1627] for more information):

- Neuroticism / negative emotionality
- Extraversion / positive emotionality
- Openness-to-experience / intellect
- Agreeableness
- Conscientiousness / constraint

There are many other suggestions as well, such as a dominance trait[1451] linked to testosterone, p.554; and defence style, p.305.

Temperament (p.561) is a term used to describe individual characteristics in infancy; it has much in common with personality[268]. Both systems describe liabilities to psychopathology (Figure 3 in[1161]).

Personality disorder ♣

This is defined in DSM as "inflexible, deeply ingrained, maladaptive patterns of adjustment to life that causes either subjective distress or significant impairment of adaptive functioning". The named characteristics are often not permanent in adults (contrary to common belief, see [935]) and even less so in children. Use of the term becomes increasingly inappropriate as you move further below age 18, and is often experienced as pejorative. Diagnoses of personality disorder are inadvertently encouraged by our inbuilt *fundamental attribution error*, p.18. Nevertheless, there is some continuity from characteristics of temperament seen in infancy, to patterns of behaviour in adulthood.

The most commonly used system to categorise personality difficulties is DSM. Within this, individual personality disorders are grouped into three clusters. The broader categories (clusters) probably have more long-term validity than the specific named disorders; for example Cluster A have more avoidant attachment and Cluster B have more aggression[335].

Multiple Personality Disorder is not a PD (p.510). For the position of PD in the diagnostic hierarchy see p.15. See also *passive-aggressive*, p.525.

The DSM categories of PD (with adult prevalences[1615]) are:

Cluster A (odd or eccentric)

Paranoid PD (2.4%). (cf. paranoid, p.524).

Schizoid PD (1.7%). This term is used only in adults, describing people who are severely socially detached and restricted in the communication of emotion (very similar to the definition of Asperger's; they may be the same: see p.427).

Schizotypal disorder or schizotypal PD (0.6%). This includes odd ideas and paranoia (p.524). It is genetically related to *schizophrenia* but without evidence of long-term functional decline.

Cluster B (dramatic or erratic)

Antisocial PD (0.7%). Essentially an adult equivalent[1096] for *Oppositional Defiant Disorder*, p.519 and *Conduct Disorder*, p.249. A subgroup have *psychopathy*, p.280.

Borderline PD (0.7%). Signs include unstable personal relationships, frantic attempts to avoid abandonment, emotional instability (p.70), impulsivity, self-harm, feelings of emptiness, dissociation, pseudohallucinations (p.345); *splitting* (p.552). Many have been abused. See duration of feelings, p.285; dyscontrol causing aggression to self and others, p.69; *manipulative*, p.504.

Histrionic PD (2.0%). Egocentric (p.180) but highly social, dramatic, flirtatious and manipulative (p.504). Some have subtle cognitive deficits. Compare *histrionics*, p.479.

Narcissistic PD (0.8%). The DSM definition focuses on the grandiose aspect of *narcissism* (compare p.511). This may arise from an extreme need for praise, or it may simply be a habit learned from parental over-indulgence. It is associated with steroid abuse (p.258).

Cluster C (anxious or fearful)

Avoidant PD (5.0%). These people limit their behavioural repertoire far more than seems to be necessary given their intellectual and social abilities. Avoidant PD and social phobia (p.298) sufferers share a common genetic susceptibility, but the former adopt quite different lifestyles, perhaps because they are permitted (by the environment or other aspects of their personality) to do so[1323].

Dependent PD (1.5%). This is a combination of self-perceived incompetence, with attachment behaviours persisting through adolescence into adulthood[629]. They are often happy for others to make decisions for them. It is often more noticeable in males because it is more at odds with their traditional gender roles.

Obsessive-Compulsive PD (1.7%). The relationship between this and OCD (p.65) is debated. Both are distinct from mild obsessionality or perfectionism, which is usually a source of pride to the individual as it leads to praise in school and at work.

Preferences (Specific) ☼

Causelist 81: Acting camp

Camp is an exaggerated form of speech and gesture (a set of mannerisms, p.505). Camp overlaps with (so can be confused with) other styles including feminine, gay, thespian, foppish, American, English private school / Oxbridge, kitsch, nasal, lisping, and youthfully exuberant. Camp, however, as Susan Sontag observed, means seeing or performing "in quotation marks… To perceive Camp in objects and persons is to understand Being-as-Playing-a-Role" [1515].

Camp has many underlying motivations:

Causes of acting camp	Notes
Group membership	Being homosexual and wanting to be a member of that group and/or to be recognised as such. The *gay voice* is not simply an exaggeration of normal prosody but has many precise characteristics such as prolonged s and z sounds. It is not a reliable indicator of sexuality [885]. It can be a way of "showing fearlessness, of thumbing their noses at gay bashers." (Gay Glossary)
Expressing one's sympathy with particular role models	
Copying TV presenters	E.g. from a favourite gameshow – if the presenter uses exaggerated (camp) gestures. This is occasionally seen in autistic children, particularly ones who are good mimics and rote learners in other areas, and who repeatedly watch the same programme.
Social interaction as playing a role	This is occasionally seen in high-functioning autistic people who crave social interaction, if it does not come naturally to them. Constant self-monitoring, with awareness of auditory and visual sensations, and enjoyment even of negative responses, make it habitual.
Positive feedback from girls	Girls are intrigued and not threatened by males who act gay.
Copying particular friends / family members / character in favourite TV series.	Recognise by specific phrases or words such as "yeah-huh". More likely if he has few social contacts.
Hardwired / genetic?	Very unlikely that this could produce the whole pattern.

Causelist 82: Acting grown-up or cocky

The most common reason is to compensate for poor self-confidence. The underlying reason is often social or cognitive difficulties.

Causes	Notes
Normal	• Showing off: p.548
	• Social experiments: occasionally using big words or adult expressions without knowing their meaning
Intrinsic early maturation	Early puberty
	Being bright
	Large physical size creating expectations in self or others
☞ Low self-esteem / defence	Feeling insecure in an academic school so adopting academic way of speaking (pompous speech may disappear when his guard is down, e.g. when crying or when feeling very relaxed).
	School failure leading to joining a big-boys' gang and copying them.
Doesn't know how to be childish	Lack of practice playing with children, or socially isolated by culture / language / long-term hospitalisation
	Asperger's use of big words (knowing their meaning), combined with poor social judgment
	Poor social skills so gets on better with adults.
Early exposure to adult behaviours	Social learning (p.550) from peers, or competition with them, particularly in teenage girls.
	American-style non-hierarchical discussions between parents and child
	Only child (p.518)
	Parentification (p.214)
	Very skilled in hobby leading to mixing with adults
	Sexual abuse (p.275)
Disinhibited (p.261)	Interrupts adults' conversations

Causelist 83: Interest in weapons, gore and killing

This naturally makes family and professionals worry about the risk of violence. There are many better predictors (pp.282, 283). See also aggression, p.289; talking about death, p.309; hurting people and animals, p.279; also non-specific causes of any dominating interest, p.229.

Causes of morbid interest	Notes
Self-protection	(More a fear than an interest), e.g. carrying knives: consider inadequate supervision by parents, friends carrying knives
Social interest	
Interest shared with brother	
Dad hunts or collects weapons	
Requirement for gang membership, respect, coolness	Consider social awkwardness, ID
Focused on a particular person	In many countries the law requires that any intended target must be informed.
⟳ Revenge	Consider paranoia (p.524), gangs, bereavement, p.430 (either recent or a central person in the child's life)
PTSD (p.532)	With flashbacks
Communication	Of anger, or referring to domestic violence, p.454
Hatred of someone (p.187)	
Not driven by known people	
Violent films, cartoons, games	
⟳ OCD	Morbid preoccupations in depression (e.g. puerperally) are less resisted than obsessions (see caveat on p.517).
⟳ Seeing no other solution to overwhelming problem	E.g. in Osama bin Laden. Consider inflexibility (p.234), secondary gain (p.471), psychosis (p.537).

Causelist 84: Love of rabbits

These are small, fluffy, warm, quiet, unaggressive animals. The motivation may be revealed by careful inspection of what the child actually does when she is with the animals. Also, what does she do when she is away from them (does she zone out thinking about them, draw them, make imaginary games, get preoccupied about how to see another rabbit, or just use them in arguments). Love of hedgehogs is similar (search Google for "Hedgehog Olympics").

Love of an individual animal is common and could be called *attachment* (p.195). There are surprisingly intense examples (e.g. an African Grey Parrot[1243]).

Causes of liking rabbits	Notes
Not really liking them	
Can't think of anything else to say	Does she often say the same monotonous thing about rabbits?
Can't think of anything else to like	E.g. if severely socially anxious
Just a figure of speech	May use this to deflect demands in performance anxiety (p.298), e.g. "I'll go to school after you get me a rabbit." (if she knows her parents won't comply).
Specific benefits of rabbits	(see also non-specific causes of any dominating interest – p.229)
Academic	Veterinary interest: more interested in the facts than in the rabbits.
Imaginary friend or world (p.231)	Thinks of rabbits as much as she plays with them. Triggered by upsets. More likely in people who have difficulty making or keeping friends.
For comfort	Seeks and hugs the rabbit particularly when upset
Symbolic (p.14)	
Care: practicing a maternal role	Perhaps like horses (p.248) but without the sexuality or patience.
Other anthropomorphising	Relating the rabbits to a story recently read.
Maturation and independence	Imagining that having a flock of rabbits would make her an independent grown-up, rather than a subordinate in her impossible family

Causelist 85: Love of pink

This trait is culturally determined, pink having evolved from being a boy's colour (in USA and UK) early in the 1900s, to a girl-baby marker in the 1950s, then a sign of liberation (and homosexuality) in the 1970s, then a girls' gender marker in the 1980s–1990s [294,576].

"They are a stirringly impossible mixture of power and delicacy… They inspire fear even as they are filled with it themselves. They are wild and they are utterly tameable… Even the males are pretty, as the females are powerful, and so horses seem to bear the same secret a little girl does about her own protean qualities even if the whole world would deny them." [1255].

Causes of love of horses	Notes
Autism ☂ (p.183)	Very unlikely. Mentioned to point out that horses lack the sterility or repetitiveness of most autistic interests. Interest in an isolated aspect of horses could be autistic.
Anthropomorphisation	
Practising a maternal role: teaching, patience, caring, soothing	This is probably the main reason, but not the only one as it would apply to dogs or donkeys or rabbits (p.246): "horses are better than dogs because no sharp teeth and you can ride them". Most boys are too aggressive or competitive for this.
Sexual	May account for peak interest being in pre-teens before sexual relationships are permitted. DH Lawrence: "The horse… is a dominant symbol… he links us, the first palpable and throbbing link with the ruddy-glowing Almighty of potency…"
You can clean them and brush them	(like grooming in people)
Wanting something out of the horses	
professional	
-- transport	(but uncomfortable and slow)
-- business	
personal	
-- class/status/leisure	
-- girls' club, outdoing boys	
-- competition	(boys are more involved than girls in horse racing and rodeos)
-- elegance	Pretty faces (unlike donkeys) and "graceful sound" (neighing, unlike donkeys). "lovely colours"
-- connecting with nature	Or getting away from people.
-- freedom, power, speed, height	
-- exhilaration (like roller coaster)	Opposite view is "scary", out of control.
-- being in command	"Empowerment that comes from commanding a larger, more forceful being"
-- admiration from the horse	
"seeking a higher knowledge about horses and humans and the mysteries of their intersection"[1255]	

Breaking rules ☼

Rules in general
Some rules are much more important than others. Some change often,
others never. Some are learned implicitly, and others are taught explicitly.
Some apply just in specific places, others when a specific person is near,
and so on. Sometimes rules are broken accidentally; other times after
careful thought about whether the benefits outweigh the costs.

Children gradually increase in the sophistication with which they make
such choices, but some continue to see rules as black and white. Causes of
this include immaturity, poor education, concrete thinking, social learning
(p.550), rigidity (p.234) and the comfort of societal or self-invented
heuristics. Effects of black-and-white thinking include inter-personal
conflict (e.g. parental alienation, p.187), cognitive dissonance (p.355), and
depression (e.g. if the child believes that anyone who fails is worthless).

Firmly imposed rules, gradually loosened as the child matures, have a
major value in keeping children safe, and making them feel safe – and in
making them use their time wisely [Chapter 6 of 57]. But of course disagreements about rules often cause conflict between parents and children.

Rules in clinical situations
The DSM terms most associated with rule breaking are Conduct Disorder
☂ and Oppositional Defiant Disorder (p.519). "Children and teenagers
with conduct disorder are naughty, awkward, disruptive, aggressive and
antisocial – these are important problems that deserve help, but they are
often best thought of as social, educational and moral problems needing
social, educational and moral solutions, rather than as health problems that
require help from health professionals; a distinctive health component can
only be identified in a minority of cases." [590]. However, finding this
minority requires careful assessment of temperament, understanding,
mood, and motivations for and against the rule breaking (note values
change depending on the situation[Chapter 5 of 57]).

If a child breaks many rules, think of ID, autism (p.183), lack of guilt
(p.475), and lack of fear of punishment[1250]. On the other hand, if a child
breaks just one kind of rule, there may be a specific cause. For example,
hyperactive children (p.79) most frequently break rules requiring stillness.
There are distinct reasons for people to lie (p.255), steal (p.250), break
sexual rules (p.269), smear (p.342), or insert objects in their body (p.118).
Compare rule breaking with the notion of *criminality*, p.446.

Table 14. Change in frequency of "naughtiness" with age.

(after 445)	90th % in preschoolers	90th % in older children
Decreasing with age		
Losing temper	2-3/day	2/week
Actively defiant	5/day	2/week
Blames others	1/week	1/three months
Angry and resentful	1/day	4/week
Spiteful/vindictive	1/month	1/three months
Steady		
Arguing with adults	2/week	2/week
Deliberately annoys people	5/week	4/week
Increasing with age		
Touchy/easily annoyed	1/three months	2/week

Causelist 87: Stealing

This is one of the main criteria in the definition of "conduct disorder" ☂
(p.249) but closer inspection often reveals easily remediable causes[1337].
Occasionally stealing or shoplifting is mentioned by parents during
assessment, shedding useful light on relationships and attitudes (p.425).

Shoplifting is almost universal, so not by itself developmentally worrying.
However it is serious if they can't stop even after being caught, or if there
is an underlying cause (see list below). It can be a game (me versus shop),
a gang sweep of the shop, or "I've nicked more than you". In its mildest
forms it is akin to taking money off the kitchen table. *Severe* shoplifting
by teenagers seems to be more often caused by mania than by depression.

Causes of stealing	Notes (some causes can be distinguished by asking what the child does with what he stole)
Normal	*Obvious* stealing occurs up to a few times each year in schoolchildren. Most people steal small amounts when they think they're unlikely to be caught. In some fairly normal situations, 40% of children will steal, but this can be greatly reduced by adult observation or even the presence of a mirror[122]. In adults, such dishonesty is almost eliminated if they have recently read or made ethical statements, or if the opportunity involves actual cash. [Chapters 11-12 of 57]. Some *superstimuli* (p.558) are so attractive that most will succumb
Immaturity	In the first few years of life children do not understand ownership. Preschoolers generally cannot resist the temptation to take something they want. Jealous siblings may hide favourite toys
Deprivation (real or imagined)	Particularly if pocket money is less than peers'. Exacerbated if pocket money is reduced as a punishment for stealing (see *perverse effects of training*, p.528)
☞Family problems	Steals mainly from family, to compensate for lack of affection. Like comfort eating (p.257)
Peer influences	Particularly shoplifting or marauding in a group. Testosterone (p.554) fuels competitiveness which is useful in most contexts but counterproductive when the friends are antisocial[1387]
Obeying parent	Daring exploit to improve status in group (p.172); or to ally with someone
Compensatory/ symbolic (p.14)	Steals from the person he feels rejected by (e.g. parents or peers). Possession is not the point, so may, e.g. bury it
Self-esteem or social inadequacy	May try to buy friendship.
Substance misuse	(p.267)
To annoy or hurt someone	
Mood disorder	(see above)
Collecting	(to complete a set)
Kleptomania ☂	This term is hardly used before adulthood

The group dynamics are crucial (as with gangs, p.472; bullying, p.219; vandalism, p.572; football hooliganism; shoplifting / stealing, p.250; other infectious behaviours, p.490). The group's "behavioural unity [occurs] with cognitive diversity" in the individual participants[1675]. The participants' behaviours have both rational and irrational elements, and vary from moment to moment and between people. However there are special characteristics of group action, described below. These are not found in solitary rule-breaking, such as psychopathy (p.280) and most fire-setting (p.466).

Some young people follow gang members, who are in turn organised by gang leaders (often adults). In intergroup conflict, the lead may be taken not by general neighbourhood gangs but by specific relevant groups (e.g. racial, political, or sporting). Generally the people lowest in the mob hierarchy are likely to have simple, short-term, ill-thought-out motivations. In contrast, premeditation is indicated by concealment of faces, wearing gloves, sending texts, coordinated travel, and carrying hammers. Mobs can be organised rapidly using mobile phones, in top-down or devolved "viral" manner, or both.

Causes of group mayhem: Situational factors Propelling	
brief excitement or novelty, versus chronic boredom	Any exciting event, such as a concert or film, can give young people energy to burn off[394]. Participating in a crowd rioting can be empowering, extremely friendly and even joyous[1675].
anger	e.g. after one's sports team loses.
the feeling of anonymity, and of being hidden in the crowd,	
a momentary error / experimentation	i.e. it may not be characteristic of the child.
on a power trip; the fun of causing chaos	"tyrant kings", can be indicated by confident leadership, and sometimes a swagger
needing possessions, shopping without money	(or feeling deprived, p.250) This is more likely if they confine their looting to relevant shops.
to earn money	more likely if unemployed, poor, or drug abusing, p.257
rebelliousness / desire to annoy	
Restraining / diverting	
expectation of punishment	More likely in neighbourhoods with "zero tolerance" policing. Less likely where good police-community relations are valued more highly than tight control.
exercise	Are there local youth clubs or sports clubs?
Individual characteristics	Note the *fundamental attribution error* (p.18) makes us subconsciously suspect long-term individual characteristics rather than situational factors.

Propelling	
male, teenage, poor[1645]	These personal characteristics tend to be associated with many of the other risk factors in this table[675]. Furthermore, in some societies risk factors are concentrated in a subgroup, so for example black teenagers were disproportiontely involved in the riots and looting in the UK in 2011.
unemployed	i.e. they may feel powerless and deprived.
illiteracy, lack of prospects,	These often cause chronic frustration and directionless anger.
impulsivity	(p.489)
long-term habit of minor lawbreaking	e.g. gang members
belief in redistribution	This can be noble if the goods are for others, but this is unusual in a riot. People who steal may not feel that they are guilty or greedy, because of the belief that they are righting a wrong. This belief can be encouraged by parents, popular media, and/or riot leaders.
Restraining / diverting	
female, middle class, doing well in school	

Social factors

Propelling	
presence of peers	showing off or overexcited by friends (p.263). Also feeling a sense of duty, or leadership.
copying peers	desire to fit in (see discussion of what is "cool", p.172) Disadvantaged neighbourhoods bring a young person into contact with many adverse peer influences[675].
negative role models	e.g. popular music glorifying violence and materialism. However, note that this music has been selected by young people as a multinational consumer group, and also to some degreee by themselves as individuals[1675].
resenting authority, such as teachers, employers, shopowners or the police	especially if there's unnecessary destruction, beyond just taking goods. Has control been over-harsh?[394]
Group identity[1675]	When in a group, one can become more aware of values and emotions and experiences of the group rather than of oneself.
Restraining / diverting	
positive role models, moral / religious values	e.g. paternal role model (absent in most single-parent families.) See also discussion of influences on *stealing*, p.250.
involvement in positive family activities	less likely in single-parent families (p.213)
supervision (parental or club). Police presence. Local community groups / effective community leaders / property-protecting adults.	Lack of supervision can be brief or longterm (sometimes allowing prettens to be "feral"). Parents may be single, at work, watching TV or drunk – or, worse, there may be no parental figure if the child is moved between carers who do not exercise authority. Police presence may be prevented by engagement rules, training, or intentional diversion of police by rioters.

Causelist 89: Disobedience ☼

This is a common complaint of parents and teachers taking the moral viewpoint that they *should* be obeyed. This is not a route to understanding the situation. The type and size of the infraction, and the time delay from adult warning, are key. For broader discussions see *non-behaviours*, p.515; and *impulsivity*, p.489.

Causes of not doing as he is told	Notes
Normal	
Single antisocial act	
Curiosity	Healthy naughtiness: (p.511)
Provocative wind-up	*Often* reinforced by attention from parent. Occasionally, wind-ups may be a useful way for an autistic child to elicit responses that he can perceive (because simple), enjoy and eventually understand.
Forgot the rule	Especially after a time delay, or when excited.
Insufficiently motivated to comply	
Ineffective discipline	The child will weigh benefits of doing as she was told, against the benefits of not doing so. Changing rules, inconsistent enforcement, and worthless sanctions are the commonest causes of disobedience. As an extreme example, children can become totally desensitised to their mother shouting commands at them, if it is frequent and not followed through.
Unreasonable or impractical request	"Don't do that" is impractical without a clear alternative. Family dynamics (p.211) are often important at home, and unrecognised cognitive difficulties at school (p.27).
Poor relationship	With the person giving instructions
Desire to do something regardless of whether or not it is wrong	
Boredom	(p.322)
Impulsivity	I.e. poor self-control (p.79)
Superstimuli	(p.558) Few children can resist sweets when hungry.
Epilepsy	Odd or occult epilepsies: p.76
Many disorders	Following their own rules rather than society's: OCD, p.65; tics, p.101; sexual deviance; autism ✝, p.183. Both fire-setting (p.466) and sexual offences are slightly more common in Asperger's (p.424)[1119]: see discussion of psychopathy, p.280.
Not told anything	
No standards, "Feral"	Consider psychopathy (p.280), or unsocialised due to neglect.
◉Deaf	Or not listening, p.130.
Incomprehension	Preoccupied, or doesn't understand
Has learned to do specific wrong things	
Wrong standards	Aggression (p.289), learned from parents fighting.
Learned escape behaviour	e.g. misbehaving in order to be sent to the Learning Support Centre, or to be sent home.
Too little *or too much* adult attention	Opposite effects are seen in socially avoidant v. attention-seeking children [1591].
Desire to conflict with the request	
Psychopathy	Rare. non-empathic sociopathy / psychopathy: p.280
Teenage rebelliousness	Exploration of social options and self-images in adolescence. In isolation, this does not cause dysfunction in family, peer group or school.
Oppositionality	The common meaning for this is to habitually and deliberately act against others (see also p.519). This implies that the child expends effort to upset people, or to resist minor or irrelevant changes, or changes which he would welcome if he had been the one to come up with the idea. If oppositionality is allowed to continue long term, disengagement from class and parental interaction lead to major social problems (✝ "conduct disorder", p.249).
	Avoiding using the term too broadly
	The key in assessment is to be sceptical about his parents' or

teachers' certainty that he is purposely trying to annoy them.

- It is important to see whether he is happy to cooperate with conversation, hand games, physical examination, hopping, etc. If he is only oppositional with particular tasks or situations or when tired, it is not correct to say that he is an oppositional person.
- If the child is depressed and irritable (p.494), and/or has poor social skills, these may be causing his oppositionality plus other problems, so should be addressed first.
- If a child is only oppositional with one parent, or with teachers, then he's either temporarily wound up by them, or this is a characteristic of his relationship with those people, i.e. *he himself* is not oppositional.
- When a child isn't speaking much (p.151), his failure to explain why he isn't complying with a request can feel oppositional to teachers & parents even if it isn't.
- Combative repartee is a rewarded behaviour in some cultures and families (p.162).

Reactive and proactive oppositionality

- If a child when bored taunts or pushes people to get a reaction and make life more interesting, this is due to a lack of more productive or pleasant things to do. The child is not opposing someone else's command or idea (reactively), but creating the ideas and the conflict himself (proactively). This is quite common in children with developmental problems. It arises because it is easier to obtain big reactions with negative behaviours than with positive behaviours. A fairly convincing sign of this (not very common) is the child giving in *very quickly* when the person she wants attention from gives it in ways other than "stop that" or "go away."
- *Reactive oppositionality* can sometimes be identified by the persistence of oppositionality during desired activities. A useful trick is to join the child in a task he is already enjoying, or better, to push him to do something that you know he enjoys (such as playing with his game computer or drawing his favourite thing). The purely hyperactive child will not object; the oppositional or unsocial child will soon refuse to cooperate.

Transient oppositionality
A child can be momentarily overwhelmed, particularly if tired, by the combination of surprise, and trying to understand a request, and needing to drop what he was doing. Such actions are often regretted almost immediately, i.e. brief impulses can be much more oppositional than longer-term attitudes (p.425; see *unliked actions*, p.353).

Can't do the right thing	
Dyspraxia (p.89)	And other disabilities
Rigidity	Has difficulty changing what he's doing (p.234)
Caught in a dilemma	When OCD rituals are thwarted (p.65). When told different rules by the same or different parents. When told to do something that conflicts with previous personal rules or misunderstood parental rules (e.g. an autistic boy who can't pick up a crisp from the table, but can when it has been put on a paper). Or becoming angry and aggressive when caught in an approach/avoidance conflict (as in confined cats[418] despite the conclusions there). See cognitive dissonance, p.355.
Depression (p.309)	can present with antisocial behaviour of recent onset.
Aggression	Has many underlying causes (p.289)

Causelist 90: Telling untruths

Lying implies intent to put wrong information in someone else's mind.
Almost always, lying is a learned behaviour maintained by rewards.
There are causes in the person, the situation, and the culture.

Forty per cent of children regularly lie, but this increases to 80% from age
5 to 10[1418]. Lying is rarely serious anough to justify much clinical effort in
its own right, but it is a very useful sign of important issues such as
inconsistent parenting, inflexible parenting, or impossible demands being
put on the child.

Consider the motive: attention-seeking, careless, self-protective, harming,
or altruistic. Also consider the level of cognition: dissociative, p.453;
denial; complete fabrication, p.359; partial fabrication, p.357. For tips on
observable signs of deception, see[1763]. See also cheating, p.439.

Age	Expected deceptive abilities (after [1418])
0–4	Mainly denials
5–6	Simple lies ("He did it"), not sustained over time
6–12	Able to plan, then instill false beliefs in others, and to resist probing questions.
12+	Ability to role-play including altering facial expression. Ability to malinger, p.503.

Causes of telling untruths	Notes
Might be untrue for most people, but true for him now	E.g. "I can't find it", "The water's too hot," "I can't understand this question."
Normal lying	Very common (see text and table above)
White lie	To protect someone else (normal occasionally after age 8)
Sarcasm or joke (p.495)	(expecting to be detected). e.g. if real answer is too boring
Not addressing the question	E.g. perceiving implications, possibly wrongly, and answering those rather than the actual words
Cognitive	
Not knowing the question	Didn't hear / thinking of something else / zoning out or absence (p.75)
Not knowing the answer…	…and not knowing how/when to say "don't know". Or may have misunderstood information from another source. See also *confabulation*, p.443.
Not knowing they should say the truth	They might think they're supposed to say what they wish is the truth.
Mixing up reality and fantasy	Tells you the truth about what happened in their imagination. Related to thinking they *ought* to be able to tell you why they did something, but not actually knowing so giving what seems like a reasonable answer [1780].
Just learned the possibility of lying, and is practising	Now needs to learn the next lesson, i.e. consequences of lying.
Not interested in the answer	e.g. "Why did you do that?" → From the child's point of view, the answer is an irrelevant mystery.

Blurts out answer before checking (see also blurting, p.433)	If concentration is too poor to allow the answer to be checked (e.g. in hyperactivity/impulsivity, p.79), *short interesting* questions with *brief* answers should be answered more reliably. With low IQ *simple* questions should be similarly protected.
Misheard question	Auditory / anger / preconceptions / different knowledge of context or background
Odd ideas	Psychosis (p.537), familial beliefs, folie imposee (see p.347)
Cognitive errors	These are common in children, adults, clinicians, and scientists: for examples see p.534
Self-deception	
Unable to face the truth	"We can still be a couple after I go to university". Denial of prejudices.
To preserve self-esteem	"I'm near the top of the class" (in the bottom set)
Over-motivated to lie	
Demands felt to be excessive	"Have you done your homework?" (p.481) "Did you do your 3 hours piano practice after school?"
Wanting to please parent or friends.	E.g. forging school marks (see *cheating*, p.439) or trying to impress.
Not having another way to obtain praise.	Group membership can produce false statements and change of views[3].
Preserving relationships & esteem, avoiding punishments	A milder version is the semiconscious dilution of information to avoid upsetting people – this happens many times in a social hour. Perhaps more common in girls because social relationships more important to them, and they are less rigid than boys in thinking about concepts[1144].
Wind-up	Said with taunting tone, monitoring the listener's reaction.
Learned from parents / friends	
Substance abuse and behavioural addictions	(p.257)
Fabricated, induced or exaggerated problems	These often involve lying. Some of the motivations are listed on p.359. Pseudologia fantastica (living complex deceptive lives[609]) is only partially achievable while living with parents.
Under-motivated for honesty	
Carelessness	Exhaustion, inadequate discipline, not caring what this particular listener thinks or knows. One of the meanings of *bullshit*[519] is indifference to how things really are; the word can also refer to attempts to impress or to lying in general.
Oppositional	(p.253) Long-term inadequacy of positive feedback.
Poor training	Parents have not praised his honesty in difficult situations, or shown him that they value it [chapter 11 in 1144].
Social learning (p.550)	Deception and corruption are universal, but they are more pervasive in some schools, universities, companies, industries, and even countries, often for quite rational reasons such as examples from leaders, and the likelihood of punishment[94,992,1500].
Psychopathy	(p.280). Also called trait-based lying.

Special Topic 9: Is this child abusing drugs?

This is the unseen epidemic in young people. We often neglect to ask about it, feeling that it is normal, or that we are powerless to change it. However detection does improve outcomes[880]. Detection can be maximised by ensuring confidentiality from parents; using screening questionnaires; and repeating enquiries after a therapeutic relationship has been established.

Pre-teens take readily available substances, e.g. alcohol, glue, cough syrups, and prescription medicines left lying around. Hospital admissions and attendances at casualty are good times for laboratory drug screening (hair drug screening is better than urine, except for detecting alcohol). See also *toxic substances*, p.566.

In some areas it is more common for *parents'* drug abuse to affect their children, for instance through violence, poverty, and neglect (e.g. failing to get their children to school). Teachers are often aware of these problems.

Any use of illicit substances has the potential to grow along this path:

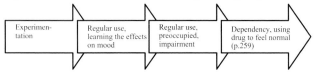

Rates are highly culture dependent, but the lifetime prevalence of *experimentation* with alcohol, tobacco, and cannabis each increase approximately linearly from age 12 (0–5%) to age 18 (60–90%). Experimentation with other substances is much lower, reaching 30% by age 18. For all substances, *dependence* affects about 10% of experimenters, except for tobacco to which about 25% of experimenters become addicted by age 18[1812].

Symptoms (independent of drug type)
Sudden deterioration (p.41) in schoolwork, behaviour, and mood.
Stealing, p.250; or selling possessions.
Parents don't know how he can afford so much.
Tremor, p.61; weight loss, chronic cough, red eyes.
Suddenly starts hanging out with drug users.
Secretive behaviour, starting to wear dark glasses or long sleeves.

Underlying causes that are worth looking for:
➢ Seeking any of the following:
- relaxation
- pleasure, "being high"
- something to do (look out for undiagnosed ADHD)
- to become more outgoing
- to fit in with the group (conversely, strong religious convictions, warm family relationships, and success at school all reduce drug abuse)
- to have more energy, be more productive, have more ideas.

➢ Self-medication of comorbidities and related subclinical states. This requires the other state to have preceded the drug misuse.
- Comfort eating improves mood in some people[320].
- A large minority of people with anxiety or hyperthymic states use alcohol or sedatives to regulate their mood[192]. Examples are PTSD, p.532; and following abuse, p.271.
- Many people with problems of aggression use cannabis to reduce this[55].
- Nicotine is used for cognitive enhancement and to relieve the negative symptoms of schizophrenia[888].

Drug use in young people in England in 2001[197]:

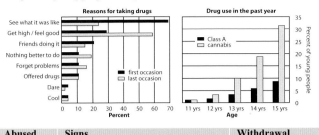

Abused drug	Signs	Withdrawal
Amphet- amine (see *Stimulants*, p.555)	Paranoia (p.524), aggression, depression, hallucinations, dry mouth, tremor, sweating (p.558), anorexia, weight loss, dilated pupils, tachycardia, switching between high and low states, reduced sleep	Fatigue, p.323; hunger; depression, p.309
Cocaine	Euphoria, paranoia (p.524), increased activity, decreased fatigue, tachycardia, weight loss, runny nose	Lethargy, p.323; reduced consciousness; fountain crying, p.316
LSD	Exhilaration, unpredictable behaviour, depression, panic (p.301). LSD can cause immediate & delayed visual hallucinations (flashbacks).	Mood changes
Solvent sniffing (including glue, petrol)	Poor concentration, disinhibition, ataxia, Chronic intermittent polyneuropathy[1629], liver & kidney damage, runny nose & eyes or rashes around nose & mouth. Aerosol cans, tubes of glue	(None)
Heroin (see *opiates*, p.519)	Drowsiness, euphoria, hallucinations, constipation (p.444), tears, pinpoint pupils, needle marks, weight loss	Diarrhoea; pains; fountain crying, p.316 insomnia; psychosis (see *noradrenaline*, p.516)
Cannabis	Slow thought, poor concentration, loquacity, euphoria, sleepiness, ataxia, hallucinations, wheezing or cough, delayed secondary sexual characteristics. Long-term use can cause "amotivation". Cannabis smell. Paranoia(p.524).	(None is certain)
Barbiturates	Irritability (p.494), aggression, confusion, and fits	Tremor, vomiting, fits, DTs (as alcohol)
Benzo- diazepines (p.430)	Sedation, respiratory depression	Seizures, p.73; paraesthesias; psychosis, p.537; fountain crying, p.316
Alcohol (see also p.420)	Ataxia & slurring of speech, smell, false ID card.	Tremor, anxiety. ‼ In chronic alcohol abuse (rare in teens): beware of delirium tremens as this needs urgent medical support. Signs: excitement, fear, visual hallucinations, fits
Anabolic steroids[1268]	(Often used intermittently) gynaecomastia, aggression, mood changes, psychosis (usually mild paranoid & grandiose delusions)	Depression

Special Topic 10: Is this child addicted?

Addiction (or dependence) is defined as the loss of control over a behaviour, or the compulsive performing of that behaviour despite adverse consequences.

Addiction to drugs (substance dependence)

Effects of repeated drug use (p.257) include:

- tolerance/habituation to some effects, so that the person experiences a diminished effect, and usually tries to compensate for this by taking more.
- dependence: i.e. an adapted state, so that return to the drug-free state entails *withdrawal* with specific signs (listed on p.258)
- life becomes oriented around obtaining the drug; there is rapid reinstatement after abstinence.
- drug use becomes highly motivated but often not pleasurable, i.e. the drug is wanted but not liked (see discussion of unliked actions, p.353)
- sensitisation to some effects, e.g. severe craving can be triggered even by reminders of drug use.

The effects of drugs are diverse (see table on p.258). In addition the effects differ between people. This is in part due to there being at least five genes involved in most drug addictions, and eighteen involved in addiction to at least one of the main drug classes (alcohol, cocaine, nicotine, opiates)[951].

See also: drug screening, p.257.

Pseudo-addiction

This is the situation following inadequate pain management, when a patient escalates his analgesic demands and adapts his behaviour in an attempt to convince prescribers that he needs more medication (especially opioids). This can cause a crisis of mistrust between the patient and his carers[1735].

Addiction to behaviours

There is much debate about whether non-drug behaviours pursued despite adverse consequences should be called *addictive behaviour*, or *behavioural addictions* – or whether they are just normal choices.

Mechanisms

Although there is some evidence for reinforcement mechanisms being similar to those in drug addictions[706],that is also true of normal, socially sanctioned pursuits such as sports or homework. Excessive behaviours in real people involve multiple factors in the person and his environment[589], including rapid reinforcement[553], habit formation, lack of alternative behaviours, and sometimes predisposing clinical and subclinical difficulties (p.257). In this book they are treated as having diverse underlying motivations (p.63), of which the following are especially problematic: behaviours performed to reduce painful feelings (much like OCD, p.65); superstimuli, p.558; and behaviours that cause additional angst as they are *unliked behaviours*, p.353.

Indicators of severity

Loss of other interests (depression can coexist, p.313). Wanting to do less but unable to. Deteriorating self-care (eating, washing). Continuing through one or several nights. Weight loss or severe weight gain. Not attending school or work. Sores on back/legs from pressure of chair. Keeping bottles by the activity to avoid the need to go to the toilet. Tingling fingers and anxiety due to vitamin D deficiency (lack of sun – p.328). Also consider signs that the behaviour is *not* out of control, such as good attendance at school, keeping network of friends.

Examples include:

- *Computer addiction* and *internet addiction*. These terms are too vague, and a more precise formulation is essential (pp.224,492 and[934]). Computer games (p.573) can overwhelm people's other interests.
- Overeating is sometimes classified as a substance abuse[375], but it and its associated bulimia (p.337) and anorexia nervosa (p.334) have major learned components. Comfort eating (p.257) may be related.
- Gambling (fruit machines, lotteries or online) satisfies and reinforces various sensation-seeking and social drives (pp.124,168), using a combination of continuous and partial schedules, usually with several distractor elements to reduce clear thought[921].
- Work[1269] and even schoolwork (see examples in[1356]).
- Shopping, buying
- Stealing (p.250)
- The reduction in behavioural repertoire seen in addiction may be related to that in autism[805] (see *monotropism*, p.509)
- People may complain of sex addiction due to obsessionality, general dislike of self, religious beliefs, or lack of distractions ([99]; see also [1572]).
- Imaginary friends (p.231).
- Nail-biting (p.511).
- Excess exercise. Exercise releases opioids and can become an addiction, p.259.

See also: relation to gratification phenomena, p.115; addiction to endogenous opioids in headbanging and other self-harm, pp.126 and 317; perpetuating factor in anorexia nervosa, p.334; in bulimia, p.335; addiction to killing, p.282; in emotional abuse, p.278; possible role in attachment, p.195.

Causelist 91: Disinhibition ☼

This is an aspect of motor function. Some limits are inbuilt; others have to be learned. If a child is highly intolerant (p.125) or immature or does not know the norms of behaviour in this culture he may act in an extreme way without this indicating disinhibition. Some acts have multiple reasons not to do them, all of which have to be overcome to allow the act (e.g. p.342). In general, the severity of disinhibition is indicated by how public it is, how unfamiliar the people involved, how frequent, how extraordinary the behaviour, and the amount of damage done.

If a child is disinhibited in one area from the list below, the other limits need to be assessed as well, to clarify the extent of the disinhibition (which helps elucidate the cause). Most children can temporarily inhibit behaviours that are embarrassing or painful or likely to be reprimanded. Some never can; others can't when they're sleepy or ill.

Limits on normal behaviour	If this specific area is disinhibited, see:
Safety	
Protecting oneself, avoiding pain	p.317
Not harming others	p.279–282
Eating only appropriate foods	pp.336, 331
Limiting food and fluid intake	p.335
Not interacting with / touching adult strangers	p.173
Protecting self-esteem	
Avoiding being criticised or told off	p.253
Acting one's age or above	pp.244, 237, 261, 161, 115
Privacy	
Keeping sexual behaviour private	p.269, 115
Masturbation being only a minor interest	p.474
Being calm	p.79-69, 125
Being gentle; avoiding anger	p.286-289
Not imposing on others	
Regulating physical space/contact/noise	
Minimising mess	pp.340-342
Being polite	p.161
Sharing	p.179
Conformity	
Talking only when people are interested	p.163
Limiting your individuality (value of individuality is culturally dependent). When people are unsure, they accept other people's judgments, with little or no justification[1471]. Even when the correct answer to a question is obvious, people will change their answer if three or more people give a different one[64].	pp.231-238 of 57
Keeping social values and financial values separate	Chapter 4 of 57.

Causes of disinhibition	Notes
Not really disinhibition	
Strong motivation(p.365)	Overcomes normal inhibition
ID	Doesn't know the norms.
Poor self-monitoring	Inadequate monitoring of the environment or people's responses, e.g. talking loud when wearing headphones.
With elation	
Happy event	Normally wears off within a day. Surprisingly, this is very unlikely to pecipitate a manic episode[32].
Hypomania / mania / hyperthymia	(pp.263–264). See also *treatable causes of hypomania / mania*, p.265.
Without elation	
Very confident	• Normal above-average (social) confidence: willing to separate from parents, but having no other unusually disinhibited behaviour, either with or without parents. This can be innate or arise from having had lots of carers. • Inadequate trait anxiety (p.423)
ADHD ⬆ (p.79)	Onset can be at head injury (p.477), especially frontal (p.512).
Autism, autistic spectrum ⬆ (p.183)	Often related to overriding interests, or treating people as objects (e.g. playing with their earlobes or hair). Unconcerned with social norms (e.g. thumb-sucking).
Tourette's (p.101)	Normal behaviour, plus tics. Can be temporarily suppressed but then needs to be "released", e.g. in 5 minutes outside class.
Disinhibited / disorganised attachment (p.195)	Most worrying are *physical* interactions with strangers (talking to them does not imply any attachment problems).
Learned grandiosity	• In a child – can be copied from parents' attitude, or learned from the way parents and others treat him. • In parents – can be useful in a parent engaged in strenuous efforts to obtain help from social services, education, CAMHS. Can be reinforced and perpetuated by a very dependent spouse.
In order to be the centre of attention	(Being the centre of attention is exciting and simplifies the child's interactions)

This should be considered in all cases of overactivity or disinhibition. Elevated, or high, mood is often overlooked in children, perhaps because ADHD is so much more common. Evidence for high mood can be collected by observation, school report and parental report. Home videos are of course objective, but they are so highly selected that they can be very misleading.

Hypomania is the extreme of normal mood. The term *mania* is used if there are also psychotic features (p.537); this is much less common. A third of manic patients have simultaneous depressive symptoms, called *mixed mania*.

It is useful to assess mood using standard cognitive, biological, and affective signs (see table below). Also consider whether there is a crescendo of behaviour in the session (which would be more characteristic of ADHD ☞: p.77 and p.79). Adults' level of risk taking is not usually affected by the presence of friends, but adolescents tend to become much more impulsive and take risks when friends are present[542], presumably in part because of elevated mood and a desire to impress.

	Signs of mania/hypomania (the most helpful signs are in bold)	Easily confused with…
Emotional/ affective signs	• **Elation**, e.g. smiling even when looking at a computer or toy (not fixed grins). • Irritability • Increased sociability • **Grandiosity**: announcing his arrival in the room. "call me awesome!", calling everyone else lazy. Ask him where is is on a scale of superness from 1 to 10.	• Inappropriate affect in autism. • Other causes of irritability (p.494) and rages (p.71).
Physical/ somatic/ vegetative signs	• Delayed sleep onset, **reduced need for sleep** • Increased libido	• Other causes of poor sleep (p.199)
Motivational signs (also called behavioural signs)	• Increased loudness, rushing around • **Overly jocular** (telling jokes in clinic) • Overproductivity, taking on extra jobs	• Excess energy is often the parents' complaint in ADHD, in which condition the behaviour is usually more variable and less directed. • Difficulty interrupting child with autism or ADHD
	• Disinhibition, exclusions from school	• Other causes of sexualised behaviour (p.269)
Cognitive signs	• Poor judgment, distractibility (p.453)	• There are many other causes of these (see e.g. p.79).
	• **Racing thoughts** / flight of ideas (e.g. lots of unrelated questions without waiting for an answer). • Increased spending	
Psychotic signs	• Hallucinations or delusions (pp.343–348). These are uncommon but important to consider	• Talking to himself (p.560)

The longer term: Temporal patterns of elevated mood or irritability

There are good graphing methods that allow a teenager or parent to reliably record changes in mood over months to years[1164]. Such graphs usually clarify whether the triggers are emotional, with the commonest patterns listed below, or biological (see pp.61, 63, 265).

Bipolar affective disorder (BPAD)

BPAD (previously called manic depression) is rare before puberty. Its key signs are elation (or irritability, p.494), grandiosity, and episodicity. Most European authorities require the episodes to last at least several days. The episodes are often followed by depressions of similar duration. If you are seeing the first episode, there should have been a gradual worsening of symptoms over days to weeks. Most episodes arise spontaneously, but first episodes are most likely to arise within a few weeks of a *negative* life event[32] (see p.499).

Signs strongly favouring bipolar affective disorder over ADHD are: reduced sleep and appetite; hallucinations or delusions, jocularity, rage (p.71), hypersexuality, overproductivity, and racing thoughts[1233]. Bipolar disorder usually has some family history. It usually has a clear age of onset, whereas ADHD has "always been there". For a comprehensive list of subjective feelings associated with high and low mood, see[29].

The most widely used definitions:
- *Bipolar I*: has had at least one episode of full mania.
- *Bipolar II*: has had at least one episode of hypomania (never manic), and one depressive episode
- *Bipolar III*: can mean cyclothymia. Another meaning is solely clinical depressive episodes in people who have a relative with at least some hypomanic symptoms.
- *Cyclothymia*: numerous episodes of hypomania and of *subclinical* depression
- *Rapid cycling* is defined as four episodes of depression or hypomania within one year. Lay people use this term (or *bad temper*) to refer to multiple mood swings during each day, but it is important to consider whether it is more a control problem (dyscontrol, p.69) or an emotional one (irritability, p.494) and in the latter case to consider the polarity (angry feelings 287; overexcitability, p.520). Consider Kleine-Levin syndrome, p.496.

Hyperthymia

In contrast to BPAD, this is not episodic; rather it is an aspect of temperament (p.561) that is noticeable from infancy. The child is overtly upbeat, energy-driven, strong-willed, overconfident, and generous[19,271]. Unlike bipolar disorder, there are usually no depressive episodes, though these may develop later in life. Hyperthymia is not impairing so it should not be called a disorder (though it is sometimes called chronic hypomania), but it is essential for understanding some children's behaviours. Hyperthymia is occasionally familial, and there is also an increased rate of bipolar disorder in relatives.

ADHD

Outbursts of anger, elation, or frustration, happen in all children, but are often more severe in ADHD, in which they are often called *emotional instability* (p.69). It is not common to find persistently elevated mood and ADHD in the same child because ADHD tends to lower self-esteem (but see *exuberance*, p.464). Overexcitable or disinhibited behaviours before puberty are usually not precursors of mania. However a worsening at puberty, or episodes lasting weeks to months, necessitate consideration of BPAD.

Atypical patterns

These are seen in some autism[831,832] or ID, e.g. Prader-Willi, p.533, Kleine-Levin, p.496. Consider also *cycloid psychoses*, p.449.

Investigation Planner 6: Treatable causes of hypomania/mania

The first step is a thorough examination and careful consideration of the causes in the previous table. Following this, tests can be selected from the following list[1033].

See also the *general approach to medical investigations*, p.373.

	Signs	Initial tests	Excluded clinically or to Order?	Date ordered	Result
First line					
Sleep deprivation	History (p.257)				
☞Intoxication (especially amphetamine, cocaine, phencyclidine, inhalants, ecstasy)		Drug screen (p.257) alcohol			
☞Medication	History • SSRIs (p.552). Mild cases have just silliness and social intrusiveness. • benzodiazepines and associated disinhibition (p.430) • steroids (pp.258,554) • asthma medications, p.424 • stimulants, p.555				
General baseline tests		FBC, UECr, LFT, urinalysis, glucose			
Hyperthyroidism	(p.484)	TFT			
Second line					
Cushings	(p.449)	(p.449)			
Infections, p.490					
Encephalitis	(p.461)	(p.461)			
☞HIV	(p.479)	(p.479)			
Metabolic					
Wilson's disease	(p.575)	(p.575)			
Porphyria	(p.532)	(p.532)			
Third line					
Epilepsy	e.g. TLE, p.562	EEG			
Brain tumours	(p.569)	MRI			
Multiple sclerosis	(p.510)	(p.510)			
Kleine-Levin syndrome	(p.496)	(p.496)			
Others	see[1555]				

Special Topic 12: Is this sexual behaviour worrying?

This includes several questions:
- How common or normal is it? → addressed here.
- Is it dangerous now or in the future? → briefly addressed here.
- Does it indicate something wrong in the child? → see pp.269, 474.
- Does it indicate maltreatment (sexual or otherwise)? → see p.271.

It can be difficult for staff, parents, or children to discuss this, and using the Child Sexual Behaviour Inventory (CSBI, see[527]) can make it easier.

A. Sex-related behaviours (for more details see[716])

Remember some children do apparently sexual behaviours because they were put up to it, or are curious. Sexual behaviour and information that could not have been obtained from films are generally more worrying than other sexual comments or drawings. See the motivations for stealing, p.250; consider impulsivity, p.489; and intoxication, p.566. See also *erection*, p.462.

Behaviours"sometimes often/daily"from age 3 to 6[909]	%Boys		%Girls	
	At day-care	At home	At day-care	At home
Wants everyday body contact	46	97	74	98
Uses sex words	17	15	0	9
Puts tongue in other's mouth when kissing	0	3	0	3
Masturbates with object	0	3	1	4
Pretends to be opposite sex in play	12	3	1	2
Tries to touch men's (other than father's) genitals	0	0	0	0
Tries to touch women's (other than mother's) breasts	5	--	2	--
Imitates sexual intercourse in doll's play	0	1	0	0

The following extract from[1439] is for European children screened to exclude most sexual abuse:

Items from the CSBI performed at least once in the past 6 months, on parental report	Prevalence (%)		
	2–5 years	6–9 years	10–12 years
Dresses like opposite sex	16.2	9.0	2.9
Wants to be opposite sex	9.8	1.0	2.2
Touches sex parts in public	30	16.1	8.8
Masturbates with hands	9.2	6.1	5.2
Scratches anal/crotch area	53.4	36.0	20.6
Masturbates with object	3.2	0.3	1.5
Imitates the act of sexual intercourse	2.3	8.7	5.9
Puts mouth on another child's/adult's sex parts	0.2	0.3	0
Uses words that describe sex acts	3.6	24.4	27.9
Pretends to be opposite sex when playing	13.8	2.9	1.5
Makes sexual sounds	2.3	6.8	7.4
Asks others to do sex acts	0.9	1.6	0.0
Rubs body against people or furniture	5.3	3.5	2.9
Imitates sexual behaviour with doll/toy	2.6	3.5	2.9
Talks flirtatiously	16.0	12.9	3.7
Undresses other children	4.9	1.3	0.7
Shows sex parts to children	13.2	7.1	2.2
Playing with opposite sex's toys	59.4	38.3	20.6
Stands too close	8.9	5.8	4.4
Touches animals' sex parts	2.6	1.0	0.0
Draws sex parts	4.9	12.2	8.1

Gender Identity Disorder is rare, complex, and heterogeneous[1005]. It is distinguished from acting like the opposite sex (e.g. tomboys, p.566), by severe dysphoria. In Canada, about a quarter become bisexual or homosexual[430].

B. Intercourse

Estimated percentage of American females age 15–19 who had ever had intercourse by exact age x (after[1819]).

Exact age x	Current ages 15-19 in 1976	
	White	Black
12	0	0
13	1.1	4.8
14	2.6	10.3
15	7.1	22.4
16	16.8	39.1
17	30.0	58.1
18	43.6	73.0

Risks of intercourse vary by age, sex, and culture; but generally include sexually transmitted disease, cervical cancer, pregnancy, and associated mental health risks (which are not necessarily causative). About 15% of teenage girls have had anal sex, mostly during menses or under the influence of alcohol or cannabis[687].

C. Pregnancy

The rate of teenage pregnancy depends strongly on cultural group, age, and year. For example, in the USA in 2004 there were 42 pregnancies per 1000 girls aged 15–17 [1667]. Rates are several times higher in some social groups.

Risks of pregnancy depend on age and culture. Consider incest, p.489.

D. Motherhood

Rates and risks vary by cultural group as some South Asian ethnic groups have high rates of teenage childbearing within marriage.

Risks of motherhood depend on age, support, and any previous mental illness. Risks of teenage childbearing are strongly debated[722].

E. Child and adolescent sexual offences

Sexual assault
- Forcing someone to have sex was admitted by 5% of males and 1.3% of female adolescents [199]
- 20–40% of all rapes are committed by under 18s[721]

Non-violent sexual offending (the law varies between countries)
- Sex with an under 13, or 4 years younger than the perpetrator. Exposure to intrafamilial violence increases this[1491].
- Bestiality or sex with animals is somewhat more common on farms and sometimes associated with violence to humans[688]. Zoophilia is a paraphilia, illegal in much of the world (contrast *touching animals' sex parts*, above; attachment to animals, p.246; cruelty to animals, p.279).
- Sibling sexual experiences (incest, p.489) are recalled by 15% of university students, prevalence of onset steady from age 5 onward. About 2% recalled intercourse or attempted intercourse, mainly from age 9 onward[498].

Hands-off offences
- Exhibitionism, voyeurism, obscene calls, stealing underwear[1406].
- Stalking by children is generally non-sexual/non-romantic; and in adolescents tends to take over their lives less than in adult stalkers. Motives include love, hatred and predation. Stalkers often have poor social skills or personality problems and some stalk a previous partner, unable to deal with the separation[929,1642].

Causelist 92: Sexual/sexualised behaviour

Sexual behaviour includes adopting a gender role and interest in potential sexual partners, as well as sexual stimulation of self and others. The term *sexualised* behaviour implies that the child's behaviour has been *made* sexual, probably by exposure to adult sex. The term should therefore be avoided unless other factors in the list below are minor in comparison.

If the behaviour is indiscriminate but not actually sexual, see p.173. For touching of people, see p.132.

Any sexualised behaviour has several aspects, which should be assessed to understand what is happening. One system includes the following aspects: "shamelessness", "sexual interest", "boundary problems", "gender identity problems", "sexualised play", "sexual intrusiveness", and genital handling[1439].

Conundrum 14: Sexualised or hypomanic

Try to avoid the question of choosing *between* hypomania and abuse as a cause of sexual behaviour. Instead, consider them separately. Measure hypomania by presence of rest of the syndrome (overactivity, grandiosity, poor sleep, undereating, etc., p.264). Sexual abuse sequelae do not have such a well-defined syndrome, but the question can still be considered *separately* on the basis of multiple signs, as listed on p.275.

Causes of sexual / sexualised behaviour	Notes
Normal behaviour	*Sexual* behaviour occurs in normal children from infancy onward, though its form varies with age and sex. Sexual interest and urge increase around puberty. See p.267 for population statistics.
Learned from friends	
Learned from inappropriate videos or computer games	Probably because of these influences, sexualised behaviour is considerably more common than decades ago, and not as good a sign of abuse as it used to be. Common influences are music videos (e.g. on MTV) and films belonging to older siblings, borrowed and watched repeatedly because the music sounds good, or the behaviour is so mysteriously different from normal life, or it looks grown-up. Children who go to bed late watch unmonitored TV; some non-Western TV channels show extreme violence in news footage.
Non-sexual behaviour that sounds sexual	Children can learn a family's idiosyncratic ways of living (e.g. drying their genitals with hair dryers) and by clumsily explaining it, give completely the wrong impression of who is doing what to whom. Careful questioning is needed to avoid severe misunderstandings.
Attention-seeking	Extreme boredom (p.322) will eventually make children try anything in any context, and they will eventually learn that sexual behaviour gets a strong reaction from adults. This is not the explanation if he is not making contact (physical or eye contact), or if it happens *less* when he is bored.

👁 ‼ Child sexual abuse	"Scientific evidence confirms the relationship between sexual abuse and sexually problematic behaviour in children. There is no particular symptom that is characteristic of victimized children. However, sexualized behaviour is a common symptom and has been found to occur in about one-third of sexually abused children. Abuse, on the other hand, is seldom the explanation of sexualized behaviour in clinical cases…" [895,citing] [908]. On the CSBI, in comparison with the normative group, sexual behaviours were *somewhat* more common in children with mental health problems, and *much* more common in children who were known to have been sexually abused[527] (the only exception was the item "dresses like the opposite sex"). Rarer behaviours or any other concerns would merit a careful search for supporting evidence (as listed on p.275).
Masturbation	(p.474)
👁 Hypomania / mania	(p.264)
Kleine-Levin syndrome	– But sleepiness is a more pronounced symptom (p.496).

In disability

Autism 🔺 (p.183)	Interest in the way parts of the body move (e.g. arms, toes). Lack of understanding of admonitions. He may do this in public because he has learned that it makes mother take him home.
ID	Occasionally an over-protected or learning disabled child can give a worrying impression, if he has an incorrect understanding of sexuality or the meaning of words (e.g. a 16-year-old boy who asked when his periods would start, meaning when would he become a man). Because cuddles are usually welcome but sexual advances from a child are not, it can be difficult to establish boundaries that are completely clear to child and parents.
👁 ‼ Child sexual abuse	The risk of abuse is increased in ID (see also above).
Masturbation	(p.474)
Klüver-Bucy syndrome	(p.496)

Special Topic 13: Is this child being abused? ☼

Definitions:
Abuse: This means a child has been treated in an unnaceptable way by
           an adult in a given culture at a given time." However, you can
           see all aspects of emotional cruelty occasionally in ordinary
           families. Abuse is when it is persistent or extreme.
Maltreatment: Term used mainly in USA for sexual, physical, and
           emotional abuse (to distinguish them from neglect, which is
           seen as different because it is a failure rather than a wilful act)
Disclosure: This means the *first* description, i.e. breaking the secret (see
           p.452).

Categories of abuse
The main forms are physical, sexual, emotional and neglect. Sometimes
other forms are recognised, such as financial, overprotectiveness (which is
really emotional abuse), and discriminatory. Abuse is often
multiple/polymorphous, i.e. of more than one type.

Abuse can be graded as emergency; possible emergency; fostering
definitely justified; probably not as risky as fostering; minor; none. Abuse
is sometimes categorised by the relationship with the perpetrator , e.g. peer
abuse (bullying, p.219), parental abuse (often particularly damaging),
sibling abuse (e.g. by an aggressive child), medical abuse (p.206), and
institutional abuse (in which the child's needs are inappropriately
overridden by the institution's needs).

Sequelae of abuse
You can to some extent predict the severity of its sequelae (e.g. distress,
self-harm) from factors in the abuse, such as number of kinds of abuse,
duration, frequency, use of force or penetration – versus the child's
resilience (p.541).

Common errors in diagnosis
Over-recognition…
- mislabelling cultural practices that are not cruel
- calling over-mothering abusive, when the child is developmentally
  under 3 years old.
- missing medical causes of symptoms (see e.g. *fractures*, p.468)
- calling poor attachment to mother abusive, when either (a) the child is
  autistic, or (b) there are excellent protective attachments to father or
  other relatives
- "recovery" of unreliable memories of abuse [210].

and under-recognition…
- going along with other statutory agencies that see no physical risk so
  close the case
- accepting traditional cultural practices that harm children, p.448.
- ignoring abuse of mother or of other children you haven't met.
- not doing enough physical examinations of children.

	Risk factors in child	Risk factors in parent	Risk factors in environment
Physical (including Munchausen by proxy, p.206)	Unwanted, low birth weight, neonatal separation, handicap, unattractive, crying +++	Single, young, abused as child, punishment-oriented discipline Recent LE's	Poverty Social isolation Various crises Large family
Sexual	Female sex	Stepfather. Female: multiple psychopathology	
Emotional	(as physical abuse, p.273.)	(1st 3 as physical abuse)	
Neglect			Poverty

Principles for initial assessment of abuse

- Document everything including phone calls.
- Experienced interviewers are more reliable. Pressure and forced choice questions must be avoided as they can produce false information (see *confabulation*, p.443).
- If you personally have any suspicions whatever → discuss all concerns with a colleague. No professional should ever intervene on their own. The "named doctor for child protection" should be involved (www.rcpch.ac.uk/publications/misc_documents/Named_paediatrician. pdf); check the At Risk Register; check other family members' notes.
- If the two of you have any significant worries → report to social services. This is the theory, but in practice you may together decide to take extra measures to clarify the situation, such as by admitting the child to hospital for a few weeks, to see if she improves away from her parents.
- "if a disclosure of sexual abuse is made about a named person the police should interview that person before any other professional." [247]
- Obtain parental consent for further investigation unless it is against the child's interest to do so. Mother may be able to give child direct permission to disclose.
- Social services will arrange a paediatric examination if appropriate, and will decide whether to take the matter further.

---

continued ▶

Physical abuse
(see also fabricated/induced illness, p.359)

Sequelae

Short term:	injury, death
Medium term:	unhappy, wary, angry
Long term:	cognitive delays

Physical abuse: Level of suspicion [after 247,1138].
Consider all columns in deciding level of suspicion

Parental signs	Behavioural signs	Physical signs		Parallel risks
Account of injuries is inconsistent with their appearance	Frozen watchfulness (especially important if directed at specific people – p.470)	Multiple fractures (p.468) at different stages of healing	High suspicion	
Lack of parental concern – or unusual hostility to staff		Cigarette burns		
Discrepant accounts of events		Human bites (esp. if adult size)		Suspicion increased by any evidence of neglect or emotional abuse.
Late presentation, by non-parent, to unknown doctor	Over-friendliness			
Unusual refusal of mother to leave the bedside	Very aggressive play	Bilateral black eyes		
Symptoms only occur at home, or coincide with parental visits to hospital	Major preoccupation with own health	Fingertip bruising		
		Burns, scalds		
High level of demand for investigation, without physical signs.	Dissociation (p.453)	Bruising in sites not easily injured	Medium suspicion	
Previous convictions.		Unusual cuts or marks		
Threatened female circumcision or similar.		Hypernatraemia, hypothermia or cold injuries without explanation		
Parent hostile to child, especially if severe & intermittent		Frequent accidents		
Social isolation; domestic violence, p.454; frequent use of physical punishment; alcohol and drug abuse; unemployment, p.570		Head injuries in infancy (under 2 years)		
		Any injury	Low suspicion	

Neglect

Neglect is the commonest and longest-lasting form of abuse. It has a poorer prognosis than other categories. Emotional neglect (neglect of a child's basic emotional needs) is classified within Neglect rather than within Emotional abuse.

Neglect: Level of suspicion [after 247,1138]. Consider all columns in deciding level of suspicion.				
Parental signs		**Behavioural signs**	**Physical signs**	**Parallel risks**
Failure to comply with necessary medical treatment.	Severe neglect	Hoarding, stealing from dustbins	Drop in height or weight, or failure to grow (with no organic cause found).	Suspicion increased by any evidence of emotional or physical abuse.
Drug abuse, mental illness ID Parents who never experienced proper parenting themselves.	General neglect	Severe withdrawal Ingrained dirt, p.483 Failure to achieve potential in school, socially immature	Hypothermia Starvation, p.553 Multiple accidental injuries (if caused by poor supervision)	

Guidelines for leaving children unsupervised: www.loudoun.gov/dss/children.htm . Factors to consider: duration (increases with age and companions); inside/outside; on balconies; in the car; on the internet; when ill or crying…

Categories of ill-treatment within Emotional Neglect

Failing to promote the child's social adaptation
- Being denied contact with peers, including carer not facilitating school attendance.
- Promoting mis-socialisation, e.g. child allowed or encouraged to misuse illegal drugs; or to engage in criminal activities.
- Failure to provide adequate cognitive stimulation, education, and/or experiential learning.

Emotional unavailability, unresponsiveness and neglect
- Extremely little emotional interaction between carer and child (unavailability).
- Failure of carer to respond to child's attempts to interact (unresponsiveness).

continued ▶

Child Sexual Abuse (CSA)

This is "the involvement of dependent children and adolescents in sexual activities they truly do not comprehend, to which they are unable to give informed consent, and which violate social taboos of family roles." This includes incest (p.489) and involvement in pornography. Practices tend to escalate over time.

1% penetrative by adulthood; 15–30% any contact; 30–60% if include non-contact sexual experiences. More within family (more repeated, more loss of trust, more family dysfunction, more damaging).
Sequelae include anxiety, aggression, PTSD (p.532), poor self-esteem, difficulty with sexual relationships, tendency to sexualise relationships, prostitution, drug abuse, and having a sexually abused child of her own. Some sequelae appear to be due to factors leading to the CSA rather than to the CSA itself. [856]

40% of female rate. More by strangers, usually by men.
Subsequently doubt their sexuality more than do girls.

Fewer, but a *higher proportion,* of stepfathers commit CSA.

Major aetiological factors in the psychological damage of sexual abuse
Secrecy
Denial: this is perhaps the most important factor of all. Lynch mobs & increased sentences make it more difficult for offenders to own up, so make things worse for the children.
Disbelief
Vulnerability to further abuse because of sexual experience.

Presentations: Disclosure to a trusted adult (p.452); crisis (self-harm, p.317, running away from home); direct questioning by an adult alerted by e.g. unexplained pregnancy; vaginal discharge; STD; highly sexualised behaviour (p.269); inexplicable change in behaviour or schoolwork; dissociation (p.453).

Reliability of history given by child depends on age (at event or at recall), level of stress, schema within which child could place the information, *nature of elicitation of recall*[210]. The following may be meaningless to a child: "Did anyone hurt you", "…touch you where they shouldn't", "We want to protect you." Better: "How does your dad show that he loves you?"

☞ **Mother cannot and will not protect the child if she doesn't believe that it happened.**

Sexual abuse: Level of suspicion [after 247,1138].
Consider all columns in deciding level of suspicion.

Parental signs	Behavioural signs	Physical signs		Parallel risks
Relationship with adult becoming closer after puberty	Child hints at sexual activity or uncomfortable secrets. Disclosure is more likely to be valid if 1) consistent when repeated; 2) detailed (especially details that could not otherwise be known); 3) accompanied by obvious emotion.	Semen around genitalia Pregnancy under age 13 Pregnancy especially where the father is unknown. Postnatally acquired syphilis or gonorrhoea	Certain abuse	
Poor sexual relationship between parents; maternal depression (p.174) or physical illness				Suspicion increased by any evidence of neglect or emotional abuse.
Mother sexually abused in childhood		Injuries to sexual areas, e.g. breasts and genitalia. Vaginal foreign objects[691] Herpes simplex esp.type 2 (see[715]) Fingertip bruises on knees & thighs	High suspicion	
Father/abuser inadequate or rapacious. Previous convictions.	Inappropriate & repeated sexual play and talk, especially with adults (p.267)	Medically unexplained or treatment-unresponsive perineal itching, soreness, pain on micturition, discharge.	Medium suspicion	
Family disorganised and primitive or close-knit and socially isolated	Severe eating disorders in older children (p.334) Self-harm (p.317), fire-setting (p.466) Running away (p.210) Dissociation (p.453)	Pregnancy at age 13–15 Anogenital warts, Hepatitis B, HIV, gonorrhoea or other STD (for details of ages & law see[1138]) Gaping anus on examination, without a medical explanation such as neurological disorder or severe constipation.		
Parentified daughter (p.214) takes over mother's role		Occasional UTIs Recurrent abdo. pain, headaches (p.135)	Low suspicion	

continued ▶

Emotional abuse

This is the persistent emotional ill-treatment of a child such as to cause severe and persistent adverse effects on the child's emotional development. The threshold for recognising it cannot be met by a single act: rather, the threshold is the *relationship* being characterised by pervasive, harmful, non-physical interactions. Importantly, perpetrators of emotional abuse and emotional neglect rarely try to conceal the abuse (fabricated / factitious illness being an exception, p.359). The hurdle is not disclosure but professional recognition.

There are several systems for categorising emotional abuse based on what the parent *does*, but the following system has the advantage of focusing on the *effect in the child* [571]

1. Emotional unavailability, unresponsiveness, and neglect
- Includes parental insensitivity.

2. Negative attributions and misattributions to the child (p.426)
- Hostility towards, denigration and rejection of a child who is perceived as deserving these.

3. Developmentally inappropriate or inconsistent interactions with the child
- Expectations of the child beyond her or his developmental capabilities
- Overprotection and limitation of exploration and learning
- Exposure to confusing or traumatic events and interactions.

4. Failure to recognise or acknowledge the child's individuality and psychological boundary (see *identification*, p.237)
- Using the child for the fulfilment of the parent's psychological needs
- Inability to distinguish between the child's reality and the adult's beliefs and wishes.

5. Failing to promote the child's social adaptation
- Promoting mis-socialisation (including corrupting)
- Psychological neglect (failure to provide adequate cognitive stimulation and/or opportunities for experiential learning).

If someone is wondering whether a child's poor behaviour at school is due to bad parenting (e.g. witnessing or experiencing violence), you should try hard to find other convincing observable reasons for the violence – and still you need to remain uncertain. You cannot rationally be certain either of what happens in private or of the effect that it has on his behaviour in school, unless the behaviour is bizarre and he could not have learned it from TV, friends, or experimentation.

| Emotional abuse: Level of suspicion [247,1138] | | | | |
| Consider all columns in deciding level of suspicion. | | | | |
Parental factors	**Signs in parent-child interactions**	**Behavioural signs in the child**	**Physical signs**	**Parallel risks**
Serious physical or mental illness, drug addiction (p.259), or involvement in seriously deviant lifestyles (note "abuse" does not always require culpability). Breakdown in parental relationship (p.191) with chronic, bitter conflict over contact or residence Major emotional rejection of the child and parental inability to perceive his needs with any objectivity Major and repeated familial change, e.g. separations and reconstitutions	See the table above, "Categories of ill-treatment". Lack of response, or extreme response, to separation from parents. Young child excessively comforting carer. Parent hostile to child. Frozen watchful-ness (p.470) Running away (p.210)	Induction of child into bizarre parental beliefs. Psychiatric disorder esp. depression Over-compliant behaviour; dominating and aggressive behaviour with no concern for others. Rejection of friendship. Poor achievement and concentration. Age-inappropriate responsibilities. Repeatedly scavenging or hoarding food (p.480). Rocking / self-soothing (p.61) Oppositional (p.253) School non-attendance	Unexplained pains. Onset of bedwetting over age 5. Encopresis (p.341).	Suspicion increased by any evidence of neglect or sexual or physical abuse.

Causelist 93: Hurting others while fairly calm

Violence or cruelty to people and animals have much in common [reviewed in 1076]. Its importance depends on:

- What kind of animal (insects are less worrying)
- Age: cruelty by boys halves from age 6 to age 12.
- Trend of severity, frequency, victim type
- Duration
- Likely sequelae (e.g. is the victim known to the perpetrator)

Sometimes helpful: Who they look at, or what part of the victim is hurt, and attempts to conceal. Contrast with causes of killing, p.282; and violence while angry, p.289.

The causes in the following list are at a superficial psychological level. Genetics and long-term environment probably underlie most cases. For example, among abused boys and girls, 35% and 27% respectively were cruel to animals, but among unabused children, only 5% and 3% [6].

Causes of hurting people or animals while fairly calm	Notes
Normal	Many of the causes below can be seen in normal people, so normality is often determined by the severity or frequency. The phrase "I had a bad day so I came home and kicked the dog" describes behaviour that is abnormal in our society – but shouting at spouse or kids is common.
Non-volitional acts	
Accidents	
Tics	(p.101)
Automatisms	(p.427)
Being unaware of hurting people	It is not known whether lack of empathy can be an isolated problem.
Profound ID	E.g. sitting in dad's lap enjoying whacking his back
Autism ☂ (p.183)	Severe autistics may hit people for the sound of the impact or to elicit interesting responses. They may enjoy the feeling of tugging hair and/or collars. Other autistics hit a specific relative because they find the result intriguing, or to go home. If they are expressionless, it can be difficult to know whether they are feeling aggressive, in which case consider what preceded the violence (with an ABC, p.365). For example, if it only happens during loud noise or heat, or when they are denied something or restrained, it probably is at least partly aggressive. If it was truly out of the blue they may well have been bored.
Hurt as a byproduct (i.e. undesirable but unavoidable or unimportant)	
Social gains	Active bystanders / some participants in bullying. Gang initiation rites.
☞Habit, or knowing no alternative	Religious or cultural practices, punishment of children. Eating meat, sacrificing animals, exorcism, smacking. Multigenerational cycle of physical violence.
Sexual gratification*	Consider the first time, reaction or feeling then (like a fetish). Erotic slapping (whether consensual or not).
Attention-seeking	This is included here only to point out that it is an unlikely cause of *persistently* hurting others, because there are

usually so many other (less energetic and less resisted) ways to get attention or to relieve boredom (p.322).

Competitiveness	Male competition, testosterone linked (p.554)
Curiosity	
To rob	
Wanting to be like someone	Copying a parent or peers or the media. Imitating witnessed cruelty.
Wanting to cause pain	Causes here are often accompanied by an effort to hide the act.
Immaturity	Normally developing children learn first not to hurt themselves, later not to hurt others. Self-control and distraction techniques can be learned from role models, just as violence can be.
Retaliation	Against the victim or someone who cares for the victim.
To shock people	
Bolstering self-esteem (bullying)	Can include hurting animals.
Hurting a proxy (see *displacement*, p.305)	• Being angry at cute/small things: e.g. hurting a rabbit as a proxy for baby sister in major sibling rivalry. • Being angry at a person so hurting his pet.
Psychopathy ♠*	This term describes the combination of certain affective signs (callousness and lack of remorse), interpersonal signs (grandiose, arrogant and deceitful) and an irresponsible lifestyle (parasitic, impulsive,and needing stimulation)[1456]. (Distinguish from *psychopathology* which is a general term for all psychic problems; *hyperthymia*, p.264; *inadequate anxiety*, p.423; *pseudo-psychopathy*, p.423.) The behavioural pattern is generally clear by age 8.

Nomenclature in this area is complex. To start with, the term can be used in a categorical or continuous sense. In addition several subtypes have been described, with the non-anxious or "callous unemotional" individuals often held to have more severe or "core" psychopathy. These "true psychopaths" experience reduced autonomic arousal (p.424) in response to environmental events. This may be due to deficient fear conditioning[169]. These "primary psychopaths" experience less anxiety than adaptive ("secondary") psychopaths[923]. A comparable system distinguishes controlled-predatory aggression from impulsive-affective aggression[1680]. Finally, the term *sociopathy* is often synonymous with psychopathy, but sometimes is reserved for the people with antisocial personality disorder (p.242) who are not unemotional.

The term is used much more often in adults, and often used in a judgmental rather than therapeutic way. It is best avoided if an alternative description can be found (as is also true for *sadistic*, p.281; and *personality disorder*, p.241).

Adult psychopaths have increased rates of autistic traits (p.388), ADHD (p.83), and bipolar affective disorder (p.264) but they also have several traits that do not map well on to standard psychiatric classifications[1509]: dominance-seeking (p.455), manipulativeness (p.504), grandiosity (p.474), deceitfulness (p.255), and impaired social reasoning[470]. They may also have impaired

continued ▶

reasoning about risks and precautions[470] (this may only apply to those who are caught, and could result from the fear conditioning deficits described above). In severe adult cases, defects have been found in the orbitofrontal cortex, amygdala, and their connection, the uncinate fasciculus[332] (but see[862]). See also fire-setting, p.466 and the eye contact of psychopaths, p.177.

☞Psychotic ideas	E.g. morbid jealousy, misidentification, paranoia, p.524; command hallucinations, p.344.

Verbal cruelty

Misjudged humour / teasing / banter / friendly competition.	If the child is unaware of another's feelings, he may carelessly hurt them. Conversely, if he has low self-esteem and misunderstands the other's intentions, he may be hurt by inane comments (see *Causes of being bullied*, p.219). If the child misjudges the social relationship, or hasn't mastered the subtleties of cultural norms, he can use teasing when it is unexpected so seems like cruelty.
Immature expression of anger	A child can say "I hate you" when the issue seems enormous to the child, particularly if the child is impulsive or carers have previously rewarded this (i.e. given hugs or given in). The child may indeed feel hatred briefly, particularly if the carer was expected to be more compliant but isn't.

* *Sadism* has both these meanings. This word is much more pejorative even than *personality disorder* (p.241) and should not be used unless the desire to inflict pain endures for many years, includes strangers, and is present even when the child is calm (see also p.279).

Causelist 94: Killing or aiming to kill

This is a common concern.

Seven per cent of murders in the United States are committed by young people between 10 and 17[69]. On the receiving end, "in 2003, an estimated 9.3% of all US students in grades 9 through 12 had been threatened or injured with a weapon in school… ." [1731].   (For hurting people or animals see p.279.)

Outcome
With appropriate care the majority of children who have killed achieve good social adjustment[1785].

Causes of killing (or aiming to kill) others	Notes
Accidental	
Recklessness (calculated or not)	(p.539)
Collateral damage	is the killing thought to be unavoidable while pursuing another goal?
Intentional	Note that several of these factors are present simultaneously in many cases, e.g. in suicide bombing[996].
Coercion	Even mild authority can induce people to be violent [1075,1492]
Obedience to authority	Including command hallucinations, p.344
Dehumanisation of the enemy	Including hatred (p.187), cognitive dissonance (p.355), psychosis (p.537)
Social bonding	
Indoctrination	
Survival	Including *perceived* dangers as in paranoid psychosis (p.537)
☞ Altered states	Alcohol/drugs/mental illness, rituals/warpaint, dark glasses
Addiction to killing	Rare, erotic
Purging inferiors	Genocide
Lust for power	
Revenge	E.g. following abuse
☞ Perceived necessity	E.g. murder/suicide by parents who see no future for their children.

Special Topic 14: Is the risk of harming others great?

The best available way to estimate the risk is by careful clinical assessment, with consideration of all risk factors and all protective factors [1101,1469]. A long-term view of the child's offending is much more useful than a cross-sectional assessment, and requires good record keeping and communication.

In emotional arousal (including sex and anger), people's values change in predictable ways, so that lessons they have learned when calm can become irrelevant [Chapter 5 of 57].

Risk factors
Many adolescents develop violent or macabre preoccupations (p.245). However identifying the tiny minority who pose a major threat is usually impossible. The youngster will often reveal useful information if asked to draw himself or his family/friends, or to complete open-ended sentences. "In a student who is obsessed with violence, the theme is likely to emerge no matter what the nature of the discussion." [1731].

!!Estimating risk requires precise details of the threat: the level of realism and specificity, preparatory steps (even ideas of place or time), the intensity of threat preoccupation, and access to weapons. A history of being teased, particularly with accumulating retaliatory thoughts; social isolation or immersion in a copycat interest / culture of violence; ideas of self harm; paranoia (p.524), and emotional disconnection during interview are worrying. Previous witnessing violence or being a victim or perpetrator all increase risk. In the UK, 72% of young people who kill or commit serious violence have been abused, and 53% have lost someone important (through death or separation)[69].

The risk varies around the world. The main variable is the availability of guns, but another in some areas is the willingness of adults to do the planning and even pay the child to commit a murder.

Multiple homicide at school/college
Threats are important, at least in attacks with lethal means at school: "A key finding… was that school shooters indicated their plans before the shootings occurred, through direct threats or by implication in drawings, diaries, or school essays. … in more than three fourths of incidents, at least one person had information indicating that the attacker was thinking about or planning the school attack… Most attackers did not threaten their targets directly before the attack… ." [1731].

Sexual homicide by children and adolescents
This is extremely rare, happening about once per year in an all-age population of 40 million. All of the young people who do this have at least six of the following ten factors: impaired capacity to feel guilt, neuropsychiatric vulnerabilities, serious school problems, child abuse, family dysfunction, history of interpersonal violence, prior arrests, sadistic fantasy, psychopathic personality traits, and a personality disorder diagnosis (particularly schizoid or schizotypal, p.242)[1130].

Most important risk factors
Access to weapons
Alcohol and drug use
Persistent anger and psychopathy
Hyperactivity
Previous violence (especially with cruelty, sadism (p.281), or high frequency)
Are the situations or the triggers still occurring?

Other current risk factors
Access to potential victims (e.g. children, women)
Neurological impairment or ID
Violent fantasies (note that if a specific planned victim is identified, professionals have a duty to warn that person, overriding confidentiality. In such a situation, children are probably more at risk than adults. However, imagery of sexual violence is endorsed by the great majority of men, and is usually accompanied by no intentionality at all. The degree of preoccupation with the fantasies is crucial (for detailed discussion see[551])).

Other risk factors in the past
Number of arrests, cautions, and convictions, plus self-reported offences.
A trend of increase over time.
Cruelty to animals and children
Violence, self-harm, and fire-setting
Family deviance, harsh erratic parenting
Witness or victim of abuse.

Psychotic conditions
Psychotic symptoms increase the risk of violence if they make a person feel in danger, or if they override proscriptions against violence. More specifically, passivity delusions (p.95), thought insertion, and persecutory delusions definitely increase the risk of violence, but only slightly[965].

Protective factors
Positive achievements in school or job
Good relationships with positive peers.
Stable relationships

Anger

Three important types of difficult behaviour are non-compliance (or "not doing as he is told", p.253), temper loss (anger, p.287), and aggressive behaviour (p.289). For *all* of these types, occurrence in two or more contexts is much more indicative of severity than occurrence in just one[1700]. The only aspect that is very worrying even when it occurs in only one context is direct aggression toward adults, which is surprisingly unusual[1700].

Individuals differ in the *strength* of various emotions they feel. In some people, negative feelings last *longer* as well, e.g. startle following negative emotions in women [540]; and self-rated anger in borderline personality disorder [756] (p.242).

Signs of the rumbling stage [1131] These can be idiosyncratic to an individual child. Recognising them can allow a rage (p.71) to be prevented.

Fidgeting	Refusing to cooperate	Increasing/decreasing voice volume
Swearing	Rapid movements	Verbal threats
Making noises	Tears	Tapping foot
Ripping paper	Tensing muscles	Looking down or sideways
Grimacing	Name calling	

For assessment of risk, see pp.283, 542.

Causelist 95: ANGER – Tantrums

Tantrums are angry outbursts in children. Some of them are true out-of-control rage attacks (p.71) but children gradually acquire the ability to exaggerate, shape, or suppress tantrums to get what they want. Signs of such pseudo-rage include pausing for a rest then starting louder; or looking around for mother's reaction (as with pseudo-crying, p.316, and other pseudo-behaviours, p.363). See also *screaming*, p.544.

Causes of tantrums	Notes
Factors in others	
Normal	Up to 10–15 minutes, 1–2 times a day
Discipline inadequate	• If the parents can describe several behavioural techniques that actually *did* work for them, or tell you about something that they did wrong before, then their parenting is probably better than average. If there are major problems with this child but not with an older sibling, then differences between the children are more common than differences in parenting.
	• It is easy to fall into the trap of noticing the parenting is imperfect, and concluding that this is the problem needing resolving. However the child may well have other problems (e.g. temperamental rigidity, p.234; autistic spectrum disorder, p.388) that make normal parenting ineffective.
	• In preschoolers, totally absent discipline is abusive (p.274)
Discipline inconsistent	• Dads often ignore the family's rules, especially after they get home tired.
	• This is also what the child will perceive at the start of a behavioural programme, so parents need to be warned: "It will get worse before it gets better."
☜ Parental unavailability (recent onset)	E.g. distress in parent
Social learning (p.550)	• Display of tantrums by others (preschoolers particularly copy their parents' behaviour)
	• Covert encouragement to have tantrums, e.g. in marital discord, p.191
Feeling of unfairness	(E.g. if a sibling or peers get something). Usually normal, but the most severe cases are emotionally abusive (p.277). Throughout life, rewards are judged relative to others'
Factors in the child	
expressive difficulties	Delay in language (p.145) causes frustration (p.291).
Developmental delay	E.g. unable to do something his sibling can, or something that his parents/teachers expect him to.
Inflexibility	(p.234)
Discomfort or distress in child	(See section on headbanging for some causes: p.119)
Other physical	(See section on aggression for some causes: p.289)

All people feel angry sometimes (for causes of pair friction see p.172).
Anger can become impairing through its frequency, severity, duration, and
resulting behaviours such as violence. Timing is important in several
ways. A worsening trend justifies greater clinical attention. The
periodicity or timing of the anger may reveal its cause (pp.61–69). The
onset of angry behaviour may not be due to its causes, but to the person
feeling stronger, more exhausted, or placing reduced value on a
relationship that has been held together for external reasons.

Anger, like violence, can be highly focused, or directed at the whole
world. A child can be angry at people, walls, and the world yet only direct
it at mum, simply because she is there and hitting her doesn't hurt (see
overflow of arousal, p.292; displacement, p.305). Specific behaviours
often contain more information than the general feeling of "anger" does.
So it can be more productive to look up the causes for the behaviours, such
as violence, p.289; self-harm, p.317; disobedience, p.253; irritability,
p.494; oppositionality, p.253. *Hatred* is a long-term form of anger, with
some distinct causes (p.187).

Situations provoking many feelings simultaneously

Some difficult situations combine many of the factors from the table at the
right. If the eldest girl is required to fill her evenings with housework, she
is likely to feel unfairly treated, coerced, deprived of freedom and social
time, and trapped in a conflict between working for school and working for
her family. A teenager who has been sexually abused may be fearful, feel
coerced, trapped in longstanding dissonance between guilt and valued
relationships, and confused that different adults follow different rules. A
mother whose son has ID may enjoy caring for him when he is happy and
she has had enough sleep, but at other times feel trapped, unfairly
deprived, and fearful of having another similarly affected baby. People
who are paranoid (p.524) often simultaneously feel fearful, got at, and
coerced – as well as confused by cognitive dissonance. Other examples
are a separated mother's feelings about her ex-partner (p.187); or a patient
unable to get through to you on the phone.

Ambivalent feelings
This means having both positive and negative attitudes to something. It is
a common phenomenon because we can have different attitudes to
different aspects of a person, or to the way they behave at different times.
Describing a child's attitude to something as ambivalent requires one to try
to discern what elicits the negative feelings, and what the positive. After
this has been achieved, the word *ambivalent* is hardly useful.

A child who hates being shouted at can simultaneously enjoy parental
closeness. Another child may approach his mother warily because that
sometimes pleases her yet sometimes leads to his being hit (see
disorganised attachment, p.195). An anorectic can feel extreme hunger
but simultaneously a moral prohibition against eating. A shy child may
conceal her eyes behind her hair but carefully monitor what is going on:
this could be described as ambivalence to people but that adds nothing.
The eye-gaze of some children with Fragile X (p.176) is an extreme
variant of this. Uncertainty about what one wants or believes is common
in schizophrenia and in other conditions[891].

A child can vacillate between two opposing attitudes (e.g. in parental
alienation, p.187); but sometimes the word *ambivalent* refers to cases in
which the person is preoccupied by the contradiction, i.e. feels
"conflicted"[1779] (also called *cognitive dissonance*, p.355). Such
complications of attitudes can be unconscious (p.570) to varying
degrees[1779]. See also *unwanted behaviours*, p.353; *perverse effects*, p.528;
attitudes, p.425.

Some contributors to feeling angry
– or giving the impression of being angry.

Learned behaviour	• A child may have learned that shouting or crying often gets what he wants (see *tantrums*, p.286).
	• The ability to inflict costs (e.g. via strength or attractiveness) is strongly correlated with proneness to anger, and to experiencing more success in interpersonal conflicts, and to feeling entitled to better treatment[1450].
To communicate	E.g. to show the depth of our feelings about something.
Dogmatism, Self-righteousness	• Belief that the world should follow rules …or that everyone in it should follow the same rules.
	• Expressing anger to others can make us feel we are in the right. Many cases of parental alienation (p.187) include this.

Upsetting situations
(NB imagined events can occasionally be as upsetting as real ones)

Coerced / loss of will / feeling trapped	Violent or non-violent protest at being forced to do something. Forced to go to bed, prevented from playing, etc.
Unfairness (frustration is the acute version of this)	• Ignored, rejected (look for poor peer relationships).
	• Best friend stole boyfriend.
	• Child with OCD (p.65) unable to make family comply with rituals that he sees as crucial.
	• Deprivation is much more upsetting if the sibling got more.
Illness, pain, fatigue	These can make people very short-tempered (see also irritability, p.494; pain, pp.135-141).
Humiliated, loss of face, inadequacy	Humiliated, embarrassed, inadequate (many young people feel permanently humiliated by their poor ability to understand what other people are saying. When they feel miserable or persecuted, they are much more likely to misinterpret people's facial expressions or intentions.
Feeling got at	When we hear drilling next door or tapping in the library, or even laughter, it is far more upsetting if we feel there is malicious intent[605], i.e. that the other person takes pleasure in our suffering.
	Such feelings can arise from assuming other people know much more than they really do, e.g. that they know the sound goes through the wall and that other people are having difficulty concentrating. Similarly, when a car swerves in front of us, we feel it was an intentional, malicious attack – but the person may not even have noticed us (see *attribution error*, p.426)
Fear	Fearful/anxious, vulnerable, insecure, threatened, out of control in the situation, powerless
Cognitive dissonance (p.355)	Told to do something impossible, or something that conflicts with another rule.

Causelist 97: Violence while angry ☼

Violence has many definitions. Here it is used to mean acts that cause physical damage or pain. The feeling that often leads to violence is called *anger*. The phrase "he has a lot of anger in him" is common but misleading; it should be replaced by "he gets angry easily" or "he's constantly angry" which of course have many causes. Rages are the most severe angry episodes (p.71). *Aggression* is used variously to mean anger (p.287), violence, or both[see 1681] (though American non-psychological usage of *aggressive* includes the positive sense of being proactive).

For violence while fairly calm, see p.279; for violence to self, see p.317; for displacement of aggression see p.305; for angry speech, see p.161.

Angry violence is one of the most common presenting problems of young people. Violence in a 2-year-old is usually called tantrums (p.286) and is very likely to go away[1621]; but the most violent boy in a school class of any age is likely to keep that distinction for many years[892]. It is worth thinking about how a child compares to what would be normal for their age and sex, in:

- Type of provocation
- Level of provocation needed
- Behaviour
- How long it lasts (seconds implies emotional instability (p.69); minutes implies learned; longer implies mood)
- Their attitude to it afterward (e.g. remorseful)

From the 16th birthday in some areas violence from teenagers can be assessed (and managed) by domestic violence teams (p.454).

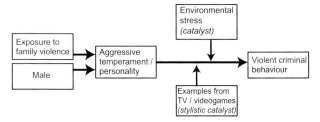

Figure 20. Causes of violent criminality.

(from [491]; see also [415]).

For a comprehensive summary of risk factors for adolescent violence, see[1645].

Mild violence

The following often indicate *lower* degrees of aggressive feelings:
- briefer outbursts
- the careful targeting of body areas, avoiding sensitive areas such as faces
- the child keeping his distance and monitoring the reaction
- using just one limb rather than swinging whole body
- hitting once rather than repeatedly
- lack of facial expression
- limited autonomic responses. If less than expected for the degree of violence, may be described as psychopathic in adulthood,p.280.
- with strangers, milder hits or a gradual escalation (e.g. starting with a mild tap).

In some families and cultures, some violence is considered an appropriate everyday behaviour. Most families consider it acceptable when it is about an important issue (mainly injury to self or family), is proportionate, defensive, all other solutions have been tried, it has a reasonable chance of achieving its goal, and injury to bystanders is minimised. Most of children's violence does not meet these criteria – but when it does, many parents support it.

Extreme violence

When all the above mild signs are absent, the child is out of control, and the term *rage* (p.71) is appropriate.

continued ▶

Causes of repeated angry violence	Notes (NB These can summate to produce greater violence or even uncontrolled *rage*, p.71)

Primitive reaction	When aggression is first used in a situation, it can be either experimentation or a *primitive reaction*. Primitive reactions are much more likely if other responses have not been learned. They can be triggered by:
	• Frustration is caused by the child's not obtaining what he wants and expects[35]. The frustration can be expressed as aggression to others or to self (e.g. self-biting, some flapping, most headbanging). Examples:
	  ○ Tantrums (p.286)
	  ○ Abuse, especially if he can't talk about it (see sexual abuse, p.275)
	  ○ Refusal to comply with child's rituals in OCD (p.65) and autism (p.183) can be particularly difficult.
	  ○ Departure of familiar staff upsets an autistic child.
	  ○ Children with selective deficits have experienced some success so are very frustrated in their poor subjects. Specific language deficits often cause this (p.145).
	• Fear (normal in threatening situations, and in many of the physical and mental states listed below)
	• Predatory, inter-male, territorial, threat to status [1121,1681]

Mood	Irritability (p.494), anger, jealousy (whether diagnoseable or not). Irritability is a key part of DSM's depression under age 18 (p.309) & mania. In mania (p.264), outbursts can be very sudden.
Compensatory	People often use aggression, or at least an aggressive tone and body language, to compensate for low self esteem and poor self-confidence. Aggression also increases in autistic people when the environment is unsettled, or when people around them are intrusive.
Threatened	The threat can be physical or emotional (see narcissism, p.511; fight-or-flight, p.466). Occasionally it results from paranoid feelings (p.524).
Sleep problems	Aggression is strongly related to sleep problems and improving sleep can improve daytime behaviour [289].
Physical abuse	Parents or carers may have resorted to aggression because they knew no other ways of controlling the child. Rarely, they perform such complex, unusual acts that the child's re-enactment is almost pathognomonic. For example, one abused autistic girl spread her fingers on an adult's forehead with thumbs touching the adult's eyelids.
Learned	Learned from parental or peer violence[100] • Learned way of obtaining something. • Learned method of expressing anger (strong association with harsh physical punishment) • Learned way of behaving (e.g. if praised by other gang members, p.472 or by father) Or not having learned to negotiate.

Violent TV & video games	In the general population the effect is very small[491] but in violent individuals, especially innately aggressive males, it can be important [226]. Mechanisms include priming, imitation, arousal and desensitisation. See figure on previous page and *video games*, p.573.

Pathological mental conditions

Psychosis	(p.537, or paranoia, p.524) These can cause fear; or command hallucinations, p.344.
Tourette's (p.101), ADHD ⟐	(These can act via several of the other listed mechanisms) Impulsivity (as in ADHD) allows aggression to emerge unchecked, but in both disorders the need for stimulation is usually assuaged by other means than major aggression.
PTSD	(p.532) Reliving a fearful experience can cause violence.
ID	With low ability youngsters, many of the other causes of aggression coexist with: • not knowing what will happen later, so constantly getting unpleasant surprises. • difficulty with affect-regulation. The impression of aggressiveness can be given by interest in other people's faces combined with clumsiness; or by closeness due to visual impairment or failure to understand personal space, p.527. Distance, speed, and complexity of movements (e.g. of throws, slaps, and dance steps) reduce accuracy and make injury less certain, so in retrospect reduce the likely degree of intentionality. A lot of what you see is not winding-up but self-entertainment (p.545: e.g. echolalia, p.459; and casting, p.103). This can also be learned behaviour imperfectly copied (particularly if the child is often hit at home, or witnesses violence: see *physical abuse* above).
Frontal deficit	Damage can reduce self-control. See frontal lobes, p.513; frontal signs, p.469; inadequate anxiety, p.423.
Emotional instability or dyscontrol	(p.69)

Physical conditions (see also p.293 for acute conditions)

Pain	(pp.135-141)
High ambient temperature	Annoyance or "arousal" overflows (p.520) to things that did not cause it [37,1383]. For example, violent crimes (more than non-violent ones) are increased by heat. Contrast *displacement*, p.305.
Hormones	Adrenaline, p.420 (cf. hypoglycaemia, p.82); testosterone increases at puberty, p.554
Other	E.g. hypothalamic hamartomas[1734] (p.76).

Investigation Planner 7: Emergency assessment of violence

Consider performing these tests if the child's anger is much more severe than usual, much more long lasting than usual (e.g. hours rather than minutes), or if it started without provocation.

Find out from carers what usually upsets him and what upset him this time. What was the last thing that anyone did before the outburst? Does he have a rigid understanding of social rules that he thinks have been transgressed? Find out from staff, from records and from the family what calmed him down last time. Is there a person who can usually calm him, by their gentleness, predictability or merely their reassuring presence? Ask him what he needs. Has he previously stated that certain interventions are unthinkably awful for him (e.g. being held still or put in a room alone)?

☞Red flags that should encourage the search for a physical cause include:

- new disorientation in time, place or person (pp.97,400,451)
- fluctuating level of consciousness (p.97)
- visual hallucinations (p.344)
- focal neurological signs
- ketotic or recent weight loss
- pain anywhere; he indicates or protects a part of his body
- In ID and non-verbal children, beware of missing medical conditions.

Obtain a full medical history as previous illnesses may be re-occurring. Enquire about his developmental level or long-term emotional state or flexibility of thinking, as it may suggest a better way to approach him.

Many of the following investigations can be performed in an emergency setting[579]. Some of the tests remain abnormal for just a few hours so considerable effort is justified to obtain them. See also the *general approach to medical investigations*, p.373, and the suggested investigations in catatonia/stupor, p.99; and hypomania, p.265. The section on repeated, long-term causes of violence (pp.285–291) is also relevant in some emergency situations.

If restraint or seclusion is used, medical assessment needs to continue regularly to minimise risk of self-harm, respiratory depression, asthma attack, asphyxia, dystonia, seizure, or arrhythmia. Pulse oximetry should be performed regularly if possible[377].

Category	Disorders	Suggested actions and tests (see[386])	Excluded clinically or	Date ordered	Result
!! ☞Risk		Search for weapons, and risks in the immediate environment. Also assess the risks to self (p.319) and to others (p.283). Minimise risks in any way possible.			
☞ Environment		Do not forget the possibility that some aspect of the environment may be keeping			

		him angry, e.g. bright lights, being talked about, being criticised; restraint, people too near or above him; people touching him even reassuringly, heat, or unfamiliarity. Is the bad behaviour being reinforced because all the attention is rousing or fun? Is his favourite person, who can always calm him, absent? Are staff and parents inadvertently upsetting him because they are so upset? Does he have nowhere to escape to (at home he may escape to his room when he is overwhelmed)? Is he better when left alone?
Basic medical tests		Has he eaten? Can he hear and understand you? Full physical examination. FBC, LFT, CRP, ESR, urea & electrolytes, calcium, phosphate
Endocrine	Hypoglycaemia, p.82; hyperthyroidism, p.484; steroids, p.554	glucose, thyroid function, pre-menstrual, p.506
Pulmonary	Hypoxia	Cardiovascular examination. pulse oximetry
Metabolic	(p.381)	ammonia, lactate
Neurological	Epilepsy, p.75; head injury, p.477 stroke, p.556; brain tumour,p.569	Look for signs of head injury. MRI brain Epilepsy is rarely violent (but see p.75 and consider EEG)
Psychiatric / psycho- logical	Rage, p.71 OCD, p.65; anxiety, p.295; bipolar disorder, p.264	History, observation, and interview for all these. See also the page numbers given.
Auto- immune, p.427	SLE, p.560; HIV, p.479	ANA, cardiac enzymes
Pain	Toothache (more on p.135)	History, examination
Infection, p.490	Earache chest infection; ☞ encephalitis, p.461	temperature; look in throat and ears; listen to chest. History of tropical travel? uristix, throat swab, ASOT, chest xray
☞ Drug induced	Substance abuse, p.257; steroids, p.554; benzodiazepines, p.430	Full physical examination including signs of drug abuse, p.257; hair/urine drug screen. Particularly antidepressants, antihistamines, amphetamine, carbamazepine. See also other toxins, p.566. If the behaviour becomes more outrageous after benzodiazepines consider paradoxical effect of benzodiazepines, p.430.

Anxiety

Causelist 98: ANXIETY (General) ☼

Anxiety is concern about *possible* danger, whereas fear is a response to a *present* danger (p.307). Indicators of severity include the number and ubiquity of triggers, and the amount of impairment (p.17).

Parents with substantial anxiety can be very observant of their anxious child's problems, and this plus a family history sometimes indicate a primarily genetic causation for the child's anxiety. On the other hand, a diagnostic pitfall exists in the practice of relying on parents for information on a child's anxiety, as on this topic self-report is generally more reliable. Furthermore, an anxious parent may believe the child to be more distressed than he actually is, even to the extent of keeping him unnecessarily off school, or arguing for him to repeat a year.

Anxiety is experienced by everyone and is crucial for safety; it is an important feature of life. It is even more central to mental health, so all professional groups concerned with children will see and treat causes (and effects) of anxiety. These are protean, as shown in the following diagram.

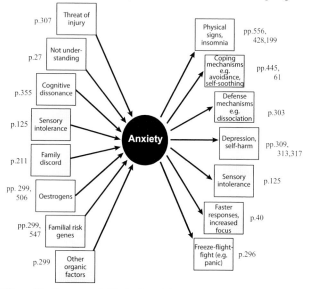

Figure 21. Causes and effects of anxiety.

Causes of anxiety (Figure 21; see p.299 for details)

These are usually classified as bio-, psycho-, and social, as on p.299. They can also be divided into life long, episodic, and immediate (also called triggers). However episodic manifestations are often accompanied by milder anxiety between episodes.

Triggers often change with age, from separation and surprises (falling, loud noises) in toddlers; to monsters, animals, and the dark in preschoolers; to teasing and being told off in the early school years; and in adolescence social acceptability and exams. Some of the triggers for anxiety tend to be associated with particular behaviours. Examples are given throughout the text.

Effects of anxiety

Simple effects of anxiety

Signs of anxiety include simple avoidance (p.429), focus on the object of anxiety, staccato movements, fast answering (e.g. rapid head-nodding), gulps, tremulous voice, forehead wrinkles[113] and sympathetic signs (p.556) such as tremor (p.61), heightened startle responses (pp.552,107), dry mouth, tachycardia, urge to micturate, dilated pupils, damp palms (p.558), and vomiting (p.337). Small children often experience tummyache when anxious. The ramifications of continuous anxiety can be remarkably limited, for example in a bright child whose only concrete *impairment* was his inability to graduate from tricycle to bicycle.

The subjective feeling of dread is not often a cause of complaint to professionals. However it is often used by children to obtain privileges from parents (e.g. school refusal, p.217), and in older teens can be a ticket to talk about problems.

Behavioural inhibition to the unfamiliar is both a behaviour and an aspect of temperament (p.561), defined as the reduction in behaviours that is produced by uncertainty or novelty[310,515]. The term is usually used when referring to infants, because their behaviours are more accessible than their thoughts. It may also be a "possible precursor" or "risk factor for anxiety disorders"[165,1320]. It is a mild version of the freezing and hypervigilance described below.

When the object of fear cannot be avoided a range of responses are characteristically used in the following order:

    freeze on guard, or hypervigilance (e.g. frozen watchfulness, p.470)
        → flight
            → fight (or minor violence, which is common in children)
                → extreme passivity (e.g. learned helplessness, p.96)
                    → syncope[205] (p.74).

of which another version ([1010], see also[204]) is:

    fear, discomfort
        →avoidance
            →panic (p.301) or screaming (p.544)
                →physiological and cognitive signs

Complex effects and sequelae of anxiety

- Children often manage external fears with simple observable behaviours (see table on p.126 and discussion of *coping mechanisms* on p.445) whereas internal fears have numerous cognitive remedies (e.g. defences, p.303).
- Some people learn to enjoy aspects of fear (e.g. the arousal and the renown), and seek out the scariest rollercoasters in order to experience these.
- Fears can lead to habits so effective that they almost completely eliminate the arousal, e.g. in the selectively mute child (p.153) who *knows* that he will not speak in school so he no longer needs to fear his accent being laughed at. For related examples see *non-behaviours*, p.515.
- Behaviours (e.g. anorexia, tantrums) can improve family dynamics, thereby indirectly rewarding and maintaining the behaviours[1091].
- Dissociation (p.453) may be the cognitive component of simple evolved behavioural responses listed above, such as freezing, submitting, or appeasing[877].
- In OCD (p.65), compulsions are an attempt to neutralise a fear; anxiety builds when a compulsion is not performed.
- Anxiety can counterbalance hyperactivity and impulsivity (p.207).

continued ▶

Nomenclature for common patterns in anxiety

Anxiety is usually classified by the cue for fear (e.g. spiders or open spaces), but sometimes by the resulting behaviours (e.g. selective mutism, school-avoidance or panics). Categories are broadly similar from preschool to adulthood, though somewhat less differentiated early in life[1523].

Anxiety is subdivided into categories as shown in the following diagram, but the fine subdivisions are not clear[1010]. For example, if a child has just one circumscribed symptom within one of the phobia clusters (see figure), it may be more useful to call it a "specific phobia" rather than using the name of the cluster[p.7 of 1010]. Also it is not clear whether panics are best seen as an indicator of severity of anxiety and depression, or whether they have a special role in aetiology, especially for agoraphobia[1010]. Even though DSM-IV classifies claustrophobia (fear of enclosed spaces) as a specific phobia, clinically it has more in common with agoraphobia (fear of crowds or open spaces where escape may be impossible, or help may be unavailable).

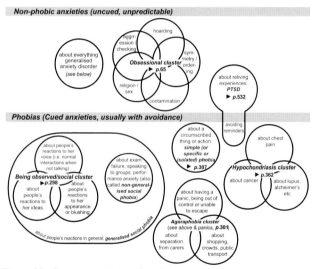

Figure 22. Common patterns of anxiety.

(after [1010]). Note that, despite having distinct names and definitions, the conditions are highly comorbid and share similar causes[1304].

Notes for Figure above:
- Phobias are handicapping irrational fears of objects or situations. The phobias generally have external cues, which can be avoided.
- GAD (Generalised Anxiety Disorder) means excessive worry about several distinct things. Symptoms can include restlessness, poor concentration, irritability, muscle and psychological tension, sleep disturbance and fatigue, p.323.
- Separation anxiety (p.197) is related to panic.

- **Social anxiety (also called social phobia)** has several components, including self-doubt, embarrassment, fear of strangers, and fear of negative evaluations by others. It is said to arise typically in adolescence (unlike normal childhood fears), but it contributes to selective mutism, p.153, which starts much earlier.

  Normal social anxiety is needed for the development of attachment behaviours. It has a moderate stimulus threshold and moderate response: 4% of all adolescents are nervous of social events or of eating and drinking in public; 2% of adolescents have felt an unreasonably strong fear of writing while someone watches[1784]. Social fears start about age 5, perhaps because of the development of the realisation that other people's opinions do matter. They then increase linearly, plateauing in young adulthood[1784].

  The overall prevalence of diagnoseable, impairing, social phobia is usually said to be about 5%, but there is debate about the threshold for formal diagnosis, because a degree of social anxiety is perfectly understandable and even useful; yet "nondisordered social anxiety can nonetheless cause enormous suffering"[1699]. Some place the threshold for diagnosis at avoidance, though anticipation is also used. Social anxiety contributes to selective mutism and to related selective behaviours (p.153). At the severe end, a few children avoid doing anything that interacts with non-family-members; this is obviously impairing.

- **Performance anxiety.** Eighteen per cent of adolescents have had what they feel was an unreasonably strong fear of exams even though well prepared, and a similar proportion are frightened of speaking to a group in class[1784]. If these are the only symptoms, and the person is impaired by them, it is sometimes described as a *non-generalised social phobia* (despite most exams not being very social events) whereas more general interactional fears are called "generalised social phobia"[835].

- The term **exposure anxiety** is sometimes used to describe the way in which a (very few) people avoid doing anything that can be seen by other people. Some very severely affected children won't even move or make facial expressions when they can be seen. Some of these have ASD.

continued ▶

Causes of anxiety	Notes
Psychological	
Sequelae of other problems	There are many such causes (social, cognitive, physical). Some are listed under school non-attendance (p.217)
Learned	E.g. dental fears acquired from parents[972].
Sensory intolerance (p.125)	It is not social anxiety (p.298) if he is comfortable in groups as long as they are quiet (see p.307).
PDD	Anxiety increased by new situations or strangers.
☜Cognitive dissonance (p.355)	Suspect this if: Inflexible personality (p.234); strong personal or family beliefs (cultural, religious, career ambitions); sexual abuse (p.275). Feeling he should be able to do a task can contribute to task-induced anxiety in postconcussion syndrome, p.477.
Simulation / exaggeration / pseudo-anxiety	Some children say they are afraid in order to get parental attention or hugs, or to avoid challenges, dirt, or exercise. Only happens when parent is around (see p.363). See also *pseudo-stranger-anxiety*: p.43.
Depression/ mania	Irritability (p.494), insomnia, poor concentration, somatic complaints
Psychosis (p.537)	Social withdrawal, decline in functioning
Social	
Family discord	p.211
bullying	p.219
☜Organic	Suspect this if (a) timing of anxiety is related to physical problems or medication changes; (b) sudden onset not related to social stressors; (c) any severe medical condition; (d) absence of family history of anxiety.
	Reasonable initial screening in such cases includes FBC, UECr, thyroid, glucose, ESR, CRP, lead.
Genetic	The heritability of individual anxiety disorders is in the range 0.2–0.5, and of anxiety disorders as a group is over 0.5[1583]. The heritability increases greatly through adolescence[143]. In rare families a single genetic defect causes anxiety in all carriers, sometimes together with other symptoms[1014]. See also serotonin, p.547.
Neurological	• Migraine, p.141; epilepsy, p.73; PANDAS, p.522; lead, p.330; tumours, p.569 • Ataxia can look like or cause anxiety. • Autonomic hyperreflexia: with headache and hypertension. Flushing above the lesion; pallor, motor & sensory deficits below it.
Cardiac	Cardiac arrhythmia, angina
Respiratory	E.g. asthma attack, p.424; hyperventilation, p.484; hypercapnia; hypocalcaemia, p.485; anaemia, p.421
Medication	Commonly methylphenidate especially under 5 (plus other stimulants, p.555), cold medicines, steroids including OCP, antipsychotics (akathisia, p.114), antihistamines. Also withdrawal of sedatives.
Drug abuse	(p.257). Also withdrawal.
Hormonal	• Premenstrual p.506; female or having a female twin[348]; see also p.506 • Hyperthyroidism, p.484 • Phaeochromocytoma, p.529.

Maternal stress in pregnancy	The effect of maternal stress during pregnancy on the developing child is difficult to separate from other factors such as inherited genes and postnatal depression, but has been very clearly demonstrated in animals[447]. In humans, the effect size depends greatly on 5-HTTLPR (p.547).
Other	• Sleep disturbance • Hypoglycaemia (p.82) • Occult chronic illness, e.g. coeliac disease, p.441

Causelist 99: Panics

Panics are episodic paroxysmal anxiety, typically lasting minutes at a time. DSM-IV defines a panic attack as including at least four of the following: dyspnoea (perceived shortness of breath), heart palpitations, trembling, dizziness, chest pain, perspiration, derealisation, paraesthesia, hyperventilation (p.484), nausea, vertigo, lightheadedness, choking sensations, fear of dying, fear of losing control or going crazy. (ICD also mentions nausea and stomach churning.) Panics vary enormously in severity.

Attempts to avoid panics generally include voluntary restriction of activity, e.g. avoiding non-stop train or motorway journeys because the situation is inescapable if a panic were to start. This can progress to avoiding even stopping trains, then avoiding buses, then avoiding walking far from the house, then staying in the house or even (rarely) in bed[1010](compare regression, p.44; pervasive refusal, p.527). Panics occur in normality and in many psychiatric disorders, especially agoraphobia (p.297).

See also startle syndromes (p.552).

Causes of panics	Notes
Normal panics	Tachycardia, sweaty palms (p.558), feeling of doom, but no real interference with life.
Agoraphobia	(See discussion on p.297).
Panic Disorder	A formal diagnosis of *panic disorder* should be used in people who get panics out of the blue (i.e. without situational triggers). The diagnosis refers to people disabled by the fear of another attack, rather than people primarily frightened of other things.
Generalised anxiety disorder (p.297)	Anxiety is present between attacks
PTSD (p.532)	Rarely volunteered by children unless asked (like obsessions in OCD, p.65)
Depression	(p.309)
☞ Physical	Paroxysmal tachycardia, mitral valve prolapse, carcinoid, phaeochromocytoma (p.529), hyperthyroidism (p.484)/thyroid storm, hypoglycaemia (p.82), labyrinthitis
☞ Medication	Sedative withdrawal

Defence mechanisms are essentially internal ways of relieving anxiety[240]. They can be helpful or counterproductive, with respect to the internal anxiety or external performance[1115]. So many defence mechanisms have been named that they span much of psychopathology, as do psychiatric and psychological terminologies, so the three are often related (see[979],[1660]). However, defence mechanisms in general can be broadly classified as self-deception, self-distraction, or distorting the situation[1115].

A distinction is often drawn between *coping* mechanisms (p.445) which are conscious, and *defence* mechanisms, as their unconscious counterparts. Even if the border between conscious and unconscious (p.570) were clear (which it often is not – p.359), this distinction is an oversimplification. Mechanisms to manage anxiety vary along many continua, such as externally visible/invisible; innate/learned; aware/unaware; effective/ineffective; and productive/counterproductive for external performance.

Evolving views

Defence mechanisms are sometimes neglected, perhaps because they are unfairly grouped together with outmoded Freudian ideas. They are also out of step with the prevailing trend of seeing people as rational creatures; they are not easily accessible to objective assessment; and they have no DSM code. However, they are reasonable hypothetical constructs[989] that can be carefully operationalised (see e.g.[457]). Their neglect is unfortunate as they describe some kinds of irrationality more convincingly than any other system.

Fortunately, other scientific areas are now catching up with psychoanalysis in this area – and in some respects have come to similar conclusions (see [806]). Defence mechanisms can often be described in terms from other fields, as "scripts" or "games people play" in stressful situations, or indeed as DSM disorders[pp.38-39 of 1643]. There is widespread acceptance of dissociation, p.453 predictable irrationality, p.534 and cognitive dissonance, p.355. The principle of defence mechanisms is becoming mainstream.

Development

"Immature" defence mechanisms are normal in young children but become much less common later. Projection and identification become more common in later childhood and adolescence. "High adaptive" defence mechanisms often appear later or not at all.

Defence mechanisms become so habitual, and so central to how other people experience us, that in adolescence or adulthood they become an important part of our *personality* (p.241).

Assessment – challenges

There is in practice no absolutely reliable way of knowing whether defence is really why a person did something. It is essential for professionals not to leap from the observation of a behaviour, to the conclusion that the behaviour is used as a defence (this is unfortunately common, both in research and clinical work).

Self-report is not adequate, because defence mechanisms are largely (some would say always) unconscious[1660].

Assessment – partial solutions

One must consider other possible causes for the behaviour, for example by consulting the lists in this book and doing a functional analysis (p.365). Other explanations for a child's behaviour have to be preferred when they are neurologically simpler (as is also true for symbolic causes, p.14).

Defence can only be a realistic explanation if the symptom occurs more when the child is anxious. If the behaviour disappears and reappears when the hypothesised cause of anxiety does, this supports the attribution. This test is necessary but not sufficient: it includes simple non-defensive byproducts of anxiety.

To convincingly demonstrate that a behaviour is actually functioning as a defence mechanism in a particular child, one needs to demonstrate that it reduces anxiety. This cannot be assumed from the fact that it works in other people or is called a "defence mechanism" or that the person thinks it helps[1115]. Definitive demonstration requires interventional investigation in the individual. This is usually not possible in the presence of unchangeable causes or with behaviours that have become habits (p.475).

Several assessment methods are available for use in young people[333], though none is perfect[1247]. People who are younger or of lower IQ tend to have fewer defence mechanisms[334]. People who use the most immature defence mechanisms generally have a mental age under 6 or are very seriously ill.

Table 15. Defence mechanisms that contribute to behaviour

"Level" of defence mechanism	Defence mechanisms Adapted from DSM-IV	Relevance to children (For a related list see[p.39 of 1643])
Action	Acting out (p.418)	Tantrums (p.286)
	Apathetic withdrawal	Depression (p.309), some insecure attachment (p.195), some autism
	Passive aggression (p.525)	Damning with faint praise. Parent stifling development by over-caring.
Major distortions of ideas	Autistic fantasy	Schizoid personality (p.242) imaginary friends (p.231)
	Projective identification (p.535)	
	Splitting (of self/others) (p.552)	
Disavowal	Denial	Not accepting the risks of addiction. An anxiolytic effect has been demonstrated[917].
	Projection	Claiming that his brother stole something, when he himself did it.
	Rationalisation	After he loses a hat, saying he didn't like it anyway.
Slight distortions	Devaluation	Component of selective refusals (p.540)
	Idealisation	Believing that dad or teacher knows everything
	Omnipotence	Protecting self from feeling inadequate – can be component of selective refusals (p.540)
Mental inhibitions (preventing problems from reaching awareness) (see also *inhibitions*, p.490)	Displacement (of aggression)	The classic example is kicking the cat after being told off[397]. There is good evidence for this in children and adolescents[396]. However, rather than a redirection it may be a simple overflow of annoyance, p.292.
	Dissociation (p.453)	Imaginary worlds (p.231)
	Intellectualisation	Common in parents, especially of children with rare problems. Focusing on details to distract oneself from the overall picture. Very effective in intellectually minded people[917].
	Isolation of affect	Child cutting himself off when *steeling* for a blood test
	Reaction formation	A child claiming that mother works incredibly hard, when she does nothing. A mother may overemphasise the strengths of her child, partly because she cannot face the child's difficulties, or because she is trying to balance something negative about him that she thinks is about to be said. Anxiolytic effect has been demonstrated[917]
	Repression	(p.421)
	Undoing	Waving wand to fix a broken toy
Defensive deregulation	This refers to extreme versions of other defence mechanisms in this table, with a clear break from reality. Examples are delusional projection, psychotic denial, and psychotic distortion (see *psychosis*, p.537).	

High adaptive level (permitting most problems to be dealt with consciously)	Anticipation	Prematurely but realistically experiencing forthcoming dire events.
	Affiliation	Relying on others for support
	Altruism	(p.420)
	Humour (p.495)	Expressing painful feelings without directly experiencing the pain or inflicting it on others. An example would be, after a parent has died, making a weak joke about how worthless parents are.
	Self-assertion	Expressing one's feelings directly, without intending offence.
	Self-observation	Thinking consciously about one's feelings and motivations
	Sublimation	Directing urges into useful (or at least socially acceptable) activities
	Suppression	(p.421)
Immature	Blocking	Interruption of a train of thought; or a transient version of repression (see p.433)
	Hypochondriasis	(p.362)
	Introjection	Child believes he is good (or evil) when parent says he is.
	Regression	(p.41)
	Somatisation	Tummyache before school
Neurotic	Controlling	Managing the environment ro minimise anxiety; perfectionism. Compare OCD, p.65.
	Externalisation	To perceive other people (or things) as having one's own characteristics. (contrast p.463)
Mature	Asceticism	Obtaining moral gratification by renouncing base pleasures
"Manic defences"	Identification with superego	The idea that mania is usually a defence against depression is now outdated.
	Manic triumph	People with bipolar disorder use many defence mechanisms[881]. It is sometimes
	Manic idealisation	argued that the presence of subtle depressive symptoms during elevated mood states is evidence for a manic defence[984], but this can equally be explained as due to distinct timecourses of various aspects of mood (e.g. insight, habit, reactivity, and biological factors) rather than a mechanism used to defend. Related processes are seen in: (a) people replying quickly to avoid a deeper more painful discussion; (b) children becoming more active at bedtime; (c) *rarely*, intentional hyperactivity used by children to prevent difficult discussions, p.81.
(Various levels)	Identification	(p.487)

Causelist 100: Fears (Specific) ☼

Fear is the unpleasant arousal experienced *in the presence of* danger whereas anxiety (p.295) is a more diffuse state of apprehension[376] (the distinction is probably more complex than this simple rule suggests[1087]).

Simple phobias are persistent fears of specific, circumscribed, objects or situations. Working out whether a phobia is really circumscribed requires careful history taking, which is most efficient if it is based on knowledge of the origins of fears, described below.

Origins of fears[1124,1304]

- *Innate fears*: snakes, spiders, height, dark.
- Social learning, p.550.
- Negative information transmission.
- *Amalgam fears*. These are constructed from their innate intolerances, which are usually fairly non-specific (p.125) and obviously have no identifiable moment of onset. Based on his innate tolerance levels, a child develops through *classical conditioning*, p.440, a general fear of situations that combine factors that he knows he will not be able to tolerate (often called "sensory overload"). This can start at a particular moment if the child is frightened (e.g. by a very loud noise) or develop gradually. They can give the impression of being specific, or they can actually become specific. They are most apparent in children with trait anxiety, autism (p.183), or other neurodevelopmental problems. They are the aversive counterpart to amalgam *superstimuli*, p.558.
- *Prototype-based fears*: A child can be frightened of one specific stimulus. These fears usually start at an identifiable moment. In almost all such cases the fear is graded, i.e. it depends on how similar a situation is to the worst one (see PTSD, p.532 and flinching, p.107).
- Intrusions and beliefs about them (p.493)
- Rare: brain lesions (p.97).

For all these types of fear, treatment can be more focused and efficient if you work out which aspect is most feared. This can be done by examining patterns of avoidance (p.429; and see table on the right), competing drives (e.g. ice cream can overcome this fear but not this one), and what the child recalls first about a difficult situation. If a child has several apparently unconnected fears (e.g. school and ice-cream vans) listing the characteristics of each may reveal commonalities.

Feared objects that are predictable but rare (such as thunder and flying) are worth distinguishing as they may need distinct treatments.

See also the opposite of fearfulness: *recklessness*, p.539.

Apparent feared object	Consider whether the feared object upsets him/her via these common underlying intolerances							
	Noise	Bore-dom	Sur-prise	Pain, risk	Embar-rassment ***	Losing posses-sions	Eye con-tact	Stran gers
a baby	√		√					
dogs	√		√	√				
a bully	√		√	√	√	√	√	
all children	√	√	√		√	√	√	
parties	√	√			√		√	
thunder	√		√					
toilets **	√	√	√	√				
blood tests			√	√	√			√
dentistry		√	√	√	√			√
horror films	√	√	√	√	√			√
Consider using the following standard amalgam descriptions if none of the more specific aspects above predominate.								
social anxiety	√		√		√		√	√
performance anxiety			√		√		√	
school-avoidance p.217	√				√			
agoraphobia, p.297	√				√			√

** Toilets have loud flushes, unpredictable "pssssst" deodorisers, and loud surprising air dryers. They can also be smelly, dark, dirty and associated with painful defecation.

*** E.g. academic difficulty, or being told off, or wetting self.

Negativeness

This term is used to include behaviours done less, or less energetically, or more miserably than the norm.

Causelist 101: Misery

This is more common in adolescence than in childhood, though it is probably under-recognised in children due to their rapidly changing emotional states. Signs of depression are described on p.313.

Depression affects about 5% of teenagers at any time[214]. It is also more common in girls. By far the most common causes are difficulties at home or school or with peers.

In a complex child living in a complex family with numerous changes of school and home, it can be a challenge to work out which are the important contributors to misery. Some methods are:

- What happens on a good day? on a bad day?
- How much fun do you have with X (work through all family members and teachers, using a visual analogue scale or scoring from 0–10).
- What was happening, and who was he living with (a) when school noticed misery; (b) when his sleep or eating worsened; (c) when he started talking about death?

Distinguish situational *relief* of low mood (which implies a persisting negative state or trait), from situational *causation* of low mood (which suggests a simple remedy).

Things that look like depression	Notes
Crying	see p.315
Self-harm	see p.317.
Talking about death or self-harm	These can be depressive ruminations (p.543), or the child can be intrigued, mystified, or obsessed. The reason for the fascination can be the extreme effect that a particular death had on someone else. A vague flitting between different people who have died suggests that none of them is particularly causative. Contrast with interest in killing (p.245).
Being in love	Smiles out of the blue, gazing into the distance, loss of energy, loss of interest in other activities. They can also be depressed because they cannot be with the object of desire.
Autistic Spectrum ↗ (p.183)	These children have had tenuous emotional connection to other people for most of their lives, starting before age 3. Children with (life-long) ASD can obviously become depressed: they become increasingly isolated, quiet and downcast, with reduced appetite and disturbed sleep. There is usually a clear social or environmental cause.
Irritability (p.494)	Depression can cause irritability, but most irritability occurs outside depression. (ICD allows substitution of irritability for low mood in the diagnosis of childhood depression). Tiredness, boredom (p.322)

Zombie effect	This term refers to medicines making people temporarily interact less, or be less sparky, even when they are fully awake. It occurs in several situations in children:
	• The most common cause is an excess dose of stimulants (p.555): the child typically becomes *more* repetitive and less spontaneous; he may also be more alert than usual. Note that methylphenidate even at low doses can also cause true low mood, e.g. with tears and withdrawing from people.
	• The above effects are quite different from those of antipsychotics, which are sedating rather than arousing (psychomotor slowing, p.537; fewer repetitions; sitting or lying, sometimes yawning) and when severe is parkinsonism (p.525)[964]. This is also different from depression – there is no insomnia, irritability, or guilt.
	• Anticonvulsants, some antihistamines, and other medicines with a sedative action, can produce a similar (but milder) effect[1278].
	• The SSRIs (p.552) can blunt emotional experiences[1282]. With other antidepressants there is often sedation, and sometimes blurred vision and dry mouth.
Urea cycle disorder (p.571)	Late-onset forms have insidious onset, usually by age 15.
Pseudo-depression	Acting babylike or inadequate, or acting like a depressed parent he identifies with. In rare cases combined with autism, the behaviours can be extreme. This is very similar to pseudo-regression (p.43).
Depression	Even if the child has any of the above problems, he may also be depressed – see signs of "true depression" on p.313
Abulia (p.97)	Complete lack of initiative.

continued ▶

Causes of true depression	Check for self-harm risk (p.319)
Genetic predisposition	The risk for depression is carried by numerous genes of small effect[946]
	The heritability of depression is about 40%[1563], but much of this may be due to inherited risk for other characteristics that increase the risk of depression (e.g. neurodevelopmental problems, physical diseases or propensity for risk taking)[440].
	The heritability increases greatly through adolescence due to the emergence of age-specific heritable causes of depression[518]. In rare families a single genetic defect causes depression with mendelian transmission, sometimes together with other symptoms (e.g.[681]). In children (and adults) the impact of life events and abuse depends very much on genetic predisposition (e.g. 5HTT-LPR, p.547).
Social difficulties ☂	Consider if mood worsens during term time, or after relationship problems. Tangible challenges cause most depression: bullying, p.219; academic difficulty at school, p.27; abuse, p.271; disrupted care, poor social skills, p.169; parental discord, p.191; parental rejection of sexuality/homosexuality. In children, schemata governing thinking about life are *much less important* in aetiology and in treatment.
Abuse	Especially physical or sexual, pp.273–275 (see above also). Habitual physical chastisement, or being constantly told off by parents or teachers. Sexual abuse can have sleeper effects, i.e. effects delayed until after puberty.
Life events (p.499)	In the main, these affect children via life changes, and via effects on the parents (see above also).
Parental loss and low parental warmth	Severe depression lasting months has many causes, but preoccupations about loss of mother are particularly severe and long lasting, e.g. when mother has died or is ill or in danger, or the child has been taken into care. Low parental warmth (e.g. when mother is mentally ill) has can have effects as severe as those of bereavement.
Cognitive factors	Academic difficulty can contribute to depression – which can itself cause a gradual or sudden decline in school performance . Also consider long-term characteristics such as poor set-shifting or a tendency to ruminate[1767].
Anxiety	Anxiety increases the likelihood of depression[1449].
ADHD ☂	In ADHD, depression can be secondary to social difficulties. In children under 5 it is a recognised side-effect of stimulants.
Seasonal affective disorder	(p.314)
Sleep disturbance	(p.199)
Inadequate exercise	Exercise can ameliorate depression and panics[1559]. It also increases pain thresholds, sense of control and well-being[1769].
Early bipolar	i.e. before the first manic episode (see p.264)
Early psychosis	(p.537)
Kleine-Levin syndrome	Episodic; usually more sleepy than depressed (p.496)
Drug abuse	(p.257) or withdrawal

Medical causes

☞ Physical states

Suspect this if:
➢ timing of fluctuations is related to physical problems or medication changes;
➢ sudden onset not related to social stressors
➢ any severe medical condition
➢ absence of family history of depression.

Reasonable initial screening in such cases includes FBC, UECr, thyroid, glucose, ESR, CRP, lead.

Physical causes of depression include:
• Side effects of medicines (e.g. antipsychotics, p.422; methylphenidate, p.555; clonidine, p.441; benzodiazepines, p.430; beta blockers, isotretinoin)
• Anaemia (p.421), low B_{12} (p.328)
• Diabetes (p.451), renal failure
• *Endocrine*: Hypothyroidism, p.485; hyperthyroidism, p.484; premenstrual syndrome, p.506; Cushing's, p.449; Addison's, p.419; OCP/other steroids
• *Inflammation* (via *cytokines*, p.450)
    o autoimmune, p.427
    o infections: mononucleosis, other viral/post-viral
    o occult chronic illness e.g. coeliac disease, p.441
    o malignancy, p.569
• Epilepsy (p.73)
• Wilson's disease (p.575)
• Mitochondrial disorders (p.508)

The Beck Depression Inventory, used from age 13 upward, places considerable weight on physical symptoms such as fatigue and loss of appetite, so it can give wrong answers when patients are physically ill (BDI-PC and Hamilton Scale reduce this problem).

Causelist 102: Not opening presents

(see also *Holidays*, p.480).

Causes of not opening presents	Notes
Depressed	(p.313)
Angry	Did she open the presents from some people but not others?
Never got good presents	Or disdainful of recent offerings?
Afraid of disappointment	
Insecurity	Likes being reminded that people like her, by looking at the package.
Enjoys the anticipation	Very unusual pre-pubertally
Autism ☝ (p.183)	Consider if odd special interest excludes all else from life.
Forgotten	Consider if learning difficulties and in unusual place
Obsessionality	May be reluctant to spoil the wrapping

Depression is often missed in children, because clinicians expect to see the full adult pattern of anhedonia, anergy, early waking, and negative cognitions. Don't forget to rule out mimics of depression (p.309). Consider the many causes of depression (p.311), including working out whether any adverse life events were timed to the onset of difficulty.

The DSM criteria can be a useful guide, but a few children are profoundly impaired by a small numbers of symptoms yet they fail to meet the "number of symptoms" criteria in DSM/ICD[45,1254]. Most clinicians recognise this so the "number of symptoms" criterion is often ignored – or intentionally overruled.

Depression in children who have never talked is recognised by the emotional, physical, and motivational signs in the list below, together with a clear history of deterioration. Regression (p.41) should be carefully excluded. OCD (p.65) can cause or can result from depression.

	Signs of depression
Emotional/ affective signs	• Sadness • Irritability (p.494) (or defiance and disagreeableness), • Suicidal thoughts, or even preoccupation with art and poetry that is haunting, sad, and bleak[256] • Mood worst in the mornings • Downcast eyes (p.175) • Depressed appearance, especially in preschoolers[256] • Self-touching is increased in depression, possibly as a self-soothing behaviour[786] (p.61). It normalises after recovery
Physical/ somatic/ vegetative signs	• Early morning waking (especially in adolescents) • Somatic signs such as tummyache and headache are seen in almost all younger depressed children • Reduced appetite and interest in sex
motivational signs (also called behavioural signs)	• Loss of enjoyment of previously enjoyed pursuits (anhedonia) is a useful indicator of severity in children (contrast behavioural addictions, p.260) • Recent onset of psychomotor retardation (p.537) and social withdrawal (similar to learned helplessness, p.96). This only affects a minority of depressed children and adults[256]. • Fatigue • Drop in school performance (see also p.41)
Cognitive signs	• Beck's triad: Negative thoughts about the self (low self-esteem / worthlessness and guilt), the world, and the future. • Poor concentration • Inability to make decisions
Psychotic signs	Persecution, unpleasant hallucinations (p.344)

Don't forget the possibility that a parent, especially mother, is depressed. If she answers "yes" to *either* of the following screening questions, signs in the table above should be sought and treatment may be needed. (1) "During the past month, have you often been bothered by feeling down, depressed, or hopeless?" (2) "During the past month, have you often been bothered by little interest or pleasure in doing things?"[1755].

Variants of depression

Combination states

- *Mixed depression* and *agitated depression* refer to people who simultaneously have features of both depression and mania (p.263). There is not yet a consensus on methods of diagnosis or treatment[136].
- *Anxious depression* describes the condition of people who are both depressed and anxious at the same time. Compared with people who are only depressed, these people are more impaired for longer, and are more likely to commit suicide[486].

Subtypes

- *Atypical depression*: In the past this term has sometimes referred to the combination states listed above, but nowadays it is usually short for "depression with atypical features", i.e. some symptoms the opposite of those characteristic of depression. Examples are hypersomnolence (rather than early morning waking) and overeating (rather than loss of appetite).
- *Seasonal affective disorder*: This can present as bad behaviour in the winters. The diagnosis is usually difficult to confirm in children, because of confounding factors altering with the seasons, including school, infections, exercise, and one-off events. However, it can usually be distinguished from school-related problems by the effect of weekends, rapid response to light therapy, and carbohydrate craving.
- *Melancholia* consists of an unremitting mood of apprehension and gloom; psychomotor disturbance such as agitation or reduced movements; vegetative signs (see left); and sleep abnormalities or abnormal cortisol levels. There is debate about whether it is a severe persisting form of depression, or quite a different disorder[1592]. It becomes much more common in older adulthood.
- *Adjustment disorders* are defined in DSM as distinct from longer-lasting anxiety or depression, but they are more logically viewed as mild forms of these[695].

Patterns of depression over years

Each individual has a temperament (p.561), one aspect of which is his mood *set-point*, i.e. the long-term degree of his tendency to be happy. In some people this adjusts to ongoing life circumstances and life events (p.499) and in others it apparently does not[410]. Some of the interindividual variation is genetic (see serotonin, p.547) and some is due to the quality of coping strategies (p.445) that the person uses.

For long-term low mood which is not actually impairing (p.17), the word *dysthymia* is occasionally used.

Double depression is a shorthand for depressive episodes superimposed on a milder depression that typically lasts for years. This is a common pattern.

Diagnoses of recurrent depression in children and teenagers quite often have to be revised to bipolar disorder (p.264) when the child has his first hypomanic or manic episode.

Crying includes tears, sobbing, vocalisation, and mouth opening, all to
varying degrees. Crying sometimes merges into whining, a pattern of slow
speech with raised pitch and exaggerated pitch contours that is especially
effective at getting attention[1510]. Grizzling and whingeing are variants of
this. Moaning is quieter, wailing is louder. The onset can be sudden (in
surprise or pain) or take a minute or more (with hormonal causes). See
also screams, p.544; breath-holding spells, p.434.

Crying is sometimes assumed to directly indicate suffering, but it occurs
mainly when other people are nearby, showing that it is usually an attempt
to *communicate* suffering. The less overt crying is, the more likely it is to
indicate misery; conversely, loud crying is usually an attempt to enlist
help. Crying is especially useful before speech has developed, in order to
express pain, fear, needs and frustration. Teenage boys cry about half as
often as teenage girls: this difference is established well before puberty.

Thought catching means noticing the flitting ideas that people have when
they are feeling bad (or good). These can be useful in talking therapies.
Thought catching can be useful in crying whereas it is not practicable in
screaming (p.544).

High-pitched cries are heard in premature babies, *intracranial
hypertension*, p.493; meningitis, and in cri-du-chat syndrome. For other
unusual-sounding cries and physical causes, see [743].

Tears on their own can indicate onion-chopping, local eye problems
(p.108) or can be part of crying. *Unilateral or bilateral tears* can be
caused by migraine, trigeminal neuralgia, or lachrymal duct blockage (e.g.
in upper respiratory tract infection).

Causes of crying	Notes
Babies	
Discomfort	Hunger, fear, hot/cold, noise, boredom / being alone
Pain due to physical illness	Earache, teething, dirty nappy, blocked nose, cow's milk protein intolerance, colic (p.137), severe constipation (p.444); reflux (GORD, p.472), injury, headache (p.139). Rare: torsion of testis; Meckel's diverticulum[1308].
	Whimpering (weak sobbing or moaning) is a sign of severe illness in a baby.

Toddlers
Sleepiness

Parental mistraining	Rewarded for crying in bed by hugs, or delay of bedtime, or being moved into parents' bed.
Pseudo-crying (cf pseudo-behaviours, p.363 especially pseudo-rage, p.286)	More regular than authentic crying, and with longer syllables. Depends on who is within earshot. There may be furtive looks to assess response. There are brief breaks rather than quiet sobbing. Parents give in to demands, e.g. because of tiredness, embarrassment, or concern. Very inaccurate pseudo-crying can be as simple as fast blinking with eye contact. A common form of pseudo-crying is *crescendo crying*. This involves successively louder stages of whimpering, quiet crying, loud crying, roaring, choking, and sometimes vomiting (which is the only one requiring immediate attention). Parents naturally worry that crescendo crying indicates something terrible happening to their baby, but a full-throated roar can only be produced by a healthy baby with energy to spare.

Older

To obtain sympathy	Crying when a difficult subject comes up in conversation, to emphasise the severity of a problem
Hormonal	e.g. gynaecological (p.506); Cushing's disease (p.449).
Methylphenidate	Dose related
Illicit drug withdrawal	"Fountain crying", defined as at least one tear dripping off the face, is three times as common in people withdrawing from cocaine, benzodiazepines, and opioids, compared with other psychiatric patients[1817].
Loneliness	(p.500)
Cultural	e.g. to express grief publicly following bereavement.

Any age

Misery	(p.309). Severe depression may prevent crying[1227].
Child abuse	(p.271)
Temperament	(p.561) and response to mother's anxiety
Infectious crying	Empathic (p.546) or depressed people can cry in response to others' crying. If a child only does this when *mum* cries, then the relationship, or the trigger of mum's crying, or triggered associations, have special importance for the child.
Manipulative	(p.504)
Tears of joy	Weddings
Surprise, shock	As after a fall
Physical causes[1227]	• Post-stroke emotional lability, p.70; see also pseudobulbar crying (p.537) • Unilateral crying face: facial nerve compression or maldevelopment, or abnormal development of facial muscles. • Crocodile tears: crying when eating because of abnormal nerve regeneration • Dacrystic seizures, p.76

In the parent

Help-seeking	Difficulty coping with child (normal or abnormal)

Causelist 104: Self-harm

Intentional self-harm (DSH, deliberate self-harm) is one of the most common presenting problems, particularly in casualty. Parasuicide is DSH that the individual thought was life threatening, or that actually could be. Thoughts about self-harm are far more common than actual self-harm but they share contributory factors. Thoughts of death are seen in 25% of healthy adolescents over any 3 months (but not plans, nor other signs of depression).

Suicidal *ideation* means thinking about suicide, which in its mildest form is a fleeting consideration among many options; like actual self-harm it is not just a sign of misery but also of lacking other attractive options. It is communicated more readily when young people are excited or disinhibited (e.g. on SSRIs, p.552), or have close confidantes, whereas *actual* self-harm is more likely when no confidante is available.

Self-injury usually refers to the use of violent means, leaving a mark. It is important to rule out bullying and child abuse (pp.219, 273–275), either causing self-harm or causing injuries that become attributed to self-harm.

For risk assessment see p.319. See also hair pulling, p.117; headbanging, p.119; hand-biting, p.113; skin picking, p.549; fabricated symptoms, p.359; and adopting an unusual persona, p.237. It is important to identify underlying contributory factors in self-harm as some have distinct remedies (e.g. communication difficulty in the family; or for ID see[1396,1690]).

Causes of self-harm and threats	Notes	
Common impulses		
Anger (p.289)	E.g. slapping one's head if work is too difficult. Isolation, confinement, and physical restriction may be specific triggers, e.g. in frustrated animals and prisoners[1781] and in intensive care[311] – especially when there is no other outlet. Prevalence increases with degree of ID, up to 30% in Profound ID.	
Grooming excess	Hair pulling (p.117), zit squeezing and nail-biting (p.511)	
Desire to focus on external rather than internal feelings	• Distraction from physical pain, e.g. in reflux (GORD, p.472) or otitis media (see discussion of headbanging, p.119). Location of the injury may help in identifying the cause. • In autism ☂ (p.183), distraction from extreme upset is the motive for much of the self-biting, headbanging (p.119), and even groin hitting. • Re-realisation, relief from anger. Poor tolerance of anxiety or anger.	Typical quote: "When I'm self-harming, I want to relieve the emotional pain and keep on living. Suicide is a permanent exit [whereas] self-harm helps me get through the moment."[399]
Addiction to the relaxation that *follows* self-harm (see also *opiates*, p.519)	This may be more common with congenital partial analgesia[1396] (p.136). For a 3-year-old with self-biting, self-hitting, and headbanging treated with naltrexone, see[1749]. Relaxation after cutting can last 1–2 days in adult: associated with suicidal ideation but not with suicidal intent[1027].	
To damage self		
Desire to punish self	• Consider parental criticism (p.512) • Chronic self-harm and depression (p.309) should raise suspicion of abuse (p.275). These symptoms, plus self-harm and flashbacks, often worsen if the person is considering disclosure (p.452). There are recurrent thoughts of guilt, anger, and fear[1657]. The most frequent injuries are to skin, e.g. cutting, scratching, burning.	
☞ Considered but irrational wish to harm self	Depression, p.309; psychosis, p.537; intoxication, p.566.	

☞Rational wish to die	Chronic illness. Early stages of schizophrenia, mania. Desire to join deceased relatives.
Brief catastrophising Symbolic (p.14)	("impulsive wish to die") Interpersonal crisis within the past day or two, with emotional instability and impulsivity
Expression of frustrated need to communicate	Interpersonal crisis within the past day or two, combined with communication difficulties in the family. Signs are overdosing in front of someone specific, making sure they find out; or collecting mobile phone to take to place where she plans to harm herself. Cutting boyfriend's initials.
To damage a particular body part	E.g. severe male genital mutilation or blinding (rare, usually psychotic)[1229].
Identification with someone else	Self-flagellation in religious sects. Imagining oneself as another injurer? or injuree? (see *identification*, p.237).
Rewarded	The damage can lead to reward, or the damage can be a by-product of behaviours performed for reward
Boredom (p.322) Removal from noisy/busy areas	Institutionalised, in prison, or ID [see 1190 pp.83-87]
Help-seeking or sympathy-seeking	Repeated threats delivered face-to-face, sometimes to parents who are unable to help.
Competition	In the game of "chicken" the winner is the person who rubs the skin longest, or makes the most cuts[933].
Attention-seeking	• This is often suggested, but is unusual because (in most environments) there are easier ways to get attention. Making cuts on the face, or dressing so as to reveal cuts, support this suggestion. • It is sometimes a very effective way of getting attention from a parent with psychological interests. If this is the cause it won't be done (or will be done more rarely) with other relatives, teachers, or peers. • Medical attention-seeking: Munchausen's (p.362).
Anorexia nervosa, bulimia	These have many causes (p.334).
Erotic	E.g. auto-asphyxia
Self-treatment	E.g.can't afford a dentist; transsexuals, infestation delusions
Showing machismo	Carving name in skin, burning self with cigarette
Social	E.g. substance abuse with friends, p.257; ear piercing; tattoos, p.561.
Cultural	Many healing, spiritual and order-preserving rituals involve self-mutilation[487].
Special impulses	Several named syndromes have more self-harm than other ID, often in rather specific stereotypies (p.553) suggesting abnormal sensations or abnormal reward mechanisms
Mental retardation	Prader-Willi (p.533), Rett (p.541), possibly Cornelia de Lange (p.445), Tourette (p.101), familial dysautonomia, Smith-Magenis (p.550), neuroacanthocytosis (tongue- and lip-biting, p.514). Sensory neuropathies (p.136) increase self-harm. **Lesch-Nyhan**[301]: ballismus, self-biting of fingers and lips, and many other methods apparently directed at causing pain. Onset of violent actions is characteristically sudden (age 1–10, most often onset at teething) rather than gradually emerging as in other developmental problems. May have profound ID or near normal intelligence, with fear and physical attempts to prevent the egodystonic self-harm (e.g. right hand trying to control left hand). Also negativistic utterances to others, sometimes apologised for (as are coprolalic tics, p.161). Various mutations of the HGPRT gene produce diverse combinations of dystonia and choreoathetosis (pp.86,439), neonatal hypotonia, mild ID, orange crystals in urine, and self-mutilation[797]. Initial screening is for uric acid in serum or in 24-hour urine.

continued ▶

Special Topic 17: Is the risk of suicide great?

Completed suicide is very uncommon and nearly impossible to predict, even with lists such as that at the right. However it remains important to try to identify those young people at greatest risk, and to alleviate risk factors where possible.

When assessing a young person who has self-harmed, be thorough. Be sympathetic, keep detailed records, and reassess regularly. Asking about the person's wishes, ideas, and plans in explicit detail does not increase the risk of suicide.

It is sensible to encourage every young person who has self-harmed to spend the night in hospital. This allows their behaviour on the ward to be observed, allows them to be consistently calm before discharge, and allows them to collect their thoughts and make appropriate plans for the day (which you can ask about if concerned).

When a person has harmed himself, it is prudent to think not only about preventing repeat self-harm, but also to reduce other risks, such as abuse (p.271), family or parental discord, and difficulties at school or with friends[1520].

Table 16. Risk factors for suicide

-- in the person
> Previous attempts
> Any psychiatric illness, drug abuse, or impulsivity
> Victim of abuse
> Male
> Recent bereavement (p.430), especially a suicide; desire to be with a loved one
> Recent exposure to news stories about suicide
> Serious or painful medical illness

-- in his/her current mental state
> Depressed (p.313), hopeless (p.482)
> Poor rapport with clinician
> Regrets being rescued
> Inability to accept a contract to not harm himself for a week, or to phone a friend if feeling suicidal
> Has positive beliefs about death
> Psychotic (mania causes special risk[1000])
> Still intoxicated

-- in their social supports
> Social isolation, unemployed
> Family wishes to be rid of child
> Family not taking child's problems seriously
> Family unwilling to take responsibility for supervision

-- in the act
> Has a plan
> Violent plan
> Put affairs in order, gave away possessions or wrote a note
> Has visited the location or handled the pills/gun.
> Access to method (e.g. farmers, doctors, vets)
> Precautions against rescue
> Attempt performed in isolation

Risk factors for suicide *attempts* are somewhat different. If a depressed teenager endorses four or more of the following, then she has a 90% chance of *attempting* suicide[838]: (a) recent weight gain; (b) recent loss of energy or feeling fatigued; (c) father lives away from home; (d) was ever on the verge of attempting suicide; (e) thinking there is a reasonable chance that she will end her life; (f) pessimistic attitude to the future; (g) situation feels hopeless.

Languor

Sleep duration
Two-year-olds generally need 10½ to 12½ hours of sleep a night, and this reduces by about 10 minutes each year. Two-year-olds also have a day-time nap of 1–3 hours, which gradually reduces and disappears by age 5.

Arousability
Pre-pubertal children usually require far louder noises to wake them than adults, and even when they briefly rouse their EEGs usually continue to indicate sleep[238]. Arousability increases as the night progresses, and as they mature[239]. Children with nocturnal enuresis are much less rouseable than children without, possibly because of delay in this aspect of maturation[1786].

See also effects of sleepiness:
    causing inattention and hyperactivity, p.79; causing passivity, p.95; causing masturbation, p.115; causing headbanging, p.119; causing repetitiveness, p.228; causing crying, p.315.

See also: *Insomnia*, p.199; absence of sleepiness following pseudoseizures, p.74; effect of illicit drugs, p.267; sleep, p.200; chronic fatigue, p.323; sleep difficulty, p.199.

Causes of complaint of daytime sleepiness	Notes [see 17 pp.656-7]
Up late last night	Especially in teenagers
Nocturnal insomnia (p.199)	There are many causes, the most common being social/organisational problems, p.199. Consider obstructive sleep apnoea, p.518.
Overeating	(Especially if sleepy after lunch)
Heat	
Sedatives	Licit: antipsychotics, benzodiazepines, antiepileptics, other sedatives. Illicit: p.257
Atypical depression	Unlike most depression, this has increased sleep and appetite (cf. p.309)
Parental monitoring	Some children with severe ID are continuously physically active and, in the absence of speech, their parents come to rely on this as a sign of happiness and health. If the child's activity level is normalised by medication, these parents then think he is sleepy, ill, or depressed.
Narcolepsy	(p.72)
Kleine-Levin syndrome	(p.496) Brief insomnia after severe hypersomnia
Prader-Willi syndrome	(p.533)
Smith-Magenis syndrome	(p.550) with night-time insomnia
Other physical causes	If onset was rapid consider encephalitis, p.461; trauma; stroke, p.556. Other causes include tumours of third ventricle; nerve and muscle diseases affecting respiration

Causelist 106: Boredom

Boredom is a major complaint of children and teenagers, but referrers hardly ever use the term because our society considers it beneath consideration. It has always existed, but the concept was introduced in the 18th century[1521].

In many young children it contributes to chaotic stimulation-seeking (p.123), but a few children become lethargic when bored (this may be a learned skill in some). With increasing maturation children acquire complex self-entertainment skills (p.545). Related to these are self-discipline skills that enable one to complete unpleasant or painfully repetitive tasks, e.g. in re-starting; forcing oneself to concentrate when angry; self-calming; over-coming the normal *inhibition of return*; ways to alert oneself quickly (e.g. shaking one's head or hand) that allow the onerous task to be restarted well; the ability to regulate perfectionism so one doesn't give up when one hasn't found the answer instantly or has used a dirty rubber or wasted a little time so cannot "win" (see[1428]). Children can use the word *boredom* for all of these.

In school, boredom occurs most often in children who cannot follow the lessons, through poor concentration (p.79), low IQ, language problems (p.145), etc. (p.27). Bright children (see *gifted*, p.473) can get bored, of course, but they usually find a way of entertaining themselves (so the problem becomes naughtiness rather than boredom). At home, boredom occurs if there are too few toys, friends, or outings, or inadequate space. People with strong interests are often bored if those interests cannot be pursued (e.g. extroverts lacking people to interact with, as in Down's, p.455).

Causes of complaint of boredom	
Environmental	
Not liking what one has to do	Or feeling forced to do something so it becomes unattractive.
Finding life or current company distasteful	
Lack of competition	Sports, wrestling, and prizes have been an important part of adolescent life for centuries, now diminishing.
Insufficient stimulation	This is the basis of the "dopamine appetite" theory[1771].
	• Many children with ADHD perform cognitive tasks better with the radio *on* [2,1508].
	• Similarly, hyperactivity is *reduced* by TV[48].
	• Music can improve arithmetic in ADHD[2]
	• Part of methylphenidate's action is to make maths more interesting ("salient")[1687].
Cognitive	
Unengaged because uncomprehending	The most boring tasks are those that are well beyond his ability (and unisensory).
Overfamiliarity	The most engaging tasks are those that engage the child at several levels, or in several modalities, and/or are novel and/or near the limit of his ability.
Not having enough to do	Limited repertoire of self-entertainment skills (p.545), so none are useable in the current situation. Lack of friends, sex, cars, shopping, etc. [See 1682].
Emotional	
Ennui	A malaise, "a state of the soul defying remedy, an existential perception of life's futility."[1521]
Depression	(p.309)
Inability to relax/sleep	
Repetitiveness	(If it exceeds one's need for novelty)

Fatigue describes both a use-related decrement in function, and the subjective feeling of this. It can be divided into physical and mental fatigue. Brief physical fatigue is normal following exercise, and increased fatigu*ability* is common in illness or as a medication side-effect. See also slowness/passivity, p.95 and muscle weakness, p.87.

Mental fatigue includes difficulty concentrating or recalling or thinking clearly, increased slips of the tongue and word-finding difficulties, and reduced interest in previous activities[278]. It is akin to sleepiness (p.321) but in most cases recovers much faster (e.g.[166]). It can usually be overcome with sufficient motivation[1726].

Chronic fatigue

Chronic fatigue is very contentious, perhaps because it is diverse and usually multifactorial[546]. It has been authoritatively diagnosed from age 2 upwards, though the great majority of cases are post-pubertal[374]. The term *myalgic encephalomyelitis* is often preferred but is only accurate if the presence of brain inflammation has been demonstrated, which is rare. A common, perhaps central, feature in CF is post-exertional malaise, which is a lowering of pain threshold following exercise[1658] (compare fibromyalgia, p.466; central sensitisation, p.436).

A common pattern is a major stress or self-limiting illness that leads to long-lasting cognitive, emotional, and behavioural changes; there is then ample room for disagreement about whether the lasting symptoms are physical or mental (see p.14 and p.325). Debate on whether a particular child's symptoms are physical or mental can itself be clinically counterproductive, as it pushes the young person into the position of defending one view or disproving another (by her words and/or actions). Similar problems can be produced in the relationships between clinicians, and between clinicians and family members.

Even though the standard diagnostic criteria for "chronic fatigue syndrome" require that physical causes be excluded, this is often not achieved. For example, in one large series, most of the children diagnosed with CFS had musculoskeletal pain or migraines or sore throats with lymphadenopathy[1028]. In such groups, which are obviously defined more broadly than the standard diagnostic criteria, the large number of physical problems might be taken to support a somatic causation. However this sheds no light on the question of whether there is a medical cause in cases satisfying standard criteria, i.e. in whom no medical cause has been found despite a thorough search.

Consider any current depression (pp.309–313), anxiety (p.295), and deficits in memory or attention[409] (p.79) *as well as* the question of physical problems, as they may need separate treatments. If the patient was never depressed before the physical illness, then any current depression is likely to have been caused by the physical illness and its sequelae[1408].

It is crucial to collect reliable information about the child's baseline activity level, most usefully from school or from a distant family member. It is pointless to ask "do you often feel fatigued" as this is true for most people. Open questions and attention-shifting questions can be useful ("What do you generally do at weekends", "What do you do with your friends?"; "What's the best film you've seen this year?"). Similarly, motor functioning can be tested as part of a developmental check (p.91). You will want to establish a baseline to monitor treatment progress, and this needs to be done (a) using reliable sources, (b) over at least a week to allow for fluctuations.

See also *comorbidity*, p.442; *non-behaviours*, p.515.

Causes of chronic fatigue	Notes
Conditions that should not be labelled as chronic fatigue	
Insufficient sleep	
Orthostatic hypotension	
Kleine-Levin syndrome	(p.496) Severe episodes of sleepiness lasting days.
Pervasive Refusal	(p.527)
Actual chronic fatigue (psychological and physical causes)	
Depression	(pp.309–313)
Puberty	Also particularly at age 2–5.
Postviral	Common, with a sudden onset, usually lasts just weeks. Rare cases last years but still have a better outlook than chronic fatigue in which no cause is identified. Common after glandular fever.
Other medical	See suggested investigations, p.325.
Secondary gain for child (p.471)	Pseudo-tiredness: The child enacts (his idea of) a sick role, in order to get out of a predicament. Common as a mild form of school-avoidance lasting a week or two (see p.363).
Childhood trauma (p.567)	(with disrupted cortisol function, especially after sexual and emotional abuse and neglect[680]). See also abuse (p.275).
Self-fulfilling prophecy	This can be a side-effect of the act of diagnosis[731]. See *feedback loops*, p.526
Secondary gain for mother	Consider excessive parental expectations [574] or Munchausen by proxy (p.206) (very unusual).
Change in values	Change in self-identity (p.237) and values can occur during chronic fatigue[63]. This can obviously be a coping strategy or, conversely, a perpetuating factor.

continued ▶

Investigation Planner 8: Medical causes of chronic fatigue

Aim to confidently dispel specific fears rapidly. Demonstration of raised antibodies unfortunately persuades families irreversibly that a physical cause exists and that there is therefore no psychological contribution.

Many clinicians reserve investigation for severe cases, on the assumption that mild cases are psychological in origin. It is certainly true that the risks posed by non-investigation are much greater in severe cases. However many mild cases have physical causes and some of the most severe cases are essentially psychosocial.

☞ Red flags that should encourage search for a physical cause include[644]:

- weight loss
- lymphadenopathy (e.g. a non-tender progressively enlarging supraclavicular or axillary lymph node)
- features of malignancy (haemoptysis, dysphagia, rectal bleeding, breast lump)
- focal neurological signs
- arthritis or vasculitis
- heart or lung disease
- sleep apnoea.

Initial tests include FBC, blood film, LFT, CRP, ESR, glucose, B_{12}, urea and electrolytes, calcium, phosphate, magnesium, CK, TFT, uristix[644,1315]. Others may be indicated, as shown in the table at right.

The following list of suggested investigations is after[1315]. See also the
general approach to medical investigations, p.373, and[703].

Category	Disorders	Suggested tests
Endocrine	Diabetes, p.451; hypothyroidism, p.485; Addison's, p.419; hypopituitarism, p.531	Glucose, thyroid function, morning and evening cortisols, Synacthen test
Gastro-intestinal	Coeliac disease, p.441; Inflammatory bowel disease, p.490	Coeliac serology (p.441), jejunal biopsy, endoscopy
Immuno-deficiency	Hypogammaglobulinaemia	Ig's
Miscellaneous	Connective tissue disorder, p.483; fibromyalgia, p.466; postural orthostatic tachycardia syndrome; malnutrition, p.504; hypercalcaemia, p.483	Hypermobility assessment, p.483; tender points score; lying and standing pulse & BP
Neurological	Multiple sclerosis, p.510	MRI, VEP (p.462), CSF (Ig's)
	Wilson's disease, p.575	(p.575)
Neuromuscular	Myasthenia, p.510; muscular dystrophy, p.510; glycogen storage diseases, p.556	EMG, ACh antibodies, Tensilon test, CK, muscle biopsy
	Mitochondrial disorders	(p.508)
Occult malignancy	Lymphoma, neuroblastoma, brain tumour, p.569	Biopsies, VMA, MRI brain
Psychiatric / psychological	Anxiety, p.295; bipolar disorder, p.264; depression, p.313; school refusal, p.217, eating disorders, p.331; fabricated/induced illness, p.359	(See other sections in this book)
Sleep disorder	Obstructive sleep apnoea, p.518; narcolepsy, p.72	Multiple sleep latency test, polysomnography
Anaemia (p.421)	Haematinic deficiency, menorrhagia, leukaemia, autoimmune, p.427	Ferritin, folate, B_{12}, bone marrow, direct Coombs test
Auto-immune disease, p.427	SLE, p.560; HIV, p.479; dermatomyositis, vasculitis, hepatitis	ANA, cardiac enzymes, muscle biopsy, ASOT
Chronic infection	p.490	ESR/CRP, throat swab, EBV, ASOT, chest X-ray, Mantoux test, Lyme serology (p.501), other specific tests
Drug induced	Substance abuse, p.257; medications, e.g. anti-epileptics, beta-blockers	Toxicology, drug levels, trial of withdrawal of medication

Digestive / excretory ☼

In developed countries, aberrant nutrition is very unlikely to be the cause of a child's unusual behaviour. Most nutritional advice is not based on hard scientific evidence, though we have attempted to collect some exceptions below.

Isolated deficiencies are more common than general malnutrition, p.504. Clinical and subclinical deficiencies of vitamin A, iron, iodine and zinc probably affect a quarter or more of children in most continents of the world[1299]. In the first world, the only common micronutrient deficiencies are of iron in menstruating females, vitamin D in breast-fed babies and in dark-skinned people with little sun exposure; and after abdominal surgery. Deficiencies of micronutrients are common in vegans (p.572) and in anorexia nervosa. Restricted eating in autism can cause severe deficiency of vitamins D, A[1031] or C.

Parents naturally seek out advice on products or therapies their children need. There is a long history of diet supplements and exclusion diets to aid development or health (see *Treatments*, p.567). The field of nutrition may be specially susceptible to false claims, due to lack of regulation, lack of immediate effects, and most people's suggestibility and ability to metabolise almost anything[372,577].

The following is a list of nutrients, most of which are essential, i.e. needed in the diet.

	Deficiency (aspects related to behaviour)	Excess (aspects related to behaviour)
Protein	Kwashiorkor, p.504	
Energy	Marasmus, p.504, anorexia nervosa, p.334	Obesity, p.335
Essential fatty acids		
Omega-3 fatty acids, e.g. docosahexaenoic acid (DHA), eicosapentaenoic acid (EPA)	Omega-3 FAs are important in development[584] but dietary deficiency is unusual in children with a normal diet. Omega-3 deficiency may contribute to depression[693,962], and to inattention and reading difficulties[783,1339] but apparently not to autism[141].	n/a
Essential amino acids		
Phenylalanine	n/a	(Must be kept extremely low in PKU (p.529) to minimise ID)
Arginine (in children), histidine (in children), isoleucine, lysine leucine, methionine threonine, tryptophan valine	Dietary deficiency or imbalance is an uncommon complication of total parenteral nutrition (p.333). Metabolic defects leading to deficiency are also rare. As well as being building blocks of proteins, all these amino acids have distinct cellular functions[1802]	
Minerals		
Sodium	Hypotension (see p.338)	Hypertension
Potassium	n/a	
Chloride	n/a	

Calcium Phosphorus/ phosphate	(p.485) (Refeeding syndrome) confusion, coma, muscle weakness	(p.483) Ectopic calcification, secondary hyper- parathyroidism, p.525
Iodine	(p.494)	
Cobalt	(No known role)	
Magnesium	(Cofactor for many enzymes; "nature's calcium inhibitor", blocks NMDA, ACh release.) Weakness, athetosis, jerking, upgoing plantar (p.56), confusion, seizures, tetany	(Occurs only with renal failure)
Molybdenum	XO deficiency type 2, p.555	
Selenium	Deficiency probably worsens mood and general health[1314].	
Sulfur	n/a	In the air, sulfur dioxide contributes to asthma.

Fat-soluble vitamins

• A (e.g. retinol)	The best indicator of deficiency, because very sensitive, is night blindness (child cannot find mum in the room, late in the evenings), but Bitot's spots on the sclerae are also useful[16]. See also *photophobia*, p.529.	Nausea, headache, dizziness, blurred vision, ataxia
• D D2 (ergosterol), D3 (e.g. calcitriol), D4	Deficiency is seen mainly in dark-skinned people, not drinking vitamin D-fortified milk, at the end of winter in northerly countries[1167]. Signs are those of hypocalcaemia, p.485.	Nausea, irritability, fatigue, anorexia
• E (e.g. tocopherol)	Ataxia (p.86), neuropathy and anaemia	Mildly increased bleeding[1618]
• K (e.g. phylloquinone)	Easy bruising and menorrhagia. Has many causes. Neonatal supplements are commonly given especially if breast feeding, to reduce strokes (p.556).	
• Coenzyme Q10	(Inadequate production in inborn error of metabolism, p.508)	

Water-soluble vitamins

• B$_1$ (thiamine)	Beriberi (weight loss, neuropathy); Wernicke-Korsakoff, p.574; thiamine-dependent maple syrup disease, p.505, insomnia	

continued ▶

• B_2 (riboflavin) precursor of FAD, which is a cofactor for many enzymes.	Cracked lips and reduced growth.	
• B_3 (niacin) →nicotinamide:	Pellagra (dermatitis, diarrhoea and dementia), red swollen mouth and tongue, seen with isoniazid; Hartnup disease, p.477.	Massive overdose can cause abdominal pain and dangerous hypotension[1122].
• B_5 (pantothenic acid)	Paraesthesia	
• B_6 (pyridoxine)	Causes seizures or ID. Can result from dietary deficiency, poor absorption in the gut, or inborn errors of pyridoxine metabolism[1570].	Large-fibre sensory neuropathy, ataxia, and weakness seen with megadoses or long-term readily available doses[362,948]
• B_7 (biotin)	(p.32)	
• B_9 (folate)	(p.467)	
• B_{12} (cyanocobalamin)	Deficiency can be due to vegan diet (p.572), pernicious anaemia (p.421) or bacterial overgrowth (p.502). Rare inborn errors of cobalamin metabolism can prevent use of the B_{12}. This causes anaemia, ketoacidosis; methylmalonic aciduria, white matter disease, p.574; and coccasionally psychosis before any neurological symptoms[1390].	(n/a)
• C (ascorbic acid)	Scurvy (bleeding gums, joint pains and weakness) is quite common in children with very restricted diets, e.g. due to autism[1167].	

Below is a list of other substances sometimes ingested (see p.566)

Non-nutrients

• "Additives"	n/a	E.g. food colours and sodium benzoate (preservative). Several of these often increase activity level[1032]
• Medication	n/a	Numerous side-effects, see *BNF*.
• Odd items	n/a	p.336

Toxic or heavy metals

Iron	Anaemia (p.421), pica (p.336), brittle nails	Haemochromatosis (genetic, dietary, or transfusions). Acaeruloplasminaemia (genetic: degen. of retina and basal ganglia; DM)
Lead	No metabolic role.	Headache, p.139; fatigue, p.323; constipation, p.444; gingival lead lines; mental state change. Even very low levels can impair development[903].
Manganese		Excess probably causes hyperactivity and cognitive impairment[1059].
Copper	Deficiency can cause fractures, p.468. Genetic: Menkes disease (defect in copper transport): ID, hypotonia, sagging facial features, short twisted lustreless hair coloured white, silver or grey[755]. Partial form is occipital horn syndrome, p.32.	Genetic: Wilson's disease (p.575).
Nickel	No major metabolic role.	(Allergy to nickel in enuresis alarm can cause alarming rash[645])
Chromium	Probably no metabolic role[1537]	Effects not clear[1497]
Zinc	Zinc deficiency probably impairs cognitive development[179]. Severe deficiency also causes acrodermatitis enteropathica.	Correction of iodine deficiency can cause hyperthyroidism[1822]. Moderate excess can cause rash and gastric upset, and can induce copper/iron deficiency. Severe excess can cause coma.
Mercury	n/a	Abdo. pain, bleeding gums, metallic taste; history of exposure such as folk remedies or eating marine mammals[361,771]. Many thermometers, sphygmomanometers, and aged electrical equipment contain mercury which is released by breakage or children's experimentation. Cleaning must be very thorough to avoid release of vapour over months; vapour can cause pulmonary oedema, mood change, tremor[922]. Mercury in thimerosal-containing vaccines does not cause developmental problems[1281].
Arsenic	n/a	Numb extremities, impaired development, inattention, history of living near metal works[1497,1641]

Causelist 108: Fussy or inadequate eating

Feeding means getting nutrition into people. The term *feeding problem* is usually used in infancy and early childhood, when the carer is expecting to be able to decide what and when the child eats. Feeding clinics typically focus on under-5s who are not putting food in their mouths, chewing, and swallowing. Feeding problems are conventionally distinguished from *eating disorders* (p.458) which occur later, when the child or adolescent has considerable autonomy[1151].

Feeding difficulty is seen in a quarter of all children, and in most children with developmental problems, at some time. There are effects on the parent-child relationship, but also short-term and long-term medical complications. The main short-term effects are hunger, lethargy, and sometimes hypoglycaemia (p.82). Long-term effects depend on the quantity and type of nutrients obtained (p.327). They include malnutrition (p.504), e.g. scurvy (p.329); dehydration; and delay in growth and development. Failure to gain weight should trigger investigation.

Feeding difficulties occur over a range of severity/pervasiveness:
1. slow eating
2. selective refusal of a few specific foods (and/or retching)
3. food selectivity by taste (e.g. rejecting spicy foods, p.128)
4. food selectivity by type or texture
5. refusal of solids
6. pervasive refusal (p.527)

The following signs increase the likelihood of a substantial environmental or social contribution to poor feeding: willingness to accept only one type or texture of food; abnormal parental feeding practices; onset after a clear trigger; and presence of anticipatory gagging at the sight of food, a spoon, or a bottle[944]. Part of the assessment of very fussy eating includes consideration of its physical sequelae. As well as physical examination, and tracking the height and weight trajectory (p.55) the following are useful: FBC, B_{12}, B_6, folate, ferritin, calcium, TFT. See also investigations in anorexia, p.334. For more general discussion see *non-behaviours*, p.515.

Development of eating and self-feeding

Weaning: Most children will take pureed foods from 4 to 6 months; soft chewable foods from 6 to 9 months; lumpy pureed foods from 9 to 12 months; most textures from 12 to 18 months; chewable fruit, vegetables and meat from 18 to 24 months, and tougher solid foods from 24 months[1141].

Self-feeding should begin with finger foods at about one year, and by two years of age the child should be totally self-feeding.

Sensitive periods: New tastes should be introduced from 4 to 6 months. New textures should be introduced from 6 to 7 months. It is sometimes suggested that there is a *critical period* (i.e. an inflexible sensitive period, p.447) for the development of chewing at 6–12 months[744,1141] but the effect is only partial [969,1490]; there are alternative explanations[231,1025] and irreversibility has not been demonstrated. Other aspects of eating may also have sensitive periods, such as the number of foods accepted, which is greatest from age 1 to 3 (as is the risk of accidental poisoning)[267]. This period is therefore important in learning about foods and about how to eat; roughly at the end of this period children become able to identify what is disgusting to them.

Causes of complaint of poor intake under 7	Notes (Severe cases often combine several causes[1370].)
Lump or texture intolerance	Usually due to fear of choking or vomiting. More likely with oromotor dyspraxia and in anxious children (p.309)
Picky / faddy	• This occurs in 15% of preschoolers[1341,1342]. If severe it may indicate a narrow/rigid child who dislikes new experiences (neophobia) or training errors (see below). Food neophobia is partly genetically determined but can be reduced by various training strategies[858] (see also inflexibility, p.234). • Children with autism eat on average half the usual number of different foods[1443] (see *malnutrition*, p.504). As an extreme example, an autistic child who is usually a fussy eater may become totally unable to eat for days after a major environmental change such as being admitted to hospital.
Training errors	• Sudden exposure to textures or lumps or spicy food • Introduction of multiple foods simultaneously, or while ill • Use of food in games, or as reward or present • Food forcing[944] leading to food refusal. Child may be bribed to finish dinner, or punished if he does not. Causes of this should be sought in the child (e.g. passivity, physical illness) and parents. • Failure to keep the unwanted food available, and regularly to model eating it • Distractions, e.g. toys on the table
Unrealistic expectations	Was the birth weight (p.432) low? Use a growth chart, adjusting the adult target to be the mean of the parents' weights and heights: Are parents' expectations realistic?
"Infantile anorexia"	The child, from 6 to 36 months, has a high level of arousal and finds it difficult to settle to eat (or to sleep)[287]. This often leads to conflict with carers at mealtime.

continued ▶

Any age	

Temporarily sated	• Unplanned snacks – is the child secretly snacking?
	• Child drinks at the beginning of meals
	• Tube feeding: sufficient calories may be delivered to prevent any appetite. Tube feeding also has delayed effects[231] such as changing the time of day when food is expected; lack of participation in mealtimes; delaying the development of chewing skills and swallowing habits (see *critical periods*, p.447); and post-traumatic feeding problems (see below). Types of tube feeding include:
	   o nasogastric tube and percutaneous endoscopic gastrostomy (PEG, with a feeding tube through the abdominal wall). These are becoming common, and bring with them risks of deficiencies (protein, iron, calcium, zinc, magnesium, folate, p.467; and vitamins D and B_{12}, p.328)[1180].
	   o total parenteral nutrition (TPN) which is intravenous, brings additional risks of sepsis, deficiencies (e.g. copper, p.330; B1, p.328), and excesses (manganese).

Minor viral illness	Duration up to a fortnight.
Choking phobia	• There are many non-functional causes to consider[936]. See also www.dysphagia.com. Globus hystericus means feeling a lump in the throat. • In infancy, most children justifying this description (sometimes called post-traumatic feeding disorder) have had serious medical illnesses with traumatic events involving their pharynx, and the majority have been tube fed[286].
Likes a particular food	Severity or duration may be greater, and choice odder, in ASD. This can lead to severe deficiency of micronutrients (see pp.327, 529).
☞ Medication side-effects	Particularly long-lasting stimulants (p.555) which often prevent eating throughout the school day. This sometimes causes hypoglycaemia after school (p.82). Other causes are antihistamines; many antibiotics; vitamin A or D excess. Consult the *BNF*.
☞ gastro-intestinal	• Especially gastro-oesophageal reflux (GORD, p.472) • Temporary, recurrent, or long-term: toothache / traumatic mouth injury / mouth ulcers. • Intestinal disease e.g. via nausea (see malabsorption, p.502; other cause of food intolerance, p.493).
Neurological	• Oromotor dyspraxia; cerebral palsy, p.437. • Migraine (can be occult in ID, p.142) • Rarer: Prader-Willi, p.533; mysathenia, p.510
☞ Other medical	• Hypercalcaemia, p.483; Addison's disease, p.419. • Cleft lip/palate, p.440; other structural abnormalities of the pharynx • Weight loss may be due to diabetes, p.451 or *rarely* tumours, p.569 (especially craniopharyngiomas, p.446) • Urea cycle disorders (often with intestinal complaints or protein refusal), p.571

Usually in adolescence

Look for[1150]:

Anorexia nervosa (see also *Eating disorders*, p.458)	➢ Very low weight. Amenorrhoea is a useful sign of severe weight loss (see other causes of this, p.506) ➢ Determined weight loss, with food-avoidance but more specifically: increased exercise, purging, self-induced vomiting ➢ Abnormal cognitions about, and preoccupation with, weight and/or shape (for standard ways to assess these see[543]). ➢ Physical signs including eroded teeth, callus on back of hand, parotid enlargement, lanugo hair, Raynaud's phenomenon (p.562)

Most affected individuals have more than one of the following contributory factors:

- *Psychological*: Perfectionism, rigidity, anxiety, avoiding sexual maturation, needing to be in control.

- *Biological*[631,1309]: Starvation (p.553) increases rigidity and focus on food; starvation and exercise produce addictive opioids; sufferers have a genetic predisposition to depression, obsessionality, and rigidity. Being female or having a female twin[348,1284]. Enjoying some foods less, perhaps as a lifelong trait[1697].

- *Social*: Parental marital discord (p.191), adoption of society's quest for thinness; perpetuating family dynamics; difficulty expressing negative emotions; seeking self-worth from others; poor relationship with mother

- *Risk factors for any psychiatric disorder*: Rigidity (p.233), adverse life events (p.499), sexual or physical abuse (pp.273–275), any other psychiatric disorder, especially depression and OCD (p.65).

Consider testing: UECr, LFT, FBC, Ca, phosphate, TFT, urea/nitrogen (BUN), glucose, pelvic ultrasound, ECG

Indications for urgent referral:
· weight loss (>1kg in a week in people already underweight).
· dehydration
· systolic BP <90
· postural drop in BP exceeding 20/10
· fainting, dizziness, cold blue hands
· hypothermia

!!*Indications for emergency admission:*
· BMI (kg/m^2) under 13
· heart rate < 50
· poor peripheral circulation (late sign)
· arrhythmia (subjective or objective)
· prolonged QT interval on ECG

Pervasive Refusal	(p.527)
Depression	(p.309)
Psychosis	(p.537) Are there delusions about food?

Overeating is usually noticed when a child becomes obese, or when he starts to be teased about it (p.219) and his (or more often, her) self-esteem suffers. Obesity is an increasing problem in young people, bringing substantial medical risks: diabetes, p.451; obstructive sleep apnoea, p.518; cardiovascular disease; and joint problems even in children[772,1816].

Obesity is quantified as body mass index, BMI, which is kg/m^2. Obese is defined in adults as BMI over 30, and pre-obese (overweight) as BMI from 25 to 30. However in young people the significance of BMI is different: the 95th centile of BMI increases from 18 at age 5 to 29 at age 18[308]. Even these figures are somewhat difficult to interpret as it seems unlikely that the same number of children are "overweight" at each age in the sense of being at increased long-term risk to their health.

For these reasons BMI-for-age has become the standard in children. WHO calls 1–2 s.d. above the age mean weight "overweight", and "obese" 2 s.d. above[1795]. These are the 85th and 97th percentiles. WHO statistics are for healthy breastfed children with non-smoking mothers, so they are a recommendation of what should be achievable rather than what actually happens.

See also *intake-regulating hormones*, p.491, *macrosomia*, p.521.

Causes of obesity	Notes
Excess appetite	
Depression (p.309)	More common than in depressed adults. See comfort eating (p.257), and overeating as an addiction, p.259.
Medicines	Atypical antipsychotics (p.422), Epilim, etc.
Cold	(More in winter)
Prader-Willi syndrome	(p.533)
Kleine-Levin syndrome	(p.496) but sleepiness is a more pronounced symptom than overeating.
Cushing's syndrome	(p.449)
Hypothyroidism	(p.485)
Bardet-Biedl	(p.429)
Leptin deficiency	Very rare.
Other	
Parenting	Ineffective meal size regulation. Letting the child choose what he eats and when he snacks. Frequent fast fatty foods. Sugary drinks. Are the meal sizes too big in this family, so she is the only child that finishes them?
Opportunity	Excess supply of irresistible foods (see superstimuli, p.558). Free access to fridge.
Underactivity	Regular exercise of at least moderate intensity helps reduce obesity[72]. Many children have no exercise at weekends, spending the time watching TV or playing computer games. Social anxiety (p.298), Asperger's, unsafe neighbourhoods, and physical disabilities all reduce activity levels.
Familial	(Both genetic and social learning, p.550) Bardet-Biedl syndrome, p.429. For other rare genetic causes of obesity with ID, see [632]
Bulimia	E.g. addiction to feeling of fullness

Make an exhaustive list of items, time and place, ABC (p.365). What do
the items have in common? Are they sucked, chewed, swallowed, or
moved around in the mouth? Consider why normal inhibitions aren't
active (p.261).

Pica means persistently eating (and swallowing) non-foods. The term can
be used in the broad sense of eating things most people wouldn't (e.g.
beetles, grass, hair, soil), or narrowly as eating non-nutritive things that are
never in the local diet (paperclips, paint). Eating lead-containing paint
(p.330) or mud next to roads can be harmful. Another risk is parasitosis.
There are often underlying metabolic deficiencies, e.g. of iron. Regional
muds are traded in Africa and may correct mineral deficiencies.

Causes of eating odd things	Notes
Habit	Trichotillomania (p.117) which can cause hair balls.
Doesn't know what is food	Immaturity or severe ID (mental age under 18 months)
Curiosity	Doesn't apply if they eat the same thing often. Sensory acuity is greater on lips than fingers.
Self-soothing (p.61)	Things that are masticatable and don't disappear: string, cotton wool, paper, stickers (like chewing gum).
pain-relief	e.g. chewing on soft or cool things (even grass) to relieve dental pain
Metabolic needs	Pregnancy, cultural pica (can reduce diarrhoea); trace element deficiencies resulting from poor diet or malabsorption (p.502)
Enjoys the texture	May want only dry foods (e.g. cereal without milk; toast not bread) or may enjoy slippery feeling of toothpaste, handcream, etc. A few children chew even liquid in their mouths, presumably to increase the sensation.
Enjoys the taste	** Completely possible for sand, ants, etc. – rare in mature 1st world child
Enjoys the effects	Betel nut
To stimulate salivation	**
Mouth cleansing	**
Copying someone	**
To shock/annoy/hide	
Psychosis	(p.537)
Specific odd things	
Worms & insects	Cultural, immaturity, curiosity, visual problem (can't see legs moving)
Things from dustbins	Feral child, neglected, hungry, or exceptionally undisgusting dustbin.
Poisonous things	DSH, inadequate supervision or packaging. Licking the soles of shoes (e.g. in profound ID) can be dangerous.

**　(see http://www.epistola.com/sfowler/scholar/scholar-betel.html)

Causelist 111: Vomiting

Activation of the sympathetic nervous system (p.428) as part of the vomiting reflex produces the common accompanying signs of pallor and salivation.

Causes of vomiting	Notes
Normal	
Posseting in infancy	Small amount during/after feed. Not true vomit.
Motion sickness	
Voluntary manual	
Self-treatment	(Appropriate or not)
⬯ Anorexia nervosa	(p.334)
⬯ Bulimia (see also *Eating disorders*, p.458)	Look for[1150]: · recurrent binges and purges (with laxatives or self-induced vomiting) · sense of lack of control · morbid preoccupation with weight and/or shape
Voluntary non-manual	
⬯ Bulimia / Anorexia Nervosa	Non-manual methods such as throat movements can be learned (see above and p.334)
Voluntary retching	Look for secondary gain (p.471). Often only saliva is produced rather than true vomit.
Rumination	Not actually vomiting but can be described by parents as vomiting, and can appear similar (p.543).
Involuntary (physical cause)	
Upper GI irritation	Alcohol, food poisoning
Throat irritation	· coughing, or rough/irritant/lumpy foods. · hyperactive gag reflex · awkward swallowing in oromotor dyspraxia, associated with unclear speech (p.89).
⬯ Migraine	(p.141)
Pyloric stenosis	Projectile vomiting usually in first few months of life; palpable pylorus
Gastro-oesophageal reflux (GORD,p.472)	Likely if occurs when upside-down, or if child leans to reduce pain.
Medication	Ipecacuanha, SSRIs (p.552, mainly at beginning of treatment), lithium (beware toxicity)
Cannabis	
Metabolic	Hypercalcaemia, p.483. Some metabolic causes are periodic, e.g. ketotic / non-ketotic hypoglycaemia, and disorders of urea cycle (p.571) or of fatty acid metabolism (p.418).
Autonomic epilepsy	(p.76)
"Cyclic vomiting syndrome"	(p.449)
Chronic idiopathic nausea	Quite common, and does not imply any mental health problem[1186].
Intracranial hypertension	(p.493) Persistent vomiting, particularly in the morning, often with behavioural changes.
⬯ Pregnancy	Usually limited to first trimester
Involuntary (emotional cause)	
Anxiety	Any type of anxiety can trigger vomiting including social anxiety[1556], hypochondriasis (p.362), pre-exam nerves, panics (p.301).
Abuse (p.271)	
Fabricated (p.359)	Exaggeration of quantity or frequency; presenting parent's own vomit as child's
Induced (p.359)	Via many of the other categories above.

Drinking too much, or *polydipsia*, can go unnoticed if a child has free access to drinks. A medical cause is more likely if the child is willing to drink anything: he may drink from puddles or dishcloths; interrupts enjoyed actitivies to seek water; and wakes in the night to seek a drink. Organic causes can precipitate a habit of drinking too much, which exacerbates or perpetuates the problem.

Initial investigations include blood urea and electrolytes, and an early morning urine for glucose and osmolality. For further details of investigations see[259].

Water intoxication occurs if fluid intake greatly exceed's the body's requirements, causing hyponatraemia[745]. Coexisting kidney disease makes this more common, as well as more likely to become severe enough to cause headache, confusion, myoclonus (p.511), dystonia, psychosis, seizures or coma (see central pontine myelinolysis, p.436).

Causes of polydipsia	Notes
Not actually excess	E.g. if the child is sweating a lot in sports
Medical (in most of these the patient is dehydrated)	
Diabetes mellitus (p.451)	Signs are polyuria, polydipsia, weight loss and elevated blood glucose.
Diabetic ketoacidosis	With nausea, abdominal pain, elevated blood glucose, dehydration, and ketonuria +++. Sometimes there are signs of the precipitating systemic infection.
Central diabetes insipidus / syndrome of inappropriate ADH (SIADH)	• Congenital causes include cerebral malformations and Wolfram syndrome, p.575. • Acquired causes include ethanol, medicines (phenytoin, alpha-adrenergic agents), head injury, p.477; autoimmunity, p.427; stroke, p.556; tumour, p.569; encephalitis, p.461; stress.
Nephrogenic diabetes insipidus	Can be familial or acquired. Acquired causes include hypokalaemia, kidney disease, medicines (lithium, rifampicin, clozapine) and postobstructive uropathy.
Rare	• Phaeochromocytoma can be detected by hypertension. May have family history of multiple endocrine neoplasia, p.569. • Hypothalamic lesion, p.485, e.g. craniopharyngioma, p.446 • Renal artery stenosis
Other medicines	E.g. carbamazepine; dry mouth due to antipsychotics.
Social and psychological	
Attention-seeking Habit	If asking for water only at bedtime or in the night.
Increased salt load	E.g. overfeeding by parents, or infant milk prepared with inadequate water; or excess salty foods. Conversely, infant milk made too dilute can cause water intoxication.
Anorexia nervosa (p.334)	To suppress appetite, or to pass a weighing test.
Nutrition in the drinks	Children obtaining most of their calories through drinks (e.g. delayed weaning or unavailability of appetising food)
Oversupply of fizzy drinks	These are so attractive to children that they drink too much. Also the excess sugar produces an osmotic diuresis and medullary washout syndrome, i.e. a secondary diabetes insipidus[259].
Inadequate nurturing	Children taken into care, into a family with less emotional bond or less monitoring of intake than they are used to, have to re-regulate their intake and may drink and eat erratically or in the wrong amounts[4].
Abusive punishment	E.g. a child forced to drink from a hose[1116].
Schizophrenia	Including early-onset schizophrenia[420]. It may be a stereotypy, self-soothing, or result from a delusion[745].

Causelist 113: Night-time wetting

The term *enuresis* by itself is variously used to refer to daytime or night-time or both, so it best avoided or qualified. For example, daytime wetting is sometimes called *diurnal enuresis*, but the former is clearer.

Most children are dry and clean in the daytime by 3 years of age (p.340), and through the night by 4 years[1531].

The old distinction between primary and secondary enuresis is not as useful as previously thought, both because of children's varying intervals of dryness, and parental memory lapses.

Causes of night-time wetting	Notes
Normal immaturity (urological or general)	It affects 10% of 5-year-olds and 5% of 10-year-olds. This is often familial and may be related to parasomnias.
Emotional upset	E.g. bullying, p.219; abuse, p.271; fostering, birth of a sibling.
Urinary tract irritation	It is usual to perform urinalysis but infection is only rarely found. Bubble bath or sexual abuse can cause urethritis.
Epilepsy, e.g. night-time fits (p.76)	Unusual but important cause. Suspect this if parent has witnessed a fit in bed.
Polyuria	Usually due to excess drinking (enjoys drink or bottle, either before bed or in the night). For other causes of polyuria see p.338.
Not enuresis at all	Rarely there can be secondary gain (p.471), e.g. for foster carers claiming compensation for night-time care. Signs include not knowing nappy size, not having incontinence nurse on rapid dial, and not having a waterproof sheet on bed. Wetting in any part of the bedroom is sometimes a protest against e.g. harsh punishment – or may reflect limited access to the toilet.
Rare	Neurogenic bladder, small bladder, genitourinary abnormality, urinary obstruction, sickle (see p.549). The wetness may be rain, or may be deposited by a sibling.

Daytime "accidents" are obviously more likely if the child has not aquired independent toileting skills. These require training and cannot be fully learned before the child has several other abilities: walking, removing clothing, being aware of the sensations of needing to micturate or defecate, and usually expressing an interest in the toilet or the potty[1531]. However, intensive conditioning approaches used in some cultures can achieve useful toilet training even earlier than these other skills (e.g.[405]). In industrialised countries this intensive approach has almost disappeared over recent generations[92].

Causes of daytime wetting (after p.310 of[743])	Notes
Normal immaturity	(Until about 24 months mental age)
Can't tear himself away from activities	
Delayed maturation	Usually familial, accompanied by delayed night-time dryness.
Attention-seeking	Common in toddlers, and obvious
Mismanagement of toilet training	E.g. ridiculing/punishing wetting
Anxiety (or fear), autonomic arousal (p.424), (hypo)mania	
Anger	Intentional voiding
Avoidance	E.g. finds the toilet frightening
Giggle incontinence in girls	Appears before puberty, and often disappears in a few years.
Likes the feeling, or experimenting	Especially in autism.
☞ Severe constipation	(p.444)
Institutional rearing	
Organic causes	When bladder control has recently been acquired, polyuria (e.g. due to polydipsia, p.338; or diabetes, p.451) and frequency can cause wetting.
• ☞ Urinary tract infection	
• Obstruction of bladder or urethra	
• Urinary system abnormalities, e.g. ectopic ureter, ectopia vesicae.	
• Meningomyelocele & other abnormalities of spinal cord	Constant dribbling & dribbling just after micturition usually have a physical cause, unlike intermittent enuresis. Needs MSU.
• Injury	
• Epilepsy (p.73)	
• Medication (e.g. antipsychotics (p.422), sedatives)	Routinely check for spina bifida (p.551).

A related problem is going to the toilet too often. Reasons include urinary infection, wanting peace and quiet, avoiding chores, enjoying looking at books there, listening to music on their MP3 player, enjoying the sound of the flush, and (in public/school toilets) meeting other people. Sitting on the toilet for a long time suggests any of these behavioural reasons; or diarrhoea, nausea, or constipation (p.444).

Causelist 115: Faecal misplacement

Encopresis (below) and smearing (p.342) are two overlapping subtypes of
faecal misplacement.

Varieties of faecal misplacement	Notes
By motivation (pre-passage). Causes are additive, not mutually exclusive.	
No motivation	Diarrhoea may indicate overflow incontinence or bowel pathology
Concentration	During activities the child can't tear himself away from, such as games or TV programmes.
Immaturity	16% of 3-year-olds are not fully faecally continent. This is the likely cause if child has been in nappies since birth, or with delay in other areas too.

☞ "Toilet phobias". Use specific interventions at right, then treat all these as any phobia (graded exposure, rewards).

Fear of falling in →	Add toddler seat insert.
Fear of monsters →	Ask if ever saw monster. Ask if any evidence of monster. Have parent make a rule about where monsters are allowed to be.
Fear of dark →	Ensure well lit
Fear of bullies in toilet →	discuss with headteacher.
Fear of painful passage of faeces →	Treat any fissure or constipation thoroughly. Pain may have led to retention, then overflow
Fear of punishment (can lead to hiding faeces) →	Parental training, re-orient to rewards rather than punishment, consider abuse (p.271).

Regressive (p.41)	Can appear as any of the other varieties, when child is finding developmental challenges too great. Also in child who only recently gained bowel control but is now ill or stressed.
Encopresis	The term *encopresis* is often used to refer to any faecal misplacement, but because this conflates completely different causes, it is better avoided – or reserved for misplacement of faeces for social reasons. Faeces can be smeared or placed. A pointed end indicates that the stool was passed there rather than being moved there. Many cases have autism-related problems (p.183). Consider also abuse (p.271).

- *Encopresis – attention-seeking.* Only convincing if it happens most when the child feels ignored (e.g. mother is in the bath or engrossed in conversation), *and* child brings it immediately to mother's attention *and* there are other attention-seeking behaviours. Can be done in places chosen to achieve maximum attention, such as the reception room with guests present.

- *Encopresis – aggressive.* Rarely happens without other signs of anger. Can be done in places chosen to cause maximum upset, such as the parental bed. Parents who assume faecal misplacement is aggressive can create relationship problems secondarily.

By what is done post-passage	
Smears on underwear	May be very small volumes of overflow incontinence. If not wiping properly → use behavioural approach.
Smearing by hand	(p.342)
Hiding	Hiding stool→ may indicate embarrassment, misunderstanding or toilet phobia. Hiding soiled pants → usually indicates embarrassment.

Smearing is a subtype of faecal misplacement (p.341). *Smearing* means smoothing faeces on to something, usually with the hand. The noun *smear* does not imply that a hand was used, so includes streaks, sometimes thick, of faeces inside the underwear (p.341).

Much too often, smearing is interpreted as symbolic (p.14) of severe repressed conflicts (p.421). In the vast majority of cases it is an accident, or a simple behaviour reinforced by minor rewards (p.540). However, occasionally smearing or anal masturbation can indicate deeper emotional problems[62].

Causes of smearing	Why bad smell doesn't prevent smearing	Why social prohibition doesn't prevent smearing	Notes
Developmental			
Accidental and/or attempt to clean hands	Bad smell already in toilet/bed. Or he keeps on walking so doesn't smell it.	Half-asleep, impulsive	Poor hand cleaning, small volume, a few simple smears, between waist and eye height, near toilet. More at night. More with poor self-control, as in ID, ADHD ☂
Severe ID	All the above reasons (and may not connect the smell with its source)	Unaware of prohibition	
Autism ☂ (p.183)	(See at right)	Uninterested or unaware of prohibition. (see at right)	Autistic child may be focusing on the feeling of the faeces. Often ID as well.
Likes response	Other motivations outweigh this	Other motivations outweigh this	May have enjoyed the extreme reaction the first time he did it.
Anosmia	Can't smell.	Confusion / immaturity	E.g. in severe upper respiratory tract infection
Anger (or emotional insta-bility, p.69)	Anger overrides	This is the purpose	Rarely on people or in wounds. Subtype of encopresis (p.341).
Non-developmental			
Delirium			(p.451)
Attention-seeking	Anger / desperation	Anger / desperation.	This also is a subtype of encopresis (p.341).
Art	Ventilation, mask, etc.	This is the purpose	
After anal masturbation "in-and-out" with stool	Child is excited, and has strong positive associations with stool.	Done in private or the child has suppressed his knowledge of prohibition.	(p.115)

Bizarre experiences and ideas

Colloquially, bizarre means very strange, or outlandish (see p.520). In psychiatry it has the additional meaning of ideas that could not possibly be true, as distinct from ideas that are just very unlikely (for examples see *Bizarre delusions* , p.348).

Causelist 117: Hallucinations

This means a perception not triggered by a stimulus. Objective signs of hallucination include talking to, looking at, smiling at, or gesturing towards empty space. Descriptions of symptoms should be factual, avoiding florid interpretation.

Are the psychotic experiences trivial, or isolated, or pervasive?

Hallucinations are surprisingly common: 8% of all 12-year-olds claim on self-report to have had auditory hallucinations in the past 6 months; and 4% have on careful interview[720]. For visual hallucinations the corresponding figures are 6% and 1.5%. For both modalities, 20% of the hallucinations are hypnopompic/hypnagogic (p.345) and 4% may be caused by high temperatures. The larger the number of modalities affected, the greater the clinical severity (e.g. lower IQ, earlier onset)[370]. Hence general function is the key to working out whether the child has a serious pervasive condition. For example, has the child regressed (p.41) or is she doing everything in a daze, moving at a slower pace, or looking through you? Signs that can be quantified are especially useful for assessing severity, progress, relapses and the effectiveness of treatments. They vary from child to child, but can include:

Reassurance-seeking	Notice clinging on to the hand of staff, even staff she does not know, apparently for reassurance. When is she actually fearful? What of?
Change of personality (p.241)	Note signs of disinhibition (p.261). In a very timid child, even disobedience or swearing can indicate illness.
Regression	See signs of true regression, p.42.
Screaming	E.g. out-of-character screaming for several hours in a day
Hitting peers out of the blue	Is she just cross or hearing command hallucinations (p.344)?
Odd/angry voices	Other children may say "stop speaking in that silly voice".
Intrusive episodes	Count the number of separate episodes lasting up to 5 minutes during which she responds to bizarre experiences. Can she continue with an enjoyed task through the intrusion, or is she distracted or cross?
Throwing things (p.103)	At the time, is she complaining about what real people are doing, or imaginary people?
Stereotypies (p.553)	Does she have any behaviours that may indicate tension (tics, trichotillomania, self-biting, rocking)?
Idiosyncratic behaviours	Anything the child only did during previous ill episodes will be a useful indicator of future episodes.
↓↑Sleep (p.200)	Note typical sleep pattern and recent changes
↓alertness	Is she doing everything in a daze, moving at a slower pace, looking through you?
↓Talking	Note number of times per hour, to self or others.
↓Participation in class	Spontaneously enlisting engagement from people passing in class? Having back-and-forth conversation? Interacting long enough to be tested?
↓Reading	Note periods during which she loses interest
↓Drawing	Including complexity, topic, concentration, intrusions. Observe this in clinic and keep examples with dates.

Working out the cause of the hallucinations

The prognosis depends on the cause of the hallucinations, and associated features. Working out the cause can be greatly helped by:

- *Prevalence*. Schizophrenia is rare before puberty (see p.543). Imaginary friends (p.231) and misunderstandings about what the child is describing are far more common.

- *Which sensory modality is affected*. Auditory hallucinations can have any of the causes below. Visual hallucinations are most often hypnagogic or hypnopompic (p.345) or caused by imaginary friends (p.231), but otherwise usually have a biological cause[1002,1350] – such as pressure on the eye *(phosphenes)*; or centrally, in which case they appear most often when sleepy. They should be drawn and compared with published drawings (in[1440]). Tactile hallucinations can be due to cocaine (p.258) or alcohol withdrawal or schizophrenia (p.543). Olfactory hallucinations can be due to temporal lobe pathology (p.73) or schizophrenia (p.543) or depression (p.122).

- *Content of the hallucination*. Imaginary friends (p.231) are always welcome. Voices repeatedly saying terrible or wonderful things to the person usually indicate mood disorder. Voices that consistently describe a risk if the child fails to do something, indicate OCD (p.65). In adults with recurrent psychotic episodes, about 30% have hallucinations whose content is related (specifically or thematically) to previous trauma, especially sexual abuse and bullying[651].

  Command hallucinations usually cause distress and can be dangerous. They are more likely to be acted on if the command hallucination is viewed as positive; if the person wants to do what they say (e.g. if delusions agree with the hallucination); or if there was low maternal control in childhood[1464]. Conversely, risk of obedience to hallucinations is reduced by antipsychotics, and perhaps counterintuitively, by traditional predictors of violence (e.g. male sex, high levels of anger, or a history of violence)[1464]. If the command is to harm herself or others, sexual abuse leading to PTSD (p.532) should be considered: it can occasionally be so severe as to cause psychosis[1744].

  In contrast, hallucinations with no emotional content for the individual have biological rather than psychic causes, and are often exacerbated by sleep disturbance[1002]. In the visual realm, such symptoms fall on a continuum of complexity, from the simple shapes of migraine (p.141), to bubbles or broccoli floating in space in occipital damage, to horses with movement, sound, and smell with more diffuse causes (e.g. drugs and sleepiness). Auditory hallucinations lacking in emotional content include tinnitus (p.565) and the hearing of voices without being able to identify what they are saying, which has various causes, such as basilar migraine.

- *Timing and duration*. If it occurs only at bedtime or on waking it is a commonplace hypnagogic or hypnopompic hallucination (p.345). If it occurs only when very tired it may be a partial sleep symptom, or an exacerbation of an underlying biological predisposition[1002]. If it lasts just 15-120 seconds, interrupting enjoyed activities, consider hypothalamic hamartoma (p.76). If it lasts just a few hours or days see p.449.

- *Associated symptoms*. If it is associated with anxiety (p.295) or headaches (p.139) they may indicate a treatable cause[1063,1444]. If it starts following a bereavement (p.430) and lasts for a few months, it is a normal post-bereavement hallucination (this is sometimes called a pseudohallucination, defined below, but the principle is similar to imaginary friends). This can be auditory and/or visual. People with acquired blindness sometimes develop Charles Bonnet syndrome[1002], i.e. visual pseudo-hallucinations (p.345) analogous to those seen in bereavement. The auditory equivalent is musical hallucinosis following acquired deafness.

Causes of "hallucinations"	Notes
Not really hallucinations	
Imaginary friends	Can be visual and/or auditory and are always welcome (p.231). Caused by sensory or social deprivation.
Immature description	He may say "a voice made me do it" as a description of an impulse, obsession (p.517), or other thought . Check his vocabulary; give him clear options to choose between (not "Why did you do that?" which can be mystifying).
Misunderstanding of adult speech	E.g. if child has heard parent saying he is "away with the fairies"
To avoid being told off	Child can learn that saying "the voice (or granddad) told me to take that biscuit" is useful.
Mimicry	A very social child may mimic the mannerisms and mouth movements of someone speaking, as an enjoyable role-play. This can happen even in children with very little language (e.g. a child with Down's syndrome), in which case the mouth movements are simple and there may be no sound.
Pseudo-hallucination	• Pseudohallucinations can be vivid, but they are not experienced as well placed in space. Adults know them to be unreal, but children often do not. They disappear when something interesting happens in the real world (e.g. the end of TV advertisements).
	• Visual parahallucinations are fleeting, in the peripheral visual field, and disappear when looked at (see bereavement, p.430; Charles Bonnet, p.133).
	• *Pseudohallucination* can also mean malingered hallucinations, i.e. pseudo-psychosis (see below)
Pseudo-psychosis	This is identified by recognising internal and external *inconsistencies*. Inconsistencies are more likely to be detected if a wide range of information is available, including careful history and observation, use of alternative sources of information, observation with and without parents, and knowledge of patterns of disorder. For example, malingering (p.503) should be suspected if questions about symptoms are followed by a long pause or "I don't know"; if hallucinations are continuous, vague, or use stilted language; or if delusions are inconsistent with behaviour [1333]. Simulation of symptoms can precede real psychosis [671].
Physical causes (see p.349)	Note causes can be additive, e.g. a bereavement hallucination only occurring while taking antiepileptics.
Sensory organ problem	E.g. tinnitus (p.565)
Migraine	(p.141)
Other	
Extreme fatigue, sleep onset or end	Hypnagogic and hypnopompic hallucinations are commonplace (at the start and end of sleep respectively). They are usually visual but occasionally auditory. Daytime hallucinations can be hypnagogic hallucinations (*daymares*) caused by narcolepsy (p.72). In families with partial sleep syndromes there is increased prevalence of hallucinations when extremely fatigued.
Bereavement	(p.430)
Anxiety	(See previous page)

Depression or mania	In both, hallucinations are mainly talking to the person, i.e. *second person*, and the content is mood congruent.
Dissociation, p.453	E.g.intrusive recall of a trauma in PTSD (pp.493, 532, 452)
Schizophrenia	(p.543)
Schizotypy	An important consideration if a first-degree relative is psychotic. Can precede a schizophrenic prodrome (p.544).
Folie imposee	(See also odd ideas section: p.347)

Causelist 118: Odd ideas, including delusions

On self-report, a quarter of all 12-year-olds claim to have had ideas of these types in the past 6 months: being spied on, persecuted, thoughts being read, reference, control, grandiose ability, thought broadcasting, thought insertion, or thought withdrawal. On careful interview only about 2% have actually had delusions[720] (see also[190]). Unlike hallucinations, very few are related to sleep or to temperature.

If a child has one odd idea, it is important to know whether he has others. In order to elicit such abnormal thought *content* in children, one standard battery uses stories about a friendly ghost, an ostracised little boy, the Incredible Hulk, a witch, a good or bad child, and an unhappy child[254]. These are good topics to ask about because if a child has important or odd emotionally laden ideas, chatting about these topics often reveals them.

See also *Telling untruths* (p.255) and *Hallucinations* (p.343).

Are the delusions important?
See the discussion regarding hallucinations, on p.343.

Categories of odd ideas
Cognitive deficits
‖ Miscommunication (e.g. culturally appropriate errors), mismodelling
Confabulation (p.443)
When rules have been superficially learned, without the deep knowledge (underlying reasons, role hierarchies, etc.) that allow most people to work out when rules don't apply (e.g. when a more important person can override a rule, or an adult in their own house, or when another rule is more important). For example, an autistic boy couldn't pick up a crisp from the table because he had been told not to eat off the table, but could after it had been put on a paper.

Unusual background information
Odd experiences, whether one-off or continuing, e.g. abuse (p.271).

Inadequate judgment, knowledge, or exploration, to allow the right answer

Folie imposee: An important consideration if parents are psychotic or odd. May be impossible to distinguish from primary psychosis, without several weeks of full separation from the family, though much briefer separations should be tried first. Unless trivial (e.g. a dad who taught his child that her elbow was called a nose), this is emotional abuse (p.277). See parental alienation (p.187).

Autism can create bizarre preoccupations and communications[424]. Was the child socially cut off even before the psychosis? See some home videos

Motivated
‖ Motivated cognitive errors induced by defence mechanisms (p.305) / cognitive distortions or biases (p.534). These include wishful thinking and other
‖ motivated irrationality – [see 1106]

Persisting fantastic beliefs, such as claimed memories of past lives, occur in cultures in which they are encouraged, and the children tend to be attention-seeking and anxious[649].

Spritual experiences can have Schneiderian content (p.544), but the individuals are not functionally impaired or suffering, there are few or no comorbidities, the experiences are controllable, and the beliefs are culturally appropriate [1110].

Malingered: see pseudo-psychosis (p.345).

Delusions. These are ideas that have arisen through pathological thinking.

They are like assumptions, in that they feel completely real, are not questioned, and the person has to stop and think to work out why he believes them, just as you have to come up with reasons why you know your name, or the fact that you are sitting on a chair.

A classic definition of delusion is a belief that is fixed, false, and culturally inappropriate. However, this definition is flawed: they are not always fixed [1487, p.142] and they can be culturally appropriate and true *by coincidence*. Often more useful in understanding the idea, and the person, is the *source* of the idea (which affects its form), or the *motivation* for it (which affects its content). Severity is graded by bizarreness, persistence, complexity, influence on actions, and lack of insight (p.491)[43].

Bizarre delusions are accorded great weight in the diagnosis of schizophrenia. They indicate a radical change in the very conditions of experience, with alterations in self-consciousness or changes in the temporal and spatial structure of the world (e.g. "A rat is living in my shoulder and talks to me")[276]. In contrast, non-bizarre delusions have fairly ordinary, world-related content, usually with with some emotional significance (especially suspicion) and with practical implications for what the person must do (e.g. "I have won the lottery, I must find my ticket.").

It may be that *all* delusions relate to the self[1487]. Sims [1487] describes Jaspers' subtypes of *true delusions*, i.e. those which have not emerged understandably:

- autochthonous delusion (out of the blue *delusional intuition)*
- delusional percept (a normal percept is interpreted as having delusional meaning)
- delusional atmosphere or mood (p.544): "something funny is going on"
- delusional memory ("retrospective delusions" – a memory (which can be true or false) given delusional meaning

Some of these probably arise due to cognitive dissonance (p.355).

Depression (p.309) and mania (p.263)

Schizophrenia and brief psychoses (p.543)

Biological causes (next page)

Dissociation (p.453)

Investigation Planner 9: Medical causes of hallucinations and delusions

Bear in mind that most hallucinations are medically benign (p.343). Worrying signs suggesting that they are not include increasing social isolation, disorganisation, or regression, or intrusion of bizarre unreinforced hallucinations into enjoyed activities. Consider also the causes of regression, p.47. See also the *general approach to medical investigations*, p.373 and[508,1502].

☞ Precise diagnosis is achieved only in a small minority, but is nevertheless urgent as it can allow treatment that prevents irreversible disease progression[1448].

		Excluded clinically or to Order?	Date ordered (or tick each test)	Result
Basic tests	Signs		Thyroid/T3, renal, FBC, LFT, ESR/CRP, B6, B$_{12}$, folate, physical exam[1034]	
Genetic & Metabolic				
Velocardiofacial	(p.572) Relatively common		Genetic tests	
X-chromosome abnormality	(see [1200]). E.g. Klinefelter's, p.496		Chromosomes (p.439)	
Fabry's disease	(p.464) with painful *Fabry crises*		Serum alpha-galactosidase	
Niemann-Pick type C	(Psychosis *before* ataxia, p.552)		(p.552)	
Prader-Willi	(p.533) Obesity, atypical bipolar disorder, extreme hypotonia in infancy		Genetic tests	
Citrullinemia	Mental state change. Type 2 (Citron defect, asp-glu carrier defect, can make kids very psychotic)		Citrulline, ammonia	
Tay-Sachs	(p.502) Cherry-red macula, progressive deterioration and ataxia.		Genetic tests, MRI	
Hartnup disease	(p.477)			
Cobalamin C disease	(p.329)		MMA and homocysteine in blood/urine	
Homocystinuria	(p.481) Progressive ID, epilepsy		Plasma amino acids; urine homocysteine	
MTHFR deficiency	(pp.468,481)		(p.468)	
Cystathione-β-synthase deficiency			(as homo-cystinuria)	
Maple syrup urine	(p.505)		(p.505)	
Leukodystrophy	(p.498) progressive ID		(p.498)	

G6PD deficiency	Haemolytic anaemia / jaundice precipitated by some medications, moth balls, broad beans, some infections. Occasionally causes recurrent psychotic mania[187]	FBC, blood film, bilirubin
Gilbert syndrome	This is debated[1679]. Look for jaundice (yellow sclerae).	Conj. & unconj. bilirubin
Marfan syndrome	(p.505) Slight increased risk.	
Fahr's disease	(p.429)	MRI
Mitochondrial disorder	(p.508)	Plasma lactate
Urea cycle	(p.571) Acute confusion	
Peroxisomal defects	(p.526)	
Lysosomal defects	Various, e.g. lipofuscinosis, p.502; mannosidosis[997]	
	Sanfilippo: p.502	Urine GAG
Congenital disorders of glycosylation	(p.474)	Transferrin Glycoforms
Lysinuric protein intolerance	(p.379)	
Cerebrotendinous xanthomatosis	(p.32)	(p.32)
Nonketotic hyperglycinaemia	Movement disorders triggered by fever[1448]	amino acid chromatogr. (urine+blood)
Succinic semi-aldehyde dehydro-genase deficiency	ID, hallucinations, anxiety, aggression[1448]	urinary β-hydroxy-butyrate, MRI
Other genetic	If there are *also* any of the following classes of problem, see[914] for a list of congenital causes: Abnormal body size, ataxia, bone/connective tissue, cardiovascular, skin, dysmorphism, endocrine, hearing, blood, ID, movement, neuropathy, genitourinary, seizures, spasticity, speech, liver, vision. If there is also deafness, consider Usher, Wolfram, velocardiofacial and Coffin-Lowry syndromes; Norrie and Darier-White disease; and familial hemiplegic migraine.	

continued ▶

Endocrine & Haematologic		
Hyperthyroidism	(p.484)	T4/T3/TSH
Hypoglycaemia	(p.82)	Glucose
Thymoma / myasthenia gravis	Fatiguability of individual muscles. Shortness of breath (p.510)	Anti-AChR
Porphyria, p.532	Intermittent abdominal pain	(p.532)
Infections (see [262])		
Viral encephalitis, p.461	Fever, headache (p.139), changed mental state	
Epstein-Barr virus, p.478	Fever, sore throat, adenopathy, fatigue (p.323)	
Lyme disease	p.501	p.501
Malaria	p.503	
Typhoid fever		
Mycoplasma pneumonia	Fever, mental state change; even without pneumonia	
Rabies	History of exposure	
Neurologic		
Confusional state / delirium	• Chronic confusional states • Delirium: p.451	MMSE (p.400)
Migraine	(p.141)	History
Seizure (esp. temporal lobe epilepsy, p.562)	Paroxysmal periods of sudden change in mood, behaviour, or motor activity, with no apparent trigger. Also interictal psychosis, p.449, post-ictal psychosis, p.532	EEG
Central pontine myelinolysis	(p.436)	Na, MRI
Moyamoya disease	Paresis, peripheral numbness, headaches, syncope/TIA/stroke.	MRI
Narcolepsy	(p.72)	MSLT
SSPE	(p.557) Decline over years.	Anti-measles
Head injury	(p.477)	MRI
Wilson's disease	(p.575)	(p.575)
Huntington's chorea	(p.482)	(p.482)
Multiple sclerosis	(p.510)	MRI
Neurofibromatosis	(p.514)	MRI
Oncologic		
Tumours	(p.569)	MRI
Nutritional		
Pellagra	(p.329) Dermatitis, diarrhoea	B3

Toxicologic (p.566)		
Lead	(p.330)	lead
Mercury	(p.330)	mercury
Carbon monoxide	Shortness of breath, mild nausea, headache (p.139), dizziness	Carboxy-haemoglobin
‖ Illicit drugs	(p.257).	Urine drug screen
Medicines	• Stimulants (and other dopamine agonists) especially after rapid dose increase. More likely in children at risk of schizophrenia. • Withdrawal of sedatives including alcohol, opiates, benzodiazepines (p.430), barbiturates • Steroids (p.554), ketamine (p.474), anticholinergics, antihistamines, antidepressants (p.552), antiepileptics, salicylates, non-steroidal anti-inflammatory drugs, many others (see BNF)	Levels.
Autoimmune		
If there are heart problems in the family		• Anti-cardiolipin • Anti-phospho-lipid • Lupus anti-coagulant (citrate tube)
SLE	(p.560)	(p.560)
PANDAS	• Anti-basal ganglia & ASOT, see p.522	
anti-NMDA	• Anti-NMDA receptor (can cause treatable psychosis, and the youngest so far was age 6)	
Vasculitis	• ANCA & IgA ANCA	

Contradictions

The manner in which parents contradict each other, or avoid doing so, reveals a lot about family functioning. Similarly, one of the most efficient ways of assessing a person's thinking is to listen and look for apparent contradictions (surprises or non sequiturs) in what he or she says or does. Some of them will turn out not to be contradictory at all within the person's value system – which then itself becomes the object of interest. Other apparent contradictions indicate gaps in the clinician's knowledge of disease or the world, offering good opportunities for learning.

Contradictions between patient and professionals are especially common in psychosomatic states. This is often because there are both physical and emotional contributions to the problem, but each individual focuses on just one of these (for an example see p.323).

Causelist 119: Unwanted behaviours

This means things people do that they wish they didn't, when both the wish and the unliked behaviour persist together. Sometimes this causes no problem, as with trivial habits, or Andre Agassi's winning Wimbledon despite saying "I hate tennis with a dark and secret passion, and always have." Sometimes, though, unwanted behaviours cause confusion or distress, which contributes to psychiatric disorders (see p.355).

Much recent behavioural research has focused on the distinction between the impulse to to do something, and the degree of pleasure experienced when it is obtained. Animals often do things they don't enjoy or "like" or which don't feel like *rewards*, because of habit or other complexities of behavioural control. In such research, "want" (or *reinforcement*, p.540) refers to what makes them do it[1357,1358]. However, in the current book we use "unwanted" in the more subjective, overseeing sense described in the previous paragraph.

For unliked *thoughts* and *images*, see *intrusions*, p.493.

Unwanted *non*-behaviour (difficulty starting)
This section is about children who want to start an activity but can't. For other kinds of non-behaviour, see p.515.

Difficulty starting is seen in disinterest, sleepiness (and other causes of inattention, p.79); perfectionism; stuttering, p.157; Parkinsonism, p.525. Many children (and adults) leave starting a job until the last minute, when urgency will help them to focus.

Rigid children (p.234) can insist on a ritual before something is done; the most common example is bedtime rituals. A child may want to go to school but be unable to get through the preparatory rituals. Extreme versions of this are most common in autism, p.183; and OCD, p.65.

Tourette's (p.101) often includes an intermittent need to obtain a "just-right" feeling before doing something such as going through a door. When this is combined with extreme rigidity, as in autism, it can produce the surprising situation in which the child wants to start an activity (such as having a bite of food) but to allow him to start he needs someone else to do something in just the right way (e.g. to say "Jim, eat!" in exactly the right way). He may ask for the ritual, or if he is non-verbal, signal desperately with eye contact that he needs this help. This situation can be distinguished from simple rigidity or rituals by the varying way in which the "just right" feeling is achieved.

Causes of unwanted behaviours	Notes
Not really unliked	
Confabulation	(p.443) Or disconnection/dissociation (p.453).
Pseudo-passivity ("I didn't want to do it!")	A child, usually with a disorder, learns that mother is sympathetic and never tells him off if he says he couldn't help it, so he starts experimenting:
	• he tries *abnormal* behaviours, labelling them as part of the disorder, i.e. they are pseudo-behaviours (p.363). Parents are easily taken in by this.
	• he tries *normal* behaviours (naughty or not), labelling them as part of the disorder. A common example is a child with ADHD, running in class: teachers often become unsure whether they can use discipline. An unusual example is a child saying "Mom, I have this American accent, and something's wrong, I can't stop it!" in order to get a hug.
	This happens in young children whereas the *made actions* of schizophrenia occur in adolescence and adulthood (p.537).
Egosyntonic motivation	I.e. wishing there were an alternative action. This is common in self-harm (p.317).
Unliked conflict	(See *cognitive dissonance*, p.355)
Anorexia	E.g. sometimes a battle of control v appetite (p.334)
Sexual	Some homosexuality, fetishism, philandering, particularly with religious beliefs (see p.355).
Unliked motivation	
OCD	Compulsions attempt to reduce egodystonic fears: p.65.
Impulse control	See both drug and *behavioural addiction*, p.259; impulsivity, p.79; boredom, p.322. Skin picking (p.549) is liked during but not after[1764].
Unliked impulse	
Tics	Touretters sometimes apologise after swearing (p.161)
Alien hand syndrome	This is a motor release phenomenon, caused by frontal damage[53]. Patients are perplexed when they see their hand making movements over which they feel no ownership or control. It is a rare type of *utilisation behaviour*, p.572. See also corpus callosum, p.445.
Lesch-Nyhan syndrome (p.318)	May be unilateral, e.g. one arm resisting self-harm by the other arm. Biting fingers in Lesch-Nyhan: patients were "terrified of their hands, and screamed for help even as they bit them." [1279]
Subconscious / subcortical / low-level behaviours	
Automatic behaviours	(pp.61, 63). It is commonplace to do something quickly "without thinking" then realise within seconds that it was a mistake (e.g. impulsive children who cry after hitting people; transient oppositionality, p.254). There are also children who snarl and start a punch (or scratch) but who manage to stop the fist mid-flight. Presumably one sees this less in adults because the stopping is so quick that it precedes any movement. See *utilisation behaviours*, p.572.
Aggression	(p.289)
Habits	E.g. idiosyncratic movements (p.99)

Special Topic 18: Is cognitive dissonance involved?

Holding strong contradictory beliefs can be a source of severe behavioural problems or psychopathology. When a person becomes aware of a contradiction (i.e. a *cognitive discrepancy*), the unpleasant feeling called *cognitive dissonance*[654] (CD) drives him or her to resolve the discrepancy, typically by revaluing or revising one belief (see figure).

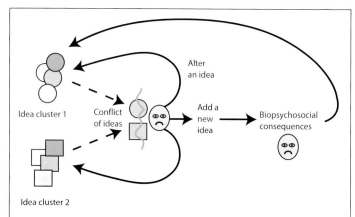

Figure 23. Cognitive dissonance can cause odd ideas and behaviours.

Cognitive dissonance (jagged line) arises when contradictory ideas are considered together (dashed lines). It is unpleasant so people adopt various strategies to reduce or avoid it (solid black lines).

Widespread relevance of cognitive dissonance
Cognitive dissonance may contribute to some of the transitions between Piagettian developmental stages, p.530. It may also account for the simultaneous occurrence of unpleasant emotion with apparently counterproductive ideas (or behaviours) that characterise many psychiatric disorders (p.511). For example, if a person realises he is doing something inexplicable or feeling very strange, he will feel confused (anxious, dissonant) and this exacerbates many symptoms (for examples, see[240]). To reduce the CD, he is likely to eventually come up with a strategy (see figure) that follows a standard pattern in his society, and which may make other aspects of his life worse. If the initial problem was wrong *ideas*, the best solution may be simply to realise the error, i.e. to drop those ideas (see *bubble bursting*, p.435).

Cognitive dissonance in clinical conditions

Anxiety states can be caused by conflicts, though they are not often described as CD[240].

CD increases the risk of various behavioural and psychiatric problems. For example, there are well-developed theories linking CD to anorexia nervosa (p.334), OCD (p.65), hatred (p.187), dissociation (p.453), abuse (p.271) and psychosis (p.537).

CD is closely related to Bateson's 1956 idea that repeated exposure to conflicting emotionally loaded information could cause schizophrenia (the "double bind" hypothesis[119,1532]). This turned out to be an overstatement of CD's usual impact. However it is clear that the related concept of negative expressed emotion (p.512) does increase the risk of schizophrenic relapse (p.544).

Parental alienation is a clear example of CD whose effect changes as the child's social awareness increases: for example, the cognitive *discrepancy* has little emotional impact below age 7 or so (see table on p.187).

As another example, a teenager's knowledge that her "consensual" sex with an adored older adult could lead that adult into prison and would shatter her religious parents can be ignored by her – the ideas can be kept separate until it is found out. At that point there arise major conscious conflicts between self-worth and self-blame, and between treasured memories and guilt (p.475).

See also examples of disobedience caused by dilemmas, p.254.

Recognising and using cognitive dissonance clinically

Clinically it can be difficult to be establish a link from CD to a behavioural symptom, because the conflict can be concealed and the symptom may have little obvious relevance to the conflict. The symptoms may be of severe anxiety or cognitive adjustments (as in the figure), arising at the time when the person confronted the discrepancy. Once suspected, a trial of treatment is appropriate: the contradictory ideas can be discussed and the child helped either to deal with the contradiction, or if that is not possible to make the contradiction less important[240]. CD can also be used as a therapeutic tool: it is one of the central processes of Motivational Interviewing[899] and the placebo effect, i.e. people will change their behaviour to avoid the feeling that they are living a contradiction.

Causelist 120: Approximate answers

Literally, this means answers that are almost right: obviously an everyday occurrence (e.g. baby talk, p.43; *word-finding difficulty*, p.149; immature conjugations). Some such approximations can reveal preoccupations, e.g.

- Freudian slips – mistakes thought to reveal subconscious influence.
- Spoonerisms (switching sounds around, e.g. "a blushing crow").
- Malapropism (substituting a similar-sounding word, e.g. Hannibal "rode elephants into Cartilage" – Mike Tyson)

However the term usually refers to answers to direct questions. In conventional psychiatric usage, *approximate answers* (or *Ganser symptoms*) must show that the general aim of the question was understood, e.g. that the correct answer would be a number or a country or a spelling. The term refers to answers that are obviously different from the correct answer, rather than drawn towards another subject. So imprecision can be imposed *after* the right answer has been obtained (i.e. vorbeigehen, or going past the correct answer: What is 7x7? → "48"). Alternatively the imprecision can be imposed on the question (e.g. *How do you spell "world"*→ GLOBE) or on both the question and the answer (→ GLOBF).

A person's behaviour when *not* confronted with a question, or not interacting, will often be a more reliable indicator of his actual ability than his answers when confronted, stressed or self-monitoring.

Ganser syndrome is the motley combination of approximate answers (no such errors in spontaneous speech), dissociative somatic symptoms, clouding of consciousness, and perceptual disturbances. Many partial forms exist [1624] so its main use is as a reminder that cognitive, neurological, and emotional causes must all be considered in assessments of symptoms.

Causes of approximate answers	Notes
Without hesitation	
Preoccupied thinking about something else	The answer given can be a mixture of the appropriate answer and the preoccupation (see examples at left).
Cover-up	Rarely, a child who often cannot find the answer peers want (e.g. due to language difficulties) may develop the habit of producing nonsense answers. This is sometimes akin to selective mutism (p.153).
Inadequate checking	As in listing all the colours (he repeats himself). Exclude STM problems (p.555). Can indicate elevated mood.
Cognitive deficit	There are many signs of this (p.55). For example, a child can demonstrate the ability to use two rules separately, but is unable to use them together (e.g. when instructed "write the alphabet, in lower case").
Language problems (p.145)	This is most likely in immigrants, in ID, or if parent(s) had language deficits in childhood. Signs include: • The child's answers are relevant to one or two words in the question, especially the concrete words such as nouns, but the order of the words, or the meaning of connecting words, is ignored. • The replies fail to answer the question – or, worse, would not actually answer *any* question properly.
Poor teaching and role models	Never learned to question self, or to be unembarrassed about this
Failure to leave topic	An attempt to produce a wrong answer fails because the patient is unable to suppress the pre-potent correct answer completely.
Many other conditions	Depression, schizophrenia, early dementia, toxicity, oppositional, or following traumas.
With hesitation	
Word-finding difficulty (p.149)	It is difficult to diagnose this if the person has some of the above problems too.
Boredom (p.322)	A child can produce nonsense (or partially sensible) answers because it is too boring to give the right answer.
Anxious	Social and performance anxiety (p.298)
Avoidance of subjects	Increases in anxiogenic situations/topics, e.g. autistic person referring to people in the vaguest possible way (saying "people" rather than man, girl, etc.)
Malingering (p.503)	Appears in some test situations (rare in children).
Joking	Consider the numerous motivations for joking (p.495)

Special Topic 19: Is this symptom fabricated, induced or exaggerated?

Classification difficulties

Fabricated, induced, and exaggerated are useful terms. However, all of them are a matter of degree [1709], and it is wise to avoid being too categorical on the questions of physical versus psychological, false versus true, and conscious versus unconscious (p.570). It is usually unrealistic and counterproductive to assume there is a single underlying motivation, and thence to categorise it as malingering (p.503: external motivation), factitious ("intentional with internal motivation", "to acquire sick role") or somatised ("other internal motivations"). These categories all have similar features, such as age of onset, chronicity, comorbidities, and poor treatment response[548]. Often multiple causes need to be identified, as when children exaggerate real symptoms because they feel adults aren't taking them seriously enough (and see[1463]).

How patients tolerate the inconsistency

Mild distortions of reality

Exaggerations are common, especially when seeking care from carers. It is particularly common when real illness has allowed a child to experience increased care (complaints of pain elicit help very quickly, at least in children), or reduction in anxiety (pp.295, 217).

A small step up the hierarchy of severity is to normal aches and pains which become interpreted, by the child or parent, as pathological or worrying. Unexplained symptoms seem to occur more in people who pay more attention to their body in general, and symptoms in particular[225] – which itself is more likely if there has been serious related illness in the child or family.

Severe distortions of reality

These, on the other hand, demand more explanation because most children cannot persist with them. For most children and teenagers, to persistently malinger is impossible due to the effort needed to present the same version to different people (see *malingering*, p.503; *cognitive dissonance*, p.355).

Severe cases (e.g. psychosis, p.537) are unusual and it is probably unrealistic to look for a full explanation in normal mental processes. In most such cases the sufferers were themselves unusual before the symptoms arose. It is wise to perform detailed cognitive testing in people with frequent unexplained physical complaints because ID or NVLD (p.28) can prevent a person from testing his own ideas (e.g. in magical thinking, p.502). Similarly, autism spectrum conditions should be carefully considered[1394]: if an autistic child talks about agonising pain from a demonstrably normal finger, one has to wonder whether it is a real pain, whether it is a phrase with an idiosyncratic meaning to her, whether she has any concept that whether it is true or not matters, and indeed whether she has any other way of starting a conversation on a subject she's happy to talk about, and eliciting this finely calibrated level of intimacy.

History-taking problems	Notes
Tendency for clinicians to regard patient as a time waster	Try not to do this, because the underlying psychopathology is probably more complex and unpleasant than the symptom he is complaining of.
Patient has mistaken views about normality	Responds to simple education.
You think he is making a physical complaint but really he isn't, or he isn't sure he is.	Example is "heart feeling heavy" in an Pakistani adolescent, feeling so bad following his father's death that he thinks he may die too. Or using phrases he heard a sick relative use.
Worries expressed in a guarded way	There's often a connection between the site and the underlying anxiety, e.g. penis size, BDD, sexuality
Side-effect of other intention	E.g. wants to speak about something else but can't. You can talk respectfully about that issue, then ask whether there's anything else he needed to discuss.
Misconstruing the referral	If the referring paediatrician asks for your opinion on "whether psychological factors could be involved," it is important to realise that they do not mean this literally (the answer would *always* be yes). The referrer actually needs a reply mentioning relevant psychological factors, the evidence for how important they are in this case, and ways in which they appear to be interacting with physical factors.
Clinical confusion	Letters, emails and comments may have been misinterpreted, e.g. regarding the likelihood of specific diagnoses. Letters that corroborate the patient's story may have been lost or simply not looked at.
Physical disorder not fitting into pattern known to referrer so referred	• Referred for, e.g., "faking symptoms": pains, slow recovery, medication side-effects, Guillain-Barré (p.87) – and all the ☞ in this book. • Anxious juniors sometimes refer normal behaviours (or innocuous psychosomatic behaviours) that they haven't encountered before

Practical approach

It is not enough just to decide whether the patient is faking or not. Prepare yourself for a big assessment, because for most medically unexplained symptoms, a good formulation will need to include many of the following: physical factors, operant conditioning, intelligence, personality, beliefs and family functioning[735]. Added complications are that motivations (and physical problems) are *changeable*, *interacting* and *incompletely known*.

A hunch is not sufficient. It is always possible to invent a formulation involving external motivations such as school-avoidance or the desire for care, or symbolic significance of that part of the body (p.14) – but this does not make it true. As in any assessment, plausible medical and behavioural factors have to be carefully considered and excluded.

Collecting enough information
A multidisciplinary assessment is usually needed (p.21). Information should be gathered from several sources, and distinct situations can be created in clinic as well. The reason is that the child's guard may drop in some situations, or the trigger for the odd behaviour may not be present in some situations. Normalising the situation, and the gentle use of open-ended questions, often allows young children to reveal the truth, but older adolescents tend to maintain secrecy until faced with concrete evidence[953].

Recognising inconsistency
Observe whether a serious problem depends on apparently minor factors:
- a behaviour occurs only with one parent
- it happens when she is denied chocolate, or stops when she is given chocolate
- when a parent asks "Are you sure?" in a jokey way, the child smiles
- a child develops life-threatening illness when her parents argue.

Common patterns are abdominal pain, p.135 chronic fatigue, p.323; hyperventilation/panic, p.484; and neurological symptoms, p.364.

Fabrication of symptoms is considerably more likely if several of the following apply, though all these have exceptions: overendorsement of rare symptoms, endorsing too many symptoms, implausible symptom combinations, fluctuations (especially relief when distracted by another task), lack of objective clinical signs, non-anatomic sensory loss, hesitant explanations, sudden onset, delayed onset after injury, variability of symptoms, the presence of anxiety or depression, exaggerating severity, claiming severe but not mild symptoms, discrepancy between observed and reported symptoms, and sudden cure[672,1363].

The degree of realism of feigned symptoms will depend on the patient's age, intelligence, social skills, general education, and specific knowledge of disease. Inability to answer very simple questions (e.g. counting forward in schoolchildren, or backward in teens), and amnesia (p.421), are very common in malingering[1624] but of course also in many organic brain states. Such questioning forms the basis of objective effort testing which has so far been applied only to cognitive testing[183].

What doesn't help
The presence of secondary gain (p.471) rarely helps in understanding the situation, because there is secondary gain in many or most cases of physical illness, and because people with physical illnesses often perpetuate or exaggerate their disability for secondary gain[672]. Similarly, *la belle indifference* may simply indicate stoicism or ID (see p.423).

One cannot rely on the old rule that fabricated symptoms are all-or-nothing, or that they don't conform to known functional/anatomical patterns. This is because many children have learned symptoms from a visibly similar disorder in self, family, or friend (or heard described, or seen on TV). For example, pseudoseizures (p.74) are more common in people who have had real seizures.

Causes of such symptoms	Examples	Signs
Operants (Creation or exaggeration of symptoms)		
Moving closer to something	Wanting to be with mother (p.197). Wanting to be in caring environment.	Varies with proximity, or expectation of separation
	Enjoying mother's expressions of sympathy.	Disappears in the absence of people. More pronounced in the presence of particularly responsive people.
Actions to elicit a reaction	Enjoying shocking people, or getting attention.	Looking at adult before major symptom. Baby talk (p.43)
	Munchausen syndrome	Can involve fabricated or induced symptoms – the term traditionally also includes the seeking of help for oneself, in multiple hospitals
Avoidance	Avoiding school. Avoiding discharge.	Varies with proximity, or expectation of approach
Acting like someone close	Copying same-sex parent. Likely to cause problems if dad is a criminal or mentally ill.	That person comes up often in thoughts or undirected interaction.
Family dynamics	A child's illness can keep parents together	Physical symptoms worsened by parental arguments or threats of separation[1091]
Non-operant		
Mass psychogenic behaviour	An odd smell making an entire class of schoolgirls dyspnoeic	See p.505.
Habit		
Symbolic (see previous page and p.14)	E.g. physical pain as an expression of fears, preoccupations, or mental pain.	Sometimes related to cognitions about traumatic events. More likely if there is mental illness or chronic depression (p.309).
Related problems		
☞ You haven't found the physical basis yet	Unlikely but important to keep in mind. The problem may have changed, or the clinical picture may have become clearer (or the opposite). A classic paper discounting hysteria as a cause of neurological symptoms was misleading, because based on major selection bias [337].	• Incomplete assessment. • Lack of differential diagnosis. • Lack of record of change. • Specialist not consulted. • Views shared by a team are particularly persistent, as are views following injury to staff. • Assessors primed by previous assessment, particularly their own or close colleagues'. • No problems with family, peers, or studies. • Don't forget delirium (often fluctuating, p.451).
Hypochondria-sis (see diagram, p.297).	Abdo. pain, back pain, and difficulty swallowing are common. More in[111].	Look for anxiety, preoccupation. The child focuses more on the belief that she has a serious illness, than on a particular symptom or disease. Fear of several distinct illnesses, either simultaneously or over time, distinguish this from a simple phobia[1010] (p.307). Repeated self-checking or requests for reassurance suggest OCD[1010].
Exaggeration by others	(p.205)	

continued ▶

Specific pseudo-patterns

Pseudo here is used to mean **not what it seems**. *Quasi* would usefully avoid implying fakery but *pseudo* is standard usage. Note that patients prefer *habit*, *stress-related* and *functional* to *pseudo* or *psychogenic*[1549].

Except for mimicking behaviours seen in other children, pseudo-behaviours are rare below age 9. The following patterns are listed because they can be identified more rigorously than the factors listed in *Recognising inconsistency* above.

Pseudo-behaviours

Occasionally these have non-volitional causes but more often this is a subtype of *acting* (p.418). Even acting does not require intentionality, as it can be habitual or dissociative (p.453) to varying degrees. Some pseudo-behaviours are much more suggestible than the corresponding organic behaviours (e.g. pseudoseizures, p.74) – but common tics (p.101) are also suggestible.

Many behaviours have both a natural form and several pseudo-forms[931]. Demonstrating that a particular child has the pseudo-form does *not* require showing that he does not have the natural form, as many children have both. A convincing identification of behaviours as *pseudo* requires not just observation of the behaviours themselves[503] but demonstration of *means, motive, atypicality and reversibility*, i.e.

> ➤ that the child has a source of information about what he is acting (a peer, relative, TV, or his own physical illness, or it is a universal experience)
> ➤ that there is motivation for doing this (such as attention, if he only does it when mother is present but not paying attention)
> ➤ that some aspects are atypical (without this they could just as easily be real behaviours) and
> ➤ that symptoms repeatedly start and stop when an emotional/social motive does (this often cannot be established, e.g. because the symptoms have been continually present; so this criterion acts as a reminder that the diagnosis of a pseudo-symptom remains uncertain).

Even when all these criteria are met, detailed and continuing organic assessment remain crucial[1791].

Pseudo-experiences

These are less exposed to the gaze than pseudo-*behaviours*, so are more difficult to identify. Like those, they are most common in children who also have the real symptom: real but minor symptoms can be exaggerated, copied, or focused on. Also, one should demonstrate *means, motive, atypicality and reversibility* (discussed on previous page). Fortunately, some of the most common pseudo-experiences have signs that are recognisable but not widely known in the general population. See other related terms defined on p.359.

Appendix A: Functional analysis ☼

by Imogen Newsom-Davis

The functional analysis approach to understanding children's behaviour, widely adopted in the practice of clinical psychology, is founded on the idea that behaviour does not occur in a vacuum. Instead it is the result of a complex, bi-directional transaction between the individual, his or her inherent traits, and the environment[690]. More specifically, it is hypothesised that a significant proportion of a child's behaviour is learned, maintained and regulated by its effect upon the environment, and the feedback it receives regarding those consequences. Indeed, the same types of learning (operant and classical conditioning, observational learning, cognitive and social learning) are seen to underpin both the acquisition of socially approved, adaptive behaviours, and the development of maladaptive or problem behaviours.

In simple terms, if you take any target behaviour, there are factors in the antecedent environment that are likely to increase the probability of that behaviour occurring, and a further set of factors (consequences) that positively reinforce the behaviour, thereby increasing the likelihood that it occurs again in the future. (Conversely, of course, there are also antecedents and consequences of behaviours that reduce the likelihood of the behaviour taking place.) Functional analysis is designed to un-pick these learned associations and processes, so that the factors contributing to target behaviour(s) can be identified. Usually, the primary aim of this process is to allow the development of a programme of intervention, either to reduce the frequency of an undesirable behaviour, or to increase the frequency of desirable ones. The factors influencing the likelihood of a behaviour occurring fall into three main categories:

- Intrinsic variables
  - non-learned component
  - age, sex, temperament, cognitive factors, i.e. the characteristics of the individual that predispose them to behave or react in certain ways
- Antecedents
  - factors in the environment prior to the behaviour occurring, that **precipitate the behaviour**
  - may include both the general setting/context, and distinct trigger events, which can be distal or proximal
- Consequences
  - contingent events occurring after the behaviour has taken place, that **perpetuate** it
  - consequences of the behaviour may be immediate (most commonly), or distal.

Methods

The key to an effective functional analysis is the quality and quantity of information gathered. Information gathering is typically carried out by questioning (interview, usually with parent/caregiver), record-keeping (parent/caregiver and others if possible, e.g. teacher) and by direct observation (in clinic and in target-setting, usually home and/or school). In general, the larger the number of different sources of information that can be used, the better the outcome, and it is important to use both direct and indirect methods. This is because accounts of behaviour may vary considerably, according to the perspective of the individual, their capacity to remember (which may be particularly compromised or biased if the situation they are describing was stressful), and their level of awareness of their own behaviour. It is also important because a child's behaviour may differ greatly (or very little) across different settings. Either way, this information is vital to the analysis of its function(s).

1. Initial interview

a. Explain general principles of functional assessment of behaviour.

b. Identify problem(s): a "broad brush" approach is most helpful at first, to give an idea of the full range of strengths and difficulties. *Use open-ended questions; ask about all aspects of behaviour and the home/school situation ("talk me through a typical day" can be a productive start).*

c. What has been tried so far to tackle the behaviours, if anything, and what was the outcome? *NB: Don't be put off by parents telling you they have "done" various interventions and they haven't worked. Often behavioural strategies will have been picked up but applied inappropriately or inconsistently, hence the failure to effect change.*

d. Identify priorities for intervention, and desired outcomes. *List all problem behaviours but usually advisable not to choose more than one or two to tackle at one time. Others can be dealt with subsequently, if necessary.*

e. More detailed description of target behaviour(s). In order to keep records (see 2, below) it is necessary to have very clearly defined targets. *It may be necessary to move parents away from emotive and over-generalised statements at this point, e.g. "she never eats her dinner", "he's always attention-seeking". Ask about specific and recent examples of behaviour and build up a clear description, checking back frequently that it is accurate.*

f. Obtain preliminary measure of severity (asking for an estimate of how frequently the behaviour occurs, and getting the parent/caregiver to rank the average severity on an appropriate scale).

2. Record keeping

This is the core of the functional analysis, allowing compilation of detailed and comprehensive data about the behaviour, its antecedents and consequences, for eventual analysis and formulation. This includes:

- frequency of behaviour (a simple daily tally for infrequent behaviours, for a period of 7 days; time-sampling or interval recording techniques may be required for high frequency behaviours)
- severity of behaviour (appropriate anchored rating scales must be selected; ask about intensity and/or duration if parents find it difficult to rate severity)
- description of each behavioural event
- settings and antecedent events to the behaviour recorded
- consequences of behaviour logged.

continued ▶

Ideally, the clinician should carry out some direct observations of the behaviour *in situ* first, as this may help to inform the design of the ABC records.

Depending on the nature and frequency of the target behaviour(s), it may be possible to combine the collection of data regarding frequency and severity, with the functional data (antecedents and consequences). If not, then severity and frequency data should be evaluated first.

NB: As the first record-keeping episode is generally used as a baseline measure (for comparison with future episodes to evaluate efficacy of intervention) it is very important that parents/caregivers are reminded NOT to change the environment or their own behaviour during this phase.

ABC (Antecedent – Behaviour – Consequence) **Diaries**, or their variants (e.g. STAR, Setting – Trigger – Action – Results) are the recording tools used for this data collection[1560]. As the name suggests, these record antecedents, behaviours, and consequences, with their date and time, and provide the basis for determining precipitating and perpetuating factors[1560]. Such diaries are particularly useful for behaviours that occur up to five times per day, and records should ideally be kept for a minimum of four consecutive days, usually to include weekdays and weekends. For behaviours occurring several times an hour, an ABC record of each event is not practicable. Instead, sampling techniques may be used (recording ABC data for each tenth event, for example). Alternatively, the clinician may rely on more detailed descriptions of the general pattern and setting of the behaviour, possibly including other recording techniques, such as discrete videoing. For behaviours that are performed privately, *response products* (e.g. marks on arm) can be used at the time, then transferred later to paper records.

3. Problem formulation and hypothesis-testing

Once a comprehensive data collection has been completed, the process of causal formulation of the behaviour is carried out. The following stages may be used:

(i)   Quantify the frequency or "overall rate" of the behaviour at baselines. Look for clustering of behavioural events, or evidence that they are episodic. Be aware of variability in the data (which may reflect a response to variation in the environment, but could just represent a natural characteristic of the behaviour).

(ii)   Calculate average severity ratings, and/or ratings of intensity and duration, over the baseline period.

(iii) List the total number of problems displayed by the child over the baseline period. Sometimes interventions aimed at one target behaviour can improve other non-target behaviours, so this measure becomes relevant.

(iv)   Assess contingencies: identify common antecedent and consequent events, i.e. those that reliably precede and follow the behaviour. Settings can be identified by looking at whether the behaviour occurred more often in certain places, or at particular times, or with particular people. (Conversely, does the behaviour tend *not* to occur in certain contexts?)

(v)   Identify reinforcers. Although some are relatively universal, e.g. social attention, there is also a great deal of individual variation. Knowing a child's reinforcement history can help.

(vi)   Is there a sense or meaning to the behaviour: does the behaviour have a pay-off for the child, or for the family?

Things to remember:

➢ A behaviour may have different functions at different times.

➢ Behaviours can be reactive to observation, i.e. the picture obtained may not be reliable. Using parent/caregiver observers minimises this risk however.

➢ A behaviour can have an internal function (e.g. reducing pain or relieving boredom), and some have no motivation at all (e.g. reflexes, flaps, tics, night terrors).

➢ Complex situations can involve both an intermittent drive and and intermittent relaxation of inhibitions (see list on p.249).

In the vast majority of cases, triggers and reinforcers for the target behaviour are very quickly apparent from ABC records (or indeed from the initial interview stage). However, if they are difficult to identify, or to ensure that you have not missed any, you may consider:

- consulting a standard list of common reinforcers (p.540) of behaviour (e.g. sensory stimulation, task escape, tangible reward). These can be recorded using the Motivational Assessment Scale at:
  http://www.ssisd.net/specialservices/downloads/MOTIVATION%20ASSESSMENT%20SCALE.doc
  or Questions About Behavioural Function at
  http://blogs.stjohns.k12.fl.us/depts/behavior/wp-content/uploads/2008/06/qabf.pdf
- if the behaviour has a list of causes in this book, they can all be checked.
- there may be a book chapter or paper on the functional analysis of a specific class of behaviours (e.g. self-injury in ID:[1690])
- the list of drives (p.456)
- one of the sub-lists within the catalogue of causes can be used (p.393).

General considerations

Behavioural techniques are commonly used when working with young children, or those with developmental delays or disorders. In these cases, the majority of the work is carried out in close liaison with parents (or caregivers), and sometimes teachers or other co-workers as well. As such, the therapeutic alliance or partnership that you manage to develop with the parent/caregiver is absolutely central to the success or otherwise of your analysis, and any subsequent intervention.

➢ Be aware of parental sensitivity to blame/guilt. Many parents will sense that you are trying to tell them they are the cause of their child's behavioural difficulties and may become defensive, or feel depressed and defeated. The alliance formed with parents/caregivers is crucial to helping them understand their role in their child's behaviour, without feeling they have failed in their parenting.

➢ Before parents/teachers complete ABCs, they need to have a good preliminary understanding of a functional approach to behavioural assessment, i.e. accepting that the behaviour is the product of an interrelationship between the child (their

continued ▶

temperament, etc.), the situation they find themselves in, and feedback from previous experiences.

➢ Parents must understand and trust your explanation of what you are doing, and have sufficient resources and commitment to persevere. Record-keeping, in particular, can be difficult for parents to adhere to and sustain. Some creativity may be necessary in order to make this feasible for parents, e.g. using other recording media, such as video/audio, or helping them to arrange extra support during the record-keeping phase.

➢ It is also useful to warn the family that when an effective intervention is implemented, it often results in the problem getting worse before it gets better (this is an *extinction burst*, p.120).

Addendum

A functional assessment usually leads directly to a behavioural or environmental intervention, but occasionally it concludes that such interventions are impractical or inadequate. This often happens with hyperactive children, p.79, in which case medication would then be considered. Functional assessment can also guide the choice of medication (e.g. for self- harm[1396]).

Appendix B: Further investigations / assessments

These depend very much on the availability of time, treatments and clinical assessment of risks.

Obtaining information from school

The school often has far more information than parents realise, e.g. from the blurtings of the child and his peers, the behaviour of the parents, and what the school bus driver has seen. Reports from school are not usually considered as investigations, but they have a higher yield than most and should be requested routinely. Rather than asking teachers to assess symptoms, it is far more effective to ask them to describe his friendships and his typical behaviour, and to send you standardised results and examples of his written and drawn work. Whether the teacher turns out to be right or wrong on any of these matters, her opinion is an important part of the assessment because it has been shaping the child's school experience for months or years.

To: Mrs L Chapman
Class teacher
Red Woods School

Dear ,

Re: (child's name, d.o.b., address)

We are writing with the parents' permission. XXXX is being assessed in the XXXX clinic and we would be most grateful if you could contribute to the assessment by sending us any standardised assessment results, examples of his best work done alone (written and drawn), any EP reports, and your own comments on his academic, behavioural and social progress.

Please find enclosed a Strengths and Difficulties questionnaire [and a Conners questionnaire] regarding the above named person. We would be grateful if you could fill it in and return to us as soon as possible in the stamped addressed envelope enclosed.

If you have any queries about this matter please do not hesitate to contact us at the above address. Thank you for your cooperation.

Yours sincerely,

Team Administrator

Blinded teacher-rated dosage trials, in which several doses are tried in predetermined random sequence, and the school rates behaviour each week without knowing the dose, are very useful in working out whether stimulants (p.555) help or not.

When you have completed your report, be especially careful not to disclose confidential information to the school (information about the family tends to be especially sensitive). If the school disagrees with your conclusions, listen carefully as they may be right. Alternatively, if you disagree with the school's opinions, and want to redirect them positively, this is sometimes more easily accomplished by face-to-face contact rather than by letter.

The most time-consuming interaction with school is usually the school observation.

School observation

Direct interaction with the teacher is invaluable if parents and teachers give divergent views of the child. Teachers are often willing to say things they are reluctant to put in writing, especially about the parents. Talking to teachers is done most efficiently by phone, and this will often clear up a misunderstanding, and elicit a sensible overview of what the child typically does in class. However, teachers may miss children's behaviours that don't bother the class; and they often have little information about what goes on in playtime unless people complain about it.

If staff time and distance allow, the ideal is to have an unknown member of the clinic staff observe the child at school. During the school visit, the child should be observed in class (unaware that he has been singled out, if possible); and he should be observed in the playground (ideally from a strategic viewpoint behind an upper storey window). It is sometimes claimed that an observer in school makes it an abnormal situation, but in practice this is rarely insurmountable. A minute-by-minute handwritten account of what the child does is invaluable. In some countries, with permission of the school (and parents) it is possible to film a child's unusual behaviours for later analysis, but in most cases this would be regarded as over-intrusive, as well as provoking changes in the child's behaviours.

Observation of play
The observation of play can reveal a great deal about a child's cognitive and social development. It is usually most revealing at school, where the child can be unobtrusively observed with peers. It can also be useful at home (if problems there are major) or in the office (particularly in long assessments with lots of space, so the child can forget he is observed).

Note especially whether the child is a loner, or a leader, follower or bullied, and any unusually repetitive behaviours. Consider doing a functional analysis (p.365) of any behavioural problems in play time. If there are intractable social difficulties at school, consider making a sociogram (p.550).

Standardised toys are used to see their effects on interaction in the ADOS. More numerous toys in a sandpit are used in the Erica method of sandplay assessment[1488]. In this, normal children may place the toys indifferently (at age 2–3), categorise them (about age 4), accidentally juxtapose categories (age 4–5), make conventional groupings; or meaningful scenes (about age 7). Further work is needed to understand symbolic, chaotic, bizarre, or closed arrangements.

The system shown below (from[1393] described in[1238]) has a vertical *social* axis and a horizontal *cognitive* axis. In it, "functional play refers to cases where children are manipulating an object seemingly to determine its properties and what the object does. Construction refers to behaviours that are directed towards a goal of building something." The idea is to mark (or describe) behaviour in the appropriate place, each 30 or 60 seconds, by the clock.

	Functional	**Constructive**	**Dramatic Play**
Solitary			
Parallel			
Interactive			

Playground behaviours can also be marked using the following categories: Passive/Non-interactive; Passive/Interactive; Adult Directed; Adult Organised; Aggressive; Rough and Tumble Play; Vigorous Behaviour; Games; Object Play; Role-play[1238]. See also types of play, p.221.

Physical assessment (For further discussion see[89])

Routine
- Knowledgeable clinical history and examination, p.409.
- GPs often have a good overview of the family, and can also supply a detailed medical history (as well as social observations).

General approach to medical investigations for behaviour
The more medically based specialties (e.g. paediatrics, audiology, ophthalmology) are highly driven by physical investigations. When first introduced investigations are typically used in a local ad hoc way, then after a few years they are incorporated into peer-reviewed lists of suggested investigations (as cited in this book). In a few cases (e.g. audiology) these have developed into nationally agreed protocols, which have some force to drive professional activity and funding.

For behavioural and emotional problems, the return from comprehensive endocrine and imaging studies, used as screening without specific reasons, is probably too little to justify them economically (e.g.[8]). However this of course depends on the cost of the tests (which is coming down fast) and the value of identifying the cause (which may be greater to the family than to the government). An additional problem is that if a hundred tests for exceedingly rare conditions are performed, each with a good false positive rate (say 2%), there are likely to be several incorrect "positives". What is certain is that a staged approach to investigation is relatively efficient, with the more common, clinically plausible, dangerous, testable and treatable disorders tested for first, and other disorders later (see also[508,644,703,1002,1502]). It is not yet useful to automate the sequencing of developmental tests[1417,1453].

The psychosocial impact of screening depends on the result. If the result is that the child is not affected and is not a carrier, the impact is positive. If the result is that the child is affected or is a carrier, many children and parents regard this as a useful outcome, especially if they already knew something was severely wrong (see[1696]). This is not always the case in the few most severe and untreatable disorders (see *Huntington's disease*, p.482). See also the psychosocial implications of *genetic testing*, p.380.

Common situations
- Relevant investigations are listed throughout the book. Investigation planners are supplied for the medically more complex situations, see list on p.5). These planners help you decide which tests are clinically reasonable, and then keep track of which results you have obtained (as inevitably some samples are lost for various reasons).
- In social, language, academic, and attention problems: consider audiological assessment.

Special situations
- When treatment has failed, reassessment should be considered (possibly by a consultation or second opinion). Second opinions are sometimes more useful if obtained from a different specialty, e.g. psychology, neurology, genetics, metabolic, rather than someone more senior in your own field. Rarer causes (e.g. from the lists in this book) also need to be considered, e.g. all the physical causes, and abuse, exaggeration, etc.
- When facing long-term educational placements, inpatient stays, or other major family adaptations. These are so disruptive that even tests with tiny yield are justified.
- If it is not possible to obtain blood from a child, many tests can be done on urine, cheek swabs, saliva, or finger-prick blood. Consult your local laboratory. Also consider giving the parents a list of blood tests that would be useful if the child needed sedation in the next few years, e.g. for dentistry. However, some crucial tests can only be done on blood. In such cases, many hospitals have a staff member who is known to be specially good at blood tests in children. Psychologists can also usefully provide desensitisation, confidence building, modelling, etc.
- For investigating pseudo-symptoms, see p.359 and e.g.[904].

Trial of medication as part of assessment

Trials of medical treatments are not routine but can be invaluable in specific diagnostic difficulties. Examples include:

- analgesic or antacid to see if behaviour was affected by pain.
- decongestant or inhaler/spacer for asthma or discomfort of upper respiratory tract infection.
- use a trial of various doses of stimulants to optimise dose in ADHD. Defer his stimulant until the clinic so you can see him on and off it. Use a longer trial to see if lack of friends, p.181, is due to hyperactivity.
- lorazepam for catatonia, p.98
- dopa for Segawa disease, p.458
- antiepileptics for cognitive benefits, p.73
- clonazepam for myoclonic hereditary dystonia, p.86
- steroids for occult inflammatory causes of psychosis or regression
- naloxone to confirm suspected opiate overdose (pp.519, 258).

If patients cannot communicate clearly or reliably, doses of short-acting medicines can be given on alternate days (or random days) and the behaviours written in a diary to see if they are reduced by the medicine.

Imaging

Scans are often requested by parents. It is worth asking why because their views affect the child, and furthermore their reason can often be satisfied in a more useful way.

It is important to consider not just imaging, but other tests as listed in this book, ideally in a hypothesis-driven way (if this is possible). In most cases when brain imaging is considered, it is sensible to have a paediatrician involved and to have a thorough physical examination first, as examination results can guide imaging.

In order of expense the imaging methods in clinical use are:

- X-ray
- CT (computed tomography)
- MRI (magnetic resonance imaging). This produces excellent images and does not expose the child to any radiation. However the MRI machine is noisy and frightening, and the child may be unable to stay still for the half hour or more needed (may need general anaesthetic).
- The following are not yet in routine clinical use:
  - ○ fMRI (functional MRI)
  - ○ SPECT (single photon emission CT) – useful in dementia[1824] and perhaps in general psychiatry[1466].
  - ○ PET (Positron Emission Tomography), MEG, tensor imaging

Indications for brain imaging in children and adolescents (after[1579,1613])
Traumatic brain injury (see p.477)
Seizure disorders with psychiatric symptoms
Movement disorders (see p.86)
Focal neurological signs
Delirium (p.451)
First psychotic breakdown (see pp.349, 544)
Regression (see p.47)
Catatonia (see p.99)
Sudden severe personality changes (see p.237)
Psychiatric symptoms with unusual presentation or course
Inadequate response to treatment (as part of a thorough reassessment)
If other investigations have been inconclusive in severe conditions.

Neuropsychological assessment

The most detailed research in this area is from brain-damaged adults, but good reviews are available regarding children[597]. It is important not to assume that testing methods that work for adults are useful for children (e.g. p.267 of[719]). When planning the assessment of a child, it is worth considering whether you want to have a standard test battery administered to all your puzzling patients[1620], or whether you want to probe individuals' deficits in great detail, with multiple individually chosen tests[1050] (or even individually tailored tests to explore and delineate difficulties, much as is done in a Functional Analysis, p.365). The latter approach can probe more deeply in a given amount of time, but it is difficult for any staff member to become expert in infrequently used tests.

It is important to realise that informal observations during neuropsychological testing are sometimes even more useful and revealing than the numerical results of the tests. In part this is because the way a person gets a question wrong or right is generally much more informative (and relevant to real life) than a mere score[1074] (see also pp.33, 37).

Progress through the following hierarchy until the overall picture is clear enough to guide management:

1. Developmental screening (e.g. Griffiths, p.451)
2. Formal IQ testing (p.59)
3. Further more focused tests (see diagram at right).

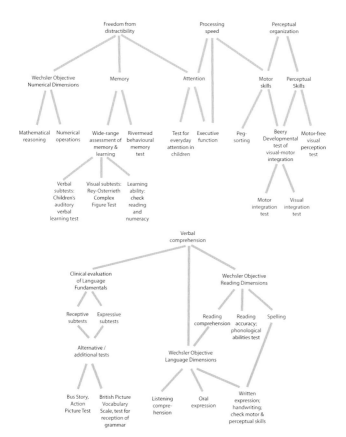

Figure 24. Hierarchy of cognitive investigations.
(Redrawn after [293].)

Social assessment

- Additional information about a child and his family can be obtained by seeing them for several appointments spread over a few weeks, ideally seeing the whole family and various subgroups at different times of day.
- Prolonged observation of the family is often useful (see p.23).
- A school visit provides detailed information about a child's behaviour away from his family.
- A home visit often provides useful information about poverty, organisation, risks, and illness in family members.
- When abuse is a possibility:
    - o enquiry of social services is essential. Ideally they do a police check on other family members. They will only reveal information if there is either consent, or a reason for significant concern.
    - o School usually have social information they will share verbally, though often not in writing.
    - o Consider also: GP, Health Visitor, Google, Facebook.
    - o Consider obtaining information from previous areas of residence. Some countries have a central computerised "contact point."
- Mother-and-baby units provide professional assessment of parenting.
- A child's change of beliefs, behaviour or mood during an inpatient stay can clarify the effect of the home environment.
- *Professionals' meetings* can be held with or without parents (though some use the term to mean parents are excluded). In social services, *Strategy meetings* never include parents but *Team-around-the-child* meetings do.

Assessment by social/environmental intervention

Many of the common methods of assessment are rather dry and distant from the child. Examples include checklist diagnoses, classical psychoanalytical assessment, and the lists in this book. Unfortunately, these can underuse the richest source of information, the child himself.

Proxy interventions

There are several methods that avoid intrusive involvement by the professional, by getting the child's family and friends to do it. These include family therapy, school observation and assessment of the whole family together in the room (at home or in clinic). They have the big advantages of being fairly naturalistic and clarifying relationships. Free play is the simplest version of this, the child "interacting" with people, the room and its contents.

Occasionally respites, temporary fostering, or admission to hospital can be used to assess how the child is away from his parents.

Interventions by the examiner

These can be reasonably standardised. Examples that assess cognition, emotion, and interaction include:

- Functional analysis (p.365) routinely uses behavioural "experiments" to see what interventions increase or decrease the rate of a behaviour. These can be used both in the clinic, and at home with the parents as reporters.
- Similar are assessments of distractability during a difficult state, assessment of his learning a sanction or new behaviour.
- Assessment through play (p.372) can be useful.

There are many methods that are not diagnostic but they help the child relax, show you his usual behaviour, and communicate difficult feelings[1724]. The child's words, and any unusual behaviours that you see, help you to create an hypothesis – which can then be tested in more conventional ways.

1) Ignoring small children temporarily is useful if they are shy.
2) Pleasant social interactions
    a) What game shall we play?

- i) Peekaboo
- ii) Catch
- iii) Dysdiadochokinesis, p.457
- iv) Standard toys in the room
- v) Race up the stairs
- vi) Robot drawing: you draw, he draws a copy simultaneously.
- vii) Play on the computer (e.g. show her the *Paint* program)
- viii) Winnicott's Squiggle Game: I do a squiggle, you make a picture out of it. Doing the same in reverse gets them involved and stops it feeling like an assessment. This works very well in the early school years[145].
- ix) Tests of Theory of Mind, p.563
  - b) Together, make a cup of tea for mum, or squash for child
  - c) Hold a pencil the wrong way up and see what he does.
3) General social interaction
  - a) Assess flexibility, e.g. by changing the subject (more on p.234)
  - b) Call his name from behind
  - c) ADOS (p.183), flexibility during DQ or IQ testing (p.451)
  - d) Offer him crisps (after asking mum) and see reaction
  - e) Drop a pencil
  - f) Assess him with different family members (see frozen watchfulness, p.470; disclosures, p.452)
4) Slightly stressful social interaction
  - a) Handshake
  - b) Hello, how are you?
  - c) For children under 10, try a high five or give me five (offer two hands and record how many hands he used and whether not done; just touches; weak; normal; or painful). Does he grin or want to repeat? Does he just count the fingers (showing much training is going on at home)? Does he just give you a disdainful look (which would be normal in a teen but is excessively negative and streetwise under 10)? Does he look at you to see your reactions? Is he sufficiently interested in imitating others, e.g. in copying your "3-2-1" before the slap? Is he annoyed when you pull your hands away and make him miss, or does he grin, rise to the challenge, and speed up?
  - d) Behaviour during physical examination
    - i) Measuring blood pressure: shyness
    - ii) Weighing: ability to remove and replace shoes
  - e) Correct or even gently correct the child's drawing
5) Boredom, in waiting room and in the actual assessment
  - a) Initially no toys, or one simple toy
6) Provocations
  - a) Provocative interpretations (not just in psychotherapy)
  - b) If child is doing something repetitively, stop it and see what happens.
  - c) If mum says something annoys him, try it.
  - d) Ask him to be quiet or sit still for a minute.
  - e) Strange Situation Test, p.556, or just ask mum to go outside the door for a minute.
  - f) Move her so she cannot reach mum (observe mum too).
  - g) Mother and clinician remain unresponsive for 60 seconds: most toddlers will make an approach.
7) Graded stressors that can be mild or severe
  - a) Hunger
  - b) Noise
  - c) Room size
  - d) Close or open the blinds
8) Make the appointment after school when he is tired or when medicine is wearing off.

Special Topic 20: Is there a genetic problem?

Most neurodevelopmental problems are multifactorial so are inherited quantitatively (by probability or severity) rather than in a classic Mendelian single-gene way.

Some Mendelian patterns are worth being aware of in case they appear in the family histories. Recessive disorders only appear if both parents have a defective copy of the gene, which is far more common when the parents are consanguinous. Dominant disorders only require one copy from one parent. X-linked genes have different effects in males and females (because males have only one copy and females have two, of which one is partially inactivated – see *mosaicism*, p.509).

Spontaneous (uninherited) mutations are common for some disorders, especially severe dominant disorders that prevent reproduction.

Most syndromes have partial forms (p.384). See also the general approach to medical investigations, p.373.

Genetic categories of inherited alteration
- a)   point mutations
- b)   copy number variations, p.439
- c)   triplet repeat disorders, p.568
- d)   epigenetics and imprinting, p.489
- e)   microdeletions, e.g. Prader-Willi, p.533; Dravet plus, p.438
- f)   modifier genes
- g)   mitochondrial disorders, p.508
- h)   mosaicism, p.509
- i)   chromosomal abnormalities, p.439
    - i)   Down's syndrome, p.455
    - ii)   sex chromosomes, p.548
    - iii)   translocations, p.439
    - iv)   ring chromosomes[875].

Macromolecules involved[1088]
- a)   metabolic enzymes: changes are detected via small molecules (often called "inborn errors of metabolism"), p.381
- b)   channelopathies, p.438
- c)   receptors (see individual transmitters and hormones in index)
- d)   transporters: see below
- e)   extracellular and intracellular structures, e.g. neurofilaments and tubules, p.514
- f)   disorders of axons or myelin, p.510
- g)   DNA repair mechanisms, p.454
- h)   folding and processing of macromolecules, e.g. congenital disorders of glycosylation, p.474; defects in nuclear proteins and transcription.

Subcellular mechanisms
- a)   synthesis: see examples listed on p.382
- b)   transport: folate transporter, p.467; neutral amino acid transporter, p.477; serotonin transporter, p.552; iminoglycinuria (deafness, ichthyosis, and ID)[146]; lysinuric protein intolerance (severe ID, poor growth, mild malabsorption)[146]; copper transport deficit, p.330
- c)   breakdown/removal: see storage disorders, p.556
- d)   cell structure: see neurofilaments and neurotubules, p.514
- e)   cell movements.

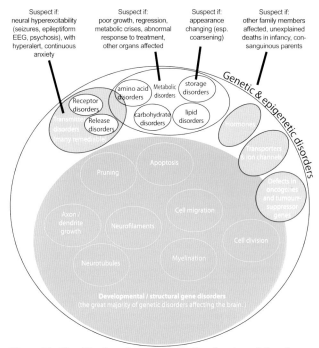

Suspect if:
neural hyperexcitability
(seizures, epileptiform
EEG, psychosis), with
hyperalert, continuous
anxiety

Suspect if:
poor growth, regression,
metabolic crises, abnormal
response to treatment,
other organs affected

Suspect if:
appearance
changing (esp.
coarsening)

Suspect if:
other family members
affected, unexplained
deaths in infancy, con-
sanguinous parents

Figure 25. Classification of neurogenetic disorders by cell function.

This diagram depicts the fact that most neurogenetic disorders (largest circle)
are developmental or "structural" (black oval). This unfortunately makes
remediation difficult in most cases (for an exception see *Marfan's*, p.505). In
contrast, successful treatments exist for many of the transmitteropathies,
metabolic disorders[299,1448], and hormone disorders, shown above the black oval.
The groups overlap, e.g. some metabolic disorders are also transmitteropathies.
The captions at the top describe the clinical situations in which genetic
disorders, or subgroups of them, should be suspected. Psychiatric disorders
such as schizophrenia and depression typically involve numerous genes of
small effect, interacting with environmental influences. There are much more
detailed taxonomies of gene disorders affecting other body systems[1499,1568].

Genetic testing

This can be broad-focus (p.381) or can test a specific gene. Genetic testing for
over 1800 conditions is now available, 400 of these direct-to-the-consumer.
However there are not yet adequate controls in place to ensure either the
technical skills of the labs or adequate explanation of results to patients[770].

Before ordering a genetic test, you should consider both benefits and risks[1146].
Benefits of identifying a child's problem include clarification, social and
financial planning, recurrence prediction or antenatal testing, support from
patients' groups, participation in research, and occasionally treatment (see
above; or at least the possibility of the family doing regular internet searches to
see the progress of research). Risks include discovering an untreatable disease
(see *Huntington's*, p.482); discovering information the child would rather not
know when he is old enough to understand; threatening the parents' relationship
(e.g. following a paternity test, or if one parent takes another partner to allow
them to have an unaffected child); and making insurance more expensive.
Tests almost certain to prove negative can be worth doing if the family or child
is preoccupied by risk. If the main purpose of genetic investigations is to advise
on the risk of a child's *children* being affected, it is often sensible to defer
testing until the child may reproduce, by which time the science of prediction
will have progressed considerably.

Special Topic 21: Is there a metabolic problem?

Metabolism means the creation and breaking down of molecules (anabolism and catabolism). In its broadest sense metabolic processes include breakdown of food and medicines in the intestines and liver; control of appetite and the basal metabolic rate; pica, p.336; disorders of electrolytes and acid-base control; and the *metabolic syndrome* of obesity, hypercholesterolaemia and diabetes. The formation of macromolecules, p.379, and their glycosylation, p.474, are generally not included.

This section focuses on inborn errors of metabolism (IEM) of small molecules (see[703]). These are mainly single gene mutations. They are not common, occurring about once in 1000 births (more in some subpopulations). They are most commonly detected in childhood, but some produce no symptoms until adulthood. "Although neurometabolic disorders are classically viewed as progressive neurodegenerative processes, many present as static or non-progressive neurological disorders. Metabolic disorders affecting small molecules, including those in which dietary treatments are effective, often show a stable clinical course."[539]

There are vast numbers of IEMs, which are not practical to recognise or to screen for individually. However IEMs should be considered in children with poor appetite (or vomiting/diarrhoea), failure to thrive, poor mental function, regression, depression, psychosis, abnormal response to treatment, or metabolic crises (described below). IEMs are more likely if other family members are affected (or there are unexplained deaths in infancy), if the parents are consanguinous, or if other body systems are affected. Fortunately, the numerous IEMs affecting a single metabolic pathway can be **screened** for by measuring the product of that pathway (e.g. ammonia, lactate). Also, **broad-focus investigations** can narrow down the diagnostic possibilities quickly. Such tests include LFT, plasma and urinary amino acids, urinary organic acids, MRI, and microarray (p.440). An **extended metabolic screen** could also include VLCFA, p.526; urine GAGs, p.382; acylcarnitine, p.508; white cell enzymes, p.572; and transferrins, p.474.

Metabolic crises can appear as epilepsy, impaired conscious level, psychosis, or cognitive regression. They can be triggered by surgery, fasting or starvation (p.553), dehydration, change of diet, immunisation, or even severe stress. For examples see urea-cycle disorders, p.571; GA1, p.32; MCADD, p.418; porphyria, p.532.

Many of the IEMs have several names, starting historically with an eponym (e.g. Tay-Sachs) or a description of symptoms or pathology (congenital adrenal hyperplasia). Later names mention the product that was measured in blood or urine (XXXuria). Usually the most precise name specifies the specific enzyme (XXX dehydrogenase deficiency). All of these are really ☂ umbrella terms until the precise mutation is specified. For further discussion and examples see *syndromes*, p.383.

If one sees behaviours suggesting a problem with a *neurotransmitter*, the underlying cause may be metabolic (synthesis or degradation) but may equally be in release, receptors, local interactions (e.g. effects of endogenous antagonists), or influence from other CNS systems.

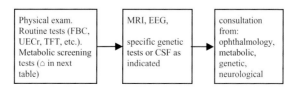

Figure 26. Sequencing metabolic investigations.

Table 17. Some inborn errors of metabolism

This lists just a few main ⬆ groups as over 1200 have been identified.

Class of molecules ▲ higher concentration ▼ lower concentration	Examples of problems of synthesis	Examples of problems of degradation	Other aspects △ = initial broad screening tests
Carbohydrate (e.g. gluconegogenesis)	diabetes, p.532 glycogen storage diseases, p.556		△:glucose, sugar chromatography
Mucopolysaccharides & oligosaccharides		▲Hunter & Hurler, p.501; disorders of glycosylation, p.474	△:urine GAG, muco- & polysacch.screen
Lipids (beta-oxidation)		▲ MCADD,p.418 ▲Storage disorders, p.556: Niemann-Pick, p.552; Fabry's disease, p.464; metachromatic leukodystrophy, p.498	△: lipids & cholesterol △: white cell enzymes**
Nucleotides (purines & pyrimidines)		▲Lesch-Nyhan, p.318	p.318
Organic acids		▲mitochondrial disorders, p.508	
A. lactate	▲Exercise		
B. oxalate			stones, p.555
C. urate		▲Lesch-Nyhan, p.318	△lactate & pyruvate, urine organic acids by HPLC
D. pyruvate	▼PDH deficiency, p.86		
E. methylmalonate	▲cobalamin diseases, p.329		
Energy (Krebs/TCA cycle)	see mitochondrial disorders, p.508		
Amino acids (including catecholamines)	phenylketonuria (▼tyrosine) p.529	▲Maple syrup urine, p.505	transmitters, p.398; essential amino acids, p.327. △: urine amino acids by HPLC
Nitrogenous (Urea cycle)	See p.571		△:plasma ammonia
Steroids			
A. Sex hormones	▲Congenital adrenal hyperplasia		p.554
B. Glucocorticoids	▲Cushings, p.449. ▼Addison's disease, p.419		p.554
Haemoglobin	▼anaemia, p.421	▲porphyria: p.532.	△: FBC, urine colour
Lipofuscin		▲Lysosomal storage disorders, p.501	△: white cell enzymes**
Cofactors & vitamins	▼CoQ10 deficiency, p.508		p.328 △:B$_6$,B$_{12}$,folate
Toxins and medication	n/a	▲G6PD deficiency, p.350; ▼▲cytochromes, p.450	

** Microscopy of vacuolated lymphocytes is used in some centres (p.572).

Appendix C: Syndromes and partial syndromes

(See glossary for specific syndromes)

Syndromes are groups of symptoms that often occur together. There are many reasons for them to do so, such as one gene (or chemical, or other influence) having multiple effects. Similarly, in the deletion syndromes, multiple genes close together on a chromosome can be deleted as a group. Symptoms are often described as essential, major, minor, or associated factors of a syndrome, depending on the degree of association.

In children's mental health the degree of diversity and comorbidity (p.442) is so high that thousands of "syndromes" could be named. It is better to restrict the term to those cases in which the unifying biological cause is known (e.g. foetal alcohol *s*; frontal *s*), or one symptom substantially predicts others (Prader-Willi *s*). There are unfortunately many exceptions (e.g. Asperger *s*; Pervasive Refusal *s*). In such cases the word "syndrome" mainly shows that the originator thinks there is one underlying focal pathology (the word "disorder" often carries the same implication). So the following are better viewed as *comorbidities* than as "true syndromes":

- Shared risk factors (e.g. Fragile X increases the risk of ASD, ADHD, and ID, but does not determine any of them nor their severity).
- Common endpoints reached by multiple aetiologies or multiple contributory pathways. For example, the multiple aspects of academic difficulty have many contributory factors (p.27) that are not shared by all sufferers, so they are not a true syndrome. The same is true for symptoms of Pervasive Refusal "Syndrome" (p.527).

Syndromes are most clear for (a) single genes of large effect, and (b) multiple visible or dangerous physical anomalies. There are also less clear syndromes, such as the common co-occurrence of tics, OCD, and ADHD.

You should be alert for the possibility of a genetic syndrome if:
- multiple family members are affected
- multisystem involvement, or multifocal within a single body system
- there are severe symptoms from early childhood
- parents are consanguinous.

When you suspect a specific clinical syndrome, request confirmatory genetic tests (labs that do these in the UK are listed at www.ukgtn.nhs.uk). Alternatively, a national expert can be found and consulted. Large reference books exist[787], but more up-to-date information can be obtained on the internet from reliable sites. Some good sites are:

Sources for both genetic and non-genetic syndromes:
http://scholar.google.com
www.wrongdiagnosis.com

Search these routinely for genetic disorders as they are kept up-to-date:
www.ncbi.nlm.nih.gov/omim (Online Mendelian Inheritance in Man)
http://www.ncbi.nlm.nih.gov/books/NBK1116/ (GeneReviews)

Others:
National Organization for Rare Disorders:
http://www.rarediseases.org/search/rdbsearch.html
Contact-a-Family:
http://www.cafamily.org.uk/medicalinformation/conditions/azlistings/a.html
Syndromes without a name: http://www.undiagnosed.org.uk/
http://www.kumc.edu/gec/support/ (Genetic / Rare Conditions)
Jablonski's Multiple Congenital Anomaly/Mental Retardation (MCA/MR)
Syndromes Database:
http://www.nlm.nih.gov/mesh/jablonski/syndrome_db.html

A clinical geneticist can be asked to advise. This is particularly important if preventive steps could help other family members, or if future pregnancies are intended. For rare syndromes, it is worth looking for regional or national clinics who can keep the family up to date with monitoring, treatment trials, and other affected families.

Partial / mild / subclinical syndromes

Textbooks usually describe the most severe cases, but for most conditions less severe symptoms are more common. The population-level term is variable expressivity. (This is different from variable penetrance which is the percentage of the carriers who show an effect.) See also discussion on p.32.

The following is a list of mechanisms by which partial syndromes appear, with cross references to examples. The number of recognised partial syndromes is increasing rapidly as a result of advances in genetics[325], and some of them are useful to treat[464].

Chromosomes, gene expression, epigenetics
a) mosaics, p.509, e.g. partial Down's and Rett, p.541
b) variant deletion syndromes: more genes (e.g. GEFS→Dravet plus, p.438); partial Prader-Willi (p.533) or *minimum critical region* of VCFS, p.572
c) length of triplet expansion, p.568
d) Fragile X premutation, p.468
e) heterozygous forms of disorders traditionally described as recessive, e.g. p.571
f) epigenetic silencing in SMA types II–IV, p.551
g) mitochondrial disorders affecting inherited subsets of mitochondria
h) variation in glycosylation of proteins, p.474

Gene products (see inborn errors of metabolism, p.379)
a) Occipital Horn syndrome (p.32) with normal IQ, shading into the same syndrome with ID, then into Menkes
b) partial form of X-linked enzyme failure syndromes found in girls, e.g. p.571
c) not picked up at neonatal screening: homocystinuria, p.481
d) GAD65 & mild Stiff Person syndrome: p.555
e) CoQ10, p.508
f) intermittent maple syrup disease, p.505
g) mild PKU, p.529
h) slowly progressive Sanfilippo A, p.502
i) Leigh and Leigh-like syndromes, p.508

Neurodevelopmental
a) *microforms* of holoprosencephaly, p.480
b) spina bifida occulta, p.551
c) mild cerebral palsy, p.437
d) Several metabolic conditions appear in mild non-specific form in children, only to become severe and recognisable in adulthood[606].

Endocrine
a) subclinical hypothyroidism, p.485

Environmental
a) dosage effects: partial Foetal Alcohol syndrome, p.467; valproate, p.572; folate, p.467; vitamin deficiencies; fatty acid deficiencies, caffeine, sleep, etc.
b) additive effects on other disorders, e.g. folate, p.467
c) marginal malnutrition with oversupply of some nutrients, p.504.
d) life events, p.499

Phenotypes/behaviours
a) Borderline Intellectual Functioning, p.434
b) partial forms of neuropsychiatric syndromes, e.g. Ganser syndrome, p.357.
c) transformation of psychological symptoms with age, e.g parental alienation, p.187
d) symptoms that increase with age, e.g. autism in infants.
e) symptoms that improve with age, e.g. autism after age 6[521]
f) satisfying only one or two of the "triple thresholds", p.17
g) variable number of symptoms, p.24
h) self-medication/drug use due to "subthreshold" disorders, p.257
i) "on the spectrum" for autism, p.519; narcolepsy, p.72; hyperactivity, p.83; bipolar affective disorder, p.264
j) occult epilepsy, p.76, and the borderlands where epilepsy merges into myoclonus, sleep disorders, syncope, migraine, vertigo, and paroxysmal dyskinesias[343]

Testing
a) SLE (p.560) without raised CRP or ANA.

Appendix D: DSM-IV behavioural syndromes

DSM, the Diagnostic and Statistical Manual[33], describes a standard set of psychiatric diagnoses, and rules for diagnosing them. DSM is currently being updated to form version 5, DSM-V. Boundaries between DSM categories are listed in the *DSM-IV Handbook of Differential Diagnosis*[502]. A major research effort has identified many factors *associated with* DSM categories (see e.g. pp.48–49 of [433]). However this research can be difficult to use clinically because common causes (such as learned behaviour) are under-researched; comorbidities are the norm in clinical populations but not in research; children differ within each category; and some children not meeting diagnostic criteria are nonetheless impaired. For other strengths and weaknesses see p.24.

Several of the DSM categories include so many diverse conditions that they are reasonably called "umbrella constructs", by analogy with an umbrella sheltering several different people[272]. This is depicted in the following figure, in which the umbrellas overlap to suggest people with multiple diagnoses.

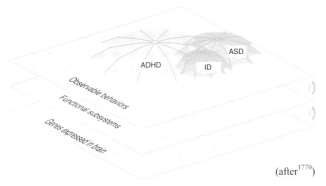

(after[1770])

Figure 27. Some DSM "umbrella constructs" in relation to science.

For abbreviations see glossary.

The following list shows most of the DSM diagnoses used in children and adolescents, with cross-references to the most relevant discussions in this book. However full DSM criteria are only given for five representative disorders (on the following pages). The individual symptoms in these five lists have many causes, and page references are given for some of them.

Disorders usually first diagnosed in infancy, childhood, or adolescence
Mental retardation, p.498
Reading disorder, p.51
Disorder of written expression, p.53
Mathematics disorder, p.457
Developmental coordination disorder, p.89
Language disorders, p.145
Pervasive Developmental disorders
- Autism, p.388
- Autistic Spectrum disorder, p.427
- Asperger, p.424
- Childhood Disintegrative disorder, p.46
- Rett's disorder, p.541
ADHD, attention deficit hyperactivity disorder, p.387
Conduct disorder, p.249
Oppositional defiant disorder, p.519
Rumination disorder, p.543
Tic disorders, p.101
Elimination disorders, pp.339-342
Selective mutism, p.153
Reactive Attachment disorder, p.390
Separation Anxiety disorder, p.391

Substance-related disorders, see substance abuse, p.257

Schizophrenia and other psychotic disorders
Schizophrenia, p.543
Brief psychotic disorder, p.538

Mood disorders
Depressive disorders, p.309
Bipolar Affective disorder, p.264

Anxiety disorders, p.295
Agoraphobia, p.297
Panic disorder, p.301
Phobic disorder, see p.295
Generalised anxiety disorder, p.297
OCD, obsessive compulsive disorder, p.65
PTSD, post-traumatic stress disorder, p.389
Acute stress disorder, p.538

Somatoform disorders, factitious disorders, dissociative disorders
Body dysmorphic disorder, p.433
Hypochondriasis, p.362
Somatisation disorder, p.359
Dissociative disorders, p.453

Identity disorders
Gender identity disorder, p.267
Identity problem, p.237

Eating disorders
Anorexia nervosa, p.334
Bulimia nervosa, p.337

Sleep disorders
Narcolepsy, p.72
Sleepwalking disorder, p.200
Hypersomnia, p.321

Impulse-control disorders not elsewhere classified
Intermittent explosive disorder, p.70
Trichotillomania, p.117

Adjustment disorders

Personality disorders, p.241

continued ▶

ADHD ⚓

For general discussion of ADHD diagnosis, see p.83

Table 18. DSM-IV criteria for ADHD

ADHD or ADD is characterized by a majority of the following symptoms being present in either category (inattention or hyperactivity). These symptoms need to manifest themselves in a manner and degree which is inconsistent with the child's current developmental level. That is, the child's behavior is significantly more inattentive or hyperactive than that of his or her peers of a similar age.

Symptoms of Inattention:
- often fails to give close attention to details or makes careless mistakes (p.37) in schoolwork, work, or other activities
- often has difficulty sustaining attention in tasks or play activities
- often does not seem to listen when spoken to directly (pp.129, 131)
- often does not follow through on instructions and fails to finish schoolwork, chores, or duties in the workplace (not due to oppositional behavior (p.519) or failure to understand instructions)
- often has difficulty organizing tasks and activities (p.27)
- often avoids, dislikes, or is reluctant to engage in tasks that require sustained mental effort (such as schoolwork or homework (p.481))
- often loses things necessary for tasks or activities (e.g., toys, school assignments, pencils, books, or tools)
- is often easily distracted (p.453) by extraneous stimuli
- is often forgetful in daily activities (pp.27,468)

Symptoms of Hyperactivity:
- often fidgets with hands or feet or squirms in seat (p.79)
- often leaves seat in classroom or in other situations in which remaining seated is expected (p.79)
- often runs about or climbs excessively in situations in which it is inappropriate (in adolescents or adults, may be limited to subjective feelings of restlessness)
- often has difficulty playing or engaging in leisure activities quietly
- is often "on the go" or often acts as if "driven by a motor"
- often talks excessively

Symptoms of Impulsivity:
- often blurts out answers before questions have been completed (p.433)
- often has difficulty awaiting turn (p.570)
- often interrupts or intrudes on others (e.g., butts into conversations or games) (p.492)

Symptoms must have persisted for **at least 6 months**. Some of these symptoms need to have been present as a child, at 7 years old or younger. The symptoms also must exist in **at least two separate settings** (for example, at school and at home). The symptoms should be creating **significant impairment** in social, academic or occupational functioning or relationships.

The symptoms do not occur exclusively during the course of a <u>Pervasive Developmental Disorder</u>, <u>Schizophrenia</u>, or other Psychotic Disorder and are not better accounted for by another mental disorder (e.g., <u>Mood Disorder</u>, <u>Anxiety Disorder</u>, <u>Dissociative Disorders</u> (p.453), or a <u>Personality Disorder</u> (p.241).

Autism

For general discussion of autism-related diagnoses, see p.183.

Table 19. DSM-IV criteria for Autism

(wording slightly shortened)

A. A total of six (or more) items from (1), (2), and (3), with at least two from (1), and one each from (2) and (3):

(1) qualitative impairment in social interaction:
- marked impairment in the use of multiple nonverbal behaviors such as eye-to-eye gaze (p.175), facial expression (p.178), body postures (p.93), and gestures to regulate social interaction (p.167)
- failure to develop peer relationships (p.181) appropriate to developmental level
- a lack of spontaneous sharing of enjoyment, interests, or achievements with other people (e.g., by a lack of showing, bringing, or pointing out objects of interest) (p.179)
- lack of social or emotional reciprocity (p.179)

(2) qualitative impairments in communication:
- delay in, or total lack of, the development of spoken language (not accompanied by an attempt to compensate through alternative modes of communication such as gesture or mime) (p.27)
- in individuals with adequate speech, marked impairment in the ability to initiate or sustain a conversation with others (p.144)
- stereotyped and repetitive use of language or idiosyncratic language (pp.156, 163, 165, 553)
- lack of varied, spontaneous make-believe play or social imitative play (p.221) appropriate to developmental level

(3) restricted repetitive and stereotyped patterns of behavior, interests, and activities:
- encompassing preoccupation with one or more stereotyped and restricted patterns of interest that is abnormal either in intensity or focus (pp.229, 553)
- apparently inflexible adherence to specific, nonfunctional routines or rituals (p.234)
- stereotyped and repetitive motor mannerisms (e.g., hand or finger flapping or twisting, or complex whole-body movements) (pp.64, 105, 104, 119, 553)
- persistent preoccupation with parts of objects (pp.134,104,36,184)

B. Delays or abnormal functioning in at least one of the following areas, with onset prior to age 3 years: (1) social interaction (p.167), (2) language as used in social communication (p.144), or (3) symbolic or imaginative play (p.221).

C. The disturbance is not better accounted for by Rett's Disorder (p.541) or Childhood Disintegrative Disorder (p.46).

Post-Traumatic Stress Disorder

See also glossary entry for PTSD (p.532).

Table 20. DSM-IV criteria for Post-Traumatic Stress Disorder

A. The person has been exposed to a traumatic event in which both of the following have been present:

   (1) the person experienced, witnessed, or was confronted with an event or events that involved actual or threatened death or serious injury, or a threat to the physical integrity of self or others (2) the person's response involved intense fear, helplessness, or horror. **Note:** In children, this may be expressed instead by disorganized or agitated behavior.

B. The traumatic event is persistently reexperienced in one (or more) of the following ways:

   (1) recurrent and intrusive distressing recollections of the event, including images, thoughts, or perceptions (p.493). **Note:** In young children, repetitive play may occur in which themes or aspects of the trauma are expressed.

   (2) recurrent distressing dreams of the event (p.456). **Note:** In children, there may be frightening dreams without recognizable content.

   (3) acting or feeling as if the traumatic event were recurring (includes a sense of reliving the experience, illusions, hallucinations (p.343), and dissociative flashback episodes (p.453), including those that occur upon awakening or when intoxicated). **Note:** In young children, trauma-specific reenactment may occur.

   (4) intense psychological distress at exposure to internal or external cues that symbolize or resemble an aspect of the traumatic event (p.307).

   (5) physiological reactivity on exposure to internal or external cues that symbolize or resemble an aspect of the traumatic event.

C. Persistent avoidance (p.429) of stimuli associated with the trauma and numbing of general responsiveness (not present before the trauma), as indicated by three (or more) of the following:

   (1) efforts to avoid thoughts, feelings, or conversations associated with the trauma (p.493)

   (2) efforts to avoid (p.429) activities, places, or people that arouse recollections of the trauma

   (3) inability to recall an important aspect of the trauma

   (4) markedly diminished interest or participation in significant activities

   (5) feeling of detachment or estrangement from others

   (6) restricted range of affect (e.g., unable to have loving feelings) (p.178)

   (7) sense of a foreshortened future (e.g., does not expect to have a career, marriage, children, or a normal life span)

D. Persistent symptoms of increased arousal (not present before the trauma), as indicated by two (or more) of the following:

   (1) difficulty falling or staying asleep (p.199)

   (2) irritability (p.494) or outbursts of anger

   (3) difficulty concentrating (p.79)

   (4) hypervigilance (p.470)

   (5) exaggerated startle response (p.552)

E. Duration of the disturbance (symptoms in Criteria B, C, and D) is more than one month.

F. The disturbance causes clinically significant distress or impairment in social, occupational, or other important areas of functioning.

Reactive Attachment Disorder ☂

For discussion of Attachment, see p.195.

Table 21. DSM-IV criteria for Reactive Attachment Disorder

Children with this mental disorder, associated with care that is "grossly pathological," fail to relate socially either by exhibiting markedly inhibited behavior or by indiscriminate social behavior.

A. Markedly disturbed and developmentally inappropriate social relatedness in most contexts, beginning before age 5 years, as evidenced by either (1) or (2):
    (1) persistent failure to initiate or respond in a developmentally appropriate fashion to most social interactions (p.181), as manifest by excessively inhibited (p.178), hypervigilant (p.470), or highly ambivalent and contradictory responses (e.g., the child may respond to caregivers with a mixture of approach, avoidance (p.429), and resistance to comforting, or may exhibit frozen watchfulness (p.470))
    (2) diffuse attachments as manifest by indiscriminate sociability (p.173) with marked inability to exhibit appropriate selective attachments (e.g., excessive familiarity with relative strangers or lack of selectivity in choice of attachment figures)

B. The disturbance in Criterion A is not accounted for solely by developmental delay A. (as in Mental Retardation) and does not meet criteria for a Pervasive Developmental Disorder.

C. Pathogenic care as evidenced by at least one of the following (p.189):
    (1) persistent disregard of the child's basic emotional needs for comfort, stimulation, and affection
    (2) persistent disregard of the child's basic physical needs
    (3) repeated changes of primary caregiver that prevent formation of stable attachments (e.g., frequent changes in foster care)

D. There is a presumption that the care in Criterion C is responsible for the disturbed behavior in Criterion A (e.g., the disturbances in Criterion A began following the pathogenic care in Criterion C).

Specify type:
Inhibited Type: if Criterion A1 predominates in the clinical presentation
Disinhibited Type: if Criterion A2 predominates in the clinical presentation

Separation Anxiety Disorder ☂

For general notes on this and related conditions, see p.197. For a discussion of subtypes of anxiety, see p.295.

Table 22. DSM-IV criteria for Separation Anxiety Disorder

Children with this mental disorder, display excessive anxiety when away from home or from those to whom they are emotionally attached (p.195).

A. Developmentally inappropriate and excessive anxiety concerning separation from home or from those to whom the individual is attached (p.197), as evidenced by three (or more) of the following:

  1) recurrent excessive distress when separation from home or major attachment figures occurs or is anticipated

  2) persistent and excessive worry about losing, or about possible harm befalling, major attachment figures

  3) persistent and excessive worry that an untoward event will lead to separation from a major attachment figure (e.g., getting lost or being kidnapped)

  4) persistent reluctance or refusal to go to school (p.217) or elsewhere (p.307) because of fear of separation (p.197)

  5) persistently and excessively fearful or reluctant to be alone or without major attachment figures at home or without significant adults in other settings

  6) persistent reluctance or refusal to go to sleep (p.199) without being near a major attachment figure or to sleep away from home

  7) repeated nightmares (p.456) involving the theme of separation

  8) repeated complaints of physical symptoms (such as headaches (p.139), stomachaches (p.135), nausea, or vomiting (p.337)) when separation from major attachment figures occurs or is anticipated

B. The duration of the disturbance is at least 4 weeks.

C. The onset is before age 18 years.

D. The disturbance causes clinically significant distress or impairment in social, academic (occupational), or other important areas of functioning.

E. The disturbance does not occur exclusively during the course of a Pervasive Developmental Disorder, Schizophrenia, or other Psychotic Disorder and, in adolescents and adults, is not better accounted for by Panic Disorder With Agoraphobia (p.297).

Specify if:
Early Onset: if onset occurs before age 6 years

Appendix E: Catalogue of causes

Introduction

A child's constructed verbal version of why he did something is often unreliable. Just like grown-ups, children usually don't actually know why they did things – but they can make up an explanation with varying degrees of plausibility[1780].

This catalogue aids thinking about most possible causes. In this book, *cause* is shorthand for contributory factors[1234]. There are many kinds of cause (p.14 and below) only a minority of which are deterministic. In most clinical situations several causes are acting together. Causes interact in numerous complex ways (e.g. pp.15, 81, 185 and figures, pp.21, 110, 355).

Some children's acts are unmotivated (such as those in reflexes, sleep, and epilepsy). Apart from these, a child's doing something is determined by the balance between pressures for doing it and pressures for doing something else. All of these factors vary between individuals and between situations (see *functional analysis*, p.365).

This appendix is a tool for thought (like a *Surgical Sieve*) listing pointers to the rest of the book. Some of the categories below could be ordered into a hierarchy (e.g. of physical size or age of onset), but some could not. Some situations have multiple facets so appear in several lists, e.g. depression in a single parent. In principle, most of the factors below could appear in most of the lists in the book, but to keep those lists shorter, only the most common or identifiable causes are included.

Timing of cause

a) disorders with characteristic ages of onset, p.43

b) genetic, pp.31, 379

c) in utero
  i) medication: see foetal valproate syndrome, p.572
  ii) nutrition: see folate, p.467
  iii) toxic substances in utero, p.566
  iv) infection, p.490
  v) maternal anxiety, p.300
  vi) injuries to mother, p.454
  vii) hyperemesis gravidarum, p.483
  viii) malformations, p.503

d) natal – see prematurity and birth trauma, p.432

e) infancy – see maternal depression, p.174

f) childhood
  i) school, p.215
  ii) birth of siblings, p.213
  iii) trauma (physical or emotional, p.567; bereavement, p.430; refugees, p.540; changes in family or family functioning, p.465 and below)
  iv) poverty, p.533
  v) accommodation
    (1) overcrowded (pp.199, 207), dirty, no garden, far from transport
    (2) temporary housing; multiple moves
    (3) refuges, p.540
  vi) Family functioning, see below.
  vii) malnutrition, p.504; fasting, p.465
  viii) toxic substances, p.566
  ix) infection, p.490
  x) dehydration, p.450

g) puberty and adolescence

    i)   friendships, p.469
    ii)   sexuality, pp.411, 548
    iii)   school and school leaving, p.215

Not really that (see *complaining of normality*, p.205)
    a)   factors in the observer (e.g. unrealistic expectations)
        i)   misunderstanding of normality or of diagnostic criteria
        ii)   parents sensitive to a particular feared outcome.
    b)   factors in the child
        i)   good at learning but not at controlling himself, p.79
        ii)   fabricated or exaggerated behaviours, p.359
    c)   factors in the behaviour (see pseudo-regression, p.43)
    d)   inappropriate comparison (e.g. with ideals or sister)

Temporal relationships. A very useful classification of causes is predisposing, precipitating, p.534; perpetuating, p.526; and protective (also called resilience, p.541). There are many "two-factor theories" but clinical situations are often more complicated.

	Child	Family	School/peers
Predisposing			
Precipitating			
Perpetuating			
(Protective)			

Family members
    a)   parents, p.525
        i)   mothers, p.509
        ii)   fathers, p.465
        iii) parental mental or physical illness or ID, p.191
        iv) homosexual parents, p.481
    b)   siblings: rivalry, family size, birth order: p.548
    c)   only child, p.518
    d)   looked-after children, p.500
    e)   extended family: protective effects, p.196; as a comparator in assessments, p.201; multigeneration families, p.214

Family interactions
    a)   common family patterns, p.211
    b)   parenting, p.189
    c)   resilience, p.541
    d)   child altering family dynamics, p.211
    e)   parent-child relationship
        i)   attachment, pp.193, 207, 197
        ii)   expressed emotion, p.512
        iii) good-enough or too-good parenting, p.190
        iv) abuse, p.271; incest, p.489
        v)   attributions, p.426
        vi) unwanted child, p.571
        vii) assisted conception, p.424
    f)   parental functioning
        i)   parental discord, p.191
        ii)   domestic violence, p.454
        iii) divorce, p.454
        iv) parental alienation, p.187
        v)   single parents, p.213
        vi) prison, p.535
        vii) unemployment, p.570
    g)   child-child relationships, p.548

    h)   immigration, p.488
    i)   personality clash, p.527
    j)   chaos, p.212
    k)   trauma, p.567
    l)   parental subsystem and child subsystem, p.213.

Social dynamics. (see above for in-family.) See www.changeminds.org
    a)   bullying, p.219
    b)   social learning, p.550
    c)   dyad behaviour.   Acting like a child/adult/parent[157].
    d)   roles people play in groups
        i)   bully, victim, or bystander, p.219.
        ii)   task-oriented: chair, innovator, investigator, teamworker
        iii)   maintenance roles: elaborator, encourager, follower, tension-reliever, standard-setter / checker.
        iv)   non-functional roles: blocker, aggressor, confessor, special-interest pleader, clown, anecdoter
    e)   feedback loops, p.526
    f)   mass psychogenic behaviours, p.505
    g)   crowd behaviour, p.447
    h)   status hierarchies, pp.172, 553

Motivations (p.509; the term *drives* is closely related, p.456.) For lists of drives see Maslow's hierarchy of drives, p.505; Reiss's motivations[1328]; social drives, p.168.

a) power, pp.172, 213	k) vengeance
b) acceptance	l) romance and sex, p.548
c) status, p.553	
d) social contact, p.168	m) eating, pp.331–335
e) family, p.465	n) drinking, p.338
f) status, p.553	o) curiosity, p.124
g) order (see *cognitive dissonance*, p.355)	p) physical exercise, p.462
h) saving	q) tranquility (versus discomfort, danger, noise, etc.), p.126
i) honour	
j) idealism	

Emotions   (* indicates those thought to be *basic emotions*, see p.461). See also *rapid changes in emotions*, p.69.

a) anger*, p.287	q) enjoyment, ecstasy, bliss, joy
b) fear*, p.307; horror	r) envy (and jealousy), p.213
c) disgust*, pp.331, 465	
d) sadness*, p.309	s) excitement, p.520
e) happiness*	t) frustration, p.291
f) surprise*, p.552	u) guilt, p.475
g) contempt/hatred, p.187	v) hope
h) puzzlement/dissonance, p.355	w) interest, p.229
i) awe	x) love, p.501
j) boredom, p.322	y) pride
k) anxiety, p.295; apprehension	z) regret
l) challenge, pp.124, 554	aa) relief
m) compassion/altruism, p.420	bb) shame
n) dislike, like	cc) tension
o) distress, upset	
p) embarrassment, p.460	

Aspects of the child
    a)   developmental level: ID, p.491; gifted, p.473; specific ID, p.551

   b)   flexible or rigid, p.234
   c)   sociability: see social drives, p.168; and social skills, p.169
   d)   level of activity, p.79
   e)   personality, p.241
   f)   temperament, p.561
   g)   predominant mood, high, p.263; or low, p.309
   h)   criminality, p.446
   i)   physical problems: pain, p.135; infections, p.490; diabetes, p.451
   j)   appearance, malformations, p.503

Learned skills/behaviours

a) defence mechanisms
    i)   identification, p.487
    ii) dissociation, p.453
    iii) splitting, p.552
    iv) humour, p.495
    v) hypochondriasis, p.362
    vi) projective identification, p.535
    vii) reaction formation, p.305
    viii) repression, p.421
    ix) suppression, p.421
    x) somatisation, p.359
    xi) (behavioural) regression, p.43
    xii) passive aggression, p.525
    xiii) manic defences, p.306
    xiv) other defence mechanisms, p.303

b) coping mechanisms, p.445
c) cultural patterns, p.448
d) religion, p.541
e) pseudo-behaviours, p.363
f) adaptations to one's intolerances, p.126
g) self-soothing, p.61
h) self-entertainment, p.545
i) avoidance, p.429
j) physical self-protection
    i)   frozen watchfulness, p.470
    ii) startle, p.552
    iii) flinch, p.107
k) addiction, p.259

Learning mechanisms. (see *ideas*, below; *memory*, p.37)

   a)   operant learning
       i)   reinforcement, p.540
       ii) punishment, p.538
       iii) experimentation, p.463
   b)   classical conditioning, p.440
   c)   habituation and sensitisation, p.546; priming; arousal
   d)   declarative and non-declarative learning, p.37
   e)   reconsolidation, p.540
   f)   social learning, p.550
   g)   school, p.215
   h)   forgetting, p.468; extinction, p.463; repression, p.421; suppression, p.421; unlearning, p.571; desensitisation, p.451
   i)   perverse effects of training, p.528

Ideas. (for a long list see www.changeminds.org) Arthur Crisp said, "Ideas are more penetrating than physical injury". They get in and you can't get them out again. The difficulty of forgetting hurtful information is made harder if they are posted on the internet.

   a)   low self-esteem, pp.313,261.
   b)   hatred, p.187
   c)   delusions, p.347
   d)   attitudes, p.425

Dynamics of ideas

   a)   dominating interests, p.229
   b)   over-valued ideas, p.521
   c)   creation and fading of delusions, p.348

    d)   bubble bursting, p.435
    e)   confabulation, p.443
    f)   conflicts, p.443
    g)   self-fulfilling prophecies, see feedback loops, p.526
    h)   ideas that shape symptoms, see pseudo-behaviours, p.363
    i)   symbols, p.559
    j)   predictable irrationality, p.534

Automatic effects
    a) Automatic behaviours (innate or habitified)
        i)   reflexes: hyperekplexia, p.483; blinking, p.108; eye contact, p.175
        ii)   epiphenomena: tics, p.101; parasomnias, p.200.
        iii) primitive behaviours gradually brought under control: frontal signs, p.469; flapping, p.105; erection, p.462; central pattern generators, p.547
        iv) automatic responses to emotion: anger in general (pp.287, 282); shouting when attacked; anger at a particular person, p.253; laughing, p.111; flapping, p.105; smiling, p.549; anxiety reducing activity level, p.207.
        v)   inhibitory factors, or release from them, p.261; fight-flight-freeze, p.296; see also causes of smearing, p.342
    b) homeostasis / allostasis (p.420)
        i)   hyper/hypocalcaemia, pp.483, 485; hypoglycaemia, p.82; hyper/ hypothyroidism, pp.484/485; hyperventilation, p.484
        ii)   self-regulation: See *drives*, p.456; *allostasis*, p.420.
        iii) anxiety and inadequate anxiety, p.423.
        iv) dopamine appetite, p.322.
    c) neurological, p.85

Anatomic regions. Many subcortically controlled movements appear early in development, and become refined, variegated, or absent later, when they come under higher control. Disorders causing lesions in random locations cause highly varied neurological and behavioural problems (e.g. multiple sclerosis, p.510; neurophakomatoses, p.514; Fabry disease, p.464). Psychiatric conditions typically involve multiple brain areas[1069].

    a) muscle: weakness, p.87
    b) peripheral nerves, p.513
    c) sympathetic system, p.428
    d) parasympathetic system, p.428
    e) spinal cord, p.551
    f) brainstem, p.434
    g) hypothalamus, p.485
    h) cerebellum, p.437
    i) basal ganglia, p.429
    j) amygdala, p.421
    k) hippocampus, p.478
    l) neocortex, p.512

Neural dynamics.
    a)   electrical oscillations, p.459
    b)   evoked potentials: sensory processing, p.121; gating, p.418
    c)   epilepsy and migraine: pp.73, 141
    d)   hyperexcitability syndromes, p.483
    e)   overflow of activation, p.520
    f)   catalepsy, p.435
    g)   attractors. These are stable states that neural networks converge to. They have been used to explain OCD[1369].
    h)   inhibition of return, p.322
    i)   hierarchical control[195] of semi-autonomous central pattern generators, p.547

Cells and cell parts
a) white matter, p.574
b) synapse: see connectivity and pruning, p.444; pre-synaptic[1698], pp.441,459; extrasynaptic receptors, p.470
c) synaptic depression, p.
d) glia, p.474
e) nucleus, see ANA, p.421.
f) mitochondria, p.508
g) storage disorders, p.556
h) peroxisomes, p.526
i) lysosomes, p.501

Pathophysiological mechanisms
a) epilepsy, p.73; migraine, p.141
b) excitotoxicity, p.462
c) stroke, p.556
d) head injury, p.477
e) tumours, p.569
f) radiotherapy and chemotherapy
g) hypoxia: see *stroke*, p.556; *hippocampus*, p.478.
h) inflammation: see autoimmune, p.427; cytokines, p.450
i) infections, p.490
j) degenerative (see *regression*, p.41)
k) metabolism, p.379
l) medication, iatrogenic, p.486; cytochromes, p.450
m) body systems: renal, haematological, cardiovascular

Hormones
a) oxytocin, p.521
b) adrenaline, p.420
c) cytokines, p.450
d) melatonin, p.506
e) steroids, p.554
f) prolactin, p.536
g) thyroid, p.564
h) testosterone, p.554
i) premenstrual symptoms, p.506
j) parathyroid, p.525
k) intake-regulating hormones, p.491
l) opiates and opioids, p.519

Transmitters[1235]. Most psychotropic medications affect multiple transmitters. Linking transmitters to behaviour is complicated by the fact that "few if any brain neurons contain a single transmitter" and the presence of 50–100 neuropeptides[1505].
a) GABA, p.470
b) serotonin, p.547
c) glutamate, p.474
d) dopamine, p.455
e) noradrenaline, p.516
f) histamine, p.479.
g) substance P, p.466
h) nitric oxide (erection, p.462; asthma, p.424)
i) acetylcholine, p.418
j) glycine, p.474
k) adenosine, p.419

Electrolytes.
a) calcium, p.435.
b) potassium, see hypokalaemic periodic paralysis, p.438
c) sodium, see hyponatraemia, p.338; channelopathies, p.438
d) chloride, phosphate, carbonate, magnesium.

Appendix F: Forms for assessment or monitoring

The Mini-Mental State Examination is useful for detecting changes in cognitive level[306,510,1501], e.g. in delirium or regression.

Previous schoolwork or marks can sometimes be used to get an idea of whether the child had all these skills previously. If this cannot be absolutely established, the MMSE can only be used for monitoring changes from the first MMSE.

If less time is available, you can pick up confidence, speech, movement, cooperation, and working memory problems with:
- 20 take away 3's
- do the days of week forward and backward for practice, then ask them to do the months backwards
- digit span (p.452)
- Corsi block tapping test: put 9 blocks on a table and tap a sequence of two. If the child can copy this then try a longer sequence. This produces a Corsi span, which is a measure of spatial working memory (p.575) and usually two less than the forward digit span.

Mini-Mental State Examination

Patient name: _____   Date: _____

Tick

Orientation
Year
Season
Date
Day of week
Month
Name of hospital or building
Floor
City
County
Country

Registration
Name three objects at about one per second. Ask the patient to repeat them. If the patient misses an object, repeat them until all three are learned. (Score one point for each object named correctly)

Attention and Calculation
Subtract 7's from 100 to 65, or spell "world" backwards. (Score 1–5) **

Recall
Score one point for each of the registered objects above, that can be recalled.

Language
Point to a pen and a watch, and ask patient to name them.

Repeat "No ifs, ands or buts"

Have the patient follow a three-stage command: "(1) Take the paper in your right hand; (2) Fold the paper in half; (3) Put the paper on the floor."

Write in large letters: "CLOSE YOUR EYES." Ask the patient to read the command and follow the task.

Ask the patient to write a sentence of his or her own choice. Score correct if the sentence has a subject, verb, and object.

Copy the design printed below. Score correct if all sides and angles are preserved and the intersecting sides form a quadrangle.

← Total score out of 30

Child / Adolescent Mental Health Assessment

(NB For specialised or complex cases, it may be worthwhile
obtaining specialised checklists to ensure that nothing is missed –
e.g. a domestic violence form (p.454) or a physical needs form[1525].)

Name:

d.o.b:

DATE:

Tick when topics covered:

	CGAS
	Extra-confidential topics
	Confidentiality ends at safety
	Parents' email
	What do parents permit us to email

Who present:

Who referred and why:

Presenting complaints
(including onset, context, effect, why now, how dealt with

1

2

3

4

5

_____

Parents' ideas, concerns, expectations

_____

Long-term problems

Severity

Aetiology

GENERAL FAMILY INFORMATION
who in home, previous marriages, miscarriages, adop/fost

parental upbringing

Circumstances, financial, neighbourhood, sleeping arrangements

Family activities, weekends, paternal involvement, plays with

Signif other adults, which are confiding, which parent closest

Mother

Father

Typical day

Family tree (incl family medical & psychiatric history)

PERSONAL HISTORY
Pregnancy, neonatal,weight, Apgars, SCBU, feeding,placid/cry

Separations over 4 weeks, Prev psych history

Milestones (sat, stood, walked, talked)

PMH (asthma, headaches, fits/faints, operations / hospitalisations, major HI)

DH, allergies, vitamins

Speech therapy, child guidance

Vision tested?
Hearing tested?
Dental check?

Self-Harm / Suicidality

Violence

Puberty: hair, voice, menarche

Sexual relationships

Work

Alcohol, Illegal drugs

Smoking

Other risks (abuse, neglect) and risk behaviour(poor self-care, illness, pregnancy)

PMP/TEMPERAMENT
How reacts to new adult/child/pace/gadget/ change of routine

How show feelings/Chuckle or roar, mood before PC, affectionate, confiding, friendships

Physical regularity, reaction when animal/person hurt, reaction when had done wrong

How tidy is his room

SYSTEMIC ENQUIRY
Off school in past year

Eat, elim

Sleep: bedtime, sleeptime, settled, how wakes
Response to OSD-6 questionnaire on
Snoring
Choking/gasping for air in sleep
Stop breathing during the night
Restless sleep
Trouble falling asleep
Sleepy during the day
Difficulty in awakening

Restless/fidget/still if needed/conc how long

Speech: age-appropr, pronunciation, lisp, stutter

Clumsiness, tics, thumb-sucking/blanket, headbanging

Mood:irritable,sulky,temper, fears/school refusal

Sibs: closest, jealousy, blows

Friends (age & sex), bully/bullied, fights/gangs/clubs - ?leader

Disobedience: destruction, fire, lies, stealing, truant, police. Alone/ in group? Ran away?

Discipline: who punishes? how? Issues: bedtime, say where, restrict TV, pocket money

School: which one, likes it? progress, seen teacher, have we contacted school?

Subjects to be covered with the child directly:
Use a friendly interested style. Arrows show progression from closed to open, easy to difficult questions. School is often the best place to start.

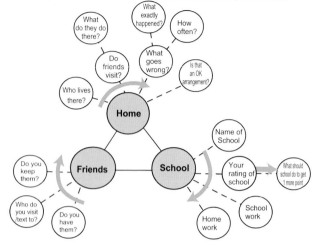

Interview in a way that is robust if anything about child protection comes up (see p.272)

What makes you happy?

If you had 3 wishes, what would you change?

School

Friends

Home

Punishment
Gently cover important sensitive topics such as punishment. Go into them in detail, but in as natural a way as possible. Oh, you do things that make your parents cross, do you? What do you do that makes them cross? When do you do this? Where are you? Why do you do that?

Suicide
With the child, be gentle: e.g. Start with "Is (school, home) fun or bad?" then if concerned, work up this series of questions until the answer is NO:

Do you think life's pretty terrible?
→Do you sometimes think it's not worth living?
→ Do you sometimes wish you weren't alive?
→ Do you sometimes think about dying or wanting things to end?
→Do you sometimes think you'd prefer to be dead?
→ Do you think you might do something to make that happen?
→ Do you have any plans?

Nightmares / worries

EXAMINATION
Appearance

(frustration tolerance, response to limit-setting or praise, disinhib)

Activity level,attention span, persistence / impulsiveness, distractibility, curiosity

voice, spontaneity, quantity, intonation, articulation, grammar, complexity

language (examples). Recep (comprehension) & expressive

repetitive behaviours, mannerisms, tics, posturings, gestures

affect (range, anxiety, panics, anger, irritability)

ideas: feels he is good at / bad at; abnormal ideas; preoccupations

halluc

obsessions/ compulsions

insight

social behaviour (eye contact, reserved or expansive, non-compliant, surly, manipulative)

interactions with others

Caregiver responses

general physical weight/height, neurol: Cranial nerves (nystag, squint), coord (finger, limb):

Construction, handedness (p.475), footedness, RL differentiation, discriminating signif people:

Opinion

Long-term issues

Short-term issues

Possibilities / concerns excluded (Down's, schiz, etc.)

Predisp

Precip

Perpet

Formulation

Risk

Plans

Record of feedback session

Screening tests to do (cross out if not needed or already done):

√ Chromosomes (p.439),
√ Fragile X,
√ UECr,
√ glucose,
√ lipids,
√ LFT,
√ FBC,
√ TFT,
√ Fe,
√ prolactin,
√ autoantibody screen,
√ lead,
√ plasma amino and urinary organic acids.
√ drug screen

Professionals involved

		Tick if for cc.
Audiology		
CAMHS		
EP		
Eye clinic		
OT		
Physio		
Preschool teaching service		
SW		
SLT		
Hospitals		
Paeds		
Other		

NAME_____ – MEDICATION HISTORY

date	(name, dose→dose) antipsychotics	ADHD-related	SSRI etc	sleep	reason	result

Appendix G: Mini-physical examination

Physical examination, particularly the neurological part, is usually entertaining for children, and can be divided into several parts, to be used when the child gets bored. The physical examination sometimes provides useful physical information, but more often the manner of the child, and the speed of his understanding, are valuable. The physical examination is always appreciated by parents, and helps to get children interacting. It is essential in many presentations, such as anorexia, delay, tics, abuse, and skin disorders. It should be performed regularly by every child psychiatrist so he/she can be fluent, amusing, and aware of the range of normality at each age. Have the parents or a chaperone in the room during physical examination.

A. Quick neurological screen in logical subdivisions

Mental status
- Alertness – Does patient seem to be aware of what is going on and is he able to communicate appropriately?
- Orientation – Does patient know who they are, how old are they, where they are, what date/day it is, what they have been doing?
- Memory – Remember three objects then later in the exam ask the patient to recall the objects
- Calculation – Count backwards from 100 by sevens

Cranial nerves
- Eyes – Can patient see, is vision normal, is eye movement normal, visual fields to confrontation?
- Hearing – Can patient hear equally in both ears (occlude other pinna while rubbing)?
- Facial muscles - Is the face equal in muscle tone and control? Have patient smile, whistle, blow out cheeks
- Tongue – symmetrical tongue size and movement
- Retch reflex (on touching uvula)
- Does the Adam's Apple move when patient swallows?
- Facial sensation – Can patient feel light touch equally on both sides of their face

Motor
- Arms: tone, power (0–5)
  Coordination in fingers, wrists, elbows, shoulders; dysdia-dochokinesis (p.457), nose-touching, catch a ball, write (p.53)
- Legs: Walking – heel-to-toe, forwards and backwards

Sensory
- Light Touch – Can patient feel light touch equally on both sides of the body?
- Sharp/Dull – Can patient distinguish between a sharp or dull object on both sides of the body?
- Hot/Cold – Can patient distinguish between a hot or cold object on both sides of the body?

B. Practical general screen, with emphasis on development. This is ordered for the child's convenience, not by body system

Organise all the parts of the examination as a walk round your room, to standardise the procedure and avoid forgetting.

---

gait (p.471): see this on the way to your room, while looking for toe-walking (plus anxiety and communicativeness). Most children enjoy the mimicry of heel/toe walking; hopping (from age 3–4); kicking a ball of paper; tiptoeing (see synkinesis, p.560).

hands (p.476)
  simian crease (*not* a reliable sign of Down's syndrome: see p.455)
  touching the thumb with all fingers in turn (some 5-year-olds can do this)
  pulse at wrist

stand, coordination (finger-nose is funny: most 3-year-olds can do it, and from age 7 most can do it with eyes closed), dysdiadochokinesis (p.457), squeeze two fingers, ask re handedness (p.475) and familiality, asymmetry of hands (if, e.g., speech problem) tremor, finger length, finger/thumb (see also other key developmental checks, p.57.)

size (look, weigh half-way through with shoes off checking for uneven wear and doing plantar reflexes gently, height, growth chart while watching how he puts his shoes and socks back on)

face – dysmorphic features
  eye movements, acuity, glasses
  unusual teeth (p.561), high arched palate (p.522)
  head circumference can be useful (see microcephaly, p.507; macrocephaly, p.502). Pull a measuring tape tightly around the supraorbital ridges and the most prominent part of the occiput. Growth charts are available at www.cdc.gov/growthcharts

speech, hearing, vision
  Hearing: whisper a toy or food at 1m distance (more tests on pp.130,90)
  Vision: Use well-lit Snellen charts.

torso: Heart rate and blood pressure (p.478), skin (with heart)

Ask permission to take a photo of the child with his family, at end of session. This is useful for identifying (and remembering) the family, and for consulting with colleagues. In epilepsy, violence and severe hyperactivity, simple photography may not be fast enough to capture diagnostically crucial behaviours. If there is a question of statementing, ask the parents to supply a video to strengthen the case; or this can be done in their presence.

If you have even mild concern that the child may be abused, start collecting information to work out whether to involve other colleagues (see p.271). Lifting the shirt (e.g. to listen to the heart) isn't enough because it would miss fingertip bruising on the upper arms; these can sometimes be seen when applying the sphygmomanometer cuff. Bruises and burns are the most common injuries and can only be picked up by asking parents to remove most clothes. In most situations this is best done by a paediatrician.

This means the physical changes, taking place gradually over several years, that lead to reproductive capability. There are several reasonable ways of determining the *start* of puberty, though all give different answers: acceleration in growth; appearance of pubic hair; testicular growth; or breast development. Menarche usually occurs later.

No single age can be specified as correct for any part of puberty, due to (a) population variation; (b) racial variation (e.g. breast development in Caucasians generally occurs about a year later than in other races[1567]); (c) differences in diet and weight (e.g. menarche is advanced by 1–2 years in well-fed girls[1218] and delayed in thin girls, see p.506); (d) effects of ill health including stress; (e) other less common factors such as high altitude and exposure to chemicals[1218].

Precocious puberty has been defined as achieving B2 below 8 years (girls) or achieving G2 below 9 years (boys). The definition governs when further investigation is usually considered. There have been proposals to lower these cutoff ages to reduce unnecessary investigation[1218,1562].

Boys
For external changes see table at right. For psychological effects of testosterone see p.554. For graphs of testicular growth in three countries see[233].

Girls
For external changes see table at right, and the following additional details:
- In USA in 2010 PH2 is reached by 6% of white 7-year-old girls and 20% of black 7-year-old girls [174].
- In USA in 2010 B2 is reached by 10% of white 7-year-olds and 23% of black 7-year-olds[174].
- For other variations in timing and order, see[1016,1017,1571].

For psychological and neurological conditions accompanying menstruation see p.506.

Age at menarche is partly inherited, but it is not clear how much of this inheritance is due to shared predisposition to diet, to exercise, etc. Harsh control by mothers predicts earlier menarche, but again it is not clear whether this is a direct causal effect, or mediated by other factors such as mood or weight, or whether it is due to factors shared between mother and daughter (see[135]). Similarly, though it is well established that early menarche in girls is strongly *associated* with a wide range of difficult behaviours and low mood[598], it is not clear how much of the effect is causal.

Table 23. Stages of puberty

Pubic hair (both male and female). This is caused by androgens produced in the testes of boys, and in the adrenal glands of girls.	Age range	
	Girls	**Boys**
PH1 No pubic hair at all (prepubertal)		
PH2 **[adrenarche]** Small amount of long, downy hair with slight pigmentation at the base of the penis and scrotum (males) or on the labia majora (females).	8.4–12.7 ††	11.2–14.3 *
PH3 Hair becomes more coarse and curly, and begins to extend laterally	PH2 + 1.5	11.8–15.2 *
PH4 Adult-like hair quality, extending across pubis but sparing medial thighs	PH2+2.5	12.7–15.5 *
PH5 Hair extends to medial surface of the thighs	PH2+5	12.8–17.0 *
Genitals (male)		
G1 Prepubertal (testicular volume less than 1.5 ml; small penis of 3 cm or less)		
G2 **[gonadarche]** Testicular volume between 1.6 and 6 ml; skin on scrotum thins, reddens and enlarges; penis length unchanged		9–14 **
G3 Testicular volume between 6 and 12 ml; scrotum enlarges further; penis begins to lengthen to about 6 cm		10.0–14.0 *
G4 Testicular volume between 12 and 20 ml; scrotum enlarges further and darkens; penis increases in length to 10 cm and circumference		11.1–15.3 *
G5 Testicular volume greater than 20 ml; adult scrotum and penis of 15 cm in length		12.3–16.8 *
Breasts (female) This is caused by oestrogens		
B1 No glandular tissue; areola follows the skin contours of the chest (prepubertal)		
B2 **[thelarche]** Breast bud forms, with small area of surrounding glandular tissue; areola begins to widen. Stage B2 may not be visible in slightly overweight girls.	7–13 in Caucasians; 6–13 in African-Americans **	
B3 Breast begins to become more elevated, and extends beyond the borders of the areola, which continues to widen but remains in contour with surrounding breast	B2 + 1.5	
B4 Increased breast size and elevation; areola and papilla form a secondary mound projecting from the contour of the surrounding breast	B2 + 3	
B5 Breast reaches final adult size; areola returns to contour of the surrounding breast, with a projecting central papilla.	B2+5	
Menstruation [menarche] (female)		
	9.5–14.0 † (US all races)	

Codes in the first column are Tanner Stages (photos are in[1016,1017]).

*	Values given are 5th and 95th centiles at stage entry[233]
**	Values given are 2.5 SD below and above mean[1562].
†	Values given are 5th and 95th centiles[1039].
††	Values given are 5th and 95th centiles[1567].

Appendix H: Confidentiality

Some information must not be kept confidential. This includes information about abuse, p.271; and about risk of harm to specific individuals, p.283. Some information is wrongly kept confidential, e.g. in some adoptions, p.419.

To other professionals, information should be disclosed on a "need to know" basis. Families are usually fairly comfortable about information sharing between health professionals, but much less so regarding sharing information with Education, Social Services or others. For example, 86% of adults are fairly comfortable with their doctor having their genetic test results, but only 18% with their employers[729]. The costs of breaking patient confidentiality (over-completeness) are:
- Loss of trust from patient, family, family's contacts, and colleagues
- Loss of trust between family members

Section 1.5 of the BPS document *Working in Teams* discusses confidentiality well. Available at www.bps.org.uk/sub-sites$/dcp/dcp-publications/general-publications.cfm. (See also reasons for people to try to keep information secret, p.166; disclosure, p.452; and methods for obtaining sensitive information, p.11.)

Writing letters about mental health often includes special aspects of confidentiality: from sane parents, from over-sensitive or mentally ill parents, and from the child after he has grown up.

- Your ***relationship with child and parents***, and the child's reaction when he sees the letter 1–20 years from now, have to be taken into account. This means that upsetting details or summaries should be avoided unless they can realistically contribute to management. *Your* judgments should be excluded from the history which should contain only facts – or, if relevant, who made which judgments.

- Harsh words can often be replaced by ***gentle words*** that will convey the message subtly to professionals. Say positive things in a warm personal way, but couch negative observations in the third person hypothetical generalities about parenting styles. Describe the parents' *style* as permissive, or give examples, rather than saying *they* cannot establish boundaries. Give them excuses; say they found it difficult to attend rather than that they did not attend for five appointments. "He was delusional on two occasions" is more precise and more acceptable than "He may have schizophrenia."

- Remind yourself that you are their servant in most cases. Even in abuse cases your life will be easier if you keep the demeanour of one.

- Some information is simply unhelpful or even damaging (e.g. paternity or Huntington's, p.482).

- Do not put the patient's or parents' words in quotation marks. This makes them feel over-scrutinised, or that someone else (the reader) has been allowed to listen in at the interview room.

- The parents will get very upset if ***sensitive family information*** is sent to other people (especially to school – parents acutely feel the need to preserve their social standing in their relationships with teachers).
  1. Warn them about privacy before they give the history to you.
  2. Allow parents to check letters and cc-lists before they go out.
  3. Put the family history in a separate letter with a shorter cc-list (each letter can refer to the other yet preserve confidentiality).
  4. Check new ideas with parents, either in person or on the phone, before you send them out.
  5. Don't send letters in haste. Have a colleague double-check difficult ones.
  6. If parents are trying to exclude all family information from the correspondence, try the letter on p.416.

Principles of information sharing

Disclose the minimum possible information, and ideally only with a confidentiality agreement in place with any recipient agency (such as Social Services or Education). Only send information if one of the following is true:

1.   the patient has capacity to consent, and has given informed consent, and disclosure is in his best interests; or
2.   the patient has lack of capacity to consent, which is likely to be permanent, and disclosure is in his best interests; or
3.   there is an immediate high risk of harm, with no other means to manage the risk than disclosure.

 "You need to consider:
1. Is there a legitimate purpose for you … to share the information?
2. Does the information enable a person to be identified?
3. Is the information confidential?
4. If so, do you have consent to share?
5. Is there a statutory duty or court order to share the information?
6. If consent is refused, or there are good reasons not to seek consent, is there a sufficient public [necessity] to share information?
7. …Are you sharing the right (minimum) information in the right way?
8. Have you properly recorded your decision?

Each of these questions is covered in more detail in the practitioners' guide" (see www.ecm.gov.uk/informationsharing).

Special situations

Confidentiality from parents
The weight given to the parents' right to know varies between countries, and between ages. In many countries specific kinds of information are specially protected if they would compromise a young person's safety or willingness to seek care, or would increase teenage pregnancies. Examples include a child's information regarding substance abuse, sexual health, or contraception she is receiving. The laws in this area are exceedingly complicated in some countries[1376].

Confidential third-party information
This can be very helpful in looking after children, but its confidential nature needs to be respected. As with interviewing families, total confidentiality can never be promised because in some circumstances the welfare of the child could override it.

Writing medico-legal reports.
It may be wise to decline to write a report if you are clinically involved. Advise the patient that this is not a normal doctor–patient meeting and that confidentiality does not apply

Vulnerable groups
The following groups may need their information kept extra secure:

- staff
- residents of a women's refuge
- child trafficking / prostitution
- serious sexual assault
- murder / manslaughter suspects
- domestic violence cases
- custody disputes
- sex offenders
- children at risk of abduction
- serious case reviews
- political / asylum children at risk
- child records of military personnel
- Witness Protection Programme
- Looked after children
- child protection
- children of parents with high public profile that places them at risk
- families of vulnerable practitioners and professionals
- fleeing forced marriage
- "honour based violence" cases

Methods of redaction

Redaction is the practice of removing sensitive, private, or confidential information from a document. You should omit some confidential information from your records, and omit even more from your letters.

If you have discovered something confidential but likely to be important in future management, be open with the patient about the benefits of recording it. If the parents tell you something that is currently secret from their child (such as adoption or embryo-implantation or the parents' histories), keep in mind that your duty of care is a balance of current care, the need for full recording, and also the child's horror when he eventually reads something. Discuss this with the parents: "What do you think I should put in the notes, bearing in mind that your son will eventually have the right to read the notes?"

Note that patients have the right to limit how their personal information is treated, and you cannot override even absurd decisions except to manage *risk*.

Level of confiden-tiality	Examples of information	Who should know the full details	Method of redaction (see also box below)	Redaction for computer databases (because of hackers, this must be extra secure)
LOW	Addresses, professionals involved	Widely disseminated but very limited content: open to all services	Information Sharing Index (see previous page)	
	Slightly sensitive family history When family have close ties to GP or don't trust GP staff confidentiality, and won't change GP	For NHS but not SSD or school Just for the trust, i.e. excluding GP		Passwords and audit trail
	Very private details that could be crucial for future carers to know (e.g. abuse, medical conditions)	"Need-to-know" within the trust. Spread is slowed rather than restricted.	Put it in a sealed envelope in notes. Have it in handwriting rather than typed (then it's difficult for computers to read).	Encryption with keys available with difficulty (e.g. on paper at trust HQ)
	Very private details with major downside and tiny upside (e.g. paternity)	Just for team	Discuss with team – if sufficiently confidential, can make team decision not to record it	
HIGH	Very unusual and sensitive. Requires personal judgment of whether sharing within team is essential. This can be risky.	Just for you	Don't even write it. Or, as psychotherapists often do, keep a separate set of notes.	Encryption with key available only to you. Hidden files with *plausible deniability* (see www.truecrypt.org)

> Vagueness in the notes is a useful tool. e.g. you can flag the delicate areas by recording "We had a conversation about a number of private issues." or "…about issues that mum wished to remain private" or "that mum wished to seek help with elsewhere." Or "Several issues are excluded from this report that we took into account but which did not influence the conclusions."

Sample letter to a parent who requests omission of family information

Dear Mr Smith,

Many thanks for your message enclosing changes to Joe's report. I very much respect your views and your confidentiality. I have made several of the changes you requested, however, unfortunately I am not able to remove all the family information from the report, as you wish.

This is because both national and international guidelines for child psychiatry make it mandatory that we consider the family almost as much as the child. As an example, it is crucial for future mental health professionals to know of Sam's father's illness. The reasons are essentially that the family create the genetic and environmental background essential for understanding any child's difficulties, and also that any treatment has to involve parents.

For example, the American Academy of Child and Adolescent Psychiatry in their "Practice parameters for the psychiatric assessment of children and adolescents" (1997) suggests that every assessment should include the following:

F. Assessment of family and community background.
   1. Parents:
      a. Strengths, weaknesses, areas of conflict as:
         (1) Individuals;
         (2) Martial couple;
         (3) Parental couple.
      b. Parental attitudes toward the child, including hopes, fears, expectations, or areas of disagreement regarding child;
      c. Parental attachment patterns toward the child over the course of development;
      d. Experiences with parents' own families of origin that influence attitudes or behavior toward child;
      e. Quality of temperamental fit between parent and child;
      f. Ethnic, cultural, religious background;
      g. Education, occupation, financial resources.
   2. Family and household:
      a. Composition of family, including nearby relatives;
      b. Composition of household, including non-family members;
      c. Boundaries and alliances within family and child's role with respect to them;
      d. Family's style of communication and problem solving;
      e. Prevailing emotional tone of family, especially as it impinges on the patient:
         (1) Supportive;
         (2) Critical or hostile;
         (3) Over- or undercontrol;
      f. Family activities, including activities of daily living leisure and recreational activities;
      g. Family expectations and discipline;
      h. Family stresses:
         (1) Moves;
         (2) Changes in family or household composition;
         (3) Unemployment, poverty;
         (4) Illnesses, accidents or other disability;
         (5) Legal difficulties.
      i. Housing;
         (1) Adequacy of heating, cleanliness, safety;
         (2) Privacy and sleeping arrangements.
   3. Family medical and psychiatric history. Inquire concerning the past and current history of physical and psychiatric disorders with potential environmental or genetic consequences for child, including history of hospitalization or symptoms impinging on child and child's reaction thereto.
   4. Community and culture, including adverse circumstances.

I enclose the report as it currently stands. I have put the great majority of family information in a separate letter, so that you can easily remove it before giving a copy to any other service if you wish. This system has been useful to other families and I hope it is acceptable to you. Please let us know if there are better ways in which we can preserve your confidentiality while working in accord with accepted guidelines on assessment of children.

Best wishes

Glossary and index

This includes symptoms and causes referred to in the main section of the book, and some additional behaviours and useful terms. More detailed descriptions of symptoms can be found in a standard psychiatric or paediatric text, in Sims[1487], in SCAN[1796] or DSM or ICD.

3di: the developmental, dimensional, and diagnostic interview for autistic spectrum disorders, p.183.

5HT: 5-hydroxy tryptamine, also called *serotonin*, p.547.

ABC: Antecedents, Behaviour, Consequences; see p.365.

Abetalipoproteinaemia: steatorrhoea and malabsorption (p.502) affecting fat-soluble vitamins A, D, E, and K (p.328). Chronic deficiency of these vitamins causes spinocerebellar degeneration (with sensory abnormalities and ataxia after age 10); acanthocytosis, p.514. Suggestive results on screening are very low LDL and VLDL cholesterol; low A, K, E; increased prothrombin time (vitamin K); elevated creatine kinase[460] (p.446).

Absence: petit mal seizure, p.75; zoning out, p.75; absence from school, p.217; absence of parent, p.194.

Abulia: p.97.

Abuse: child abuse, p.271; substance abuse, p.257.

Acalculia: see *dyscalculia*, p.457.

ACC: anterior cingulate cortex, see p.513.

Accents: variations between groups of people in spoken language. Most are geographical but others include social class, the gay voice (p.243) and the American black voice. People with autism often have idiosyncratic voice or prosody (p.148) but a substantial minority of them permanently latch on to a specific conventional accent (p.243). If a child on holiday rapidly adjusts his accent to conform with local usage, this suggests the child is both flexible and socially interested – i.e. very unlikely to have autism. Ultra-rapid changing of accent within a sentence comes in several forms: normal bilingual; camp, p.243; pedantic, p.163; and the autistic child who interacts little with people, but has learned phrases through vast numbers of repetitions (usually from a video), and communicates by stitching these sound fragments together. See also *pseudo-accent*, p.354.

Accident: a sudden, unplanned and unexpected outcome of an action. Some accidents are useful for learning of risks (and accidental achievements, p.44). See frequent accidents as an indicator of neglect, p.274; or physical abuse, p.273. See also urinary accidents, p.340; faecal accidents, p.342; accidental overdoses, p.486; accidental ingestion, pp.331, 566.

People tend to place too much weight on the long-term recklessness (p.539) of the child (this is the *fundamental attribution error*, p.18). But taking a broader view, accidents can happen for three kinds of reason:

- the situation: Accidents are more common in deprived areas, with single mothers and large families[1316]. Reasons include inadequate supervision; unsafe homes; inadequate entertainment so in desperate boredom they try absurd things; attention-seeking gone wrong (e.g. climbing on shelves to get parental attention).

- innate traits of the child: ID; autism; poor vision; poor judgments of distance; innate impulsivity[1316] (p.79). Religious people tend to take fewer risks (p.541). Some people take delight in risk (p.124).
- temporary states of the child: sleepiness; excitement; haste; aggression; thinking only about the destination so he can't think about how he negotiates obstacles on the way, buried in a book as he walks along the pavement; risk-taking increased by presence of friends, p.263.

Acetylcholine: peripherally this is the transmitter at the neuromuscular junction (see myasthenia, p.510) and in the parasympathetic nervous system, p.428. In the CNS it regulates learning; hence cholinesterase inhibitors improve cognitive function (e.g. in dementia and possibly other conditions[1810]) and muscarinic agonists may improve learning in schizophrenia[1467]. Anticholinergic agents relieve parkinsonism. The alpha-7 nicotinic receptor may have a role in sensory gating (as measured by pre-pulse inhibition, p.462), and so be responsible for the failure of this in some patients with schizophrenia[12,1189]. See also *Neuroleptic malignant syndrome*, p.514.

ACh: acetylcholine.
ACTH: adrenocorticotrophic hormone, see diagram on p.531.

Acting: trying to look or sound a particular way. Usually done to get a reaction from other people, in which case it will be done near them, usually facing them, sometimes with eye contact, and will eventually reduce if ignored by others. Occasionally done to see what it feels or sounds like – in this case, the child will be focused, usually avoiding eye contact, and ignoring it will not make it disappear. Echolalia (p.459) is a more precise term for the simplest of all acting, which is focused on one or a few words (sometimes parts of words) without consideration of what they mean or any effect on other people.
See also acting camp, p.243; acting grown-up or cocky, p.244; acting immature, p.27; acting tough, p.178; acting out (below); acting unloveable, p.303; pseudo-behaviours, p.363.

Acting out: turning feelings into actions; or acting on one's desires (id) despite being forbidden by the conscience (superego). This term is an interpretation rather than an observation; and is often misused to refer to all physical misbehaviour.

Acting young: can indicate ID or *pseudo-regression*, p.43.
Activities of Daily Living: see *adaptive behaviours*, p.419.

Acyl-CoA dehydrogenases (ACADs): a family of enzymes that metabolise fatty acids. MCADD (medium-chain acyl-CoA dehydrogenase deficiency) is the best known, as mild illness or fasting in infancy precipitates severe hypoglycaemia, which can be fatal or cause ID. MCADD is therefore part of the neonatal heelprick test, p.32. See also *mitochondrial disorders*, p.508.

Adaptive behaviours: behaviours used by a child to look after himself. The term also sometimes includes a child's ability to conform to social norms. Standard tests are the Vineland Adaptive Behaviour Scales[521] and the Living Skills Assessment. These tests can contribute to a diagnosis of ID (p.491) which is defined in terms of both IQ (p.59) and adaptive behaviours. Adaptive behaviours include:

- Feeding (p.331)
- Hygiene (p.483) – teeth, hair, bathing, menses
- Washing machine and changing his clothes
- Road safety
- Use of public transport and general orientation
- Shopping (including location of foods) and budgeting
- Cooking and preparation (including sequence of tasks).

ADD: Attention Deficit Disorder. This is the obsolete DSM-III term for non-hyperactive ADHD.

Addiction: for drug addictions and behavioural addictions see p.259. For wider aspects of drug use see p.257.

Addison's disease: adrenal insufficiency. Weakness, fatigue, hypotension, nausea and vomiting, loss of appetite and weight. Some cases have hyperpigmentation, especially of old scars, nail beds and mouth. See *glucorticoids*, p.555.

Adenosine: an inhibitory transmitter inhibitory in the CNS. Caffeine, and theobromine in chocolate, block this. Adenosine levels increase with each hour one is awake.

ADH: anti-diuretic hormone. Also called vasopressin. See SIADH, p.338; hypothalamus, p.485; and diagram, p.531.

ADHD: see Attention Deficit Hyperactivity Disorder
ADI-R: Autism Diagnostic Interview - Revised, p.183
ADL: Activities of Daily Living. See *adaptive behaviours*, p.419.

Adolescent: teenagers are age 13–19, but *adolescent* has many definitions:

Start:	1. Onset of puberty (p.411)
	2. 10th birthday (WHO; USA CDC)
End:	1. 19th birthday (WHO; Dept. for Education)
	2. 18th birthday (Children Act 1989)
	3. School-leaving
	4. 24th birthday (USA CDC)
	5. Marriage/childbirth.

Adoption: permanent legal commitment by parent(s) to a child from another family. Adoptive parents are highly screened; but there are small negative as well as positive differences in their parenting in comparison with biological parents (see e.g.[266,642]). Adopted children have more behavioural problems than children reared by their biological parents, presumably mainly due to their genetic inheritance and impaired pre-adoption parenting (see [1248] for discussion). In addition, there can be a mismatch between adoptive parents' academic expectations and the adopted child's abilities; and adoptive parents may be less accepting of severe behavioural disturbance than biological parents[1248].

There is currently a debate regarding the right of biological parents to refuse consent to disclose information, when this can be important for the care of the child[694]. Crucial medical information is sometimes kept confidential from adoptive parents, including not just the parents' difficulties but even the presence of profound ID in the child[182].

ADOS: Autism Diagnostic Observation Schedule, p.183

Adrenaline (also called epinephrine): the main fight-or-flight hormone released by the sympathetic nervous system (p.428). Compare noradrenaline (p.516) which is mainly a transmitter but also a hormone. Adrenaline is also released by some of the rare phaeochromocytoma tumours, p.529.

Adrenoleukodystrophy: p.498
Adultification: p.214.
AEA: Acquired Epileptic Aphasia, p.45.
AEP: auditory evoked potential, p.462.
Aggression: p.289.
Agoraphobia: p.297.

AIDP / CIDP: acute and chronic inflammatory demyelinating polyneuropathies, p.87.

Akathisia: p.114.
Akinetic mutism: p.97.

Alcohol: abuse, p.258; alcohol withdrawal, p.258, 344; delirium tremens, p.258; *Foetal Alcohol syndrome*, p.467; GABA receptor, p.470.

ALD: adrenoleukodystrophy, p.498.
Alexithymia: p.152.
Allodynia: p.136.

Allostasis: maintaining stability in the body, not by simply opposing changes but by changing other aspects of behaviour[1040]. Whereas homeostasis consists of graded physiological responses to change, allostasis an enhanced version of this: proactive, dynamic, and sometimes cognitive. Examples include turning the HPA axis on and off (p.485); building body energy stores when we are unstressed; reducing activity levels (by being depressed) when things have gone wrong; and increasing vigilance at appropriate times.

Altruism: liking to help other people. Altruism is distinct from wanting to help a particular person, and arguably from wanting people to be happy in order to feel a warm glow oneself.

There have been many studies purporting to demonstrate altruism. However there is much debate about whether these studies in fact demonstrate quite different factors such as non-random participant selection, unrealistic options being available, preference for fairness, and behaviour being different under scrutiny[940,941]. To some extent these behaviours seem to be innate[1713], but they can be increased by religious beliefs, the content of video games (p.573 and [552]), song lyrics [617], or wanting to be thought well of [58]. Contrast *selfishness* (p.179).

See also altruism as a defence mechanism, p.303.

Ambidextrous: see *handedness*, p.475.
Ambivalence: p.287.

Amnesia: abnormal loss of memories or of the ability to create them. Infantile amnesia is the normal inability to recall events of infancy. For organic conditions see *post-traumatic retrograde and anterograde amnesia*, p.477; *hippocampus*, p.478.

Related processes include *forgetting*, p.468; *extinction*, p.463; and *unlearning*, p.571.

Loss of memories, that starts at a moment of stress and is *specific* for stressful or unpleasant information, is often called *functional amnesia*, *dissociative amnesia*, *pseudo-amnesia*, or *repression*. This is a highly contentious area with many dubious publications (reviewed in[839]). The most common error is overdiagnosis of dissociative amnesia, caused by a failure to ensure that the child is actually wanting to think about and disclose the memory (cf. malingering, p.503); that he was sufficiently mature and awake and the event sufficiently interesting for it to be reliably remembered; that no physical condition interfered with consolidation; that new learning ability is unimpaired; and that there is no causative brain lesion[211,839]. It is probably very rare[839]; it may sometimes be a culture-bound syndrome[1267]; and it involves increased frontal cortical activity specifically timed to repress hippocampal recall[840].

The term *suppression* is sometimes used to mean a conscious version of repression, e.g. when a memory is unpleasant so a person adopts the coping mechanism (p.445) of doing something else to preoccupy herself . There is no sharp division as the level of conscious awareness is variable and generally not fully known. Many impulses can be usefully suppressed and failure to do so can be impairing. Examples include tics, anger, sexual impulses, appetite, laughter, synkinesis (p.560) and hyperactivity (p.77). In some circumstances excess suppression can be impairing, e.g. in anorexia nervosa (p.334) rational thought about weight and health can be suppressed; see also *selective mutism*, p.153.

Memory loss following trauma can extend beyond the traumatic events, to autobiographical information, general semantic information, or even to self-care (in which case it might be called pseudo-dementia). In such cases it is crucial to exclude depression, p.313; regression, p.41; and organic *post-traumatic amnesia*, p.477.

Amygdala: brain nuclei responsible for anxiety. See love, p.501; amygdalar lesions in frozen states, p.97; in *Klüver-Bucy*, p.496.

ANA: anti-nuclear antibodies. These are present mainly in people with autoimmune conditions. There are several ANAs, e.g. anti-dsDNA; anti-histone; anti-centromere; and anti-ENA (extractable nuclear antigens). The individual ANAs are partially specific to named autoimmune conditions, such as SLE (p.560) and scleroderma.

ANCA: anti-neutrophil cytoplasmic antibodies, found in autoimmune conditions, especially vasculitis.

Anaemia: abnormally low level of haemoglobin in the blood. It is important as it is easy to detect and treat. It can cause fatigue, poor concentration, and failure to thrive.

Some of the most common causes are:
- Deficiency of haematinics, i.e. ferritin/iron, p.330; B_{12}, p.329; folate, p.467. Autoimmune interference (p.427) with with B_{12} absorption causes pernicious anaemia, with mild cognitive

impairment, paraesthesias, swollen red tongue. See also malnutrition, p.504; malabsorption (p.502);

- Haemoglobinopathies (sickle, p.549; thalassaemia, p.563).
- Blood loss, e.g. menorrhagia, p.506; worms, p.576.
- Red cell destruction, e.g. malaria, p.503; G6PD deficiency (haemolytic anaemia), p.350.
- Multifactorial, e.g. malignancy, p.569; schistosomiasis, p.543.

Angelman syndrome: ID, laughing and smiling, with a jerky gait (see *imprinting*, p.489).

Anger: p.289.
Ankylosing spondylitis: p.93.

Anorexia: formally, lack of appetite. Usually a shorthand for anorexia nervosa, p.334. See also infantile anorexia, p.332.

Anticipation: genetic problems appearing earlier in subsequent generations. For an example see *Huntington's*, p.482.

Antidepressants: there are several classes of these. See *SSRI*, p.552; *ideographs*, p.487.

Antiepileptics: their most common use is to relieve epileptic fits, but they also have useful effects distinct from seizure-control, p.73. They often cause sedation which appears as sleepiness, p.321 or stupor, p.99 or chronic fatigue, p.325 or even regression, p.47. Many of the antiepileptic medications can cause blood dyscrasias or liver toxicity. Rarely they cause hallucinations, pp.345, 349.

See valproate, p.572. Occasional effects of carbamazepine include violence, p.291; and polydipsia, p.338. Effects of phenytoin are numerous (e.g. p.338) as are those of barbiturates, (e.g. pp.258, 349). See also benzodiazepines, p.430, which are used in the emergency management of seizures.

Antihistamine: see *histamine*, p.479.

Anti-NMDA encephalitis: autoimmune attack (p.427) on NMDA receptors, which in children and adolescents usually presents as a psychiatric problem involving mood, behaviour, or personality change[507]. Other symptoms include confusion; hypersomnia or interrupted sleep; opisthotonus (p.93); and dyskinesias. These progress over a variable period (weeks to months) to seizures, stereotypies, and autonomic instability (p.428). In the past these were usually diagnosed as viral encephalitis (p.461).

Antipsychotics: important medication for psychosis (including schizophrenia). Used in lower doses in children and adolescents, for aggression, self-harm and repetitive behaviours (e.g. in autism[1038]) and in autism may gradually improve language and social skills somewhat[1775]. *Typical* antipsychotics are often used in adults. *Atypical* antipsychotics have fewer side-effects and are far more often used in children; their most troublesome side-effect is weight-gain (p.335), but they occasionally cause breast enlargement and galactorrhoea; pacing, p.114; oculogyric crises, p.93; parkinsonism, p.525; cold hands, p.562; tardive movements, p.561; and dystonic tongue and jaw muscles. In some individuals, effectiveness reduces over time[1422]. Weekly drug holidays of a day or two may be useful[1330]. See also *ideographs*, p.487.

Anxiety: p.295.

Inadequate anxiety is related to the common complaint by parents that "he shows no fear". In principle, it may be one of the contributory factors in common situations such as children impulsively darting into the road, sexual disinhibition, some violence, and people with ID climbing along the sides of buildings.

The reasons why inadequate anxiety is rarely identified as a problem in these situations are that (a) the accelerators for these misbehaviours are more obvious than the missing brakes. We are used to using a short list of accelerators to account for inappropriate behaviour (ADHD, hypomania, autism, or ID; see also p.262), and an even shorter list of missing brakes (inadequate or inappropriate knowledge about those situations, or inadequate interest in social norms), (b) treatments to weaken or divert the accelerators often work. Furthermore, educative treatments can usefully strengthen the child's brakes (anxiety) in dangerous situations, even though they are obviously not called anxiogenic treatments (similarly, getting one answer wrong can create anxiety on the next question, that improves performance in some tasks[1064]).

Counter-phobic fascinations lead many people to explore their own worst fears. They read about shipwrecks, act on stage[810], experiment with drugs, ride rollercoasters, or hurtle downhill on mountain bikes. This kind of experimentation is occasionally useful. For example, most people who have overcome a fear of tarantulas have achieved this through learning about them[854]. The example shows that the impression of inadequate anxiety can be created by people who have unusual expertise, often acquired by self-administered graded exposure during which they never stray too far from comfort.

Inadequate anxiety can be confined to just a few situations, and if it is suspected its extent should be mapped (as for excess anxiety, see figure on p.297). For example, lack of social anxiety can produce behaviour that is strikingly odd (and risky) such as sitting on strangers' laps. Deficits confined to one sphere like this require consideration of other possible explanations (e.g. autism, p.183; for other reasons see pp. 261, 249). A *pseudo-psychopathic* condition has been described following orbitofrontal lesions, characterised by ignoring social constraints, and inadequate anxiety[1626]. Compare *psychopathy*, p.280; *la belle indifference*, p.361; *learned helplessness*, p.96; *Yerkes-Dodson curve*, p.40.

Apgar Newborn Scoring System: a system devised by Dr Virginia Apgar for rating the health of a baby, one and five minutes after birth[49]. The baby receives 0, 1, or 2 points for each of five areas: **A**ppearance (complexion); **P**ulse rate; Reflex responses such as **G**rimace; Muscle tone or **A**ctivity; and **R**espiration. High scores (7–10) are correlated with good developmental outcomes.

Aphasia, Aquired Epileptic (AEA): pp.41, 45.
Approximate answers: p.357.
Apraxia: p.89.

Arm swinging during walking is reduced symmetrically by self-consciousness; or by hunched posture. It is initiated by the cerebellum (p.437), a lesion of which can produce an arm that just hangs or swings randomly during walking. Arm-swinging can be reduced in one or both arms by increased tone in shoulder muscles, as in dystonia or pain anywhere in the arm, or (rarely in children) parkinsonism (p.525).

Arousal: activation of sympathetic nervous system (including alertness, preparation for fight or flight (p.466), faster heart rate (p.478) and breathing, sweating (p.558), dilated pupils, etc.). Conditioned arousal and PTSD, p.127; reduced arousal in psychopathy, p.280; reduced arousal in learned violence, p.290; arousal in sensory intolerance, p.125ff; cortisol response to novelty in autism, p.125; effect of arousal on attitudes, p.283; effect of heat on violence, p.292.

Art therapy: this is a way of exploring a patient's feelings by helping him create drawings, paintings and sculpture. It is particularly useful when specific memories are difficult to talk about. The act of creating or communicating can itself be therapeutic. These methods can be used informally to assess a child's developmental level and preoccupations.

ASD: see *Autism and autistic spectrum disorders*, p.427.

ASOT: antistreptolysin O titre. See PANDAS, p.522.

Asperger's syndrome: a subset of autistic spectrum disorder. Speech milestones are normal, i.e. onset of phrase speech before 3. They are old-fashioned, pedantic (p.163), or have flat speech (p.467). They are aloof, can't understand why other people are interested in tedious things; they desire social contact but can't negotiotiate rules. Their social awkwardness gradually diminishes: the most difficult period of life is likely to be secondary school. After a diagnosis in childhood, this can mature in two ways: either to a somewhat rigid, robotic or eccentric adulthood, or simply into slow social and emotional maturing, approaching normal adult skills sometime in their twenties. There is little or nothing to distinguish this from high-functioning autism[1205] – so all these categories are likely to be combined into *autism spectrum disorder* in the next version of DSM.

Assisted conception: there are many subtypes of assisted conception, and the effects of each of them on child outcome have not been thoroughly studied yet. Assisted conception is used more by healthier, wealthier and older parents, in stable marriages[505], i.e. bringing social benefits to the child but also slightly increased risk of genetic disorders.

After conception, on the positive side these parents are especially likely to treasure their baby; the mothers are much less likely than most to become depressed while pregnant[505].

Unfortunately, conception is more likely to lead to multiple births and prematurity (p.432), and hence somewhat more likely to lead to developmental problems[738]. In addition, these mothers have held idealised views of maternity and can have difficulty adjusting to the losses of occupational identity, liberty and social activities after childbirth[505].

Asterixis: p.105.

Asthma: the most common chronic disease of children in developed countries. In asthma, *expiration* is prolonged and effortful, but usually in psychogenic breathlessness (p.457) *inspiration* is difficult instead, the teenager struggling to pull in more air. Children with asthma, especially severe asthma, have a considerably increased rate of emotional or behavioural problems (but not of antisocial behaviour), possibly due to stress, difficulty with medication management, and extra days off school[1054].

Occasionally there can be behavioural effects of the medicines used to treat asthma, e.g. steroids (p.554) and sympathomimetics (p.428).

Asymmetry: as a preoccupation in tiqueurs (the need to match/balance touches), p.64; as an obsession in OCD, p.65. Asymmetrical growth or pain causing asymmetrical postures, p.93; gait asymmetry, p.471; hand asymmetry, p.410; asymmetrical polio, p.573; malformations, p.503; focal overgrowth, hemihyperplasia and hemihypertrophy, p.521.

Ataxia: p.88.
Ataxia telangiectasia: p.454.
Atomoxetine: p.516.
Attachment: p.195.

Attention: "how it is that the organism can effectively regulate its receptiveness to stimuli and its readiness to respond to them." [1587]. Aspects of this include:
- Intensive attention: being aroused to a purpose
- Sustained attention: persisting in a task (also called concentration)
- Selective attention: avoiding distraction
- Controlled attention: narrowing or broadening the focus, or focusing on multiple sources.

Attention Deficit Hyperactivity Disorder (ADHD) ☝: For general discussion of ADHD diagnosis, see p.83. For DSM criteria, see p.383.

Attitude: (a) In common usage, this means oppositionality (p.253) or rudeness (p.161).

(b) It is also a term from social psychology, meaning the degree of favour or disfavour with which an individual regards an object. Attitudes produce cognitive, affective and behavioural signs when relevant stimuli are encountered. The evolutionary purpose of attitudes may be to rapidly trigger approach or avoidance[1779]. Like emotions, they are created by a mixture of top-down and bottom-up processing, that can be imaged (in mainly frontal and sensory cortices, respectively)[350,1118]. People often fail to report their true attitudes when asked, but attitudes can be accurately measured covertly by the amount of arousal people experience in carefully chosen situations[263,615].

The term is usually used to reflect long-term predispositions, but an attitude can alter briefly (transient oppositionality, p.254; pseudo-regression, p.43; effect of arousal on attitudes, p.283; attitudes that vary depending on which categorising system is currently in mind[1093]). See also *ambivalent feelings*, p.287.

Examples. Attitudes shape important aspects of life such as friendship, attraction, attachment, conformity, voting, health behaviour, sociability and prejudices. They govern a child's behaviour in class and his response to bullies (p.219). They have a major influence on the amount of homework, reading and sports he does. Parental attitudes to school and the law have a major influence on his behaviour. Their attitudes to him, and to his his successes or failures, influence his mood and his attitudes and the parent-child relationship (see, e.g., p.250). The child's and teacher's attitudes to each other are crucial, p.215. A child's not wanting to grow up can result from or influence other attitudes: see *anorexia*, p.334; *tomboy*, p.566; sibling rivalry, p.213. A negative attitude to adults (or the appearance of it) can be self-protective, as in the semi-mute truculent teen who rejects criticism and some feelings of failure; but this also makes engaging with health services difficult.

Attribution: this is a term for "perception of causation"[827]. Trying to work out the causes of other people's behaviour is a major preoccupation of humans. Crucial aspects of attributions (also applying to causes in this book) are (a) who is blamed, (b) to what extent could they control what happened, and (c) whether this a long-term or a brief effect.

To some extent, people tend to make the same kinds of causal attributions throughout their lives (see *predictable irrationality*, p.534). There is a major self-serving / self-protecting bias, but this is only part of the story. For example, people in unhappy relationships tend to attribute their difficulties to long-term, general, internally caused factors. Conversely positive behaviour by others is often assumed to be a short-term specific effect, caused by something external that was going on at the time[1447].

Attributions can have major effects on long-term relationships because when a minor problem occurs the attribution can minimise or magnify it[1008].

Such patterns are often seen in a parent's attitude (p.425) to his or her child (i.e. how the parent *attributes* the behaviour). For example, misbehaviour that the child objectively cannot control often elicits the feeling within the parent that the child is intentionally winding him/her up. This can become so severe that parents describe it as brief hatred (p.187). A child's difficulties can be *attributed* to (say) a genetic inheritance from the father, which can obviously be endearing or frightening depending on the circumstances. Conversely, some parents *attribute* a child's disability or suffering to something they themselves did (e.g. separating from a spouse, or not being faithful, or giving the wrong medicine) then spend many unhappy years trying to make it up to the child.

The attribution style of a child may predispose him to certain clinical conditions. For example, children who habitually blame misfortunes on themselves will often feel shame and guilt (p.475), and are more likely to become depressed. On the other hand, people who habitually blame others (called external personal attribution bias) are more likely to develop paranoid ideas (p.524)[180].

Certain conditions, such as addiction, self-harm and anorexia nervosa, are often attributed by family and society to personal choice, i.e. that it was under their *control*, which is another aspect of attributions. These conditions elicit less sympathy and care than other conditions (e.g. ID or deafness) which are viewed by most as just very bad luck.

Attributions can be culturally determined (p.448). Appropriate attributions are one aspect of insight into one's condition (p.491). See also *fundamental attribution error*, pp.18, 241; *guilt*, p.475.

Atypical disorders: These are different from the best-recognised forms, as in "atypical depression" (p.314), "atypical autism" (p.183), "atypical eating disorders" (p.458); "atypical psychosis"[1502] (pp.537, 449). The DSM term is "NOS", as in "PDD-NOS" meaning "pervasive developmental disorder, not otherwise specified." These "NOS" disorders are highly heterogeneous, and there are frequent attempts to carve them into smaller more homogeneous pieces. This is occasionally clinically useful, though little rigorous research has been done on them.

Auditory: see *Ears*.

Autism ☝ and *autistic spectrum disorders* ☝: These most commonly refer to the formal diagnoses (p.388) but are also used more loosely to mean a child being excessively self-contained, in a world of his own. For general discussion of the diagnoses, see pp.183, 442. For DSM criteria: p.388; autism-related interests: p.229; autistic repetitive behaviours (stimming): p.64; autistic intolerance: p.126; eating behaviours: p.331. For comparison with schizoid personality disorder (p.242) in adults see[821].

Apparent increases in autism prevalence over recent decades are attributable to changes in diagnostic criteria and professional awareness[1397,1773]. Autism is not increased by the MMR vaccine (p.508) nor by thimerosal (p.330). For causes of autism see p.186.

Differential diagnosis: for distinction from compulsions: p.67; from avoidance: p.230; from psychosis: p.538; from tics: p.101; from other causes of regression: p.41; from ADHD: p.82; from other causes of deviant development: p.49; from pre-sleep stereotypies: p.200; from other causes of repetitive behaviours: p.63; from other causes of intolerance: p.125; from other causes of language deficits: p.145; from other causes of echolalia, p.459; from other causes of social difficulty: p.181; from other causes of a special interest: p.228; from catatonia, p.98.

Comorbidities: with anxiety, p.126; with selective mutism: p.156; with depression: p.309; with visual impairment: p.134; with ID: p.184; with ADHD: p.25,84.

Autoimmune conditions: conditions in which the immune system attacks normal tissue. Most are idiopathic, e.g. SLE, p.560; juvenile rheumatoid arthritis. Some are triggered by infections (PANDAS, p.522; Kleine-Levin, p.496) or by milk allergy (cerebral folate deficiency, p.467), or caused by genetic disorder (e.g. Down's, p.455); occasionally they are ☜ paraneoplastic (p.524). Other autoimmune conditions can coexist and should be searched for (e.g. p.352). See Stiff Person syndrome, p.555; Eaton-Lambert syndrome, p.459; Cogan's syndrome, p.442; anti-NMDA encephalitis, p.422; ANA, p.421. Note that interpretation of immunology results can be complex[971].

Type 1 (allergy / atopy).

Type 2 (IgG and IGM antibody-dependent cell-mediated): pernicious anaemia, p.421; myasthenia gravis, p.510.

Type 3 (immune complex): SLE, p.560.

Type 4 (cell-mediated, T-cells): Guillain-Barré, p.87; multiple sclerosis, p.510.

Automatism: semicoordinated, repetitive motor activities with impaired awareness. These occur in both focal and generalised seizures. They occur in the majority of children with absences, especially when elicited by hyperventilation[1416]. Perseverative automatisms continue behaviours that started before the seizure. Scratching automatisms can be started by light touch during an absence.

Hence automatisms vary between seizures in a single child, and many different oral and manual automatisms have been described[1416].

Autonomic Nervous System (ANS): neurons outside the central nervous system, many of which are not directly controlled by the central nervous system. These create effects that usually do not reach awareness, i.e. controlling homeostasis and acute adaptations. The ANS is subdivided into sympathetic, parasympathetic and enteric nervous systems.

Sympathetic nervous system (SNS, thoracolumbar n.s.): neurons outside the central nervous system that control the body's immediate stress response, p.556, including anxiety, p.295; and vomiting, p.337. The SNS can be activated by excitement, fright, or hypoglycaemia, p.82.

Sympathomimetics are medicines that enhance or mimic the effects of the sympathetic nervous system, e.g. bronchodilators used in asthma; stimulants (p.555); decongestants; and cocaine (p.258). Clonidine generally has the opposite effects, p.441.

Parasympathetic nervous system (PSNS, craniosacral n.s.): this exerts neural control on body organs, in a way that is complementary to, and usually slower and more focused than, the sympathetic nervous system.

The following table summarises the main effects of the SNS and PSNS (after[78]).

	SNS	PSNS
Eye – pupil	dilatation	constriction
Eye – ciliary muscle	relax (far vision)	constrict (near vision)
Eye – lacrimal gland	slight secretion	secretion (p.315)
GI – salivary glands	slight secretion	secretion
GI – general	decreased motility	increased motility
Lungs	bronchodilation	bronchodilation (sic)
Bladder – detrusor	relax	contract
Bladder – sphincter	contract	relax
Genitals – male	ejaculation	erection (p.462)
Sweat glands	sweat (p.558)	palmar sweating
CVS – heart	↑rate and force	↓rate and force
CVS – arterioles	constriction	(no effect)
Muscles – arterioles	constric. or dilatation	(no effect)
Muscles–metabolism	glycogenolysis	(no effect)

Problems involving the ANS include syncope, p.74; vomiting, p.337; cyclic vomiting syndrome, p.449; breath-holding spells, p.434; insomnia, p.199; migraine, p.141; constipation, p.444; dry eyes, p.108; self mutilation, p.317; emotional instability, p.70; psychopathy, p.280. Specific syndromes include autonomic epilepsy, p.76; sensory and autonomic neuropathies, p.136; trigeminal autonomic headaches, p.140; autonomic hyperreflexia, p.299; Fabry's disease, p.464.

Autonomic instability (a subtype of dysautonomia) includes tachycardia, hyperthermia, hypertension, and sometimes hypoventilation. It is uncommon but seen in many conditions such as neuroleptic malignant syndrome, p.514; anti-NMDA, p.422; porphyria, p.532; Lyme disease, p.501; Ehlers-Danlos, p.460.

See also *temperature*, p.562

Aversion: specific intolerances, p.127; symptom of catatonia, p.98.

Avoidance: a common cause of behavioural symptoms. There are many things that children try to avoid (fears, p.307; aversions, p.127; too much of anything, p.123) and many ways they avoid them (see intolerance strategies, p.126). Avoidance has many causes other than fear, as in a child who avoids the school hall because he hates the music there, or because he is not allowed to take his favourite toys or playstation there. When avoidance is conscious it is called a coping mechanism (p.445); when unconscious a defence mechanism (p.303) of which one is dissociation (p.453). Avoidance is an important mechanism in many named disorders (such as selective mutism, p.153) and also one of the criteria for PTSD (p.532). Avoidance can be covert, e.g. of tics or obsessions / compulsions. The degree of avoidance is indicated by the range of things avoided (pp.295, 307), their individual thresholds (e.g. avoiding unpleasant tasks is commonplace whereas avoiding pleasant tasks needs explanation), arousal (see above), and duration. There are many types of autistic stereotypy (pp.64, 229), some of which can be used to avoid unwanted stimulation; examples include headbanging, p.119; and hand-biting, p.113. Avoidance of scholastic tasks is a major problem often caused by specific developmental problems (children conscious of their difficulties, which doesn't happen in profound ID and can start as late as puberty if the impairment is mild). See also *Pathological Demand Avoidance*, p.527.

Axes: of diagnoses, p.16; of play and interests, pp.221 and 227.
Babble: See stages of speech, p.143.
Baby talk: p.41.
Back symptoms: p.93.

Balance: vestibular sense, p.122; need to balance left and right, p.64; balanced translocations, p.439; forced balancing, p.64.

Bardet-Biedl syndrome: this is a ciliopathy (p.440). It often includes ID, retinitis pigmentosa, obesity, hypogonadism, polydactyly, hypoplasia of the corpus callosum (p.445), and several other ciliopathic effects[90].

Basal ganglia: large nuclei in the centre of the brain whose main role seems to be initiating behaviours. See slowness, p.95; parkinsonism, p.525; anti-BG antibodies in PANDAS, p.522; hand-wringing, p.477; dysprosody, p.148.

Calcification of the basal ganglia has many causes[1639], of which the most important treatable one is hypoparathyroidism. A rare cause is Fahr's disease, also called idiopathic basal ganglia calcification, whose earliest symptoms can be motor, cognitive or psychiatric.

BDD: body dysmorphic disorder, p.433.

Beckwith-Wiedemann syndrome: a genetic disorder of great variability, caused by imprinting (p.489) and sometimes undetected in the parents. Most of the symptoms are examples of *overgrowth*, p.521. It generally includes two of: large tongue, weight over 90th centile, midline defects in abdominal wall, ear creases/pits, and neonatal hypoglycaemia. One side of the body or face may be larger than the other (hemihyperplasia). IQ is usually normal. Risk of cancer is increased (see p.569). See *imprinting*, p.489.

Bed-sharing: p.198.

Behavioural phenotype: behaviours associated with a genotype. *Social phenotypes* are one subtype, and can sometimes be sufficient to recognise a syndrome[490]. A broader approach is to look for behavioural patterns that help diagnostically[1628], whether or not the underlying cause is genetic (e.g. the hyperorality and hypermetamorphosis of *Klüver-Bucy*, p.496). Furthermore, some believe that behaviours should be combined with accompanying physical dysmorphology and neuro-psychological findings, to aid in linking behaviour to genes[1670].

Behavioural phenotypes can be:
- Specific, though not sensitive. Examples include the hand-wringing of Rett, p.541; the mutilating unliked self-harm of Lesch-Nyhan, p.318; the excessive interest in faces, even of strangers, in Williams syndrome, p.177; the extraordinarily ambivalent eye-gaze of Fragile X, p.176. Some would include the hyperorality (not oral exploration) of *Klüver-Bucy*, p.496; and the navigation difficulties of callosal agenesis, p.445, but though specific these are not linked to a specific genotype.
- Moderately specific. One example is the love of imitation in Down's syndrome. Others are the hyperphagia, atypical bipolar disorder and severe skin-picking of Prader-Willi, p.533. When combined these are very specific.
- Non-specific. Examples include the increase in neurodevelopmental syndromes of Fragile X, p.468; the over-sociability of Down's syndrome, p.455; the speech dysfluencies associated with ID (see *cluttering*, p.441); the assorted psychiatric problems of VCFS, p.572.

Behavioural inhibition: p.296. See also *Inhibition*.

Belching: release of accumulated swallowed air from the stomach or the oesophagus. It is usually associated with more troublesome symptoms such as gastroesophageal reflux (GORD, p.472), bloating or dyspepsia. It can also be a learned behaviour, with air-swallowing (into the oesophagus, called aerophagia) and belching up to 20 times a minute [213]. This is sometimes a sign of anxiety, in which case it is associated with features of anxiety rather than of gastrointestinal disease. Inability to belch occurs in rare conditions and can result in severe abdominal symptoms[213].

Benzodiazepines: a group of sedative medications. They are important in the short-term treatment of anxiety and epilepsy, and in the diagnosis and treatment of catatonia (p.98). In a small minority of people, small doses cause disinhibition and even violence (which of course do not settle if even larger doses of benzodiazepines are given). See also *temperature*, p.562.

Bereavement: children's normal reactions to bereavement depend very much on their age, the nature of the relationship, and whether there is a surviving carer with a close relationship[1724]. Specific problems can include certainty that the deceased person will return; feeling that they or someone else is responsible; being angry about the unfairness of the loss and about consequent life changes; and feeling that they are now different from other children. Below age 7–10, they often express these feelings most clearly in their play or drawings – which they can then talk about.

For most children, the expected effects in the year following the death of a parent are comparable to very mild depression. Surprisingly, the severity of effects is not usually affected by whether the death was expected or sudden. However children are likely to have more severe difficulties if the remaining parent is depressed; or if the death was through suicide; or if family income is badly affected[275]. Such difficulties include anxiety, depression, anger and behavioural regression.

The five classic stages of preparation for one's *own* death are shock / denial, anger, bargaining, depression and finally acceptance[883]. These five stages have been used to understand people's reactions to loss of family members – or of jobs, abilities and even expectations. Kübler-Ross emphasised that preparation for dying is an individual process, so the stages are very variable and may also include fear, relief, hope, etc[826].

See post-bereavement hallucination, p.344; bereavement anniversaries, p.62; revenge, p.245; risk factor for suicide, p.320; bereavement leading to worries about one's own health, p.360; parents' repeated bereavement in ID, p.211.

Bestiality: p.268.

Bewilderment, momentary disorientation, and repeated alerting: The child looks puzzled, stares, and looks around as if to work out who people are – or where she is (photos in[1359]). Classify as follows:

Momentary: Momentary out-of-the-blue disorientation can occur after absences (p.75) or other covert seizures.

Relaxed: Disorientation following day-dreams (p.450) usually has a clear relation to sleepiness and dozing, and the child is relaxed enough to look around more slowly.

Prolonged: In delirium (p.451) the confusion often lasts for hours or days, often fluctuating.

Psychosis: This can produce prolonged bewilderment, either due to delusions or delusional mood, p.544. Bewilderment can also be momentary, if there are brief hallucinations (see p.344).

Clarify with an EEG and consider trial of anti-epileptic medication.

BG: basal ganglia, p.429
BIF: Borderline Intellectual Functioning, p.434.

Bilateral skills: these require much more skill and planning (coordination) than unilateral movements. *Stabilising* by the non-dominant hand is progressively more difficult in holding a yoghurt pot while eating; holding paper still while drawing; and holding meat with a fork to cut it. Sequences of bilateral movements of varying complexity are used in tying shoes and piano playing; lego is less regimented. Clapping is symmetrical and works even if performed inaccurately. Skipping (skipping rope is symmetrical; skipping along is alternating). Midline stereotypies (p.64). See *Mirror movements*, p.507; *synkinesis*, p.560.

Bilingual: to be a native speaker in two languages conveys great benefits, socially and sometimes occupationally[172]. The cost of achieving this in normal children is very small: it delays language acquisition by about 3 months. However in children with extremely poor language skills, who struggle for years to learn their first few words, and who remain unable to learn that words from home don't work at school, the cost is much higher.

Bilharzia: see *schistosomiasis*, p.543.

Binkie flutter: mandibular trembling, seen as vibration of a dummy (pacifier) between bouts of vigorous sucking[535].

Biotin: p.32.
Bipolar Affective Disorder: p.264.

Birth: this can be vaginal, by Caesarean section, or using forceps or suction (Ventouse). The proportions delivered by each method vary greatly around the world.

Establishing causation of problems recognised in childhood
Even if mother reports that her child had a birth difficulty, and the difficulty is known to be *associated* with developmental problems, one cannot be certain that it *caused* the problems. For example, even if one knows obstetric errors were committed, it is not certain that the baby would have been fine without the errors, or indeed without an obstetrician. Similarly, cerebral palsy is often treated as synonymous with birth injury, but there can be preceding causes (p.437).

Generally the best one can do is (very roughly) estimate the likely effect size of each of the multiple risk factors. For example, one can estimate the risks due to low birth weight, p.432; meconium, p.506; cord around neck, p.445; prematurity (below); low Apgar, p.423; and previous stillbirths[1136]. These "obstetric" risks need to be considered together with genetic risks, p.379; intrauterine risks, p.393; and postnatal risks, p.393. Intrauterine infection by CMV or toxoplasmosis can be detected by retrospective analysis of stored heelprick samples.

Prematurity
Prematurity is defined as birth before 37 weeks of gestation. Many problems become increasingly common as gestational age decreases, including ID; retinopathy, pneumonia, feeding difficulty, p.331; and memory deficits (see *hippocampus*, p.478). Birth trauma is much more common in premature births and can result in cerebral palsy, p.437. There are very many factors, in mother, baby, and placenta, that increase the risk of prematurity, but few of them are individually decisive[1430].

For high birth weight see overgrowth, p.521.

Birth order: p.548.

Birth weight: for high birth weight see *overgrowth*, p.521.

Low birth weight is obviously on a continuum but is usually defined as below 1500 g, with *extremely low birth weight (ELBW)* below 1000 g. Improvements in neonatal care have led to increased survival of unimpaired infants, and also increased survival of impaired infants. Low birth weight babies are often premature (p.432) and have increased risk of cerebral palsy (p.437), hydrocephalus (p.482), ID and a wide range of cognitive, motor and psychiatric difficulties. Girls who were low birth weight have a 22% risk of depression in adolescence, versus 4% in those who were not LBW[323]. This increase in depression does not occur in boys.

Biting: p.113.
Bizarre: p.343; *bizarre delusions*, p.348.

Blaming: (a) A learned coping mechanism (p.445) that avoids negative sanctions for onself and shifts them on to someone else (e.g. a rival sibling). For mysterious problems, blame offers clarity, avoids disquieting explanations, and suggests straightforward solutions (comparable to the resolution of cognitive dissonance, p.355). Fear of blame is an important contributor to social responsibility. (b) A developmental stage between ignorance of causation and recognition of its complexity.

Blinking: p.108.
Blindism, blindness: see p.133.

Blocking: (a) in learning theory: when an animal has learned that CS1 predicts US, this prevents it from learning that CS1+CS2 predicts US.

(b) blocking as a defence mechanism, p.306.

(c) a form of thought disorder (p.563) in which the train of thought is suddenly lost[1487]. Also called thought blocking.

Blood tests: see *general approach*, p.373; difficult blood testing, p.373.
Blunting of affect: discussed with *flattening*, p.467.

Blurting: answering a question before the questioner has finished. This is one of the DSM symptoms of impulsivity (p.383). Doing it correctly requires carers who produce predictable sentences, good speed of understanding and speech, correct prediction of the end of the sentence, and rapid speech. Disinterest, depression, delay in learning or language, or trained politeness will all prevent correct blurting. Blurting out *wrong* answers is a combination of two signs, i.e. not waiting and getting it wrong, which is useful because you can test what needs to be changed to make the answer right (p.256).

Blushing: p.460

BMI: body mass index, calculated as mass/height^2, with the mass in kilograms and the height in metres.

BNF: *British National Formulary* (standard list of medicines and doses).

Body dysmorphic disorder: preoccupation with the idea that one's appearance is abnormal. This should not be trivialised as it is often accompanied by depression, social phobia, and OCD, and leads not only to cosmetic surgery but also to school refusal, bullying and increased risk of suicide. It usually starts in adolescence.

Screening questions to distinguish it from simple dissatisfaction with a body part include not only whether the patient's description is consonant with the degree of deformity, but also: How noticeable do you think it is to other people? How many hours do you spend thinking about it each day? How many times a day do you check it? Does it lead you to avoid social situations?[1666]

A subtype of BDD called "muscle dysmorphia" has been described[1265] in which people are preoccupied with the amount of muscle (compare anorexia athletica and reverse anorexia, p.458).

For other appearance-related issues see tattoos, p.561; anorexia nervosa, p.334; self-identity, p.237.

Body odour: odour is difficult to describe accurately, to discuss sensitively, or to compare with published descriptions. However it occasionally points to the cause of a child's behavioural difficulties.

The commonest problems are infrequent washing, dirty clothes, urinary accidents, and faecal handling problems (dirty nappy, poor wiping; smearing, p.342; anal masturbation, p.115). Other common smells are perfumes, talc, cooking smells, alcohol, and cannabis. Body odour changes at puberty. *Localised* odours are found with nasal foreign bodies, ear infections, and infected vaginal discharge. There are many causes of bad breath (halitosis) including tonsillitis, dental infection, plaque on the posterior surface of the tongue, and eating garlic or onion[1475,1754]. Rarely, breath chromatography may aid diagnosis[1754].

Poor hygiene should not be ignored for the sake of politeness, because it can lead to taunts and friendship difficulties. It is not a simple indicator of mild neglect (p.274), because the family may be subculturally different or eccentric, or the child may be using violence or stratagems to avoid bathing. The topic can be approached by asking about the child's progress toward full self-care. Like all potentially offensive comments it needs to be discussed with parents before being included in a report.

Rare metabolic causes of unusual body odours (pp.18–20 of [703]) include maple syrup disease, p.505; the sweet smell of acetone as in ketoacidosis, p.338; animal-like in PKU, p.529; acrid like sweaty feet in isovaleric or glutaric aciduria; cabbage in methionine malabsorption or tyrosinaemia; rancid butter as also found in tyrosinaemia; and strikingly unpleasant in trimethylaminuria and dimethylglycinuria (which can seem garbage-like or fish-like depending on the intensity)[1322,1754].

See also osmophobia, p.128; olfactory hallucinations, p.344; relationship to orexin, p.491; anosmia, pp.485, 342, 525.

Borderline: *Borderline Intellectual Functioning* is defined as IQ 71–84, and is sometimes called *Borderline Learning Disability* (see table of IQ, p.59). See also *Borderline Personality Disorder*, p.242.

Boredom: p.322.

Boundaries: rules regulating a child and his environment. These ensure safety, improve socialising, and make the child feel more secure. The term oversimplifies developmental tasks of learning multiple rules, their hierarchy, and appropriate ways of behaving when they conflict. The term *boundaried* describes people who follow rules carefully, particularly rules *against* doing something. See breaking rules, p.249; necessary aspects of parenting, p.189.

Bowlby, John: originator of attachment theory (p.195).
BP: blood pressure.
BPAD: bipolar affective disorder, p.264.

BPD: Borderline PD, p.242; Bipolar Affective Disorder, p.264. (also biparietal diameter, bronchopulmonary dysplasia).

BPPV: benign paroxysmal positional vertigo, p.454.

Brainstem: in sensory processing, p.121; evoked responses in anxiety, p.125; central pattern generators, p.547; flinching, p.107. See also *reticular formation*, p.541.

Breath-holding spells: there are two kinds, both involuntary, mainly affecting preschoolers. If the child has no pulmonary or cardiac disease, these spells are physically benign; but they can make limit-setting difficult. Useful to know in order to avoid mistakenly confusing them with (voluntary) temper tantrums (p.286). Also, the history of the trigger avoids incorrectly diagnosing epilepsy (p.73).

	Reflex anoxic seizure (RAS)[1752]	Expiratory apnoea syncope (EAS)[1751]
Usual colour	white/pale	blue/cyanosed
Trigger	pain such as from bump on head, or a sudden fright, causes reflex vagal cardioinhibition	fright or anger
Onset	colour drains to grey, pale, or bluish, child loses consciousness	child is crying, yet stuck in expiration, with mouth open unable to start the next inspiration
Severity	dystonic posture of arms and hands, and some irregular jerks of arms or body (i.e. like a tonic-clonic epileptic seizure).	usually mild. *Rarely*, the apnoea is sufficiently prolonged to cause an anoxic seizure.
Termination	lasts 10–20 seconds then relaxes, often with post-ictal sleep	lasts a few seconds, then ends with a gasp of air.
Investigation	if recurrent consider Fe, EEG, cardiology	none needed.

Breathlessness: see *dyspnoea*, p.457.
Bruxism: p.200.

Bubble bursting: the replacement of overoptimistic ideas with realism. This is commonplace in life, as in the financial world, and in the history of science[884]. Wishful thinking (p.534) can produce a self-consistent network of ideas, supporting one another. When new ideas are acquired that contradict the existing network of ideas, cognitive dissonance (p.355) is created, and when this becomes sufficiently severe the entire network of ideas collapses. For example, a boy whose main understanding of himself and of seduction was based on thousands of hours of video games, had a very rude awakening when he tried to treat a real girl in the way that worked in the game.

Bulimia: p.337.
Bullying: p.219.
BUN: blood urea nitrogen.
Burping: see *Belching*, p.430.

Calcium: see hypocalcaemia, p.485; hypercalcaemia, p.483; Eaton-Lambert syndrome, p.459; calcium channelopathies, p.438; parathyroid hormone, p.525.

CAMHS: Child and Adolescent Mental Health Services. Sometimes called CFCS, Child and Family Consultation Service.

Camp: p.243.
Cancer: see *tumours*, p.569.
CAPD: *Central Auditory Processing Disorder*, p.121.
Casting: p.103.

Catalepsy: prolonged delay in correcting an externally imposed posture. It is a graded phenomenon that depends on the degree of discomfort, the ease of finding a new position, the level of environmental stimulation, and the person's usual rate of movement. Unsurprisingly therefore, there are several pharmacological subtypes[1424] and distinct conditions involving it, including catatonia, p.98 and parkinsonism, p.525. Distinct from *cataplexy*, below.

Cataplexy: sudden transient collapse produced by loss of muscle tone, sometimes precipitated by strong emotion, typically laughter, joy, surprise, tickle or anger[1561]. Cataplexy is a symptom of *narcolepsy*, p.72, and uses the same mechanism that prevents people thrashing about during REM sleep[1479]. Nevertheless, when cataplexy happens in narcolepsy, it only lasts for a few seconds and the person stays awake. Knee buckling is characteristic of cataplexy[1561]. Cataplexy in children is often atypical, sometimes with a "cataplectic face" of dropped jaw and eyelids and slumped head, rarely accompanied by slurred speech[1454]. Cataplexy is quite different from epilepsy as it is a subcortical effect with sudden reduction in noradrenaline activity in the locus coeruleus[1803]. Distinguish other causes of drop attacks, p.75 and *catalepsy*, above.

Cataracts: opacification of the lens, one of the common causes of blindness, p.133. The causes of childhood cataracts are not found in the majority of cases, but if identified can shed light on behavioural problems. An ophthalmological examination can reduce the length of the following list of possible causes[116]:

Inherited (mild cataracts in relatives may be asymptomatic); injury (sometimes from physical abuse, p.273); oxygen therapy; Down's syndrome, p.455; hypocalcaemia, p.485; hypoglycaemia, p.82; diabetes, p.451; galactosaemia, p.472; steroids, p.554; radiation; eczema; juvenile rheumatoid arthritis; rubella and other TORCH infections, p.490; cerebrotendinous xanthomatosis, p.32.

Catatonia: p.98. Distinguishing from autism, p.98.
Catch-up: see *late developers*, p.496.
Causes: p.393.

CBCL: Child Behavior Checklist[5]. This lists 113 behaviours (similar to those in this book). Depending on whether they happen never, sometimes or often, they are added up into a series of summary scores. These are internalising, externalising, aggressive, anxious/depressed, withdrawn, delinquent, attention, sex, social, somatic and thought.

CD: conduct disorder, p.249; cognitive dissonance, p.355; coeliac disease, p.441.

CDD: childhood disintegrative disorder, p.46.
CELF: Clinical Evaluation of Language Fundamentals, p.51.
Central Auditory Processing Disorder (CAPD): p.121.

Central pontine myelinolysis: damage to the brainstem, especially affecting white matter (p.574), which is rare but most often results from metabolic complications of polydipsia, alcoholism, anorexia, or rapid correction of hyponatraemia. Symptoms range from hallucinations and delusions to locked-in syndrome (p.97) and death[228].

Central sensitisation (of pain): a spinal mechanism responsible for some of the increased pain in fibromyalgia[777,1793], p.466; complex regional pain[764], p.136; chronic fatigue syndrome[1163], p.323; irritable bowel syndrome, p.494; and numerous other pain-related disorders[1793].

Cerebellum: part of the brain traditionally believed to fine-tune muscle activity. It has clear roles in maintaining muscle tone (constant slight tension: for hypotonia, look for the pendular stretch reflex in a hanging knee) and muscle strength; making voluntary movements rapid and precise (failure of this at the end of movements produces the clinical sign of *past pointing*; during movements produces *intention tremor*; and in movement reversals produces the sign of *dysdiadochokinesis*, p.457); synchronising simultaneous movements at multiple joints (look for shin-heel or finger-nose incoordination); creating associated movements such as arm-swinging, p.423; and the automatisation of motor skills. Gait and saccades are also regulated by the cerebellum[710,927]. Developmental Coordination Disorder (DCD ☂, p.89) is therefore often conceived as primarily cerebellar dysfunction[e.g.1678].

However the simple "motor cerebellum" notion is in question for several reasons. Other brain areas can learn to compensate for cerebellar motor deficits[710], making it likely that responsibilities are also shared during normal functioning. Also cerebellar abnormalities are associated with many non-motor deficiencies.

These non-motor deficiencies constitute the exceedingly variable *cerebellar cognitive affective syndrome* which can be life-long. It includes many domains including visuospatial learning, emotion regulation and working memory[1009,1557]; repetitive behaviours, sensory intolerance, psychosis and social deficits[1437]. Cerebellar damage can cause or contribute to disorders such as dyslexia[1158] and ADHD ☂[273]. In addition, after cerebellar surgery or other damage, patients can be awake but mute, and sometimes refusing food[1270], for weeks or months (*cerebellar syndrome* or *posterior fossa syndrome*); children who do not suffer this complication tend also to be spared from long-term cognitive and affective symptoms[1343].

Cerebral palsy: ☂congenital motor problems. Subtypes are spastic (the majority, subclassified as hemiplegic, diplegic or tetraplegic), dyskinetic, ataxic and athetoid. Some subtypes have more associated comorbidities. If only one or two limbs are affected, there is usually no ID.

Because the processes damaging motor cortex in CP often damage other cortical areas as well, CP is *associated with* numerous developmental problems. Three quarters have low visual acuity; 30% have epilepsy, and a similar proportion have ID[1182]. Sensory problems include impaired two-point discrimination (in about half); poor stereognosis; and allodynia (p.136). Three quarters have speech problems.

Family or school may wrongly believe that CP is a purely motor problem; some websites encourage this. Problems with peer relationships are quite common in CP. General factors that cause psychological problems in non-disabled children tend to have a bigger effect than the CP itself [1220].

Despite over 80% of babies with CP having abnormal brain imaging, it is often impossible to be sure of the cause[874]. A third have had birth-related problems, and 40% were premature[562]. Many have signs of hypoxic-ischaemic encephalopathy (p.486) or perinatal stroke (p.556). Ten percent have a brain malformation[874]. Underlying these broad categories ☂ are many more specific conditions, justifying detailed history and physical examination, detailed family history, neuroimaging, and often genetic or metabolic investigations[1433].

Like Landau-Kleffner, p.45, and epilepsy in general, p.73, cerebral palsy is a problem that, through being overt, named and recognisable, attracts more attention than less overt syndromes with the same cellular pathology but in more hidden brain areas.

Cerebrotendinous xanthomatosis: p.32.

Challenging behaviour: term used to refer to aggression, destruction, self-injury, tantrums, eating inappropriate things, and repetitive movements, usually in people with ID.

There is no consensus on a threshold of severity to justify using the term[96]. Suggestions have included "behaviour which is likely to delay access to ordinary community facilities", having "at some time" caused "more than minor injury" to self or others, placing staff "in danger" at least once a week, causing "more than a few minutes' disruption daily", and even the hyperkinesis of Fragile X. Some have included not drinking, or risking exclusion from school.

The word *challenging* implies that the behaviours are voluntary, and exist in order to challenge other people – or that they are challenging to manage. Often neither is the case. It is also misleading to group together such diverse behaviours as those listed above. Furthermore, it is misleading to use a different term for these behaviours just when they occur in people with ID. See *ideograph*, p.487.

Channelopathies: (these characteristically cause paroxysmal rather than continuous symptoms, for reasons that remain unknown[343,886])

a) voltage-gated calcium channels
   i) malignant hyperthermia.
   ii) some subtypes of hemiplegic migraine, p.142.
   iii) Eaton-Lambert syndrome, p.459.
b) Voltage-gated sodium channels cause diverse conditions, especially cardiac arrhythmias (such as long QT syndrome), periodic paralyses, and epilepsy (see *hyperexcitability syndromes*). Seome examples are listed here:
   i) in severe myoclonic epilepsy of infancy (Dravet syndrome), 75% of patients have a new mutation in the SCN1A gene and are very severely affected with a high risk of ID. A more benign outcome is seen in the inherited mutations that have been selected in the evolutionary sense of permitting parents to reproduce, and which are classified as GEFS+, generalised epilepsy with febrile seizures plus[400]. In contradistinction, deletions affecting this gene as well as its neighbours cause the combination of Dravet syndrome plus dysmorphic features[373].
   ii) hyperkalaemic periodic paralysis: episodes of extreme weakness lasting minutes to hours, triggered by rest after exercise, potassium-rich foods, stress, fatigue
   iii) paramyotonia congenita – myotonia with exercise or cold.
   iv) some subtypes of hemiplegic migraine, p.142
   v) primary erythromelalgia / erythermalgia.
c) voltage-gated potassium channels
   i) neuromyotonia
   ii) episodic ataxia 1 (induced by startle, exertion, or stress).

d) chloride channel: myotonia congenita: stiff movements that loosen on repetition.

Chaos: in the family, p.212; in children's behaviour, p.84.
Charcot-Marie-Tooth disease: p.87.

CHARGE syndrome: the combination of coloboma, heart defects, atresia of the nasal choanae, retardation of development, genital or urinary abnormalities, and ear abnormalities or deafness. Seventy per cent have a CHD7 mutation. Numerous additional physical problems are associated, as well as psychiatric diagnoses of anxiety in 20%, autism-related conditions in 16%, and ADHD in 12%[1694].

Cheating: the majority of people will cheat if they want a prize and are confident of not being caught [Chapters 11-12 of 57,658]. Eight-year-olds cheat more than 12-year-olds, and low-achievers more than high-achievers[809]. Cheating on exams peaks in high school and declines after that[94]. The rate of cheating is halved by having people write something privately that could reveal they had cheated, and halved again simply by reminding them not to cheat[809]. See also *lying*, p.255; *stealing*, p.250; *homework*, p.481.

Checklist diagnoses: p.24.

Child: 1. Up to puberty (common use), p.411.
2. Up to 18th birthday (Children Act 1989).

Child Behavior Checklist: see CBCL, p.436.
Childhood Disintegrative Disorder: p.46
Choking phobia: p.333.

Chorea: dance-like irregular rapid small movements, p.85.
Choreoathetoid movements are minor writhing of outstretched fingers, like playing a piano (they can seem like tics but unlike tics they are not stereotyped). Sydenham's chorea is a manifestation of PANDAS, p.522. See also Huntington's disease, p.482; neuroacanthocytosis, p.514; SLE, p.560; pseudo-chorea, p.363. For further differential diagnosis and suggested investigations see[1703].

Benign hereditary chorea is exacerbated by excitement or stress, so is socially embarrassing. It is non-progressive or can even become milder in adolescence; there is usually a family history[173,853]. Many other conditions need to be excluded and the difficulty in doing so on clinical grounds alone means that the diagnosis of BHC is often unreliable[1442]. Genetic testing is essential as the most common cause (TITF-1 mutation) can be accompanied by hypothyroidism (p.485) and lung dysfunction[853].

Chromatography: used for separating complex mixtures into individual molecules and then identifying those molecules. Used for hair analysis in drug abuse; assessment of the metabolism of medication in individuals; detection of poisons; identification of inborn errors of metabolism; detection of drug interactions; assessment of medication compliance.

Chromosome testing: making a microscopic or molecular overview of all chromosomes (see[1207]). This is important in ID and ASD for accessing reliable information on treatment, prognosis, and genetic counselling. See also *general approach to investigations*, p.373.

Method	Size of abnormalities detected	Diagnostic yield in ID (higher when IQ under 50)	Detects copy number variations?	Detects balanced translocations and inversions?
Conventional karyotyping	over 5 Mb	5–10%	no	yes
High-resolution karyotype analysis	over 3 Mb	15–20%	no	yes
Telomere analysis	varies	6% **	no	some
Chromosomal microarray	100–200 kb	9–13% **	yes	no

** These percentages are in addition to abnormalities detected by karyotyping.

None of the methods in the table above detects point mutations, for which FISH tests (fluorescent in situ hybridisation) or sequencing are needed.

Microarray diagnosis of ID has been justifiable on cost grounds since 2007[1794]. A key benefit is that microarrays detect copy number variations, which are common in ID and autistic spectrum disorders[24,920,1534]. Currently the commonest form of microarray testing is CGH (comparative genomic hybridisation).

Chronic fatigue or *Chronic Fatigue Syndrome*: p.323.

Ciliopathies: category of genetic disease in which symptoms are caused by dysfunction of cilia. One is Bardet-Biedl syndrome (p.429).

Cingulate cortex: see p.513.

CK: creatine (phospho)kinase. See creatine phosphokinase (CPK), p.446.

Clanging: a pattern of speech in which sounds rather than meaningful relationships appear to govern word choice[43]. Occasionally seen in schizophrenia.

Classical conditioning: learning that one stimulus is often associated with another. Pavlov repeatedly rang a bell before giving his dogs food, and soon the dogs learned to salivate when the bell rang. This does not require conscious awareness of the association. Classical conditioning is important in the triggering of anxiety[1087]. Idiosyncrasies in the rate of such learning underlie much PTSD, pp.532, 127. When children learn to associate fear with an object, as when Little Albert associated loud bangs with a white rat (see[656]), the fear can generalise to other similar objects (compare *overflow*, p.520).

Cleaning: p.112.

Cleft lip/palate: one of the most common congenital malformations (for others see p.503). The lip defect is visible, and the cleft palate can cause feeding difficulties, p.331; and nasal tone, p.147. Problems with attachment, speech, social interactions, and self-confidence are common[1127]. Clefts arise within over 400 syndromes, such as *velo*cardiofacial syndrome, p.572, in which genes interact with non-specific risk factors such as maternal smoking or heavy drinking, and folate deficiency[1788]; and in holoprosencephaly, p.480. There are several milder forms including high arched palate (p.522); bifid uvula, front tooth abnormalities, lip fistulae, and ankyloglossia (tongue tie)[1788].

Clingy: see *separation anxiety*, p.197.

Clonidine: an anti-adrenergic medicine (presynaptic α_2 agonist, see p.516) that reduces the activity of the sympathetic nervous system, p.428. As a cause of depression, p.311; as a cause of dizziness, p.454.

Clothing: (see also *hygiene*, p.483; *apraxia*, p.89).

Milestones: Most 1-year-olds cooperate with being dressed. 3-year-olds can pull on clothes and do up big front buttons. Tying a bow knot on shoes appears at age 6–8.

If clothing is unusual, work out what is the significance of the clothes to the child or parent:
- sporty (p.223)
- poverty or ostentation
- grown-up (esp. pubertal girl; or a boy trying to be like dad)
- humorous slogan on the clothes ("let's just assume I know everything" or "normal rules do not apply.")
- ethnic or religious identity
- tomboyish (p.566)
- conformity: style, labels
- school uniform
- which parent gave the clothes
- very idiosyncratic (e.g. in mania, rebelliousness).

Clubbing of fingers: p.466.
Clumsiness: p.89.

Cluttered speech: This is a vague term for speech which is dysrhythmic, sporadic, disorganised, occasionally repeating phrases and often unintelligible. Quite unlike stuttering, the affected person is usually unaware of the problem, and close attention *does* improve fluency. Causes include Fragile X syndrome (p.468), Down's syndrome (p.455), and possibly most other causes of ID[1647]. However the pattern of cluttering is not specific enough to contribute to diagnosis[1647]. For a checklist of cluttering symptoms see [363].

CMS: Children's Memory Scale, p.38.
CNS: central nervous system.
CNV: copy number variation, p.439.
Coalitions: p.213.

Coeliac disease: dietary intolerance to wheat gluten (gliaden), affecting about 1% of the population. In children it usually appears within a few years of weaning. Classical symptoms include diarrhoea, weight loss, weakness, and anaemia; but in milder cases there may be no sign other than indigestion or anaemia[676]. Hence most coeliac disease remains undiagnosed. A coeliac screening test is anti-tTG with total serum IgA.

Coeliac disease and behaviour
Common "minor" symptoms include picky eating, whining, screaming, headache and itching. Nearly half of coeliac patients have developmental delay, ID, ADHD, ataxia, hypotonia, or epilepsy[1820]. Coeliac is occasionally a reversible cause of depression or anxiety[10]. Coeliac disease can mimic, exacerbate, or even ameliorate coexisting eating disorders[925]. In *rare* cases, malabsorption (p.502) resulting from coeliac disease can make a reversible contribution to autistic symptoms[10,554].

Coenzyme Q10: see mitochondrial disorders, p.508.

Cogan's syndrome: autoimmune condition of ears and eyes causing oculomotor apraxia: Jerky movements of the head, difficulty in changing direction rapidly when running.

Cognitive biases: p.534.
Cognitive dissonance: p.355.
Colic: p.137.

Collude: acting together with others for a non-explicit aim. Some people would describe clinicians who allow government finances to influence their prescribing as colluding. A more common use is to (misguidedly or not) fit in with what the patient or his family wants. Within a family, the father (for example) might give in to what the child likes in order to be loved, or to avoid an argument.

Command hallucinations: p.344.

Comorbidity: The occurrence of two or more disorders in the same person.

There are several reasons why *true comorbidity* can be found in a population[257]: disorders sharing risk factors, risk factors being associated with one another, the comorbid pattern constituting a meaningful syndrome, or one disorder increasing the risk for the other.

In addition the misleading appearance of comorbidity (*artifactual comorbidity*) can be created by referral artefact, overlapping diagnostic criteria, artificial subdivision of syndromes, one disorder representing an early manifestation of the other, or one disorder being part of another[257].

A complex example is autism, in which for many years a core problem was thought to impair three distinct areas (p.183). Two of the more influential theories were that this core problem was a defect in *Theory of Mind* (p.563), or *weak central coherence* (excessive attention to local details in a picture, pp.36, 163). However we now know that the impairments have somewhat separate causes[591,648,1371,1782], all of which can be exacerbated by ID (p.185). In other words, a child diagnosed with "autism" has *comorbidity* between the three areas, and often with ID as well; but none of these associations is close enough to justify the term *syndrome*, p.383, nor perhaps even the unifying term *autism*.

Comorbidity increases the likelihood of disability and of referral, or of relatively mild problems being impairing, p.25; and increases the complexity of assessment, p.21. The *lack* of comorbidities helps identify benign variations of spiritual experiences, p.347; or of hallucinations, p.343. See also self-medication of comorbidities, p.257; DSM and ICD approaches to comorbidity, pp.24, 385.

The most common comorbidities tend to share common causes:

- *developmental*: attention problems with dyslexia, p.51; blindness with other neurodevelopmental problems, p.66; hyperactivity with oppositionality, p.253; tics with compulsions, p.101; cerebral palsy with ID, p.437; comorbidity in CAPD, p.121; common comorbidities of autism, p.427
- *anxiety*: this has multiple overlapping syndromes (see figure, p.297). A specific example is OCD with anorexia, p.65; or anxiety with chronic fatigue, p.323.
- *somatic*: most people with one of the following disorders actually have more than one[1750] (and many are depressed): irritable bowel, p.494; fibromyalgia, p.466; chronic fatigue, p.323; temporomandibular pain, chronic pelvic pain, p.137.

- *autoimmune*, p.427
- *dissociative*: see *multiple personality*, p.510
- *malingering, factitious, or somatised*: p.359
- *infections in underdeveloped countries*: p.490
- *micronutrient deficiencies*, p.327.

Compartmentalisation: dividing up a fundamentally homogeneous area into regions that have less communication between them than within them[283]. See also *connectivity*, p.444.

A concrete example is the dividing up of neocortex into separate areas during development[1725].

Less concretely, the separation of groups of ideas helps to minimise cognitive dissonance (p.355). The separation of ideas can occur because they seem irrelevant to one another, or if the person has no tools to consider them together: for example, a person can hold complex information about science and religion, but generally does not think about the two together. Alternatively, the separation of ideas can be learned and motivated: e.g. a girl holding both her peers' values and her parents' values, but thinking about them at different times. The process of forming multiple personalities appears to be related to this (p.510). Often the term *compartmentalisation* is used in an even broader sense to include excluding specific information from consciousness[709] (see *dissociation*, p.453).

At a societal level similar dynamics can be seen in the relative isolation of religions and of academic disciplines.

Complex Regional Pain Syndrome: p.136
Compulsion: see *Obsessive Compulsive Disorder*, p.65
Computers (spending time on): p.224
Concentration: sustained attention (p.79)
Conduct Disorder ✝: p.249.

Confabulation: false recall, without intent to deceive. Such errors can be roughly graded as trivial, substantial, or fantastic.

Trivial errors are common, and include approximations (p.357), simplifications, and minor distortions. They usually remain undetected because the speaker checks what he says as much as the listener does.

Substantial errors can be increased by pressure to recall something[784]. A one-off forced answer situation can produce immediate confabulation which is then stored, i.e. it is thereafter correctly called not a confabulation but a false memory (p.465). This effect can be easily produced in preschoolers and a small effect is still present in adults[7]. Surprisingly, content-specific confabulation can also result from organic lesions[235].

Fantastic or bizarre errors indicate failure of self-monitoring and often a brain lesion, which is rare in children (see p.574). This is quite different from the holding of bizarre beliefs, in which case everything the child says is consistent with those beliefs (p.347).

Conflicts: These can be internal or external. For internal conflicts see *cognitive dissonance*, p.355; *self-identity*, p.237; *guilt*, p.475; and ambivalent *attitudes*, p.425. For external conflicts see *contradicting*, p.162; *hatred*, p.187; *violence*, p.289.

Congenital Disorders of Glycosylation: p.474.

Connectivity: connections are sometimes more important than the things connected. Ideas can coexist peacefully or can conflict (p.355). Connections between people (relationships) can be unstructured or can entail roles of various degrees of determinism (p.211).

Small world networks[1720] have a mixture of close and distant relationships, and are found in social relationships as well as interconnections in the brain. Such networks develop during normal maturation of children and adolescents, with increasing numbers of long-distance connections within the brain[478] (see also[639]).

Temporary disruptions to normal connectivity underlie some disorders. For example, autoimmunity can temporarily or permanently disrupt localised areas of white matter in multiple sclerosis, p.510. Diverse molecular events can transiently alter network function, causing epilepsy[986]. Dissociation is a learned separation between ideas, functions and/or brain regions (p.453).

Classical disconnection syndromes[274] are most often described following brain injury. They include (a) conduction aphasia, in which Wernicke's and Broca's areas are disconnected, causing impaired repetition with intact comprehension and fluency; (b) agnosias, in which objects revealed to one sensory modality can be perceived but cannot be named or used appropriately; (c) apraxia, in which spontaneous actions are normal but the person cannot perform instructions to command, cannot mime actions, and cannot copy others; (d) pure alexia, the inability to read despite an ability to write; (e) pain asymbolia, in which pain is perceived and properly located but is not aversive (due to not reaching the limbic system); (f) hemispheric disconnection, as in callosal agenesis, p.445.

Long-term connectivity disruptions are found in many other disorders. Autism may result from abnormal or deficient functional connections between brain areas[288,528], or perhaps over-connectivity within the frontal lobes combined with inadequate connections between frontal and other cortex[326]. Regional disconnections may underlie Non-verbal Learning Disability[1385] (see p.28). One of the factors contributing to schizophrenia appears to be excessive pruning of unneeded synapses during adolescence[814] (also called synaptic reduction[748]).

See also *white matter*, p.574.

Constipation: means having hard stools that are difficult to expel. Infrequent bowel movements (e.g. every 2–3 days) are not necessarily accompanied by constipation. Some mothers interpret straining as constipation, leading to over-treatment. Severe constipation can occasionally cause a child to cry, p.315, or curl into ball, p.169, or wet himself, p.340, or headbang, p.119. For other causes of prolonged sitting on the toilet see p.340.

Retention can be due to the pain of an anal fissure, p.341; unpleasant toilet-training; or other toilet-related fears. Constipation can result from inadequate roughage or fluid in the diet (or other causes of dehydration); retention as above; various psychotropic medications; hypercalcaemia, p.483; opiate use, p.258; hypothyroidism, p.485; bowel obstruction (e.g. by Hirschprung's disease); coeliac disease, p.441; cystic fibrosis, p.450; lead poisoning, p.330; or congenital absence of abdominal muscles[743].

Contradicting: p.162.

Conversion disorders: This term unjustifiably implies an underlying mechanism, so has been superseded by *dissociation*, p.453. See also *ideographs*, p.487.

Cool: p.172.

Coping mechanisms: a behavioural skill used to cope with adversity[1185]. In general, this could include writing things down to compensate for a poor memory, or using medication to reduce tremor, or indeed hunting to alleviate hunger; but in psychological use the term refers mainly to skills acting on the external world to reduce *anxiety*. The term *defence mechanism* (p.303) is similar but usually refers to the more internal ways of reducing anxiety.

> *Action-based coping*: dealing with the problem that causes the stress, e.g. study more for exam; confront the threat.
> *Emotion-based coping*: dealing with the stress itself, e.g. talking about it, relaxation/sleep, alcohol, avoidance (p.429). Perhaps the simplest, though usually not considered because they are so simple, are self-soothing behaviours (p.61). The habit of finding a different way to construe difficult situations (i.e. *reappraisal*) is associated with much better emotional and social outcomes than the habit of trying not to express one's feelings[623] (these could also be described as defence mechanisms).

Coping and defence mechanisms can help in one area of life while making another area worse. When none of these mechanisms is available a child may think optimistically about the situation or may just feel helpless[1185] (see *learned helplessness*, p.96). See also cognitive dissonance (p.355), as a type of stress which sometimes invokes specific coping mechanisms.

Coprolalia: Swearing, p.161.
Copy number variation: p.439.
CoQ10: Coenzyme-Q10, p.508.

Cord around the neck: a single coil around the neck is found once in seven births; a double coil once in 40 births; and three to eight coils once in 200 births[1327]. A single coil is usually not damaging, but multiple coils usually are. A more useful sign of foetal risk is *meconium*, p.506.

Cornelia de Lange syndrome: mild to profound ID, microcephaly, low frontal hairline, joined eyebrows, upturned nose, prominent philtrum, thin downturned lips (often bitten), delayed growth, severe limb abnormalities in 30%, various other internal and sensory problems. A previously reported association with self-harm may be incorrect, but preference for protective devices to prevent self-harm [1190] is similar to Lesch-Nyhan.

Corpus callosum: fibre tract carrying most of the fibres between left and right cerebral hemispheres. (See also *connectivity*, p.444.)

Agenesis of the corpus callosum occurs in 1:1000 and has many genetic causes[1230]. Two-thirds *of known cases* have epilepsy, and the agenesis most often comes to light when seizures in the first two

years of life are investigated by imaging. In this condition (as with postnatal damage to the corpus callosum) IQ is often normal. Naming and simple reading are generally intact, but depth perception is impaired, as are more subtle skills, e.g. understanding jokes (because they get only the concrete meaning), syntax, planning, bilateral skills (p.431) and making conversation relevant and appropriate.

Testing: simple tests for crossed signals (such as asking for the number of taps on the left hand to be reproduced by the right hand) do not usually reveal corpus callosum problems, because there are many other interhemispheric pathways, e.g. the anterior commissure, which partially compensate if the loss occurs before adolescence[1230]. In uncompensated cases, one hand can interfere with the other hand doing something (intermanual conflict). If the examiner moves one hand on top of the other, the patient may not realise that he has touched his own hand. Complex visual information (such as patterns of dots) can only be transferred between hemispheres via the corpus callosum, whereas simpler encodeable patterns (such as letters) can be transferred by the smaller interhemispheric paths[1230].

Navigation: a person with callosal agenesis and normal non-discrepant IQ may be able to navigate on paper, or give a verbal description of a path, but when standing outside her front door not know whether to turn left or right. This can be tested in clinic: can the child find the waiting room? See also *navigation*, p.512.

Corsi block-tapping test: p.399.
COS: childhood onset schizophrenia, p.538.
Co-sleeping: p.198.
Covering the ears: p.131.
CP: child protection, p.272; or cerebral palsy, p.437.
CPK: creatine phosphokinase, p.446.

Craniopharyngioma: rare benign tumours occasionally causing anorexia, fatigue, headache, dry skin, polydipsia, polyuria, weight gain or poor growth, and/or amenorrhoea. See *hypothalamus*, p.485; *tumours*, p.569.

Creatine phosphokinase (CPK, also called creatine kinase, CK): an enzyme found in heart and skeletal muscle. Elevated levels are found in blood with muscle bruising (e.g. following violence, or with ataxia, or dyskinetic movements in catatonia[1171], or modestly elevated following submaximal exercise); myositis; muscular dystrophy, p.510; myocardial infarction; neuroleptic malignant syndrome (very high levels), p.514; malignant hyperthermia; and abetalipoproteinaemia, p.417. Also raised in some cases of hypothyroidism, p.485.

Creativity: see imagination, p.488.
Crescendo: of activity level, p.77; of crying, p.316.
CRH: corticotrophin-releasing hormone. See hypothalamus, p.485.

Criminality: this word implies that a tendency to break laws is a fixed aspect of a person, like a personality disorder (p.241); this is incorrect (see below and *ideograph*, p.487). This term is a legal parallel to the use of the term *Conduct Disorder* in adolescents (p.249). Risk factors for criminal behaviour include the following:

Situational risk factors: the situation an individual finds himself in brings risks of its own, such as increased need, lack of money or availability of vulnerable victims. The great majority have used illicit drugs in the months before conviction. School-leaving itself does not increase crime, though in some studies 60% of convicted young people have left school before the minimum school leaving age (see p.215). Unemployment is the main reason for the discrepancy, as it increases spare time, frustration and poverty. (In addition, conviction for crimes increases unemployment, though only slightly, and some individual characteristics such as short temper and low intelligence probably increase both: see[483] for discussion.)

Individual characteristics: it is obvious that some kinds of offending will be associated with individual characteristics such as sex, age, physicality, risk-seeking, intelligence, and short temper. For example, hierarchically organised criminal activities usually involve adults[1655], whereas teenagers are more likely to steal, to be violent, or to commit drugs offences. People with mild ID can be led into lives of crime (e.g. as prostitutes or drug mules); they are unable to understand information supplied by the police, and often supply information or sign confessions (whether correct or not) that lead to conviction[441]. Studies showing criminal convictions to be much commoner in Asperger's than in autism are strongly confounded by the much lower IQ found in most people diagnosed with autism, the higher degree of supervision given to these people, and the reluctance of courts to convict people with severe ID (see[1119]).

Social risk factors: social relationships can smooth the road into a criminal career, or alternatively may be an incentive to keep to the straight path. The likelihood of a youth offending in one study was 15% if any one relative was convicted; 24% if the father was convicted; 35% if a brother was convicted; and 44% if three or more family members were convicted[492]. A third of sentenced young offenders aged 16–20 have been in care in childhood; another third have been physically abused; and a third of the females have been sexually abused[894]. Over half have been expelled from school or have run away from home (p.210). Other risk factors include having a young mother, and living in a rough neighbourhood[484].

Critical periods: a period of childhood during which a stage of development must be passed, or it will never be possible again. A clear example in humans is binocular depth perception (p.177). It may also be true for rapid high-frequency auditory discrimination (p.144).

Partly critical (or sensitive) periods. these are periods during which good progress is needed if final perfect outcome is to be achieved. For example, the cognitive, emotional and growth effects of early deprivation in institutional rearing show considerable catch-up following adoption as late as age 10, though the recovery reduces with increasing age of adoption[1401,1654]. Similarly, language acquisition has a partly critical period, so that perfect performance is almost never achieved by people who are exposed to a second language after age 8 (see data in[782]). Similar effects are seen for musical performance; for skill in chewing and the number of foods accepted (p.331); in the development of attachment behaviours (p.195). See also *late developers*, p.496.

Crowd behaviour: people often behave differently when they are in a crowd, compared to when they are alone or with just a few others. Mob violence (such as trampling on people or throwing rocks) is increased by feelings that become more likely in crowds, such as powerlessness, the feeling of anonymity, low personal responsibility, and excitement (see *infectious behaviours*, p.490). Groups of people can behave like a herd (or a school of fish) if they strongly influence one another, or if they are all influenced by an outside force (such as a fashion)[1291]. See also *mass psychogenic behaviours*, p.505.

Smaller groups also influence behaviour. People eat and drink more in company. *Groupthink* is a form of restricted thinking in which people avoid saying anything that could disrupt the group or their position in the group. See also bystanders in bullying, pp.219, 279; risk-taking increased by presence of friends, p.263.

Crowds: see effects of crowds in autism, p.119; hanging out with the wrong crowd, p.171; overcrowded home, pp.199, 207; sensory complexity of crowds, p.227; agoraphobia, p.297.

Crying: p.315.
CRP: C-reactive protein (a marker of inflammation).
CSBI: Child Sexual Behaviour Inventory, p.267.
CSF: cerebro-spinal fluid.
CSWS: epilepsy with continuous spike and wave during slow sleep, p.46.
CT: computed tomography imaging (e.g. of the brain), p.374.

Cultural effects on symptoms: there are several reasons for behaviours to arise or be perpetuated in some regions but not in others. These include chance; cultural and biological effects of infections and malnutrition; and cousin-marriage (itself bringing long-term cultural and biological effects).

Within DSM, specific patterns from exotic cultures are called *culture-bound syndromes*. More recently these are seen to be metaphors, causal attributions, or cultural idioms of distress[850]. Such detailed knowledge of a culture is invaluable when patient and professional come from different cultures. Related examples include pseudo-paralysis that was common in Central Europe in the early 1900s, and the Jumping Frenchmen of Maine, p.552.

When conditions have entered mainstream medical usage[731] they are sometimes assumed to be universal, even culture-free, disorders. In some cases this is right, but there are exceptions. For example, the characteristic categories of fears in OCD (p.65) have recently been joined by fears related to the internet, and recycling compulsions are increasing. Children's fears are determined by observational and informational learning (p.307). Bulimia nervosa and fear of weight gain are culturally determined, whereas the self-starvation of anorexia nervosa has been seen in all cultures over thousands of years[825]. Chronic fatigue syndrome could be called *subculturally-bound* in that most interested people cleave to one of the standard accounts of it, i.e. that the symptoms are purely physical or purely psychological[850]; the proportions differ between countries[291].

Many children continue to be given traditional remedies, including some that contain potentially harmful levels of steroids, non-steroidals or opiates. In any society, fasting (p.465) affects some subgroups more than others. Traditional practices such as frightening exorcism[201,1252] and female circumcision[50,1355,1377] are damaging and illegal in most developed countries, but continue to be practised. These are complex issues because of the wide range of procedures used, and differences in values between cultures.

More relevant to daily practice in most places, however, is the broader subject of the impact of patients' beliefs on behaviour, whether the beliefs are cultural or familial or personal, rational or bizarre. These beliefs influence their actual symptoms, their help-seeking (mainstream and otherwise), guilt, the way they describe the problem, and their readiness to question advice.

See also *race*; *tattoos*, p.561; cultural self-mutilation, p.318.

Cushing's syndrome: excess glucocorticoids (p.555). Look for obesity, striae of weight gain, buffalo hump, acne, hirsuitism, hyperglycaemia. Cushing's can cause depression, mania, or psychosis. In suspected Cushing's syndrome, check FBC (raised white cell count), discuss with endocrinologist, HPLC of urinary steroids.

"Cyclic vomiting syndrome": a heterogeneous condition of intermittent vomiting (four vomits per hour for one hour, nausea lasts 1–5 days, then well between episodes). Migraine is increasingly recognised as a cause, especially when there is a family history of migraine or the episodes are preceded by an aura[1186]. Twelve per cent have a demonstrably reversible physical cause for the vomiting, and a further 40% have an identifiable disorder that could contribute to the vomiting[949]. The 12% include oesophagitis, duodenitis, irritable bowel, p.494; duplication cyst, malrotation, chronic appendicitis, adhesions, choledochal cyst, cholelithiasis, sinusitis, asthma, p.424; kidney stone, VLC-acyl-CoA dehydrogenase, p.418; porphyria, p.532; mitochondriopathy, p.508; epilepsy, glioma, medullo-blastoma, astrocytoma, VP shunt dysfunction.

Cycloid psychosis: this term has been used in recent decades to describe episodic psychoses (p.537), usually acute and transient, often with symptoms changing every few hours or days, and with good long-term functioning[1013,1244]. It may still be a useful ☝term for psychoses that are substantially different from most schizophrenia or bipolar affective disorder, particularly in having triggers that are rather biological (and recurrent), followed by episodes lasting days at most. Examples include Prader-Willi, p.533; delusions during the sleep-dominated episodes of Kleine-Levin[61], p.496; episodic ataxia and familial hemiplegic migraine, p.142; premenstrual psychosis, p.506; monthly psychosis starting before menarche, p.506; many metabolic disorders such as urea-cycle defects, p.571; post-migraine psychosis[530]; and ictal or post-ictal psychosis, p.532. Other causes include running out of the monthly supply of tablets or money, and intoxication after receiving paychecks (for many other causes see pp.343–349). "It is patently obvious that such [specific underlying causes] should not be relegated to a heterogeneous atypical group with unspecified etiological mechanisms that would obscure the specific therapeutic possibilities…"[1104].

Psychosis and fits are complementary in some patients. For example, some antipsychotics increase fits and some antiepileptics precipitate psychosis. Also, in *inter*ictal psychosis the psychosis characteristically disappears for several days following the fit (closely related to the unusual phenomenon of "forced normalisation" i.e. amelioration of psychosis during epileptiform discharges)[1409,1672].

Cyclothymia: p.264.

Cystic fibrosis: an autosomal recessive genetic disease affecting mainly the pancreas and lungs, with malabsorption and intermittent severe infections. Life expectancy has increased in developed countries, from about 10 years before 1970, to over 40 now. Anxiety about symptoms tends to improve adherence to the arduous treatment regimes, as does cohesive family function[1748]. See *heelprick*, p.32; inadequate intake, p.331; constipation, p.444; malabsorption, p.502.

Cytochromes: liver enzymes that metabolise food and medication. They vary between individuals, and influence medicine effects and medicine interactions. For example atomoxetine reaches 5 times the plasma level in some individuals compared to others[849]. In one extreme case an abnormal cytochrome contributed to an undetected fatal overdose of fluoxetine[1419]. In future, cytochrome identification is likely to reduce such disasters and improve the effectiveness of medication.

Cytokines: diverse family of molecules (interleukins, interferons and tumour necrosis factor) that are released in inflammation, and can cause physical symptoms such as coeliac disease, p.441; illness behaviours and depression[366].

Dacrystic fits: epileptic crying seizures, p.76.
Daily living skills: see *adaptive behaviours*, p.419.

Damaged: "had something happen to it to cause a defect." The term *damaged child* implies that a child was perfect before a particular event and may never be so again. The term should not be used without good evidence for deterioration and causation (see *ideograph*, p.487).

DAMP ☞: disorder of attention, motor, and perception (meaning social). This concept of Gilberg is an even broader umbrella concept than ADHD (ADHD, dyspraxia, cognition; compare figure on p.385). It has been unkindly described as "neurodevelopmental blah".

Danger (to others): p.283.

Daydreaming: thinking about something else without visible sign (except for perhaps a smile or frown). This cannot be established by observation alone; it is only certain if the person can tell you what he was doing. *Imaginary world* (p.231) is a broader term that includes motionless daydreaming, plus moving about and talking to imaginary friends. Contrast with *absences*, p.75.

DCD: *Developmental Coordination Disorder*, p.89.

Deaf: p.130. When capitalised, this word refers to the Deaf cultural community, who sign. (see also *Ears*, p.458).

Declarative memory: p.37.
Defence mechanisms: p.305.
Deformity: see *malformation*.

Dehydration: shortage of water in the body. No single sign is reliable, but any three of the following indicate deficit over 5%: decreased skin elasticity, capillary refill over two seconds, absent tears, dry mucous membranes, sunken eyes, abnormal pulse, decreased urine output[595].

Causes of dehydration include vomiting and diarrhoea; purging or reduced intake in anorexia nervosa, p.334; sweating, p.558; diabetic ketoacidosis, p.338; large burns or blood loss; use of diuretics (including stimulants and alcohol).

Effects of dehydration: can cause delirium, syncope (p.74), sickle crises (p.549), renal stones in cystinuria, p.556; and in other urea cycle disorders, p.571; renal failure; stroke; episodic jaundice of Gilbert syndrome (possibly with mild abdominal discomfort and lethargy). Contrast *drinking too much*, p.338.

Deliberate self-harm (DSH): pp.319, 317.
Delinquency: not a diagnosis. Means law-breaking.

Delirium: sudden onset, restless, fluctuating conscious level, hallucinations/delusions, disoriented in time (then day, month, season, place and finally person), occasionally day-night reversal. Quite common in feverish children (think also of excess bedclothes or long hot baths). Causes are biological and need urgent assessment by GP or paediatrician. Consider neuroleptic malignant syndrome, p.514; delirium in dehydration, p.450; in HIV, p.479; delirium tremens, p.258; other causes of reduced consciousness, pp.97–98.

Delusions: p.348.

Dependence: see over-dependence on mother, p.43; gradual reduction in dependence, p.189; personality disorder, p.242; addiction, p.259

Depression: in children, p.313; in mothers, p.174.

Desensitisation: becoming less aroused by a stimulus, e.g. a child learning to ignore mum's shouting, p.253; desensitisation to violence caused by video games, p.292. See also *sensitisation*, p.546.

Developmental coordination disorder, p.89.

Developmental level / Developmental quotient (DQ): assessment of a child's developmental level in all functional areas. The areas tested generally include both adaptive behaviours (p.419) and thinking ability (see IQ, p.59). The developmental level is best expressed as an age-equivalent in each area. For example, the Griffiths, which is useful up to a mental age of 8, gives age-equivalents for Locomotor, Personal-Social, Hearing/Language, Eye-hand coordination, Performance, and Practical reasoning. These tests tend to be more fun than IQ tests (p.59), so are easier to engage toddlers. Locomotor levels are often unrelated to the other scores. For more information see p.55.

Deviance: p.49.

Diabetes: usually this is shorthand for diabetes mellitus, meaning excess blood sugar (diabetes insipidus causes similar symptoms but without the increased sugar, and is much rarer, see p.338).

Diabetes can reveal itself insidiously or as an acute medical emergency. Physical symptoms include polyuria, and in some types of diabetes, severe weight loss. Behavioural symptoms include chronic fatigue, p.325; and polydipsia, p.338. Blood and urine glucose are elevated.

Diabetes control has major psychological aspects, due to the importance of avoiding impulsive eating, the potency of the self-administered insulin to cause weight gain and hypoglycaemia (see p.82), and the desire of adolescents to be normal[217,1714]. "Brittle" diabetes is unstable, difficult to control blood sugar levels.

Especially in teens, many cases are due to poor diet control or poor adherence to injecting technique.

Fabricated hypoglycaemia is intentional self-starvation or insulin overdose, and can be used to blackmail parents regarding food, school attendance, or time on the computer. It can cause brain damage or death, and can also be used to force hospital admission.

Diagnostic hierarchies: p.15.
DID: Dissociative Identity Disorder, p.510.

Diet: see constipation, p.444; general malnutrition, p.504; micronutrient deficiencies, p.327; diabetes, p.451; vegan diet, p.572; dietary restriction in autism, pp.327, 329, 529; parents with ID, p.192; dietary treatments, p.327, 567; diet in hyperactivity, p.82; Omega-3 oils, p.327; diet in PKU, p.529; total parenteral nutrition, p.333; pica, p.336; metabolic crises, p.381; coeliac disease, p.441; ketogenic diet, p.465; kidney stones, p.555; urea-cycle disorders, p.571; Wernicke's encephalopathy, p.574.

Digit span: a simple test of auditory working memory, p.575 (or short term memory, p.555). The child can be asked to repeat the digits forwards or backwards. Both are correlated with intelligence, but the score backwards is more so[101]. Both measure several abilities, not one[1582].

Digit span increases linearly from age 4 to 15[549]. Forward digit span of 5, 6 and 7 is reached by 60% of 6, 8 and 11-year-olds, respectively[1423]. Backward digit span is usually about 2½ fewer than forward digit span[549].

Reliability is greatest on the first and the last digits[1423,1582]. Alternatively the child can be asked to store and immediately recall single-syllable words or non-words, though these produce lower scores[549]. For other memory tests see pp.38, 399.

Disability: any restriction or lack (resulting from an impairment) of ability to perform an activity in the manner or within the range considered normal for a human being [see 788]. Contrast *impairment*.

Disclosure: means the *first* recounting of a fact, i.e. breaking the secret. See disclosure of abuse, p.271; of sexuality, p.237; in OCD, p.65. See also disclosure of confidential information from professional to professional, pp.19, 413.

Disclosure of *abuse* is not a simple event[20], but often preceded by increasingly disturbed behaviour over weeks to months (with symptoms of anxiety and PTSD, p.532; and rarely psychosis[1744]). The person typically gives occasional hints to assess others' interest and sympathy, and makes multiple partial disclosures (partial in terms of who is let into the secret and what is revealed). The appropriate level of suspicion following disclosure of abuse depends on factors in the disclosure, pp.275–276; physical and parental signs, p.276; and discussion with colleagues, p.272.

Disconnection syndromes: p.444.
Disinhibition: 261.
Disobedience: p.253.
Disorders, specific named: see DSM, p.386. See also *Syndromes*, p.383.
Displacement: p.305.
Disruptive behaviour: Often used to refer to ADHD ↟, p.83; Oppositional Defiant Disorder ↟, p.519; and Conduct Disorder ↟, p.249. Includes aggression, defiance, destructiveness, overactivity, and

impulsiveness [1589]. "Disruptive Behaviour Disorder, Not Otherwise Specified" is so broadly defined that it can include essentially any difficult behaviour (see *atypical disorders*, p.426).

Dissociation: functional disruption of the normal connectedness of brain function, involving memory, perception, and/or self-identity. In the dissociated state, unbearable information is not experienced. There seem to be distinct subtypes of dissociation: global dissociation from the world, as in the feeling of depersonalisation or derealisation, involves distinct processes from keeping a few painful ideas repressed ([709]; see p.421), or from preventing incompatible ideas entering consciousness at the same time (see *cognitive dissonance*, p.355; *compartmentalisation*, p.443).

It is easy to identify dissociation if a severe psychological precipitant immediately precedes it (e.g. suddenly believing oneself to be swimming on holiday, when one is at a party with friends and hears of boyfriend's infidelity (an *oneroid*, i.e. dreamlike, *state*). In less clear cases an exhaustive exclusion of physical causes (p.349), and careful consideration of the possibility of pre-existing psychiatric disorder, are required. An important predisposing factor in many cases is childhood trauma (p.567) or abuse (p.271) especially if severe, repetitive, prolonged or repeatedly recalled[1287].

Imaginary friends (p.231) can be viewed as an early form of "normative dissociation"; related terms include daydreaming and highway hypnosis[1287].

DSM-IV names five dissociative disorders: Dissociative Identity Disorder (multiple personality, p.510); Dissociative Amnesia (p.421); Dissociative Fugue; and Depersonalisation Disorder. Two other named disorders include dissociation: PTSD (p.532) and Acute Stress Disorder (p.538). A few case of selective mutism may be dissociating (p.153). Dissociation may have a role in the aetiology of psychosis [1117]. Feeling numb or detached is rare in children, so diagnostic criteria need to be adapted. See also: defensce mechanisms including repression, p.421; avoidance, p.429; fabrication, p.359; conversion disorders, p.445; multiple personality, p.510; imagination, p.488; other complex effects of anxiety, p.296.

Dissonance (cognitive): p.355.

Distractibility: teachers see a child distracted by (or distracting) peers; parents see similar, plus a child being distracted from dressing by toys, etc. The clinical task is to work out the relative weights of the distinct influences on a child's behaviour[1770]:

(a) innate long-term characteristics of the child, generally described as ADHD (p.83). This is part of temperament (p.561). Contrast intolerance of distractions, p.128.

(b) the set task. Clearly if he is not interested in this task, not understanding it, not motivated to continue, or unable to remember what he was doing, it will neither prevent distractions nor pull him back after he has briefly assessed them (see *boredom*, p.322). If the child is actively trying to *avoid* (p.429) the current task, then switching to another task is not really distractibility.

(c) his internal state (for example preoccupations and sensory intolerance, which depend in turn on mood). Consider depression and, rarely, hypomania.

(d) the distractor. This can be external or internal; internal can be physical (e.g. pain, p.135) or associations or intrusions (p.493). The duration or level of upset caused by the distraction may be idiosyncratic (e.g. in PTSD, p.532).

Divergent thinking: see imagination, p.488.
Divorce: discussed with *parental discord*, p.191.

Dizziness: means the feeling that the world is turning. Consider ear infection, low blood pressure (e.g. very thin, standing up fast, side-effect of clonidine, p.441); head injury, p.477; hyperventilation, p.484; intoxication, p.566; BPPV (benign paroxysmal positional vertigo, i.e. dizziness brought on by specific position or head movements); migraine, p.141; syncope, p.74.

DM: diabetes mellitus, p.451.
DMD: see *Duchenne muscular dystrophy*, p.510.

DNA repair defects: defects in DNA repair (for many others see[1310]).
  i) Xeroderma pigmentosum: inherited deficiency of DNA repair, causing mainly extreme sun-sensitivity. Neurodegenerative risk is proportional to the DNA repair deficiency.
  ii) ataxia-telangiectasia[915]: causes cerebellar atrophy, oculocutaneous telangiectases, oculomotor apraxia (inability to move the eyes from one object to another), and increased risk of leukaemia.

Domestic violence: most definitions of domestic violence are impractically broad, including not just repeated physical injuries but also single incidents or risk of psychological harm.

If there is any cause for concern, women should be asked, using questions such as "Is everything alright at home?", "Is your partner supportive?", "Do you ever feel frightened of your partner or other people at home?", "Have you ever been in a relationship where you have been hit or hurt in some way?", "Are you now in a relationship where this is happening?"[220]. Such questions should not be asked when other family members are present, as this can lead to an increase in violence at home.

In practice domestic violence teams will establish some threshold, either informally or based on a formal risk assessment (such as the Barnardo's Domestic Violence Scale which lists events, risk factors and protective factors: http://www.londonscb.gov.uk/files/procedur es/dv/dv_risk_assessment_matrix__final.pdf). As with other thresholded services (such as individual teaching, special schools, housing benefits, and child protection), domestic violence just below threshold can end up having worse outcomes than that just over threshold, because protective procedures are not invoked. Protective procedures include refuges (p.540), involving social services, and court injunctions.

Children *exposed* to domestic violence experience both internalising and externalising symptoms[475]. Perhaps surprisingly, according to this meta-analysis, exposure at an early age is not more damaging than later exposure.

Men and women are equally likely to say they are victims of domestic violence; but women are more likely to be injured[40,436]. Only 7% of spouses claim "mutual violence"[40] but it is usually misleading to assume that one partner is the victim and the other is the perpetrator. The reason is that bidirectional violence is much more common than unidirectional[40]; they are both likely to have been victims in the past; and many perpetrators *feel* helpless, trapped and victimised.

Although extreme domestic violence to a pregnant woman can obviously damage the foetus, in practice this seems to be rare. These children have essentially the same outcome as those of unassaulted mothers, as long as maternal health and social variables are controlled for[1727] (see also *toxic substances in pregnancy*, p.566). By far the greatest risk of severe injury to the fetus occurs in car crashes; falls cause this degree of trauma very rarely[1733].

In many areas child protection services stop at the 16th birthday, in which case domestic violence services develop some expertise in 16- and 17-year-olds being injured by – or injuring – their parents. See also the broader issue of *parental discord*, p.191.

Dominance: (a) genetic sense, see p.379.

(b) For social dominance, see status among peers, p.172; testosterone, p.554; psychopathy, p.280.

Dopamine: a neurotransmitter that signals unexpected reward, and is arousing. It is increased by stimulants, p.555; and blocked by antipsychotics, p.422, and cannabis. Dopamine hypofunction is a minor factor in ADHD[1688] and the major factor in Parkinson's, p.525; and Segawa disease, p.458. It is also released by some of the rare phaeochromocytoma tumours, p.529. See also dopamine appetite, p.322; neuroleptic malignant syndrome, p.514.

Down's syndrome: Trisomy 21, the commonest cause of ID, found in 1/750 births. ID can be severe or very mild (e.g. in mosaicism, p.509). Signs include upward slanting eyes, large protruding tongue, Brushfield spots on the iris, epicanthic folds, brachycephaly, short neck, and single palmar ("simian") creases on short broad hands. Note that diagnosis based on these physical signs is *not* reliable[404].

Behaviour can be difficult to manage because of stubbornness and argumentativeness (actual violence is relatively uncommon); many of these children have an exceptionally strong desire for attention and interaction that overrides other rewards. They tend to be weaker in receptive and expressive language than in visuospatial tasks (see STM, p.555), perhaps because of deafness that has historically affected more than half, due to (largely treatable) otitis media.

Although people with Down's are characteristically social, a few satisfy criteria for an autism-related diagnosis. It is not clear how many of these are due to ID or hearing loss or mood (for case histories see[1325]; see also testing non-verbal children, p.516).

Many parts of the brain are small in Down's, but the greatest deficiency is seem in the hippocampus (p.478) which is typically half the normal volume[1384]. Chromosome 21 is one of the smallest chromosomes, but contains over 200 genes. Dosage effects in several of these are responsible for the cognitive, ophthalmic, cardiac, tongue, skeletal, and other changes in Down's syndrome. About a quarter of people with Down's develop an autoimmune disorder, especially thyroiditis, type I diabetes, or coeliac disease[901].

DQ: developmental quotient, p.451.
Dravet syndrome: p.438.

Draw-a-person test: p.56.

Dreams, recurrent: most recurrent dreams have unpleasant content[550], but some are pleasant or non-affective[1815]. The most common recurrent themes are being chased, sexual experience, falling, flying, schools, teachers, studying, arriving late, missing a train, trying repeatedly to do something, and failing an exam; the simplest of these appear from early childhood[1160]. A single theme (such as being late) may recur with varying details. Dreams can be exceptionally vivid or unusual in organic states such as fever, drug abuse and withdrawal [1414]. They are distinct from night terrors (p.200) which are unrecallable and during which the child is exceptionally difficult to arouse.

Thirty-five per cent of 11-year-olds recall a recurrent dream having taken place during the past year[550]. Sleep may actively enhance declarative memories [455], suggesting a reason why they are often "pictorial metaphors of current concerns." [1815]. A positive attitude to dreams increases the likelihood of recall[125].

Causes of recurrent dreams
- Most occur in normal healthy children, but they are more common in children with anxiety, depression, aggression, and/or stressful life events (p.499; for details see [550]).
- Worries and simple phobias (p.307).
- Desires, such as sex or food.
- Migraines (p.141): hallmarks are brilliant colours, and sometimes continuation into the waking state [967].
- Many medicines and herbal remedies cause vivid nightmares[1473,1604].
- PTSD (p.532). Recurrent dreams of the trauma are far less common than such experiences while awake[1184].
- TLE (temporal lobe epilepsy, p.562): can rarely cause the same dream for years, eventually appearing in the daytime and even evolving to be the aura of a grand mal seizure[467].
- Dopaminergic disorders such as Parkinson's, p.525; and Segawa, p.458.

Dribbling: Dribbling from the mouth usually indicates both a physical problem and a self-monitoring problem. The physical element can be hypersalivation (e.g. clozapine-induced sialorrhoea); difficulty swallowing (e.g. with tonsillitis or bulbar palsy); akinesia (e.g. with antipsychotics, p.422); fear of swallowing (as in OCD, p.65); oromotor dyscontrol (p.90); a habit of opening the mouth; or a habit of putting things in the mouth (hyperorality or large sweets). Generally the dribbling will still not be a problem unless self-monitoring is impaired by sedation (consider sedative medications), sleepiness, or long-term cognitive difficulty. If severe dribbling disappears during sleep, this may be due to mouth-breathing, or the child may be causing it while awake, e.g. collecting saliva in his mouth for a big intermittent pour.

For urinary dribbling see p.340.

Drinking too much: p.338.

Drives: The term *drive* historically referred to *tissue needs* or *biological needs* to distinguish them from psychological needs, but that distinction is now realised to be an oversimplification[1328]. For examples of *drive* in its broad sense, see: fight-or-flight, p.466; drive to reduce anxiety, p.295; defence mechanisms, p.305; drive to reduce cognitive dissonance, p.355; social drives, p.168; selfish goal principle, p.520; regulating sensory input by seeking arousal, p.124; or by seeking specific sensations, p.124; or seeking to avoid sensations, p.125. Compare *motivation*, p.509.

Drug screening: p.257.
dsDNA: double-stranded DNA (anti-dsDNA is a test for SLE, p.560).
DSH, deliberate self harm: pp.319, 317.

DSM: *Diagnostic and Statistical Manual*: p.385.
DT: delirium tremens, p.258.
Duchenne muscular dystrophy: p.510.

Dyscalculia: Poor calculation abilities ☝. This is an umbrella term for a wide variety of problems, overlapping with non-verbal learning disability, p.28. The causes and diagnostic difficulties of dyscalculia also have much overlap with dyslexia, p.51. Dyscalculia can be developmental (also called primary) or due to brain injury (often called acalculia or secondary dyscalculia)[54].

Normal development of numerical thinking has the following steps: (1) magnitude and the feeling of quantity; (2) sounds for numbers; (3) pictures of numbers, including multi-digit numbers; (4) mental number lines; (5) complex multi-step rules for calculation (see[54,1691]).

Working out the specific aspects of calculation that are difficult for a child allows remedial teaching to be well targeted[462]. Here are some of the more common underlying problems:
- Messy handwriting (p.53) or failure to line up columns can cause difficulty with written arithmetic.
- Poor STM (p.555) or poor teaching (such as moving on to long multiplication before the times tables have been mastered) are often to blame.
- Impulsive children give an answer before checking it; or fail to maintain attention during a multi-step calculation.
- Judgment of magnitudes is impaired in many people with dyscalculia, and appears to be a function of the right parietal lobe[800].
- Most infants can distinguish small, medium and large groups of dots. A few people have a specific inability to instantly know the number of dots on a page even when there are just two or three dots (see www.mathematicalbrain.com).

Dyscontrol of mood: see *emotional instability*, p.69.

Dysdiadochokinesis: difficulty with rapid alternating movements. The patient cannot rapidly alternate touching the palm then the back of his hand, on to the other arm. When testing this, label it as a game or cleaning doorknobs as a race. See *cerebellum*, p.437.

Dysgraphia: p.53
Dyskinesia: see figure, p.85.
Dyslexia: p.51.
Dysmorphophobia: previous term for Body Dysmorphic Disorder, p.433.
Dysphagia: difficult or painful swallowing. See p.333.
Dysphonia: see *speech problems*, p.147.

Dyspnoea: the subjective feeling of breathlessness. This usually indicates excess carbon dioxide in the blood. Medical examination is necessary to consider respiratory and cardiac causes, as well as acidosis, neuromuscular disease, blocked nose or severe postnasal drip, and hyperventilation (p.484).

There is often an emotional contribution to dypnoea. This can be acute as in *panics*, p.301. Fear of severe illness in oneself (or of impending death, especially following bereavements) can cause dyspnoea[817]. Asthmatics report less dyspnoea when elated, i.e. they *under*estimate problems with lung function. When apprehensive they do the reverse[1346]. See *asthma*, p.424; mass dyspnoea, p.505; psychogenic breathlessness, p.424; *heart*, p.478.

Dyspraxia: see *Clumsiness*.
Dysregulation of mood: see *emotional instability*, p.69.

Dystonia: p.85. Simultaneous contraction of agonists and antagonist muscles. Dystonia can be fixed (immobile) or varying (usually torsional). Dystonic postures and movements occasionally have the following features, which when present clarify the diagnosis of dystonia: overflow at its peak to other body parts; overflow to the opposite side of the body (mirror dystonia); elegant tricks that reduce dystonia (gestes antagonistes)[21]. Note that there are many other causes of unusual postures (p.93).

Examples of dystonina include torticollis, blepharospasm, oculogyric crises (p.93), and some parkinsonism (p.525). There are at least 14 genetically distinct subtypes of dystonia, with characteristic age of onset, triggers for episodes, transmitter involvement (dopamine, ACh and/or GABA) and associated features[212]. Focal hand dystonia in musicians (like writer's cramp) can appear just when a specific piece of music is being played; this task specificity has often led to it being considered psychiatric[961] but there is evidence of impaired GABA function[943].

Paroxysmal nocturnal dystonia. Previously thought to be a parasomnia but now recognised as usually being a consequence of an orbito-frontal seizure (so the EEG electrodes require special placement).

Dopa-responsive dystonia, or *Segawa syndrome*. Classically, leg dystonia worsens during the day and is improved after sleep[412]. The first symptom is often dystonic posture of the foot, appearing in the first decade then spreading over the next few years to other extremities[740]. Depression, OCD, sleepiness and nightmares (p.456) are common[1653]. Symptoms can seem psychogenic, e.g. with bizarre patterns such as a boy being able to run and hop, but walking stiffly with apparent scoliosis (p.93) and arms in odd positions. The same boy walked to school easily but in the evening could only walk a few paces[1226]. A trial of dopa can clarify the diagnosis[1289]. The cells of the substantia nigra have a genetic restriction of their ability to make dopamine (unlike Parkinson's disease, in which these cells die; the difference can be seen on ultrasound)[638].

Dystrophy: diseases, mostly hereditary, that affect the shape of body parts. Leukodystrophy, 498; muscular dystrophy, p.510; myotonic dystrophy, p.568; reflex sympathetic dystrophy, p.136.

Ears: see Deafness, p.130; Deaf, p.450; Deaf parents, p.191; Deafism, p.66; Covering ears, p.131; Central Auditory Processing Disorder, p.121; not listening, p.129; noise intolerance, p.125; auditory sensation-seeking, p.123; touching earlobes in autism, p.132; Fragile X, p.468; auditory hallucination, p.343; tinnitus, p.565.

Eating disorder: even though this has the broad dictionary definition of any eating abnormality that is impairing, the term is often used in a much more specific way, to mean just anorexia nervosa (p.334) – or sometimes bulimia (p.337) as well, or all eating disturbances associated with weight and shape concerns.

Many types of eating abnormality have been described. People often move between categories so they are often considered together[479]:

- Binge eating disorder. This is recurrent binge eating, akin to bulimia but without the extreme weight-control behaviours[479].
- Food avoidance emotional disorder is a term, now rarely used, for loss of appetite without body image disturbance[1149]. The child wishes he or she had more appetite.
- Other well-recognised "atypical eating problems" include selective eating, food phobias, functional dysphagia (p.333), psychogenic vomiting, and food refusal [1151].
- Less common clinically are anorexia athletica, "reverse anorexia" in people who want to gain weight, fadorexia or ortharexia in people excessively preoccupied with eating the right foods, multi-impulsive bulimia, night eating syndrome.

See also *pervasive refusal*, p.527; *pica*, p.336; *feeding*, p.331; *fussy eating*, p.331; *overeating*, p.335; *eating odd things*, p.336; *vomiting*, p.337; body dysmorphic disorder, p.433.

Eaton-Lambert syndrome: autoimmune attack (p.427) on presynaptic calcium channels, causing progressive weakness that improves with exercise[381].

EBV: Epstein-Barr virus, p.478.
ECG: electrocardiogram (heart recording).

Echolalia and echopraxia: these terms are often used very loosely to include all repetitions of self or others (whether spoken or movements, respectively). However there are numerous causes of repetitions and these terms are best reserved for echoes like those of canyons, i.e. occurring within a few seconds and having no regard whatsoever for the meaning.

Hence for types of repetitive speech see stuttering, p.157; winding up, p.157; pat phrases, p.158; palilalia, p.62 ; mitigated echolalia, p.160; delayed echolalia, p.159; (true) echolalia, p.159; vocal tics, p.102; other causes of repetitive speech, p.157.

For physical repetitions see pp.61–63; mirror system p.507; mimicry, p.507.

Eclampsia: see pre-eclampsia, p.535
EE: see *Negative expressed emotion* p.512.

EEG: electroencephalogram (brain recording). This can sometimes clarify that a behaviour is organic in origin. Because many scalp locations are recorded, EEGs can localise some kinds of brain pathology. They can be thought of as a type of brain imaging that has poor spatial resolution but records changes over milliseconds. Electrical activity is recorded mainly from the superficial layers of cerebral cortex.

Band	Hertz	Normal	Abnormal
Delta	0–4	In babies; in sleeping adults	When brain pathology reduces alertness.
Theta	4–7	In drowsiness or meditation	Various. increased in ⬆ADHD.
Alpha	8–12	Emerges in sensory cortices when they are inactive (a "default mode")	
Beta	12–30	In alertness; reduces during movement	Benzodiazepines (p.430) cause rhythmic beta.
Gamma	30–100	Synchronising neurons for cognitive functions	
Mu	8–13	Synchronous firing of motor neurons. Supressed by observing an action (see *mirror neurons*, p.507)	

Non-specific findings: changes in ID and specific learning disabilities are usually non-specific. See *epileptiform discharges*, p.73.

Suggestive findings: changes in ADHD and autism are somewhat distinct from one another[297] though in clinical practice the relationship between the two conditions is complex[161].

Specific findings[1166]: generalised 3 Hz spike-and-wave complexes in absences; other spike-wave complexes in infantile spasms and Lennox-Gastaut syndrome; regional polyspikes in focal cortical dysplasias; hypsarrhythmia (chaotic brain waves) in West syndrome; anterior temporal spikes in mesial TLE. Quantitative EEG (QEEG) is not sufficiently specific to be used as a test for ADHD[1506].

EEGs change during maturation. See also *evoked potentials*, p.462.

Egocentricity: p.180.

Ehlers-Danlos: a heterogeneous group of genetic disorders with hypermobile joints (see p.483); skin hyperextensibility; and delayed wound healing with atrophic scarring[995].

Electroencephalogram: see *EEG* above.

Embarrassment: a self-conscious wish that something about oneself were less public. The word *shame* is similar but usually implies a greater transgression; *guilt* (p.475) has a more moral emphasis (see[829]). It occurs in normal people and is exaggerated in social phobia (p.298). It prevents open communication (p.152) and can be a useful regulator of behaviour in public (p.261). It makes many people with OCD keep their symptoms secret (p.65), makes incontinent children hide their accidents (p.341), and makes illiterates pretend they can read.

Embarrassment is one of the more difficult *facial expressions* to recognise.The expression includes gaze down or shifted sideways, head away, and a smile, often with attempts to control the smile[829]. Blushing is created by sympathetic innervation[556]. Complaints of blushing do not reflect the actual amount of blushing[556]. Embarrassment is also sometimes expressed as laughter (p.111) or, less commonly, anger (p.287).

Parents often give in to their children's tantrums in public to avoid further embarrassment (p.315).

EMG: electromyogram (muscle recording).

Emotional instability or *dyscontrol or episodic dyscontrol* or *emotion dysregulation or lability*: p.69

Emotions: Brief valenced states, typically focussed on specific objects, and giving rise to behavioural response tendencies relevant to those objects. In contrast, mood is the pervasive, diffuse and sustained emotional climate that influences cognition more than actions[622]. (See list of individual emotions on p.395; facial expressions, p.465; emotion dysregulation, p.69; rapid changes in emotions, p.69.)

About 30 *distinct emotions* are commonly recognised[829]. They produce behavioural changes, as well as facial expressions that communicate the emotion to others. A few of the emotions (especially those marked with * on p.395) seem to be *basic emotions*, i.e. distinct basic neurological states (on the basis of their universality in people and other primates, rapidity, specific physiology, automatic appraisal, and other features[451,829]). Other emotions are more complex, generally with cognitive as well as physiological elements.

Emotions and cognitions influence perceptions, e.g. of pain (p.135) or of breathlessness (p.457). Somewhat similarly, an adrenaline-induced state of arousal does not have an intrinsic meaning, and can be described by subjects as either angry or euphoric, depending on their expectations[1432]. *Positive emotions* encourage play, exploration, integration of ideas, and strengthening of relationships[520].

Empathy: discussed with *Sensitivity*, p.546.
ENA: extractable nuclear antigens, see *ANA*, p.421.

Encephalitis: inflammation of the brain, often accompanied by inflammation of the brain's coverings (meningitis). Either is a medical emergency, though often the specific cause cannot be identified.

Urgent paediatric assessment is needed to consider these diagnoses following onset of seizures, decline in conscious level (p.97), delirium (p.451), vomiting (p.337), hard neurological signs (p.58), blanching or non-blanching rash, severe drop in blood pressure, or (in babies) a bulging fontanelle. The neck is often stiff in meningitis.

Tests include ESR; culture plus microscopy of blood and CSF; EEG; and imaging. See also *infections*, p.490; herpes viruses, p.478; anti-NMDA encephalitis, p.422; SSPE, p.557; Rasmussen encephalitis, p.539; encephalitis lethargica, p.522.

Encopresis: p.341.
Enuresis: p.339.
EOS: early onset schizophrenia. See *schizophrenia*, p.543.
EP: educational psychologist.
Epigenetics: p.489.

Epilepsia partialis continua: a rare form of epilepsy, with twitching of a body part, usually a distal limb, lasting any period from hours to years[303]. The twitching is sometimes aggravated by movement or sensation. In children and adolescents the most common cause is Rasmussen syndrome (p.539).

Epilepsy: p.73.
Epinephrine: see *adrenaline*, p.420.
Episodic dyscontrol: p.69.

Erection: tumescence of the penis. This is a spinal reflex involving nitrous oxide, and can be initiated by pressure or vibration, or spontaneously as in foetal erections that start before the 16th week of pregnancy[760].

> Failure of erection may be brought to attention by observant mothers or in adolescence by the boy. Erectile dysfunction can be psychogenic, neurogenic, hormonal, vasculogenic, drug-induced (antihypertensives or antidepressants) or caused by systemic disease[981]. There may be a specific association with Fragile X (p.468).

> Persistent erection (called priapism if it lasts for hours) occurs in both painful and painless forms. Many of those affected have a haematological cause (sickle, p.549; leukaemia, polycythaemia[1702]); others result from straddle injury[1095], following intercourse[1213], and in appendicitis and Fabry's disease (p.464). Urgent thorough investigation is needed.

ESR: erythrocyte sedimentation rate (a marker of inflammation).

Evoked potentials: this is similar to EEG, but rather than looking at spontaneous activity it records the responses to external stimuli. The evoked potential is usually recorded from the brain or brainstem. Most relevant to behaviour are:

> Auditory evoked potentials (AEPs). These can be used to check hearing even if the patient is a baby, uncooperative, unconscious, or dissociating. When one noise is followed by a second similar noise, the response to the second one is reduced in most people. This reduction, called pre-pulse inhibition (or *pre-pulse inhibition of startle*) is diminished in schizophrenics and their relatives[1188] and in various other psychiatric groups[209] (see *acetylcholine*, p.418).

> Visual evoked potentials (VEPs) can detect blindness in patients who cannot communicate or who are malingering. VEPs can show nerve damage as in multiple sclerosis, p.510.

Exaggeration: describing a real thing as bigger or more severe than it really is (pp.365, 359). In common use (but not DSM's use, p.389), this implies it is intentional.

Excitotoxicity: neuronal death caused by overexcitation, usually by the excitatory transmitter glutamate[1191]. This is quite distinct from arousal or hyperexcitability syndromes, p.483. In young people it can be found following hypoxia, hypoglycaemia, p.82; head injury, p.477; or status epilepticus. It may be one of the pathogenic mechanisms in degenerative conditions such as Huntington's and multiple sclerosis. Neurons in the hippocampus, p.478, are especially vulnerable.

Exercise: this usually refers to repeated large physical movements. If spontaneous and varied it is physical play, p.221. Mental exercise: see mental fatigue, p.323.

Effects of exercise
It can reduce obesity, p.335. Mild exercise can improve depression and anxiety in children[910]. It often reduces stiffness and in rare conditions temporarily relieves weakness, p.459. Exercise increases adrenaline, noradrenaline, dopamine, and lactate (p.508) – all of them much less in ADHD[1759]. Severe or unaccustomed exercise can cause musculoskeletal pain, p.93; myokymia, p.61; and other symptoms, pp.438, 464.

Inadequate exercise
Lack of exercise increases misbehaviour at home, p.207; worsens sleep, p.199; and if prolonged, causes weakness, p.87. Avoidance of exercise: pp.323, 126, 299. Exercise intolerance can be physical and/or psychogenic, see pp.323, 418.

Excess exercise
Increased exercise in anorexia nervosa, p.334; distinguishing this from OCD, p.65. The "female athlete triad" consists of disturbed eating, amenorrhoea, and reduced bone density. Exercise releases opioids and can become an addiction, p.259.

Regulation
After imposed inactivity lasting more than an hour, children let off steam (p.80) and after exercise they become less active. Children have their own individual activity levels[1175], and some studies suggest they regulate their daily activity amount[1765]. Boys take about 20% more steps per day than girls[1758]. In both sexes, activity levels reduce later in childhood.

Exorcism: see p.448.

Experimentation: there is some randomness in our behaviour, sometimes called *fundamental indeterminacy*[572]. This is crucial to learn about the world and to adapt to changes (in the environment or in people)[1772]. The word *experimentation* is often used to describe this, even though the child is usually only aware of the tangible reinforcers (p.540), not the *information* they have just acquired. All the behaviours in this book are sometimes done just as a trial, or as play (p.221). People also try old behaviours, or behaviours they have observed in others, in new contexts (see *extinction*, below). Some people are always more predictable (i.e. less random) than others, and most people become more predictable when they are anxious (see discussion of Yerkes-Dodson, p.40).

Expressed emotion: see *Negative expressed emotion*, p.512.
Expressionlessness: p.178.

Externalising: as a defence mechanism, p.306. The term is also used broadly to distinguish behaviours which affect the outside world (*externalising*, e.g. ADHD or violence) from those which cause internal effects (*internalising*, e.g. depression or dissociation).

Extinction: decline in behaviour elicited by a stimulus. This is an active process, creating a new memory, and so extinguished behaviours can reappear in certain circumstances (*spontaneously*, i.e. after time; *renewed*, when testing occurs in different contexts, or *reinstated*, when the US is presented unexpectedly)[1129]. Extinction is quite distinct from forgetting which is the gradual fading of unused memories or their accessibility over time, p.468. Extinction of children's difficult behaviours is one of the most important general behaviour management techniques, and it is also part of standard exposure-based therapies. Deficiencies in fear extinction mechanisms[1129] probably underlie many cases of phobia and PTSD (see p.127). See also *extinction bursts*, p.120; *unlearning*, p.571.

Exuberant: is an uncommon term, with several closely related meanings: (a) a *happy* temperament, unrestrained and lively, with noisy hilarity, enjoying both novelty and social interaction[1261]; (b) a persistently *active* temperament, the opposite of behavioural inhibition[516] (p.296); (c) a combination of a and b, i.e. of hyperthymia (p.264) and ADHD (p.387). It can sometimes be difficult to work out the relative contributions of the hyperthymia and ADHD (see p.264). If the most extreme behaviours are highly social or extravagant, the former is a better description.

Eyes: links to all aspects are listed under *Visual problems*, p.133.

Fabricated symptoms: p.359.

Fabry's disease: a genetic disorder with many forms[868,1020]. The hallmark is the presence of many angiokeratomas, purplish bumps a few mm in diameter, initially between umbilicus and knees, first appearing in childhood. Males get the full disorder from their hemizygous X-chromosome, but females inactivate half of their X-chromosomes (mosaicism, p.509) so experience milder disease with later onset. First symptoms are often shooting pains or chronic pain. Episodes of burning in hands and feet last several days ("Fabry crises"), often triggered by exercise, hot weather, or stress. Autonomic changes include reduced sweating, tears and saliva; nausea and diarrhoea. Disfigurement, shooting pains, and nausea combine to cause personality changes and depression.

Face-hand test: there are two of these.

   a) Simultaneous touches on the cheek and the opposite hand can be detected reliably from age 7, regardless of mild ID[878].

   b) If pseudo-paralysis is suspected, the child's hand can be dropped on his face. The idea is that, at least if he doesn't expect it, a malingerer will automatically prevent his face being knocked. This test, also called the *arm drop test*, cannot be relied on[907].

Faces:

   Receptive: includes recognising individual people, plus their age and sex and their emotions. This is done in a holistic way, in a different brain area from other recognition[1623]. Checking what people are looking at: see *Pointing*. See also *Facial expressions (understanding)*.

   Protecting the face: p.107.

   Injuring the face: of self, p.110; of others, p.290.

   Dysmorphic features: these can be looked up in[787].

Facial expressions (using): see smiles (p.549), expressionlessness (p.178) and eye contact (p.175). Some people make odd faces, e.g. when thinking or surprised. The structure of female faces leads to their being interpreted more often as happy; and male faces are more often interpreted as angry[131]. Children with autism are more neutral in their facial expression, in comparison with other children (whether ID or not); have more difficulty imitating facial expressions[368]; and they also make more ambiguous expressions[1809].

frightened   angry   happy   laughing   sad   disgusting   surprise

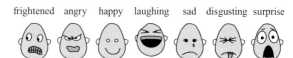

Figure 28 Faces most children use by age 5.

Facial expressions (understanding): people with autism are better at recognising happiness and sadness, than surprise and embarrassment; they are less sensitive to negative emotions such as distress, fear, and discomfort; and they pay more attention than controls to the bottom half of people's faces [reviewed in 624]. Abused children over-identify anger relative to fear and sadness [1264].

Factitious: p.359.
Faecal misplacement: p.341.
Fahr's disease: p.429.
Faking: see *malingering*, p.503.

False memory: memories for events that never occurred. This is crucial in legal cases involving alleged abuse or trauma (p.567). For possible mechanisms see *confabulation*, p.443; *reconsolidation*, p.540; *memory distortions*, p.40.

Family: see *Parents*, p.525; *Siblings*, p.548; *Looked after children*, p.500; genograms, p.203; common patterns of family dynamics, p.211; child altering family dynamics, p.211; expressed emotion, p.512.

Fantasy, Fantastic stories: see *Imagination*, p.488; imaginary and verbal / fantastic play, pp.221–222

Fasting: abstaining from food. For the predictable effects of long-term partial fasting, see *anorexia nervosa*, p.334. It can cause amenorrhoea, dehydration (p.450), cardiac arrhythmias, kidney stones (p.555), vitamin deficiencies (p.328), and many other problems[833]. Fasting can also have idiosyncratic effects, such as an episode of jaundice in Gilbert syndrome; or other metabolic crises, p.381. The ketogenic diet, i.e. a diet that forces the breakdown of fats, is an effective method for treating refractory epilepsy. For the effects of multi-day fasts, see[833].

During the month of Ramadan, observant Muslims fast from an hour before dawn until sunset and then share a family meal each evening. Several exemptions apply (prepubertal children, pregnancy, lactation, menstruation, travelling, sick, mentally ill, or needing medicines) but many adults prefer not to use their exemptions. Prepubertal children are gradually trained to fast, and doing this in a non-Muslim school is often more difficult. Babies conceived during Ramadan fasting have a somewhat increased risk of disability[30] and slightly worse long-term health[1651].

Fathers: fathers usually have less contact with the children than mothers have, but more of this is play. Fathers also have more antisocial behaviour and alcoholism than mothers.

See: children behaving better with dad than with mum, p.201; contrast between parental roles, p.201; rough-and-tumble play, p.222; modelling a dominating interest, p.229; assertive speaking style, p.162; tendency to over-indulge, p.179; protective effect for child of attachment to father, p.196; contrast with stepfathers, pp.212, 272, 275; family's belief that son will be like dad, p.212; sons copying father's treatment of women, p.212; sexual interactions with children, p.267; father of girl's pregnancy being unknown, p.276; criminal father, p.446.

Fatigue: p.323.
FBC: full blood count (in USA: CBC, complete blood count).

Fear: p.307. See also *anxiety*, p.295; and the opposite: *recklessness*, p.539.

Feeding: p.331.
Female genital mutilation: See p.448.

Fibromyalgia: widespread pain in muscle and joints, often accompanied by hypersensitivity to pain or pressure (see growing pains, p.137; chronic fatigue, p.325). There are often psychological contributors (or sequelae), and in many cases no physical cause is found. However sufferers do have enhanced pain-sensitivity, apparently increased by anxiety-proneness, low mood, and catastrophising, as well as several identified neurophysiological mechanisms. These include local spinal *central sensitisation* of pain (p.436), broader *pain augmentation*, greatly increased Substance P in CSF, and reduced descending *diffuse noxious inhibitory control*[1769]. Various methods have been used to establish a threshold for diagnosis, e.g. the number of points that are tender (from a specified list) or the number of quadrants of the body affected; but as pain is a very common experience the presence of disability is probably more clinically useful. See also *comorbidity*, p.442.

Fiddling: repetitive pointless small movements. Common in ADHD where it may be a *utilisation behaviour*, p.572.

Fight or flight: phrase coined by Cannon which infortunately leaves some people believing there are only two options and that the primary option is fighting. Both of these seem to be incorrect (p.296).

Fingers: see *Hands*, p.476.

Fingernails: the commonest problem is heavily bitten fingernails, usually a sign of trait anxiety, which when very severe can cause bleeding. Dirty fingernails are very common, even in children who are otherwise clean, so they do not indicate neglect. Over-long fingernails can indicate that the parents are too busy, or that the child resists excessively, or that parents have not been given guidance on cutting fingernails when the child is deeply asleep. Girls of any age enjoy decorating their fingernails, often as a social activity. When inspecting the nails, look for:

- abnormal nail shape, which can contribute to identification of some causes of ID[127].
- ungual or periungual fibromas, which are small painless lumps growing from the side or base of the fingernail, seen in tuberous sclerosis (p.569).
- finger clubbing, i.e. loss of the normal angle at the base of the nail (clearest when viewing the fingers side-on) associated with hyperthyroidism, laxative abuse and many systemic diseases which may require formal assessment[1128]. The proportion of cases that is benign is not known. For an assessment algorithm see[1526].

Fire: several behaviours need to be distinguished including fire interest, match lighting, and fire-setting (causing minor, moderate, or severe damage). The prevalences of these in 4–9-year-old boys are 35%, 9%, 3%, 0.4%, and less for severe damage, respectively[354,973]. Severity is indicated by repetitiveness, damage, degree of planning, lack of thought about controlling the fire, and failure to control the fire. Fire-setting by children accounts for 20–60% of forest and house fires[354].

Substantial fire-setting is generally not a child's only aberrant behaviour[978,990]: the commonest associations are with other delinquency; hyperactivity, p.79; daily smoking, perhaps because of the availability of ignition materials; substance abuse; and cruelty to animals, p.279 (compare *psychopathy*, p.280). Underlying causes of severe fire-setting include anger (e.g. following abuse), serious family problems, difficulty making close relationships, poor planning ability (especially in younger children), and in rare cases psychosis or the use of fire by parents as a punishment[978], or Asperger's (see p.253).

Flapping: p.105.

Flattening of emotion or speech:

Flattened speech is a kind of dysprosody (p.148) most commonly seen in depression (see psychomotor retardation, p.537) and Asperger syndrome. Flattened speech is also heard in Parkinsonism[340] and other damage to the basal ganglia[1656], p.429.

In contrast, *flattening of affect* is reduction of emotional responses, so they are between apathy and normality. It is especially noticeable with extreme stimuli[1487]. Flattening or reduction of the usual range of emotion is common in chronic schizophrenia, and with antipsychotics, and this of course is reflected in speech[1487].

Blunting refers to a lack of care for the feelings of others, seen in schizophrenia, autism and psychopathy[1487].

Flexibility: mental, p.234; physical: see hypermobility, p.483.
Flinching: p.107.
Flynn effect: p.59.

Foetal Alcohol syndrome (FAS): this is defined by a symptom count, with milder forms of *Foetal Alcohol Spectrum Disorder* called *Foetal Alcohol Effects* or *Partial FAS*. The symptoms include short palpebral fissures, thin vermilion on the upper lip, smooth filtrum (with the upper lip, i.e. all the flesh below the nose, being thinner than the lower lip), growth retardation, small head, structural brain abnormalities (for details see [724].) This physical syndrome is often accompanied by enormous associated problems, such as mother's continuing drinking, plus the original reasons for her having been drinking in pregnancy, and a high rate of adoption (p.419) and fostering.

Foetal valproate syndrome: p.572.

Folate: a vitamin of great importance in development, immunity, production of blood cells, and digestion[417]. Related developmental disorders include:

Gestational
- Neural tube defects (p.513) such as spina bifida (p.551). Often caused by autoimmunity to the folate transporter[417].
- Folate deficiency may increase the likelihood of a Fragile X mutation causing ID[417], or of cleft palate, p.440.

- Folate levels are lowered by some anti-epileptic medications: see *foetal valproate*, p.572.
- Down's syndrome (p.455) may be more common and more severe in the presence of functional folate deficiency[417].

Other
- Cerebral folate deficiency (irritability and slowed head growth in infancy; visual and auditory deficits from early childhood; ataxia and seizures. Probably caused by autoimmunity to folate transporter).
- Folate-responsive seizures (which start neonatally).
- MTHFR deficiency[176] causes homocystinuria (p.481) which can in turn cause psychosis and regression. Treatment is very effective if started early, so diagnosis is urgent. Check for homocysteinaemia, blood folates, amino acid chromatography[1448].
- Because folate is a cofactor for many enzymes, many genetic syndromes are increased in severity by low folate[417]. Furthermore, supra-normal levels of folate can compete with blocking antibodies at folate transporters.
- Folate deficiency (rare in countries with folate-fortified food, which include the USA, Canada and Chile, but not the UK or Europe[1198]) causes anaemia, diarrhoea, drowsiness, glossitis, and increased susceptibility to infections, plus a wide variety of neurological problems.

Football: p.223.
Forced normalisation: p.449.

Forgeting: gradual fading of information, or increasing difficulty of recall. Children with ID often seem to have learned something, but then to have forgotten it the next day. In practice this usually means that the material was too difficult and not repeated sufficiently. Forgetting is not *extinction*, p.463.

Formulation: a detailed story relating key factors and how they led to the problem. See difficulties in formulating, p.18; ways of overcoming them, pp.23–26; full, simplest, and most treatable formulations, p.14; multiple, hierarchical and serial causes, p.14; mixed physical-mental problems, p.100, 323, 361; different formulations for different audiences, p.183.

Fractures: especially following multiple fractures, consider physical abuse, p.273 (especially in preverbal children); rickets, p.485; osteomyelitis; copper deficiency, p.330; severe prolonged disuse of the limb; impulsivity, p.79; inappropriate housing; inadequate parental supervision; osteogenesis imperfecta (often with blue sclerae); primary hyperparathyroidism, p.525; congenital analgesia, p.136. For details and rarer causes see[774]. When in doubt, the following may be appropriate: complete physical examination, urinalysis, blood count, Ca, phosphate, liver function / alkaline phosphatase, serum 25-OH vitamin D, copper, caeruloplasmin, amylase, skeletal survey, head imaging, and ophthalmological review.

Fragile X syndrome : the commonest single-gene cause of ID. Includes long face, simple protruding ears, high-arched palate, hypermobile joints, visuospatial deficits, hyperactive. They have a special kind of gaze-avoidance (p.176), but are quite friendly. Postpubertal testicular enlargement is common but so is erectile failure[627,1019], and irregular menses[1019]. Cluttering speech (p.441). Associated with increase in inattention (p.79), autism (p.183), and ID (weak in auditory STM; strength in verbal LTM) and often have a large fund of stored information.

Fragile X is a triplet repeat disorder, p.568. The pre-mutation of Fragile X is much more common than "full Fragile X" and also increases the likelihood of ASD or ADHD[485]. The premutation is often present in a grandparent of a child with Fragile X, and often results in the Fragile X-associated tremor/ataxia syndrome[34].

Friction between individuals: p.527.
Friedreich's ataxia: p.92.

Friends: these are discussed with *peer relationships*, p.171. (See also imaginary friends, p.231.)

Freud, Anna: originated the study of defence mechanisms (p.303).

Freud, Sigmund: founder of psychoanalysis. One of the most influential figures of the 20th century, with many profound insights and a similar number of major errors[1552]. See Freudian slips, p.357; unconscious, p.570; Freud as a systemiser, p.560; his view of sport, p.223; view of self-identity, p.237; pseudoscience, p.537.

Frontal signs: the influence of the frontal lobes (p.512) increases gradually, as they are myelinated through childhood and adolescence (p.574). Even though the following signs are classically associated with damage to the frontal lobes they can also be seen in damage to other areas of the cerebrum[1329] and brainstem, as well as in immaturity; neurodisability[1085], and sometimes in schizophrenia (see *soft neurological signs*, p.58). The most striking difference between frontal lesions and lesions to other areas of neocortex is often the subtlety of the deficit, or indeed the lack of obvious specific deficits[1329].

Emotional frontal signs

- emotional insta (p.70)
- major change of personality (e.g. apathetic or disinhibited).

Neuropsychological frontal signs, i.e. deficits in the following functions:

- visual memory (p.38)
- backward digit span (p.452)
- reading comprehension
- similarities and differences (p.36).

Neurological frontal signs[346,618]:

- loss of integrative functions
  - stereognosis
  - graphaesthesia
- loss of sequenced movements
  - Ozeretski's test: clench one fist while extending the fingers of the other hand, and repeat this while alternating sides.
  - Tapping test: tapping twice with one hand and once with the other, and repeating.
  - Finger-ring test: alternating between flexing the arm with clenched fist, and extending it with fingers forming a ring.
  - Fist-palm-edge test (alternating these three ways of touching a table).

    ○ Piano test: touching all the fingers in turn to the thumb. This should be done on both hands simultaneously.
- frontal release signs are primitive reflexes that can be seen if they are not inhibited by frontal cortex. For details of how to elicit them see[1085,1379]:
  - glabellar tap (usually tapping on the eyebrow causes blinking that habituates after two or three taps; this habituation is lost in frontal damage)
  - utilisation behaviours, p.572 (e.g. grasp reflex on stroking the palm)
  - snout (pouting) reflex on pressing the upper lip
  - tactile rooting: moving the mouth towards an object touching the cheeks
  - visual rooting: moving the head towards, or pouting towards, an approaching object[1085]
  - suck reflex on touching upper and lower lips with a finger
  - palmomental reflex: chin muscle twitches on stroking base of thumb
  - upgoing plantar (p.56)
  - synkinesis (p.560)
- reappearance of infantile behaviours (see p.56)
- perseveration (p.527).

Frustration: p.291.

Frozen watchfulness: this is a type of hypervigilance (p.296) indicating fear of particular people; it is a useful sign of physical abuse (p.273). A crucial aspect of this sign is that it disappears when frightening people (e.g. abusers) are not in room. It can be frozen and gaze-*avoidant*, i.e. using peripheral vision for threat-monitoring. If the child has generalised his fear of the abuser to other adults, or strangers, care will be needed to work out whether he is generally anxious (p.296) or depressed (p.313) as well.

G6PD: p.350.

GABA: gamma-amino butyric acid, the main inhibitory transmitter of the brain. Its effects are enhanced by benzodiazepines (p.430) and baclofen, working at the $GABA_A$ and $GABA_B$ receptors respectively. Deficiency has a central role in many epilepsies[534,761], some dystonias, p.458 and Stiff Person syndrome (p.555). Surround inhibition in the cerebral cortex is signalled by GABA, as are major pathways in the basal ganglia. GABA receptor abnormalities predispose to alcoholism[1804], presumably due to anxiety. Deficiency of the GABA degradative enzyme SSADH is the commonest major abnormality of GABA: symptoms include ID, epilepsy, ataxia, hyporeflexia, expressive language problems, anxiety and sleep disturbance[1235].

As well as acting as a classical transmitter, GABA has an extrasynaptic tonic inhibitory effect, which appears to be underactive in Fragile X, overactive in absence seizures, and also important in the action of alcohol and in hormonal mood changes[132] (see p.506).

During embryogenesis both GABA and glycine (p.474) act as excitatory rather than inhibitory transmitters[504].

GAD: generalised anxiety disorder, p.297; glutamic acid decarboxylase, p.555.

Gag: ambiguous term, used to mean *retch* or *choke*. Also glycosaminoglycans (see p.502).

Gain: benefits obtained through behaviour (i.e. actual or hoped-for reinforcement). There are several subtypes that have been defined in various ways[1650], but the most common usage currently is:

- Primary gain, usually relief of unpleasantness or tension. This can be intrapsychic (i.e. defence mechanisms, p.303) or concrete (i.e. coping mechanisms, p.445)
- Secondary gain: additional material or social benefits, such as benefits of the sick role. This is of limited use in diagnosis as benefits accrue whether the behaviour is organic or not (p.361).
- Tertiary gain: benefits to other people[365]. See Munchausen by proxy, p.206.

When the primary gain is avoidance, there is invariably some secondary gain that guides the choice of behaviour (because there are always numerous ways of avoiding something). For example, if the problem is dislike of brocolli, not having it is a primary gain, and the alternative food provided (plus increased maternal attention) are typical secondary gains.

Furthermore, all three levels of gain can coexist[188]. For example, if the initial problem is fear of a bully at school, staying off school can be motivated by avoidance of the bully (primary gain), increased parental attention while at home (secondary gain), and benefits for mother, i.e. her worries are relieved (which could be described as a tertiary gain for the family group, and/or as a secondary gain for the child).

Gait: this is the pattern of limb movements used for locomotion. Each person has several gaits, including running, jogging, walking for quiet, walking to carry heavy objects, or while testing the ground. In mildly affected children, gait asymmetry becomes obvious during running.

Many abnormal gaits can be recognised. An antalgic gait minimises the weight put on a painful leg. A stamping gait indicates peripheral neuropathy. Cerebral palsy (p.437) has several distinct gaits. A waddling gait, with rotation at each step like a duck, can result from obesity, cogenital hip dislocation (Trendelenberg), muscular dystrophy (p.510), spinal muscular atrophy (p.551), or Guillain-Barré (p.87). Severely impaired leg control can lead to bunny-hopping (an elaboration of the W-posture, p.483). Autistic children have a wide range of idiosyncratic gaits, e.g. leaping whenever starting to walk; or flapping and crouching whenever approaching something; or a camp gait (p.243).

- Toe-walking, which means not putting the heel down first (i.e. no heel-strike), is common for the first year of walking but persists longer in some cerebral palsy (p.437) and other neurodevelopmental conditions. Unless treated, severe cases with limited passive dorsiflexion of the foot eventually develop contracture of the Achilles tendon.
- Signs of pseudo-gaits include exaggerated effort, strained facial expression, grasping the leg, excessive slowness, moaning, violent trembling, dragging a leg, postures that waste effort (though the gait in chorea (p.439) or neuroacanthocytosis (p.514) can appear contrived), give-way weakness (though this can happen in anxious people with physical problems); fixed positions of ankles or toes;

sudden buckling of the knees; "walking on ice" gait of small cautious steps with fixed ankle joints.[930] See also pseudo-behaviours, p.363.

- Rareties in children: festinant gait in Parkinsonism, p.525; unsteady gait in Tay-Sachs, p.502; fear-of-falling gait in Stiff Person syndrome, p.555. Any progressive deterioration needs investigation (p.41). If gait worsens during the day and is improved after sleep consider Segawa syndrome, p.458.

Galactosaemia: a genetic disorder (1 in 20 000 in some populations). Neonatal problems include poor feeding and growth, jaundice, and Gram-negative sepsis. Later problems include cataracts; ID; and usually primary ovarian insufficiency (POI) causing amenorrhoea and infertility[159].

Gambling: see *behavioural addiction*, p.259.

Gang: (a) a group of delinquents. Such a "deviant peer cluster" includes mainly boys who are doing badly in school, and who are not effectively monitored by their parents[415]. Membership strongly predicts later drug addiction and violence. Compare *conduct disorder*, p.249.

(b) a group of people who defend their territory, and have a shared criminal activity, typically drug-dealing. Such gangs have some internal organisation (which can be subtle[893]) and usually a way of identifying each other. They are most famously associated with American inner cities, but are found around the world under various names.

There are many reasons for an individual to join such a gang, ranging from financial ambition to fear of being attacked near home. They provide routines, supervision, exercise, discipline, competition, rewards, goals, and (relative) safety.

Signs of gang membership include hanging out with a new group of friends all of whom wear a marker (e.g. a bandana, tattoo or cap), use of hand signs, and carrying a weapon. Less specific indicators include using new private slang or a new nickname, having more money, being vague about his whereabouts, losing interest in school, and writing graffiti-style *tags*.

(c) a less common meaning nowadays is a clique, or small group of close friends.

See also *group mayhem*, p.251.

Ganser syndrome: p.357.

Gastro-oesophageal reflux (GORD): causing hoarseness, p.147; feeding difficulty, p.331; crying, p.315; self-harm, p.317; headbanging, p.119; invariant behaviours, p.63; posture in Sandifer syndrome, p.93; belching, p.430; vomiting, p.337.

Gaze following, Gaze monitoring, Gaze referencing: p.170.

Gazing: prolonged looking, also called staring. This can indicate monitoring (e.g. frozen watchfulness, p.470), wonderment, or an interest, (p.229), e.g. in the opposite sex. It can also signal aggression. Eye-gaze is sometimes used as a synonym for *eye contact*, p.175. See also *hand-regard*, p.56; *absences*, p.75.

GEFS: generalised epilepsy with febrile seizures, p.438.

Gender differences: within days of birth, girl babies have significantly more interest in faces than boy babies[313]. Girls on average learn to speak slightly before boys, both in words and sentences (p.55). Both sexes learn to sit and walk at the same age (p.55).

From age 4, boys are substantially (over one standard deviation) better than girls in rotating an image mentally[1378]. Boys also have a demonstrable throwing advantage from about age 2. This is not due to strength: boys are better at throwing balls long distances, but also at throwing darts short distances, and catching or intercepting ping pong balls[842,1719].

Boys have more early developmental problems; but after puberty (p.411) girls have more mood problems. Autism, ID and ADHD

are several times more common in boys, and activity levels are higher (p.462); but anorexia nervosa (p.334) and physical pain (p.135) are much more common in girls. Startle responses may persist longer in women than in men[540].

Many inter-individual differences in both sexes are attributed to levels of testosterone (see discussion on p.554). There are also social differences between boys and girls in their interests, p.227; education and care of younger siblings, p.215; style of bullying, p.219; crying, p.315; screaming, p.544; religious activity, p.541; rates of sexual behaviours, p.267; incidence of sexual abuse, p.275; FGM, and discipline, p.214.

Generosity: see *sharing*, p.179.
Genetics: p.379.
Genogram: p.203.
Ghrelin: see *intake regulating hormones*, p.491.

Gifted children: this has various definitions ranging from the most capable 3% to the most capable 15%[1253]. Rather than basing this purely on IQ, it may be more predictive to categorise children as supersmart, socioemotionally gifted, modestly gifted and artistically gifted – or simply to mention the areas they are best in[281]. The term *prodigy* implies a much more extreme degree of skill, e.g. in music[1053] or chess[723], often produced by vast amounts of practice from a very early age, building on good or excellent innate ability.

Gifted children have fewer mental health problems than other children, but of course they are not invulnerable. If other children in the class are not of a similar level this can cause boredom, p.322; naughtiness, or social isolation, p.181.

Giftedness sometimes gives the impression of Asperger syndrome (p.424) but gifted children are not actually impaired when given equally capable friends, and tasks or conversations that interest them. Unlike Asperger, they are happy to follow a conversational lead, and their work shows unusual creativity.

Over-optimistic parents are more common than gifted children. Do not rely on preferred drawings or videos of mathematical recitations, as you cannot be sure how much training was received. Sometimes parents' overenthusiasm can be tempered by a reminder that rapid development does not predict hyper-achievement in adult life. See multiple simultaneous activities, p.80; naughtiness, p.322; IQ tests, p.60.

Gilbert syndrome: p.350.
Give me five: p.378.

Glasgow coma scale: p.97.

Glaucoma: Raised intraocular pressure, which if sudden is a medical emergency ‼. It is very uncommon in children. Signs include eye pain (unless chronic), red eye, reduced visual acuity. Rarely glaucoma appears without red eye, mimicking migraine. It can be precipitated by tricyclic antidepressants.

Glia: small cells of the nervous system primarily providing

Glia: small cells of the nervous system primarily providing metabolic support for neurons. Glia play a part in many neurodegenerative disorders, either by producing toxins or reducing their support to neurons[97]. Glia remove excess glutamate and so usually prevent excitotoxicity, p.462. See also glia-based neoplasia, p.569.

Global cognitive deficits: see discussion of *Learning Disability*, p.498.
Globus hystericus: see choking phobia, p.333.
Glucose-6-phosphate-dehydrogenase (G6PD) deficiency: p.350.
Glue-sniffing: p.258.

Glutamate: this is the main excitatory transmitter in the brain[769] and is therefore important in excitotoxicity, p.462. It is pro-epileptogenic, and in this is opposed by GABA[207]. Psychiatrically the most important receptor is NMDA, which is important in learning (LTP) and which is opposed by GABA. Ketamine and phencyclidine are anti-NMDA and cause hallucinations. See anti-NMDA encephalitis, p.422. Fragile X (p.468) involves a metabotropic glutamate receptor[115].

Glycine: the main inhibitory transmitter in the spinal cord, brainstem, and retina[660]. Glycine is also an inhibitory transmitter in the forebrain[504], but GABA (p.470) is more important there. See hyperekplexia, p.483.

Glycosylation: the process of attaching oligosaccharides to a large molecule, typically to a protein.

The number of identified congenital disorders of glycosylation is growing fast[393,759]. Some muscular dystrophies are caused by defective glycosylation of α-dystroglycan[686]. Some non-syndromic ID is caused by faulty glycosylation of assorted macromolecules such as the glutamate receptor[686]. The same may be true of some autoimmune disorders (p.427).

Glycoprotein storage disorders are caused by inherited deficiencies in the lysosomal enzymes responsible for oligosaccharide degradation. This can be detected by urine chromatography.

Good-enough parenting: p.190.
GORD: Gastro-oesophageal reflux disease.

Grandiosity: eliciting grandiosity, p.263; prevalence of grandiose ideas, p.347; learned grandiosity, p.262; in a treasured child, p.214; in mania, p.264; in narcissism, p.511; in psychopathy, p.280; in steroid abuse, p.258; grandiose interests, p.228

Gratification phenomena: these are simple behaviours done because they feel good. They produce simple sensations, usually tactile / somatosensory. Examples are masturbation (p.115) and some hair-twiddling and thumb-sucking.

Gratification behaviours are one of the kinds of activities performed in order to achieve a specific sensation (p.124). Contrast *self-entertainment*, p.545, which is more experimental, *self-soothing*, p.61, which is more relaxing; *behavioural addictions*, p.259. (Note the term *need-gratification* was historically used to describe what we now call drives: see *Maslow*, p.505).

Gricean maxims of communication: p.143.
Growing pains: p.137.
Growth charts: p.55.
Guillain Barré syndrome: p.87.

Guilt: the feeling that one is bad because of an action (or inaction). This is common in depression, p.309. Alternative responses are defence mechanisms such as denial or rationalisation (p.303). Guilt is a perpetuating factor in many stuck situations. It is a major contributor to the adverse long-term effects of sexual abuse (p.275). Lack of guilt is especially pervasive in *psychopathy*, p.280.

Many *parents* feel guilt for their child's difficulties. Common ideas are that the parent caused the problem by having been at work too much, or not having paid enough attention to the children, or not feeding the baby well enough, or arranging the wrong immunisation, or choosing the wrong father, or driving the father away, or in some cultures belief that children's disability results from adultery or other guilt. Such beliefs are sometimes reinforced by other family members. They can prevent a parent from acting confidently and effectively.

Gums: growth of the gums (gingival enlargement/hyperplasia) is seen with medication (phenytoin and other anticonvulsants, cyclosporin, and calcium antagonists), as well as in inflammation, pregnancy, puberty, neoplasms, enlargement of the underlying bone, and in some rare genetic syndromes. See also bleeding gums caused by mercury, p.330; and by scurvy, p.329.

Habit: a behaviour that has been learned so thoroughly that it is performed even when the original motivation is absent.

Habituation: discussed with *sensitisation*, p.546.

Hair: pulling one's own hair, p.117; playing with hair, p.225; eating hair, p.336; lanugo hair, p.334; sacral hair, p.340; pubertal hair growth, p.411; drug screening, p.257; hair care as a daily living skill, p.451.

For mutations look at the distribution in the family. Blond in phenylketonuria, p.529; brittle and steel-coloured in Menkes, p.330; a white forelock (sometimes with deafness and heterochromia, i.e. differently coloured irises) in Waardenberg's syndrome; red in POMC mutation, p.491; white to yellow-brown in albinism (and similar in phenylketonuria, p.529); *red albinism* or OCA3 albinism, seen mainly in Africans. A low hairline is seen in Cornelia de Lange, p.445; and alopecia in Hartnup, p.477; phenylketonuria, p.529; Menkes; and other syndromes[755].

Hallucination: p.343.
HAND: p.479.

Handedness: most children favour one hand for tasks, which is visible in prenatal scans of the foetus sucking his thumb[689] – 90% of the population favour the right hand. The vast majority of children who write with their right hand will also hammer, throw, and toothbrush with their right hands, but a substantial minority of "writing right-handers" will use a left-handed method to perform more complex two-handed actions such as dealing cards or opening a jar. "Writing left-handers" are much less predictable: many of them use right-handed methods for some of these tasks[46].

Left-handedness can be inconvenient for standard cutlery, and it makes producing conventional cursive more difficult (hence the unusual writing positions sometimes adopted). However, left-handedness has a small association with creativity[395]. Furthermore, men apparently earn more if they are left-handed, but females earn less if they are[395].

Among children with coordination deficits, 30% are left-handed, and 13% are ambidextrous[575]. In some countries, the majority of left-handers, especially the children of less educated parents, are still required to write with their right hand[1060]. This can contribute to clumsiness and writing difficulty[1060].

Ambidextrous people have slightly lower IQs (mean 94) than left-handed (mean 98) and right-handed (mean 100)[316].

Self-cutting is usually done in places that the dominant hand can conveniently reach. See also *lateralisation*, p.497. Left-footedness can be revealed by asking the child to kick a ball.

Handicap: a disadvantage for an individual, resulting from *society's response to* an impairment or disability, that limits or prevents fulfilment of a role that is normal (depending on age, sex, social and cultural factors) for that individual[see 788]. See *impairment.*

Hand-regard: p.56.

Hands:

> *Visible problems*
> clubbing, p.466; Down's syndrome, p.455; callus in manual vomiting, p.334; cold blue hands in anorexia, p.334; Raynaud's phenomenon, p.562; hand-arm vibration syndrome, p.562; fingernails, p.466; asymmetry, p.425; thin fingers, p.505.
>
> *Movements*
> hand-wringing, below; flapping, p.105; midline stereotypies, p.64; Rett, p.541; blindisms, p.66; writer's cramp, p.458; milkmaid's grip, p.522; tremor, p.61; pill-rolling tremor, p.525; hands or fingers in mouth, pp.337, 496, 543; thumb-sucking, p.564; hand-licking, p.550; posturing hands, p.93.
>
> *Sensory*
> touching, p.132; tactile intolerance, p.128; Fabry's disease, p.464; tingling hands, p.260.
>
> *Social*
> touching, p.132; moving an adult's hand, p.167; hand games, p.254; hand signs, p.472 [and sign language, p.130; Makaton, p.502]; hand gestures accompanying speech, p.520; hands-off sexual offences, p.268; handshakes, pp.107, 132 and handshaking in Fragile X, p.176; high-five, p.378.
>
> *Tests*
> face-hand test, p.464; eye-hand coordination, p.91; dysdiadochokinesis, p.457; Fogs' sign, p.560; sequencing tests, p.469; coordination test, p.410; high-five, p.378.

Other
sweaty palms, p.558; clammy hands, p.129; hand temperature, p.562; handedness, above; hand-regard, p.56; bilateral skills, p.431; hand-biting, p.113; one hand controlling the other, p.318 (and *alien hand*, p.354; *intermanual conflict*, p.446); keeping hands too clean, p.521; hypermobility, p.483; finger length and testosterone, p.554.

Hand-wringing: may be associated with anxiety, hypocalcaemia, p.485; and/or basal ganglia calcification, p.429. See midline stereotypies, p.64; Rett syndrome, p.541.

Hard neurological signs: p.58.

Hartnup disease: one of the few treatable causes of ID, p.32. Signs include photosensitive skin rash, episodic ataxia, mental problems ranging from lability to psychosis to ID. This is an autosomal recessive disorder with many different mutations affecting the neutral amino acid transporter gene[80]. Resulting reduced absorption of tryptophan can cause secondary deficiency of niacin, p.329. Less severe mutations, and heterozygotes, interact with other transporters to determine less severe clinical states[218].

Hatred: p.187.
Headache: p.139.
Head circumference: p.409.
Headbanging: p.119.

Head injury: (more precisely, traumatic brain injury).

Information should be collected to assess severity and risk, including the date and time, witnesses, shape of the object and where it struck the head, speed of car, use of seatbelt, height of fall, on to what surface, maximum duration unattended (if injury was unwitnessed), duration until responsiveness; behaviours including vomitting, sleepiness, crying, seizures. Complications include intracranial haemorrhage and effects of other injuries sustained.

Indications for brain imaging vary from place to place, but usually include Glasgow Coma Score 13 or below (see p.97) or declining; focal neurological signs; deformation of the scalp or skull; or severe mechanism of injury[11].

Sequelae
The *post-concussive syndrome* includes: impaired attention and memory; fatigue (p.323); headache (p.139); dizziness; irritability (p.494); sensory intolerance (p.125); anxiety and insomnia; impulsivity; task-induced anxiety.

Closed head injury is very unlikely to have substantial enduring effects if the loss of consciousness was limited to a few days[277]. However, in rare cases there can be onset of symptoms such as hallucinations several years later.

The time delay between the trauma and the forming of new memories is called post-traumatic anterograde amnesia (PTA). If PTA is less than 24 hours, enduring impairment is very unlikely. Retrograde amnesia is the loss of memory for events before the injury: it does not have such prognostic significance.

See also head injury as an indicator of physical abuse, p.273; as a cause of coma, p.97; deafness, p.130; headbanging, p.119; causes of accidents, p.417.

Hearing: see *Ears.*

Heart: in healthy people, heart rate and blood pressure increase with exercise, arousal, antiasthmatics and stimulant medications. The heart rate rises about 5 bpm in mild negative anticipation[495]; about 5–10 bpm while on stimulants (including atomoxetine[1740]) and about 30 bpm for several days following major stressors[1246]. Ninety per cent of children are in the following ranges:

Age ▼	Systolic	Diastolic	Heart rate
5	<108	<68	90–130
10	<115	<75	80–120
15	<120	<79	60–100

For more details see www.nhlbi.nih.gov

Specialist opinion should be considered if the child has cyanosis, clubbing, oedema, or breathlessness at rest, especially of recent onset. Paroxysmal arrhythmias can be misinterpreted as panics, p.301. Other signs of arousal, p.424. Patients may complain of heart problems when they are actually talking about how sad they feel, p.360.

Heelprick test: p.32. For retrospective testing see *birth*, p.432.

Herpes virus family: these viruses all form long-term latent infections of nerves and brain (see also *infections*, p.490).

- Herpes simplex (HSV 1 and 2) commonly causes painful recurrent localised infections of the nerve sin skin. Herpes simplex encephalitis is much rarer, but is often very severe, so blind treatment with acyclovir and/or antibiotics is sometimes justified. Anogenital infection, especially with type 2, is usually sexually transmitted (see p.276).
- Epstein Barr virus (EBV). This is a member of the herpes family. It often causes infectious mononucleosis and (rarely) cancer. It can contribute to the aetiology of chronic fatigue, p.323; schizophrenia, p.543; and many autoimmune diseases such as multiple sclerosis, p.510.
- Varicella Zoster Virus (VZV). About 25% of children hospitalised with chickenpox have neurological complications. Three per cent acquire lasting ataxia or epilepsy; strokes affect 1%[955]. It also causes zoster (shingles).
- Cytomegalovirus (CMV).

HGPRT: hypoxanthine-guanine phosphoribosyl transferase (see Lesch-Nyhan, p.318).

Hiccups: usually a normal example of myoclonus (p.511). If intractable, this needs neurological examination. A rare cause is aripiprazole[1313].

Hierarchy: of power between family members, p.213; between peers, p.172; within criminal gangs, p.446; within the assessment process, p.15; of diagnoses, p.15; of types of anxiety, p.297; of acceptability of diagnoses to parents, p.19; of needs, p.505; of pains, p.135; of cognitive investigations, p.376; of metabolic investigations, p.381; of distortions of reality, p.359; as an aspect of sensory complexity, p.227. See also *status*, p.553; hierarchy of boundaries, p.434.

High (mania and hypomania): p.263.
High five: p.378.

Hippocampus: a small part of the medial temporal lobe, with a role in memory.

After bilateral hippocampal damage, delayed recall is impaired far more than immediate recall, and episodic memory is impaired far more than semantic memory[1665]. Verbal and topographical memories can be unrecallable even though they are easily recognised; this separation does not affect memories for faces[295].

The hippocampus can be damaged by hypoxia, caused by neonatal trauma, or neonatal pneumonia[751]. Rarer causes include carbon monoxide poisoning, near-drowning, suffocation, and status epilepticus. Separately, it has been suggested that severe stress releases glucocorticoids (p.555) that cause hippocampal atrophy, accounting for the memory deficits seen in PTSD (see discussion in [773]; other brain areas may be similarly affected[711]). See *excitotoxicity*, p.462.

Histamine: this chemical is best known for its peripheral inflammatory effects, but it is also a neurotransmitter, produced in the posterior hypothalamus and sent widely through the brain, increasing alertness and influencing daily cycles of sleep and feeding[636]. Some anti-histamine medications cross the blood-brain barrier, and hence cause drowsiness. This is a side-effect if they are being used to relieve itch; but it is sometimes useful.

Histrionics: defined as a display of exaggerated emotion; melodrama. Doing this occasionally is normal, but when pervasive it can be called Histrionic Personality Disorder, p.241.

HIV: Human Immunodeficiency Virus. This is often transmitted from mother to child at birth, though advanced medical care can largely prevent such *vertical transmission*. The prevalence varies greatly between geographical regions. Early treatment improves survival and cognitive outcome[1662]. HIV can progress to AIDS including delirium with hallucinations, delusions, catatonia, depression, and/or hyperactivity[663], plus movement disorders (chorea, p.439; dystonia; myoclonus, p.511; tremor). Testing is complex, involving counselling and, e.g., ELISA.

There are three categories of problem for people with HIV[458]:

1. Immunodeficiency permitting secondary infections. This is the main cause of death if HIV is *untreated*.
2. Direct neurotoxicity of HIV causing HAND (HIV-associated neurocognitive disorders). This builds slowly, over years to decades and varies from unnoticeable to severe dementia. It occurs even while immuno-deficiency is being adequately treated, because many HIV treatments do not cross the blood-brain barrier.
3. Cofactors. For example, if the HIV was contracted through drug use or prostitution there are far more psychosocial risks than if the HIV was contracted through a transfusion or from a long-term partner.

Similar symptoms can also result from *immune reconstitution inflammatory syndrome* after starting highly effective antiretroviral medication[663].

Maternal HIV
In the 1990s this implied that mother was dying of HIV-related infections, and that is still often the case in Africa (see skip-generation families, p.212). Nowadays, with modern therapies secondary infections are much less common, and most mothers with HIV live a full and satisfying life[815]. Women with HIV have

the same rate of pregnancy as those without, and the same motives for pregnancy[1480].

Hoarding: This means accumulating possessions to a damaging degree. It can be an isolated problem, or it can be caused by various underlying conditions (OCD, p.65; general anxiety, p.295; autism, p.183; anorexia nervosa, p.334; severe neglect, p.274; Prader-Willi, p.533; schizophrenia, p.543; dementia). When it is an isolated problem, the person generally values and is interested in the hoarded items, and is very upset when they are discarded (unlike the disinterest shown by hoarders with severe brain damage)[1026]. Hoarding may have a specific neural substrate, which is active in animals that hoard (e.g. squirrels).

The most severe hoarding is done by adults, the most troublesome being the hoarding of food or animals; but the onset of hoarding is often in childhood. It is not uncommon for parents to have to "edit" a child's collections of cans, toys, wrappers, or clothes, when he or she is out of the house. Children with major hoarding problems typically have normal reasons (pleasure, happy memories, or in case they need the item one day) to which they give excess weight[1550].

Hobbies: this word is usually used for adult-like play, especially if it is pursued for long enough to allow a gradual accumulation of skill. Examples include cleaning and adjusting bikes, p.112; football, p.223; other sports and trampolining; reading; drawing, p.56; computer games, p.224; internet, p.492; making models; lego; horses, p.248; collecting, pp.226; chess; making or listening to music; boardgames; singing; magic. Listening to music is often called a hobby but is too passive for some definitions. Playing doctor or school or shop could be a hobby, but doesn't usually last long enough for skills to accumulate. For other types of play, see p.221.

Holidays: displeasure when anticipating a holiday can be due to bad experiences in the past (cold, wet or boring) or to anxiety (about change, malaria, flying or the trip to the airport). Specific intolerances while on holiday are usually obvious (e.g. missing one's friends and the internet connection), but insistence on continuing the routines from home can result from temperamental rigidity, p.234. Occasionally holidays are rejected for the same reasons as presents, p.312. "Drug holidays" refers to planned temporary breaks in use of a medication. *Summer camps* usually provide outdoor fun, but some are designed to give an academic boost or a chance to meet other children with the same disease. They can also provide respite for parents. See also summer learning loss, p.45; accents, p.417.

Holophrastic: describes a single word that is used by an infant as if it were a full sentence (e.g. "More!"). The listener has to work out the exact meaning from the context, e.g. the child has just had a spoonful of icecream. Closely related situations are: (a) a child learning a phrase or sentence and using it without realising that it contains separate words within it that can be changed; (b) a child using a word or phrase as a shorthand for a more complex idea that he can't describe fully (many *pat phrases* are like this, p.158).

Holoprosencephaly: failure of the developing brain to form some or all of its principal fissures. This is a very variable multifactorial syndrome in which the degree of facial malformation generally predicts the degree of cerebral malformation. The most severe form has a single central eye and is not compatible with life. There are *microforms* of HPE with normal IQ and characteristic single upper incisor[1512] (note this *fusing* is essentially the opposite of a *cleft*, p.440). Holoprosencephaly is the most frequent CNS malformation in humans, having been observed in 1 in 250 conceptions, though the prevalence of the mild forms is unknown[1196].

Home-schooling: see p.215.

Homework: distractions from homework: pp.128, 30, 453; attitude to homework, p.29; *overwork*, p.521. Homework can be prolonged by inconsistent enforcement, distractions, academic difficulty, and obsessionality (in the child or parent). Aggression can be triggered by excess or incomprehensible tasks, but this can also be produced if the manner of the supervision is unpleasant, or aggression can be used by the child as a simple operant because it sometimes results in his being allowed to do something else. Teachers' attitudes to homework vary widely. Some use it as a recap of the week's learning which can be done independently by the child; others assign homework problems so hard that the most able child in the class can only get half of them right. This is presumably designed to push the most able children, and to enlist evening teaching by parents or tutors – but it has adverse effects such as parents dictating the answers, various forms of cheating, and children feeling inadequate. Evidence that homework helps academic progress remains elusive; and it can cause fierce family conflict.

Homocystinuria (rarely called homocysteinuria): one of the few treatable causes of ID, p.32. Infants appear normal; problems later in childhood or adulthood include dislocated lenses, blood clots (thrombophilia), vascular disease, progressive ID, epilepsy. Tall stature. There are many subtypes and mutations, and unfortunately the newborn screening heelprick detects only untreatable forms[767]. Some of the treatable forms affecting children are biochemically and behaviourally distinct, e.g. MTHFR deficiency (p.468).

Homosexuality: The term "lesbian, gay, bisexual and transgender" (lgbt or lgb) is sometimes preferred. The term *gay* used to mean overtly camp homosexuals (p.243) but nowadays more often refers to all male homosexuals. See also psychosocial risks of gay lifestyle, p.239; camp, p.243; coming out, p.240; internal conflict, p.353; sex in general, p.548; parental rejection, p.311; pink, p.247.

Some aspects of male homosexuals tend to be male-like (e.g. interest in casual sex and interest in visual sex stimuli) but others are female-like (preferred partner gender, neurocognitive performance, and hypothalamic structure; see[1295] for a review including related data on lesbians).

Homosexual parents
When these are functioning as same-sex couples, the adjustment and development of the children is as good as with heterosexual couples[1228]. These children have conventional self-concepts, acrtivities, and preference for same-gender playmates. Teasing seems not to be a common problem, and the children's witnessing prejudice against their parents can be upsetting but apparently not sufficiently to impair their overall adjustment. Children raised by homosexual parents are more likely to become homosexual themselves, due to a combination of genetic and environmental

factors, but the effect sizes are not yet clear, nor the question of whether the outcome is affected by the children's sex or by concordance with parents' sex (see[762,1155]).

Hopelessness: the feeling that the future will be bad and there's nothing one can do about it. This is an important risk factor for suicide attempts[130] and completed suicide[129]. Many other factors are also useful in predicting these outcomes (see p.320). See also maternal hopelessness, p.313.

The Beck Hopelessness Scale (printed in[130]) is well studied. It has 20 items describing negative feelings about the future, loss of motivation, and deciding to give up. Typical items are "I might as well give up because I can't make things better for myself" , "my future seems dark to me" and "It is very unlikely that I will get any real satisfaction in the future." Among adults (aged 15 and above) attending a psychological clinic, endorsing nine or more of these 20 items is strongly correlated with completed suicide in the next five years[129]. However in this study fewer than half with this risk factor actually completed suicide.

Horses, love of: p.248.
HPA: hypothalamo-pituitary axis, see diagram on p.531.
HPLC: high-performance liquid chromatography, see *chromatography*.
Humour: p.495.

Huntington's chorea / juvenile Huntington's disease: Signs in children include cognitive decline over years, stiffness in the legs or parkinsonism (p.525), clumsiness, oromotor problems, seizures[586], and *rarely* psychosis or depression[1335]. Chorea (p.439) is less common than in adults with Huntington's. Family history is not always present, in part because if a child inherits it from the father the child's Huntington symptoms can start before the father's, a phenomenon called *anticipation*.

The main investigation is genetic testing, but because it is almost invariably fatal, knowing the diagnosis can produce adverse psychosocial effects on the child and family[1617]. In deciding whether to test, a key issue is that confirming this diagnosis does not currently improve prognosis, though treatments under development may do so in future[1712].

Hydrocephalus: enlargement of the cerebral ventricles[1637]. Neonatally this can cause an obviously large head with bulging fontanelles, increasing head circumference, and the ‼ *setting-sun sign* of visible sclera above a cornea nearly fixed in downgaze. If the hydrocephalus starts after skull fusion, symptoms can be much more vague, such as headache and reduced concentration (which can become severe).

Causes include Dandy-Walker, Arnold-Chiari, and aqueductal stenosis (for more see[390]). However, usually the hydrocephalus itself, rather than the underlying cause of the hydrocephalus, is the reversible cause of any symptoms[963]. Hydrocephalus is the most common reason for paediatric brain surgery. Contrast *intracranial hypertension*, p.493.

Normal pressure hydrocephalus is rare in children but important as it can cause cognitive decline without headache, and cognitive abilities can often be improved by shunting[1616]. It is easy to miss but readily detected on MRI.

Hygiene: dirty clothes can result from clumsiness or from unwillingness to wear anything else. Body odour is a more sensitive indicator of washing. Consider ID (in child or parents, see p.419), neglect (p.274), depression, living conditions, soiling (p.342). Poor hand washing and dirty kitchen cloths cause illness and time off school.

Hyperactivity: p.79.

Hyperacusis: literally, hearing more. However the term is usually used to mean finding loud noises unpleasant, p.127.

Hypercalcaemia: a useful mnemonic is groans (constipation, p.444), moans (depression), bones (bone pain), and kidney stones (p.555). Also causes confusion, anorexia, cardiac arrhythmia, weakness, poor appetite, p.331; nausea and vomiting, polyuria, catatonia, p.98.

Hyperekplexia: also called hyperstartling or pathological surprise reaction [93,412]. This is usually an hereditary disorder of glycine function, p.474. Signs in infants include stiffness, an exaggerated head-retraction reflex, and a startle response elicited by a gentle tap on the nose. Older children and adults shut their eyes and raise their arms to protect their heads. Hyperekplexia is one of the *startle syndromes*, p.552. Contrast panics, p.301; flinching, p.107; and sensory intolerance, p.125.

Hyperemesis gravidarum: the extreme end of the spectrum of nausea and vomitting in pregnancy, with 1–2% of all mothers seeking medical help. When hyperemesis does not prevent normal weight gain of the pregnant mother, the outcome for the infant is unchanged. However if the mother gained less than 7 kg during pregnancy, the risk of low birth weight (p.432) and prematurity (p.432) is tripled to approximately 13% [419].

Hyperexcitability syndromes: (see also *Hyperekplexia*).

> **Central**: Stiff person syndrome (p.555) includes epilepsy. Mutations of the Na-K pump *or* the PQ Ca++ channel can cause hemiplegic migraine, plus ataxia and seizures [545].

> **Peripheral nerve**: Acquired neuromyotonia (Isaac's syndrome, autoimmune disorder of voltage-gated potassium channel [585]); myokymias, fasciculations; cramp-fasciculation syndrome; Morvan's disease. The cause can be hypocalcaemia or autoantibodies.

Hyperlexia: reading without comprehension. This is sometimes misinterpreted as a high-level ability, e.g. in autism.

Hypermetamorphosis: p.496.

Hypermobility: joints that bend unusually far.

> *Examination of joints*
> The key issues are the degree of laxity, the distribution of affected joints, and any resulting pain or disability. Abnormal joint mobility can be demonstrated by extending the fifth metacarpophalangeal joint more than 90 degrees, touching the thumb to the wrist, or placing the hands flat on the floor while standing with knees straight. Sitting on the floor with legs flat in a W-posture is a related sign, but it is a less reliable indicator of widespread hypermobility because it can be due to prolonged early practice,

e.g. when vestibular or neuromuscular deficits prevent a child's normal self-stabilisation while sitting.

Diagnosis
In about 1%, joint laxity is part of a more widespread genetic syndrome with skin, eye or heart abnormalities, e.g. Ehlers-Danlos, p.460; Marfan's, p.505; and osteogenesis imperfecta (p.468). These syndromes have a degree of overlap[995].

Benign joint hypermobility is found in 10% of children, more in females. It is also called Ehlers-Danlos hypermobility type (previously Ehlers-Danlos III) and is identified using the Revised Brighton criteria[602] which exclude the specific genetic syndromes. There is some overlap with developmental coordination disorder, p.89.

Significance
Hypermobility increases the risk of joint pain and arthritis, and is often found in chronic fatigue (p.323). Hypermobility restricted to subsets of joints is seen in cerebral palsy, p.437; Down's syndrome, p.455; Fragile X, p.468; Stickler syndrome and other syndromes[1294]. See also Occipital Horn syndrome, p.32.

Hyperorality: see mouthing, p.56; *Klüver-Bucy*, p.496.
Hyperthymia: p.264.

Hyperthyroidism: signs include tachycardia, weight loss despite increased intake, tremor/chorea (p.439), muscle weakness, sweating (p.558), heat intolerance, insomnia (p.199), diarrhoea, anxiety (p.299).

Subclinical hyperthyroidism means low TSH with thyroxine in the normal range[916]. When found, it may be a treatable cause of severe hyperactivity.[1569]

Hyperventilation: breathing in excess of metabolic requirements. This has many physical and psychological causes that often interact[544]. Hyperventilation is an aspect of DSM's panic attacks, but also occurs separately from panics and the possibility of contributory or intermittent respiratory disease should not be neglected. Asthma attacks (p.424) cause prolonged expiration; whereas anxious excess breathing usually has prolonged *inspiration*. Hyperventilation causes hypocalcaemia (p.485) which can have transient neural effects. Hyperventilation can also be used as a component of treatment[1066]. Effects on absences, p.427. See also *dyspnoea*, p.457.

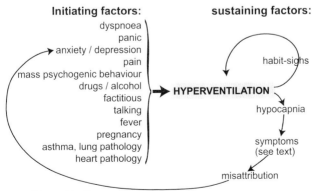

Figure 29. Causes of hyperventilation.
(after[544]).

Hypnagogic and hypnopompic hallucinations: p.345.
Hypnic jerks: p.200.

Hypocalcaemia: low calcium levels. This has many causes[1639].

> The first sign is sometimes tingling in lips, fingers or toes. Tendon reflexes are strengthened. Carpopedal spasm (*main d'accoucheur*) can develop in hypocalcaemia, hypomagnesaemia and hyperventilation. Short-term effects include fitting, p.73; tetany; anxiety, p.295; vomiting and fatigue[1639], p.323. A long-term effect is rickets (softened, curved bones). Causes include vitamin D deficiency, p.328; hyperventilation, p.484; hypoparathyroidism, p.525; velocardiofacial syndrome, p.572.

Hypocretin: a peptide found in the hypothalamus with a role in sleep and appetite. Named for *hypo*thalamus and the similarity of its sequence with that of se*cretin*. Also called *orexin*. See *narcolepsy*, p.72.

Hypoglycaemia: p.82.
Hypomania: see *Bipolar Affective Disorder*, p.264.

Hypothalamus: a tiny part of the brain, weighing 4 g, at the top of the brainstem. It regulates pulse, blood pressure, breathing, temperature, feeding and drinking, sex (see homosexuality, p.481), aggression[1734] and sleep. The hypothalamus is probably even more important in disease than the amount of evidence suggests, because of the difficulty of studying small groups of neurons deep within the skull.

> However a crucial job of the hypothalamus is to regulate hormone production, and this is well-studied. The nuclei together with the hormones they control are listed below (and in the figure on p.531).

> *Named nuclei*
> a) suprachiasmatic n.: circadian rhythm
> b) tuberomamillary n. sends histamine (p.479) throughout brain
> c) pineal gland: produces melatonin (p.506)
> d) supraoptic n and paraventricular n: together these produce the oxytocin (p.521) and ADH (p.338) for release in the posterior pituitary (p.531). It is also the leader of the HPA (hypothalmus-pituitary-adrenal) axis, producing CRH which stimulates the anterior pituitary to release ACTH, which in turn stimulates the adrenal gland to release glucocorticoids (p.555). The paraventricular nucleus also controls the release of prolactin (p.536).
> e) ventromedial n: has a role in satiety and sexual behaviours (e.g. lordosis reflex).
> f) dorsomedial n: feeding, drinking, and weight regulation (see *intake-regulating hormones*, p.491).

> *Abnormalities in the hypothalamus*
> Uncommon conditions affecting this include hypothalamic hamartomas, p.76; Prader-Willi syndrome, p.533; Wolfram syndrome, p.575; Kallmann syndrome, p.495; gelastic epilepsy, p.111; craniopharyngioma, p.446.

Hypothyroidism: signs include fatigue, cold intolerance, constipation (p.444), impaired memory, depression, goitre, hoarseness and weight gain. The severest congenital form is cretinism, which includes profound ID. In developed countries it is usually prevented by the heelprick test at birth (p.32).

Subclinical (or mild) hypothyroidism has thyroxine in the reference range but elevated TSH (discussed in[1353]). This is found in about 2% of children. Its most common symptoms are weight gain, impaired growth, anaemia, sleepiness and impaired cognitive development[1303]. It does not usually worsen, except in children with Down's syndrome or high titres of anti-thyroid antibodies[811].

Repeating the blood test after 3–12 months can be useful to exclude transient hypothyroidism[1134]. See also *iodine*, p.494; benign hereditary chorea, p.439.

Hypotonia: low muscle tone. For a test see p.437.

Hypoxic-Ischaemic Encephalopathy (HIE): HIE refers to brain damage caused by systemic hypoxia, most often due to factors outside the baby, especially intrapartum asphyxia.

There is much overlap between the terms *stroke, hypoxic-ischaemic encephalopathy (HIE)*, and *cerebral palsy (CP). Stroke* is an ambiguous term, most often (as here and p.556) referring just to localised brain ischaemia with local causes such as clot formation, but sometimes used more broadly to include the effects of HIE as well. *Watershed infarcts* (or watershed strokes, p.557) are the mechanism of much of the damage in HIE. CP (p.437) is quite a different term, referring not to any original cause at all but to the cognitive and behavioural outcome. The best-known outcomes of HIE are CP, ID, p.491; epilepsy, p.73; and *Klüver-Bucy*, p.496.

Iatrogenic: literally means problems caused by doctors. Similar problems can also be caused by other professionals. In some cases, talking therapies can have adverse effects[1174], as can *lack of* a diagnosis or excessive time off school for therapies.

Diagnostic errors include underdiagnosis, overdiagnosis, and incorrect diagnosis. Overfocus on one problem (e.g. ADHD, autism, or a single-gene syndrome) can prevent adequate attention to other issues that may be more important (e.g. anxiety, poor parenting). All these can delay obtaining the best care.

Management errors include underassessment (which can prevent finding a treatable cause) and overinvestigation – which sensitises people so, e.g., every problem from then on could indicate a brain tumour. Inappropriate advice can make parents overprotective or impose unnecessary restrictions (e.g. never to go swimming with epilepsy). Parents can misunderstand genetic aetiology to imply that normal parenting methods will not work.

Medication problems include sedation or intoxication with prescribed drugs; addiction to prescribed opioids; and pseudo-addiction, p.259. There are also hard-to-reverse long-term problems such as antipsychotics'(p.422) side-effects of obesity and the now-uncommon tardive dyskinesia. It is not rare for children to accidentally be given 10 times a prescribed dose, and very occasionally this continues for years. For other side-effects, see the entries for specific drug classes.

See also medical effects on self-identity, p.237; *treatments*.

ICD: International Classification of Diseases, describes a standard set of symptoms for each diagnosis. For strengths and weaknesses of this see p.24.

ICE: acronym for Ideas, Concerns, and Expectations (p.13).

ID: see *intellectual disability.*

Id: Freud's term for basic drives, impulses and instincts.

Ideas of reference: interpreting everyday events as referring to oneself. When severe these are called *delusions of reference* (compare *paranoia*, p.524). See also: response to hearing laughter, p.111.

Identification: see *self-identity*, p.237; *projective identification*, p.535.

Ideograph (or *loaded word*): a term that implies or encourages an underlying belief or viewpoint[1044]. For example, in politics, use of the term "family values" usually implies and encourages opposition to non-traditional relationships.

In psychiatry, the names of medication categories are "disease-centred", e.g. *antidepressants*, *antipsychotics*[1102] and *mood stabilisers*[120,593], and this creates the impression of clarity for both the diagnosis and the treatment. Many feel that as there is no direct correspondence between the drugs and the disorders, "drug-centred" pharmacological terms such as *SSRI* or *antihistamine* should be preferred.

The biological bases of most psychiatric diagnoses remain unclear, yet the very existence of a name and a definition in a rigorous or biological style increases the number of people who will consider the category to be qualitatively and biologically distinct. This simplification can be useful (see *taxonomy*, p.561; for examples of continua see *on the spectrum*, p.519; *syndrome*, p.383; ADHD, p.83; PTSD, p.532; *social anxiety*, p.298).

Sometimes people describe a behaviour using a word that is just one of the potential explanations for it, e.g. *acting out*, p.418; *collude*, p.442; *conversion*, p.445; *sadistic*, p.281; *deliberate*, p.317; *refusal*, p.540; *criminality*, p.446; *uncontained* (for *violent*).

Other examples of words that can mislead are *damaged*, p.450; *insists* and *punishes*, p.193; *sensitive*, p.546; *non-stimulant*, p.516, *learning disability*, p.498; *boundaries*, p.434; *instrument* (for a test); *challenging behaviour*, p.438; *containment*; *in care*, *looked after children*, p.500.

Illness behaviours: psychological responses to ill health. A minor degree of denial is common. Other normal illness behaviours include help-seeking, self-treatment, feeling sorry for oneself, and adopting the sick role. The sick role[1222] is a standardised role adopted by people while they are ill. It brings socially sanctioned benefits (e.g. staying off school, having special attention) but also duties such as resting, doing whatever is necessary in order to get better, and not having too much fun.

Abnormal illness behaviours include many fabricated and exaggerated symptoms (p.359), hypochondriasis (p.362), and long-term changes of identity or values (pp.237, 323).

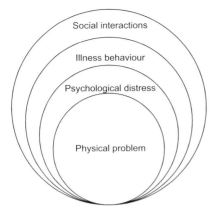

Figure 30. Glasgow model of illness behaviour.

(The diagram emphasises that the illness behaviour can be a bigger problem than the original physical ailment). After[1695].

Illusion: misperception of an external stimulus
Imaginary friends: p.231.

Imagination: the ability to temporarily believe something that one knows isn't so[305]. *Dissociation* (p.453) describes the subset that is not fully volitional. The term *fantasy* is usually reserved for the more far-fetched or complex creations. *Creativity,* the ability to create new ideas, is distinct because children can imagine a world that has been described to them by a book or a peer. *Lateral* or *divergent* thought usually underlies creativity, but not always: snippets of old ideas can be introduced randomly or in a mechanistic way.

See imagination, imaginary worlds and imaginary friends, p.231; imaginary and verbal/fantastic play, pp.221–222; imaginative swearing in hypomania, p.161; behaviour when imagination is limited, p.63; aggressive and non-aggressive outlandishness in excitement, p.520; imagining self as someone else, p.318; daydreaming, p.450; relationship to psychosis, p.537; function of transition object, p.567.

Immigrants: sweeping generalisations are inappropriate here as families that have moved for higher education are very different from those who have fled famine or war (see *refugees*, p.540; living in ghettos, p.212; generation gaps, p.212; *cultural effects on symptoms*, p.448).

Parents from poor countries often lack the skills or the confidence to advocate for their children, resulting in fewer resources being offered by health, education, or social services. Immunisations should be performed, and children should be screened for anaemia (p.421), parasitic infections (p.490), dental caries, tuberculosis (p.569), hepatitis B, and visual problems[488].

Immigrant children in school full-time become fluent within a year or two, and failure to achieve this should lead to mandatory auditory and cognitive testing. Bilinguality or disrupted early schooling are often assumed to account for school difficulty years later, to the great detriment of children with unrecognised ID.

Impairment: p.17.

Imprinting: switching off ("silencing") the copy of a gene that came from one parent, generally by methylation of cystines[1766].

> Angelman syndrome (p.422) is a microdeletion syndrome. Prader-Willi, p.533 involves the same genes but alternative genes fail to fill in the gap due to imprinting. Similar gene changes may also be involved in some cases of Rett (p.541), Sotos[879] (p.551) and autism[1766].

> Beckwith-Wiedemann (p.429) has excess methylation of genes whereas Russell-Silver syndrome has reduced methylation of the same genes, accounting for the overgrowth in the former versus the short stature in the latter[446].

> Imprinting is an example of *epigenetics* (gene effects that do not depend on the basic DNA sequence). Other examples are the partial silencing of glucocorticoid genes (p.555) that apparently depends on early environment and parental care[1047,1721]; and of genes in spinal muscular atrophy (p.551).

Impulsivity: acting without thinking properly about it first, or valuing immediate rewards over delayed ones. See p.79; recklessness, p.539; and unliked behaviours, p.353.

Inadequate anxiety: p.423
Inattention: p.79.

Incest: sexual activity between close relatives, regardless of age. How close is acceptable varies between cultures, but sexual activity within the immediate family, and between a person and his/her step-parents or foster carers is usually taboo. In some parts of the United States sexual relationships between cousins are prohibited. The term used to be used mainly to refer to father-daughter sexual relations, for which see childhood sexual abuse, p.275. Prevalence, p.268.

Inclusion: this word has the theoretical meaning of mainstream schools restructuring and adapting *themselves* to the needs of children with disabilities, so that these children belong to the school community. This is in contrast to the older concept of *integrating* these children, which means simply placing the disabled children in mainstream schools[77]. In practice, most education systems in the world find a practical compromise, adapting mainstream schools to some degree, while keeping a few special schools for children who would disrupt mainstream classes too much or be unable to learn in them.

> In practice, being included in one group usually means being outside another. *Inclusion* in a broad sense means ensuring that the child has available at least a few peers of roughly matched ability; this is often incompatible with a child with ID being "included" in a small school near his home. Similarly, for children needing highly specialised education (e.g. severe epilepsy or autism) which is not available within daily commuting distance of their home, there is a difficult choice between being "included" in a school with similar peers or "included" in their own family.

> See also: early predictors of special schooling, p.57; behaviours copied from peers in special school, pp.43,105; social isolation caused by inappropriate school choice, p.181.

Induced symptoms: p.359.

Infection: this can damage the body systemically or locally; directly or by the severity of the body's response (e.g. inflammation via *cytokines*, p.450; scratching, p.110); or by induced autoimmunity, p.427.

It is worth taking an immunisation history, as unimmunised children can experience severe complications of infections. A child may not have been immunised, usually because his parents objected or because he was born in an underdeveloped country. See MMR, p.508; viruses, p.573.

TORCH infections are important causes of congenital infection and often malformations. They include toxoplasmosis, rubella, cytomegalovirus, herpes viruses (listed above), hepatitis B, syphilis, HIV, and parvovirus B19. Diagnoses can sometimes be made by chasing the Guthrie card and doing a TORCH screen on the old card; however, note this can never prove the causation of developmental problems.

Tetanus is an immunisable condition caused by the neurotoxin produced by *Clostridium tetani*. It can cause opisthotonus (p.93) and an odd fixed grin (called risus sardonicus, with raised eyebrows and lockjaw) (contrast *smiles*, p.549).

Chronic infections
These are probably the biggest factor creating IQ differences between countries, and the steady IQ improvement from 1900 to 2000[466] (see p.59). Common sites of chronic infections in developed countries are the tonsils and urinary tract, but in developing countries many organ systems are simultaneously affected.

Infections persisting in the body can be bacterial[1100] (tuberculosis, p.569; chlamydia, helicobacter, salmonella, brucella, borrelia, p.501; streptococcus, haemophilus); viral[808] (HIV, p.479; hepatitis; all the herpes viruses listed on p.478); or parasitic (malaria, p.503; worms, p.576; toxoplasma, leishmania, trypanosomes). Chronic infections often worsen the impact of other infections[1459].

Infectious behaviours: doing something because someone else has recently been witnessed doing it. Almost any behaviour or symptom seen in a friend can be imagined or exaggerated in oneself. Examples include infectious laughter (p.111), infectious itching, infectious crying (p.316), and perhaps some religious cult behaviour. The mirror system (p.507) may be involved. See also *empathy*, p.546. Crowd dynamics can turn infectious behaviours into *mass psychogenic behaviours*, p.505.

Inflammatory bowel disease: includes Crohn's and ulcerative colitis. These increase the risk of malnutrition (p.504), via poor intake, diarrhoea and vomiting, inflammatory load, malabsorption, medication effects and surgery. Tube feeding (p.333) is increasingly used as a treatment for months or years.

Inflexibility: p.234.
Inhalant abuse: p.258.

Inhibition: forces that prevent one acting as one wishes. See normal inhibitions, p.261; motor inhibition differences in named disorders, p.117; behavioural inhibition to novelty, p.296; stopping activities when anxious, pp.296, 153; inhibitory defence mechanisms, p.305; inhibition of return, p.322; pre-pulse inhibition, p.462; surround inhibition, p.470.

Inserting objects in body: p.118.

Insight: an individual's awareness of his illness. This includes awareness of any current and past deficits, and their importance for his life; attribution of symptoms to the disorder; and the reasonableness of his beliefs regarding treatments[31]. There are obviously large cognitive/developmental components in this, but there are also social and emotional aspects. Insight is therefore an important indicator of the severity of disorder, of the likely compliance with treatment (at least after puberty), and of help-seeking behaviour.

Insomnia: p.199.
Instability of mood: see *emotional instability*, p.69.
Insula: p.513.
Interests: p.229.

Intake-regulating hormones: a family of hormones, which includes ghrelin (*growth hormone releasing factor*) and many others. Short-term intake is increased by ghrelin, and reduced by peptide YY or cholecystokinin. Long-term intake is increased by neuropeptide Y, and decreased by POMC. Hence children with POMC defects become obese; they also have red hair[170].

As well as regulating food and fluid intake, these hormones affect sleep, memory and anxiety[1507]. Hence, some patients with narcolepsy (p.72) have disturbance of sleep and olfaction, apparently both caused by orexin deficiency[86].

Intellectual disability: a term growing in acceptance internationally to describe globally low intelligence. For ways of assessing, see *IQ*, p.59; *Developmental quotient*, p.451; and *Functional level or Vineland*, p.419. See also *Learning Disability*; *Borderline Intellectual Functioning*, p.434. For gradations of ID see p.60. For treatable causes of ID, see p.32.

IQ tests are calibrated to place 2% of the population below IQ 70 (see *IQ tests*, p.59). DSM defines ID as the combination of this low IQ with functional impairment (which is almost invariably found with such an IQ). However because of complexities of testing (p.59), prevalence estimates of Mild ID range from 0.5 to 8%[1484]. In the UK, 3% of children have a Statement of Special Educational Needs[1484] though many of these are for physical or behavioural problems rather than for ID.

ID can be underestimated in preschoolers because their abstract thinking is still immature, and because the slower children have not yet dropped far behind. In young children, while there remains a chance that the child will catch up with his peers, it is sensible to use the intentionally imprecise term *global developmental delay* (see p.496).

About a third of children and adolescents with ID experience mental health problems, a figure much greater than the 8% found in the general population[155].

Developmental syndromes can include intellectual disabilities; specific learning disabilities, p.551; characteristic behavioural difficulties (see behavioural phenotypes, p.430; Smith-Magenis syndrome, p.550; Down's syndrome, p.455; Lesch-Nyhan syndrome, p.318), as well as physical problems and in some, malformations, p.503.

See also parental ID, p.191; missed ID in immigrant children,p.488.

Intermittent Explosive Disorder: p.70.
Internalising: see *externalising*, p.463.

Interpreter: an important contributor to multicultural assessments[1743]. If the local area has only two languages, it is good to have a permanent interpreter as part of the health team; but if the local area has immigrants speaking dozens of languages this of course is not possible.

Sequential interpreting is standard practice, i.e. the interpreter listens in one language then speaks in the other language. Concurrent/simultaneous interpreting is less reliable but is necessary if speakers cannot wait, e.g. due to confusion or a family argument.

Resist offers by the interpreter to summarise a long discussion into a few words. Exact literal interpretation is important in order to understand the mental state of the speaker. In addition, ask the interpreter for his impression of the family status, education, traditions, relationships, symptoms and inconsistencies, from the point of view of the home country.

Telephone interpreting loses the opportunity to observe body language but is necessary when no interpreter is available locally. Using a family member as interpreter is risky as they often add their own views without saying so.

When a whole family is being interviewed but only one of them needs the interpreter, sit those two together so that the interpreter can unobtrusively do simultaneous interpreting for the family member while the rest of the family is talking. See also p.166.

Interrupting: breaking an ongoing activity. The break can be transient or enduring. Vocal tics can appear in the middle of a sentence, but they do not destroy the train of thought if the child has become used to them (for an example see p.230). Interruption by absence attacks is often followed by resumption of the previous activity (p.75). Interrupting other people is a DSM symptom of impulsivity (p.383); however there are many causes, including disinhibition (p.261), social learning (p.162), not hearing or not understanding, disinterest or narcissism, overwhelming interest (brief such as danger, or long-term, p.229), haste or desire to provoke (as in TV interviewers), fear of forgetting a point, thinking faster than the speaker can speak, and not knowing or agreeing with the rules of a game. If the other person refuses to be interrupted, the two people talk over each other. Opening the mouth signals a desire to interrupt.

Internet: young people spend an enormous amount of time on the internet (*averaging* 23 hours a week in South Korea), and some become behaviourally addicted (p.259). Many spend time on social or pornographic websites, but the most damagingly attractive are gaming sites (p.573). The important issue clinically is not the exact number of hours, but whether it is outside their control and impairing their functioning. People who become addicted usually have other mental health problems as well[184].

Cyberbullying includes the sending of upsetting information to children (sometimes in the night-time) or the spreading of malicious gossip electronically. In a few cases the victim has committed suicide. (See also *bullying*, p.219).

Children are "groomed" online by paedophiles, sometimes persuaded to post pornographic pictures of themselves online; and sometimes to meet in person. Some websites disseminate information about how to commit suicide effectively, and others allow self-harmers to chat to each other; but it may be that the negative effect of these is more than offset by websites offering useful support[164]. See also insomnia attributed to pornography, p.115; fears/obsessions about the internet, p.448.

On the positive side, the internet enables some shy, socially phobic, or disabled people to socialise and find others with similar interests (p.229). The internet also connects families of children with rare disorders. It can be used to administer tests and some therapies. The internet is where most patients and their families (and clinicians) will obtain information on diagnoses and treaments. Assessment of young people's public postings on MySpace and YouTube often provides key information regarding risk[1275].

See also *spending time on computers*, p.224.

Intolerance: sensory intolerance, p.125; in autism and in anxiety, p.126; in migraine, p.141; caused by sensitisation, p.546; lump and texture intolerance, p.331; intolerance of change, p.126; irritability, p.494; intolerance of distractions, p.128; strategies resulting from intolerance, p.126; creation of fears based on intolerances, p.307; intolerance of people being close, p.107; intolerance of laughter, p.111; pseudo-intolerance, p.128.

Physical intolerances: food intolerances, e.g. milk protein intolerance; coeliac disease, p.441; lysinuric protein intolerance, p.379 (see also urea cycle disorders, p.571); heat intolerance in hyperthyroidism, p.484; cold intolerance in hypothyroidism, p.485. Exercise intolerance is highly multifactorial, see pp.323, 418.

Intoxication: see *toxic substances*, p.566.

Intracranial hypertension: the most common symptoms are headache (p.139), nausea and vomitting; visual loss; fatigue; ataxia; dizziness; neck pain; paraesthesias; and tinnitus (p.565). Characteristically the headache is exacerbated by activities that raise intracerebral pressure, such as bending, coughing or straining; it wakes the child from sleep; and it is often posterior. The key physical finding is papilloedema, though this is sometimes absent. There are many underlying causes, and neurological assessment is needed urgently[1331]. Idiopathic intracranial hypertension, without abnormality on imaging, is also called pseudotumour cerebri. See also *hydrocephalus*, p.482.

Intracranial pressure, raised (ICP): see *intracranial hypertension*, above.

Intrusion: unliked thoughts or images that arrive suddenly, without effort to recall them. These are core aspects of PTSD (p.532), OCD (p.65) and psychosis (e.g. hearing voices, p.343); they are also rare symptoms of epilepsy (p.76). Clinical severity is related to the extent that the experiences occur out of the blue[1070]. See also *unliked behaviours*, p.353.

Causes of *complaints* of unliked thoughts or images include:
- intrusions more frequent than previously
  - attempts to avoid thinking a particular thought makes that thought occur more frequently[1311]

- intrusions more prolonged, perhaps due to well-documented task switching deficits in OCD[626]
- intrusions more unpleasant
  - attempts to avoid thinking any thought makes that thought more frequent[1729] and more distressing[1311]
  - worry about past real traumas, or the content of traumatic thoughts, or about whether the person is going crazy (or similar), add to the distress caused by intrusions[1540]
  - intrusions causing violence
- long-term risk of flashbacks following LSD use (p.258).
- trying to focus on a task – then anything else is an intrusion that can impair performance of the task[1225].

Intuition: p.18.

Iodine: an element required for thyroid function. Deficiency can cause mild or severe hypothyroidism (p.485). Mild iodine deficiency is common, even in industrialised countries[1823]. Worldwide, iodine deficiency may be the commonest cause of ID, despite major efforts to iodinate salt[387].

IQ, IQ tests: p.59.

Irritability: having a large immediate negative reaction to a relatively small stimulus. This definition has two halves. The large reactions are often labelled as *impulsivity* (see above); violence, p.289; rudeness, p.161; or disinhibition, p.261. Having these effects caused by unusually small stimuli is *intolerance* (pp.125, 493).

Note that the small stimuli may be misleading: a child who attacks his sibling for accidentally bumping into him may be deeply resentful of the child for some reason, and just tipped over the edge by the bump, or using the bump as an excuse. Irritability is common when sleepy, ill, or preoccupied; or when hypoglycaemic, p.82. For irritability in depression, see p.309; in mania, p.263; in anxiety, p.297; with paranoia, p.524; and psychosis, p.537. For a female-specific rating scale see[198]. See also *sudden changes in emotion*, p.69; *Intermittent Explosive Disorder*, p.70.

Irritable bowel syndrome (IBS): symptoms in children usually include lower abdominal discomfort, cramping pain, and increased flatus[739]. Nearly half of children meeting adult criteria for diagnosis of IBS (which include abdominal pain relieved by defecation, disturbed defecation and bloating) turn out to have another cause of their abdominal discomfort, most commonly dyspepsia, IBD (p.490), lactose malabsorption, or coeliac disease (p.441). Nausea, epigastric discomfort, pain radiating to the chest, and regurgitation are *less* likely in IBS than in other conditions. Somatic complaints such as abdominal pain are also a common symptom of depression in children (p.313). See also *central sensitisation*, p.436; *comorbidity*, p.442.

Itch: p.110.
Jail: see *prison*.
Jargon: see stages of speech, p.143. For clinical jargon, see *ideographs*.

Joint attention: (or sharing of interests) has both responsive and proactive components, e.g. gaze monitoring and protodeclarative pointing (p.170). It usually develops between 9 and 15 months of age. Playing side-by-side allows this skill to develop.

Joking: an important social skill, p.495.
McGhee's stages of humour development[1046]:

    I. Incongruous actions toward objects. From 18 months, when make-believe starts
    II. Incongruous labelling of objects and events. From about 3 years, when language starts being used in playful ways
    III. Conceptual incongruity. From age 3 to 4 when child realises that classes of objects have key characteristics
    IV. Multiple meanings. From about age 7 when Piagettian concrete operations start (p.530). This humour includes other people's points of view, reversibility of operations, and imagined actions on objects.

An informal progression (see also[104]):
- Simply misusing names or saying "You're a girl!"
- stories of impossible events
- wee, poo and sex
- simple *riddle-wait-give surprise answer*
- telling jokes to ridicule people
- making up jokes, even on the fly
- concealing our feelings with a joke
- varying the content and style to keep people interested.

Making jokes: the main themes of jokes are mocking, resolution of incongruity, taboo feelings, and internal conflicts (see *laughing*, p.111, and chapters 4–5 of [258]). Obviously some of these are uncommon in autism. But if pursued to the exclusion of normal activities, joking can be a *stereotyped interest* (p.229) and it has been suggested that some comedians are mildly autistic (pp.129 and 169 of [258]). Girls are often uncomfortable with the rudeness and competitiveness of joking (p.154 of [258]).

Getting jokes: "The set-up to the joke is the near-side cliff, and the punchline is the far side. If they're too far apart, the listeners don't make it to the other side. And if they are too close together, the audience just steps across the gap and doesn't experience an exhilharating leap of any kind" (p.132 of [258]). Some children can't leap and others don't want to. Poor comprehension of humour is more associated with poor social comprehension than with NVLD [1452].

Kallmann syndrome: hypogonadism with anosmia, usually discovered when puberty is delayed.

Kernicterus: athetoid cerebral palsy, impaired upgaze, and deafness, resulting from neonatal hyperbilirubinaemia[1462]. With modern treatment most effects disappear by 2 years of age[1790].

Ketamine: p.474.
Killing or aiming to kill: p.282.

Kinship care: usually means care of a child by extended family. There are often advantages over normal fostering, such as staying with people they know; maintaining their culture, religion and language; and keeping in touch with parents. The term sometimes implies giving the care legal status. It also sometimes includes care by family friends. See also *looked after children*, p.500.

Klein, Melanie: a major contributor to object relations theory, p.517. Klein introduced the idea of projective identification, p.535.

Kleine-Levin syndrome: a rare condition that starts mainly in adolescence, with episodes of prolonged sleep lasting for days, interrupted only for meals[341]. Males often become hypersexual, and females often become depressed[61]. Almost all have difficulty speaking during episodes. The sleepy episodes are followed by insomnia and sometimes mild euphoria.

Episodic depression in girls with KLS can be confused with premenstrual symptoms (p.506) until the timing becomes clear (KLS usually has 3–6 episodes per year, lasting 7–15 days, and fades away after 10–20 years of these). If mood is low, the other main diagnosis to consider is bipolar disorder (p.264). For other similar conditions see[61].

KLS is probably much underdiagnosed due to great clinical heterogeneity[958], but the diagnosis is useful as it affects treatment. The cause may be autoimmunity acting in the hypothalamus, precipitated by infection in genetically susceptible individuals[61].

Klinefelter's syndrome: the most common sex chromosome disorder (XXY, p.548). Small testes and reduced fertility, and sometimes gynaecomastia, long limbs and mild neurodevelopmental difficulties especially in language. IQs are slightly below the general population, averaging 90[138].   There is predisposition to ADHD, tics and psychosis[1200].

Klüver-Bucy syndrome: this consists of various combinations of hyperorality (which is nearly continuous, and perhaps the most consistently abnormal feature; it is not always exploratory, as it can involve just holding fingers in the mouth); absence of anger; hypersexuality; visual agnosia (so his play disregards the fact that a toy car is a car); aphasia; failure to learn fear of objects (which is probably due to amygdalar damage: note that fear of heights can be preserved); and "hypermetamorphosis". This last is a misleading term (see[857]): the child has his behaviour relentlessly driven by visual stimuli. If there are many toys/stimuli available the child can move continuously from one to the next; but if there is only one of interest, the child's attention remains intently fixed on it for half an hour or more, during which he repeatedly mouths, inspects, pushes, pulls, turns or kicks it (i.e. he is fixated on the object but not on the activity; compare *perseveration*, p.527).

Hypoxic-ischaemic encephalopathy (p.486) appears to be the commonest cause of KBS in children, in which case the symptoms often appear at age 5–7. However Herpes Simplex encephalitis (p.461), tuberculosis (p.569), or anything that damages the temporal lobes can cause the syndrome[776]. The particular combination of symptoms seen in an individual child depends on the location of damage in the temporal lobes (p.513) – and which other brain areas are affected.

Kwashiorkor: p.504.
Lactate: see *mitochondrial disorders*, p.508.
Landau Kleffner syndrome: p.45.
Language deficits: p.145; see also *Speech problems* , p.147.
Language disorder ☝: see *Language deficits*.

Late developers: (also called "late bloomers"). This can affect all areas of development or just one.

Global delay

- Most of the children who are described as "globally delayed" will never catch up with their peers (see predictors, p.57). This becomes clear by age 5 or 6, so the description of them usually changes to "ID" at about that age.
- Less common is the globally delayed child who catches up. This is sometimes a family trait. Alternatively, if a cause of delay passes (such as prolonged physical illness or neglect; many others are listed on pp.32 and 41–47), then most children will largely catch up. This is true even when the cause of delay is severe, such as staying in a pre-revolution Romanian orphanage for the first few years of life (see p.447).

Circumscribed delay
Late development can affect just one aspect of a child's development, as when uncorrected deafness delays speech acquisition, p.144. If a *sensitive* period has been passed, then catch-up will be partial, and if a *critical* period (p.447) has passed, there will be no catch-up in that circumscribed area.

- In general, mildly delayed achievement of milestones in one area is associated with a somewhat lower level of final attainment in that area (e.g.[1332]). As a more specific case, delayed speech at age 2 ½ tends to catch up with peers within a few years, but *only if* receptive language is normal at 2 ½ [987].
- Late development of locomotor skills is associated with a slightly increased long-term risk of schizophrenia[754].

See also causes and effects of pubertal age variation, p.411; deviance, p.49; boys' speech delay in comparison with girls (p.55).

Lateral thinking: see imagination, p.488.

Lateralisation: hemispheric specialisation (brain-sidedness): To some extent, most people have more language function in their left hemisphere and visuospatial function in the right. The usual development of language dominance in the hemisphere opposite to the dominant hand may be accounted for by the *embodied cognition* theory[264].

Eye dominance or *eyedness* is weakly correlated with handedness[1052]. Test it by having the child fix both eyes on your finger, then move your finger towards his nose, forcing both eyes to converge gradually until the non-dominant one gives up. See also *handedness*, p.475.

Laughing: p.111.
LBW: low birth weight, p.432.
LDL: low density lipoproteins.
LE: Life event, p.499; lupus erythematosus (see SLE, p.560).
Lead: p.330.
Learned helplessness: p.96.

Learning Difficulty: this term has two meanings.

(a) When people outside education services use the term, they usually mean ID, p.491. Compare *Learning Disability*, p.498.
(b) Term from the UK 1981 Education Act, defined as meaning long-term or short-term difficulty in learning in class. However current usage in education services in the UK emphasises permanent impairments. This can be due, for example, to blindness, motor impairments, ID, ADHD, or

anxiety (for a fuller list of causes see p.27). Here is a list of
subtypes (for comparison with other terminology see p.60):

	Typical IQ	Characteristics
Specific Learning Difficulty (SpLD)	--	(see Specific Learning Disability, p.551)
Mild Learning Difficulty	70–80	In UK educational use, this indicates the roughly 10% with lowest ability, except the more severely affected groups below.
Moderate Learning Difficulty (MLD)	50–70	"Their needs will not be able to be met by normal differentiation. They have much greater difficulty than their peers in [literacy, numeracy and concepts]" (www.education.gov.uk). Similar to *mild learning disability*, p.60
Severe Learning Difficulty (SLD)	30–50	Attainments remain within P4-P8 (p.522) throughout school
Profound and Multiple Learning Difficulty (PMLD)	<30	These children have severe learning needs, and attainments remain within P1-P4 (p.522). *In addition* they have physical disability or sensory impairment. They require a high level of support for personal care, and have restricted communication.

Learning Disability: This has two meanings:

(1)   In American (and DSM-based research) usage Learning
Disability denotes a circumscribed or "specific" cognitive problem
(such as "Reading Disorder" or "Mathematics Disorder"). In the
rest of the world and in this book, these are called "*specific* learning
disabilities" (p.551).

(2)   In American (and DSM-based research) usage the term *Mental
Retardation* means global cognitive impairment (i.e. impairment in
verbal, visuospatial, working memory and processing speed; but not
necessarily in physical or motor functioning). In the rest of the
world, "retarded" is often considered offensive, so the term
learning disability or *general/ global learning disability* is used
instead. To avoid confusion, in this book the term *Intellectual
Disability* (*ID*, p.491) is used to refer to global deficits.

Compare *Non-verbal Learning Disability* (p.28), *Intellectual
Disability* (p.491), *Borderline intellectual functioning* (p.434). See
also p.27.

Left-handed: see *handedness*, p.475.
Lesbian: see *homosexuality*, p.481.
Lesch-Nyhan syndrome: p.318.

Leukodystrophy: A family of genetic disorders affecting myelin
development[321,865,1461]. Because myelination continues into
adolescence, many of these disorders reveal themselves long after
infancy. They are invariably progressive, usually starting with non-
specific problems such as skill loss of personality change, later
joined by more focal signs such as localised spasticity, swallowing
difficulty, or seizures. Because the symptoms are non-specific, the
presence of a leukodystrophy is often unsuspected until MRI is

performed (VLC fatty acids and other tests listed below are used for screening). Note there are other treatable disorders of white matter which are not leukodystrophies: p.574. Some leukodystrophies are storage disorders (see *lysosomal disorders*, p.501; *peroxisomal disorders*, p.526); others are not. Some have specific treatments. Some of the forms are:

- Metachromatic leukodystrophy can appear from age 1 to 10 as general cognitive regression (p.41) with ataxia, dystonia, and peripheral neuropathy; and from late adolescence onward as various psychiatric disorders; many patients survive for 10 years. Test for arylsulfatase A.
- *Adreno*leukodystrophy (a peroxisomal disorder, p.526) causes a progressive dementia with incoordination. It also causes Addison's disease (this is the disorder of the film *Lorenzo's Oil* which is the name of a recognised treatment in a subgroup). Adrenomyeloneuropathy is a milder form of this.
- Refsum's disease includes ataxia, night blindness and other visual problems, hearing impairment and scaly skin; elevated phytanic acid is a screening test.
- Vanishing white matter disease often comes to attention due to stepwise decline, with childhood-onset ataxia and seizures. The triggers for the decline are unusual, including fever, mild head trauma, or even severe fright.

LFT: liver function tests[480]. LFTs can be raised by many medicines, herbal remedies, anabolic steroids, oral contraceptives, viral hepatitis, alcohol, gallstones, coeliac disease (p.441) and Wilson's disease (p.575).LFTs include alanine aminotransferase (ALT), aspartate aminotransferase (AST), alkaline phosphatase (ALP), bilirubin (BIL), albumin (ALB) and total protein (TP). Gamma-glutamyl transpeptidase (GGT) and prothrombin time (PT) are sometimes ordered at the same time.

Life events: Together with long-term difficulties and temperament, negative life events contribute to low mood and anxiety.

In preschoolers and elementary school pupils, death, divorce, separation or prolonged imprisonment of a parent have the greatest effect. These continue to be very stressful in secondary school, when they are joined by getting pregnant or married, becoming involved with drugs, acquiring a visible deformity, and learning of being adopted (for many more details see[304]).

Life events have many characteristics: timing, physical location, desirability, concordance with long-term goals, degree of change required, whether the individual is responsible (often described as the event being *dependent* on the individual), and type of event (loss, disappointment or danger)[454,594].

The impact of a specific life event can be judged by its effect on mood, anxiety, monitoring, avoidance and concentration. There is specificity to a limited degree, in that loss events predispose more to depression, and danger events to anxiety[499]. Manic episodes are far more likely to be precipitated by negative events than by positive ones (for details see p.264). Individuals' resilience (p.541) varies greatly. The progress over time, of a life event's impact, is complex[410] and can be followed using formal questionnaires (e.g.[718]).

Life skills: see *adaptive behaviours*, p.419.

Lining up: this is common in early play, and is usually appropriate self-entertainment (p.545). Lining up can be increased for social reasons such as competition, copying a peer, making a bigger toy, admiring how many toys he has, or tidying the room. It becomes suggestive of autism if it is well below the child's abilities and lasts more than half an hour a day or if there are tantrums if it is disrupted (see p.229).

Lining-up of lego can symbolise cars or fences or many other things. It can be used as a memory aid in arithmetic (like fingers).

Cars can be lined up in a queue (like a traffic jam) or side-by-side (as in a parking lot). This is normal if used to represent cars (look for turns, crashes and bumps), or a train (listen for train noises). It can have various attractions: precise alignment of each car with the next, practising the difficult task of steering a block train round a corner, etc.

Indicators of complexity (that are more common in normal play than in autism) include (a) continually making and unmaking the lines; (b) the lines evolving to different shapes rather than gazed at or protected; (c) enjoying 2D patterns such as parking lots or branched shapes, or 3D constructions; (d) child being happy when distracted or interrupted from lining up; (e) presence of other interests, sometimes integrated into the lining up. Sequencing by colour or size, or extending the line from room to room, increase the complexity slightly, and have little diagnostic significance.

Locked-in syndrome: p.97.

Loneliness: this means an unsatisfied hunger for social interaction, sometimes with specific people. There are many variants of it. One can long for (a) specific people (e.g. after divorce, bereavement, change of schools, emigration, or being taken into care); (b) someone to share their private thoughts with, i.e. a best friend; (c) emotional closeness within the family; or (d) to be included in more social interactions (e.g. a bullied child, p.219; a deaf child in a mainstream school; a child whose parents find the neighbourhood too frightening to let him out, so his interactions with imaginary friends increase, p.231; a child with very specific interests who wishes he could discuss them with friends). Loneliness drives the creation of imaginary friends, p.231; the presence of imaginary friends is quite strong evidence that an unusual degree of loneliness has occurred.

Loneliness involves not only separable social drives (p.168) but other reinforcers (p.540), plus avoidance of problems that occur when alone. Loneliness may be driven by other people's effect on our own mood, self-esteem, relief of boredom, etc. The *feeling* that relationships are inadequate sometimes reflects the person's general mood, rather than indicating an objective difference between their relationships and other people's.

People differ in the amount and kind of social interactions they crave, and in how big an issue it is for them. Loneliness can be especially troublesome for teenagers as they try to create a self-identity (p.237) and a social network away from their family[682].

Looked after children: children fostered or in children's homes. Reasons for children being taken into care are abuse (62%), family dysfunction (10%), parental disability (6%), family in acute stress

(6%), absent parenting (6%), disability (4%) and socially unacceptable behaviour (4%)[1340].

Decisions regarding whether to take a child into care depend not only on whether the parenting is *good enough* (p.190), but also on the availability of extended family (see kinship care, p.495), the level of evidence, and community factors such as the proportion of allegations that are investigated in different localities[1737]; the tendency for some staff to regard neglect as less serious than other abuse[1374]; the quality and impartiality of social and legal services[144]; and the local availability of suitable carers[128].

Nearly all adolescents in residential units have psychiatric disorder, as do 60% of those in foster care. As a single surprising example, excess drinking of water (p.338) is far more common in looked after children[4].

Love: this word probably refers to the same process as attachment (p.195) but convention dictates that each word is usually used in different contexts. Whether one can love a country, a house or a toy depends on the definition. Emotional and physical warmth are key ingredients of love[652] and of parenting (p.189). Most children also adore their parents[652]. See also sexual behaviours, p.267; smiling out of the blue, p.309; oxytocin, p.521; hate, p.187.

- People "truly, madly and deeply in love" who are viewing a photo of their loved one have reduced amygdala activity[112]. Because the amygdala is activated by stress, this suggests that a component of love is stress-reduction. If so, attachment and love are closely related, or identical.

Low birth weight: see p.432.
LP: lumbar puncture.
LSD: lysergic acid diethylamide, p.258.
LTM: long-term memory. Memories lasting at least a few days.
Lying: p.255.

Lyme disease: infection with tick-borne *Borrelia*. 3–30 days after the tick bite, the pathognomonic sign *erythema migrans* usually appears, with a deep red centre inside a pink surround, over 5 cm across (there is often a lighter ring between the red and pink, creating a characteristic bull's eye appearance). The condition is seen mainly in high-risk geographic areas in the summertime. A minority develop complications such as headache, muscle soreness, and polyneuropathy. Consider Lyme disease in children who have had a headache for over a week, especially with any cranial nerve palsies. Laboratory confirmation requires isolation of *Borrelia* or specific IgG or IgM[662].

Muscle pain and fatigue can persist for months after Lyme disease, without this indicating presence of *Borrelia* in the body[91]. If laboratory tests are inconclusive other causes of chronic fatigue (p.325) should be considered[662].

Lyonisation: see *mosaicism*, p.509.

Lysosomal storage disorders:
a) Fabry disease, p.464.
b) mucopolysaccharidoses. There are several types but the initial test for all of them is glycosaminoglycans (GAG). The signs first noticed include protruberant abdomen, hirsutism, atypical

facial appearance, ID, and skeletal abnormalities[1677]. For treatments see[299].

- types I and II (Hurler and Hunter syndromes). There is multisystem involvement.
- Type III (Sanfilippo) is eventually fatal, but is highly variable in rate of progress[1068]. It often starts around age 3–5 with restless, destructive, anxious, and sometimes aggressive behaviour[1634] Words are typically lost about age 6–8, and motor function declines years later[998]. Coarse facial features (thick lips and prominent eyebrows) are found in most, as are epilepsy and periods of screaming[998,1634].

c) GM1 gangliosidosis: variable presentation and age of onset.

d) GM2 gangliosidoses: Tay-Sachs and Sandhoff syndromes, also called hexosaminidase A and B deficiency, are clinically indistinguishable and include progressive deterioration and unsteadiness of gait (p.471). Tay-Sachs is most often described in Ashkenazi Jewish infants but also occurs in other genetic groups and at later ages. All have a cherry-red macula.

e) lipofuscinoses: accumulation of pigments made from a mixture of fats and proteins. Detect by electron microscopy.

f) sphingomyelin: p.552.

g) sphingolipid: e.g. metachromatic leukodystrophy, p.498.

h) glucoproteinoses.

i) Mucolipidoses.

Macrocephaly and megalencephaly: megalencephaly means a large brain, whereas macrocephaly means a large head. Practically all children with large heads *and without other obvious abnormality* simply have large brains, without functional or diagnostic implications[976].

Heads can be large due to increased volume of skull, subdural fluid, brain, or CSF (see[390] for an extensive list of causes and a systematic approach to diagnosis). It is worthwhile screening for treatable causes such as GA1, p.32. From age 2, children with autism have (on average) slightly increased brain volume, despite having had normal brain size at birth. From adolescence the autistic brain slowly shrinks throughout life, but because the skull does not shrink, the slight macrocephaly persists[641].

Macrosomia: see *overgrowth*, p.521.

Magical thinking: reasoning about causes that is obviously incorrect. It is heard much more often from children, but this may be because adults check their ideas for rationality before speaking (see[190]). A

common example is adults thinking that if the first thing they throw in the bin in the morning goes in, it will be a good day. A simple form of *predictable irrationality*, p.534.

Makaton: a multimodal system of communication, i.e. hand signs accompanied by speech, often used together with standardised simple drawings of everyday objects such as toilet, drink, etc. This helps people with speech difficulty or ID to move towards normal English verbal communication. Its signs are taken from British Sign Language but sentences are structured as in English. There are versions of Makaton for many countries. Compare *sign language*, p.130.

Malabsorption: Defective crossing of the intestinal wall by nutrients. Similar effects can be produced by maldigestion, defined as the defective hydrolysis of nutrients. Some conditions affect all nutrients; others are specific for lipids, proteins, amino acids, carbohydrates, or specific sugars such as lactose. There are very many causes, both life-long or temporary (e.g. infection, gastritis, heart failure, hyperthyroidism)[1105]. In bacterial overgrowth, bacteria compete with the child for B_{12} (p.329). B_{12} is also unabsorbed in the autoimmune condition of pernicious anaemia, p.421. See also abetalipoproteinaemia, p.417; generalised itch, p.110; coeliac disease (and its rare contribution to autistic symptoms), p.441; inflammatory bowel disease, p.490; cystic fibrosis, p.450; methionine malabsorption, p.434; lactose malabsorption creating impression of IBS, p.494; transporters, p.379; food intolerances, p.493.

Malaria: infection by plasmodium, which is carried by specific mosquitoes. It is a major cause of death and ID in tropical areas, especially affecting small children. Malaria is so common that it has led to protective mutations, including sickle, p.549; thalassaemia, p.563; and G6PD deficiency, p.350. The main signs[1535] are fever, which can be continuous or recurrent; headache, joint pain and vomitting; occuring within two *years* of being in an endemic area with inadequate skin protection. Severity is usually greatly reduced by the partial immunity that lasts for two years following malaria infection; but children from endemic areas are often severely anaemic. Mental state change (e.g. irritability, clouding of consciousness, posturing or convulsions) indicates cerebral malaria.

Malformation: one in 50 babies has a malformation easily detectable at birth. The most common are birthmarks (of which neurophakomatoses, p.514, have special significance); hypospadias; congenital hip dislocation; cleft lip, p.440; brain malformations (listed below); asymmetry, p.93; overgrowth, p.521; and extra digits. Some malformations develop later, e.g. contractures, post-injury changes, clubbed fingers, p.466. Subtle facial abnormalities (such as hypertelorism, and lowset ears) are often only clarified by clinical geneticists. Severe rare conditions such as missing limbs, conjoined twins, and hermaphroditism will not be discussed here.

Unusual appearance can contribute to bullying, p.219. For identification of syndromes, see p.383. Compare body dysmorphic disorder, p.433.

Brain malformations often bring ID and epilepsy. They include:

- microcephaly (p.507)
- macrocephaly (p.502)
- holoprosencephaly (p.480)
- white matter defects (p.574)
- cerebral cortical malformations: agyria, polymicrogyria, focal dysplasia. Neuronal migration defects cause several syndromes that include ID, epilepsy, and craniofacial and ophthalmic defects[79].
- hydrocephalus and its causes (p.482)
- neural tube defects (p.513)
- craniosynostosis. A third of children with premature fusion of a single suture have neurodevelopmental deficits[813].
- neurophakomatoses (p.514).

Malingering: intentional actions simulating impairment with an external or obvious motivation and intent to deceive (but see discussion of related terms on p.359, and *Telling untruths* on p.255). Among criminal defendants and compensation-seekers, some measures find malingering in half of adult subjects[1709] and it is similarly common in adolescents. It is commonplace for a young child to exaggerate a pain in order to obtain more sympathy, to temporarily regress to obtain more attention, to say he can't do a task when he actually just doesn't want to, or even to exaggerate viral symptoms in order to have a day or two off school. Before adolescence, the term malingering is rarely appropriate[1418] because of children's lack of concealment, their difficulty with sophisticated role-play (p.222), and because their motivations, though obvious, are usually internal (e.g. tiredness, boredom, hunger, or wanting a cuddle). However, adolescents can feign psychotic symptoms to obtain a change of carers, and feign symptoms of ADHD in order to obtain medication to sell[1418].

Malnutrition: inadequate intake of nutrients. There are two main types. (a) deficiencies of *micronutrients* (listed on p.327). In many countries around the world, maternal health and child development (both physical and cognitive) are impaired by multiple micronutrient deficiencies[26]. (b) *protein-calorie* malnutrition. A widely used classification of protein-calorie malnutrition[1715] is:

Weight (% of expected)	oedema present	oedema absent
60–80%	kwashiorkor	undernourished
below 60%	marasmic kwashiorkor	marasmus

Inadequate diet can have major effects on mental and physical development. This appears to be one of the means by which maternal depression (p.174) impairs infant development[76]. Most children with delayed growth gain about 10 IQ points if they receive food supplements[1705]. They can show similar gains if they are given extra stimulation in childhood.

Malnutrition of the mother while pregnant affects the child's tendency to obesity, in two ways. If she is malnourished in the first two trimesters, the baby is likely to have a lifelong tendency to be overweight. Conversely, if she is malnourished in the last trimester, or he is malnourished in his first few months of life, he is less likely to become obese [1312].

Malnutrition is common in anorexia nervosa, p.334. Malnutrition and overnutrition can coexist, especially in children with autism or ID[1167]. Malabsorption or chronic nausea, or other chronic illness, can cause malnutrition. See also *malabsorption*, p.502; *placental insufficiency*, p.531; *poverty*, p.533; *anaemia*, p.421; *starvation*, p.553.

Mania: the most common meanings refer to elevated mood: see *bipolar affective disorder*, p.264; manic defence, p.306.

In the following words "mania" is used in a different sense, indicating just an excessive interest: pyromania, p.466; trichotillomania, p.117; kleptomania, p.250; erotomania, p.268.

Manipulative ☝: a common term for people who mislead or threaten others to achieve a personal end. Examples are children whose tantrums continue until they get their way (p.286); people of any age who fabricate or exaggerate symptoms (p.359); and adults with borderline personality disorder (p.242) when they harm themselves in order to obtain professional care. The term is pejorative, vague and can reduce other staff's empathy, so should be used with care[1273]. See also *psychopathy*, p.280.

Mannerisms: p.85. These are odd *ways* of doing something appropriate (a goal-directed action cannot itself be a mannerism, though sometimes the odd embellishment attached to it is called that). A mannerism can be fluidly applied to a wide variety of situations, or it may only be seen in particular practised contexts (e.g. always flourishing a handkerchief grandly before blowing the nose). Compared to stereotypies (p.553), manneristic actions are often slower and more complicated[1487]. The term is sometimes used to imply that the behaviour was odd on purpose, in order to have an effect on other people (acting camp is an example, p.243); but this does not apply to the mannerisms of autism.

Maple syrup urine disease: an autosomal recessive defect in the breakdown of branched-chain amino acids, leading to their accumulation. The best-known form is catastrophic neonatally, but milder variants are classified as intermittent, intermediate, thiamine-responsive[167] and symptomatic[506]. Symptoms include ID, autism, seizures and dystonia. Diagnose by characteristic smell of urine, and plasma amino acids.

Marasmus: p.504.

Marfan syndrome: connective tissue disorder with a fibrillin mutation causing dislocated lens and aortic pathology. Signs include long limbs, thin fingers, scoliosis (p.93), and high palate (which can contribute to speech difficulty). Teasing often leads to introversion and to mood problems[1663]. The risk of psychosis is somewhat increased. This is one of the first structural (non-metabolic) genetic disorders with effective treatment for complications. See also *hypermobility*, p.483.

Maslow's pyramid depicts the importance of satisfying basic, continual life-support needs, before occasional quality-of-life needs or desires. The hierarchy is not fixed, and the priority given to each need varies between people and between situations (such as time of day). Human needs and desires are very numerous: Fifty-eight *categories* of them are listed in[1024]. See social drives, p.168; drives for sensation, p.124; *superstimuli*, p.558.

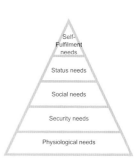

Figure 31. Maslow's hierarchy of needs.

Mass psychogenic behaviours (or mass sociogenic illness; previously called mass hysteria): almost any behaviour or belief can spread through a group. This is most likely in groups of females who have a lot in common, have been exposed to a novel situation, are aware of a potential mechanism for this situation to be harmful (whether chemical, biological, radiological or spiritual) and if the symptoms are subjective (e.g. dyspnoea, p.457)[1212]. It happens most in schools and healthcare facilities[1212], and like most psychic problems may be more common during major population disruptions such as war[1135]. The process at an individual level is that of *infectious behaviours*, p.490. An additional process occurs in a group: Once one peer is affected, the likelihood of other peers becoming affected increases, so the symptom rapidly spreads through the whole group.

Massively multiplayer online role-playing games (MMORPGs): p.573.
Masturbating: p.115.
Maternal: see *Mothers*, p.509.
Matching: p.64.
MBP: Munchausen by proxy, p.206.
MCADD: medium-chain acyl-CoA dehydrogenase deficiency, p.418.
MD: muscular dystrophy, p.510; medical degree.
ME: myalgic encephalomyelitis, see p.323.
Meares-Irlen syndrome: p.52.

Meconium: foetal faeces. When this is passed in utero, it stains the amniotic fluid. If the baby gasps for breath he may inhale it. This occurs in 10–20% of births, depending on the population and obstetric management. It is much more common in post-term pregnancies. Of babies who are admitted to a neonatal special care unit due to meconium aspiration, more than half will have long-term neurodevelopmental problems[133].

Medicines: discussed with *treatments*, p.567.

Melatonin: chemical released during hours of darkness. This timing is disrupted in Smith-Magenis (p.199).

Memory: p.37; also *working memory*, p.575; *memory distortions*, p.40.
Meningitis: discussed with *encephalitis*, p.461.
Menkes disease: p.330.

Menses, premenstrual symptoms: menstrual bleeding typically lasts 2–7 days each 21–34 days, with a mean volume of about 30 ml per cycle.

In amenorrhoea consider pregnancy; anorexia and other causes of weight loss, p.334; excess exercise, p.462; *prolactin*, p.536; *polycystic ovaries*, p.531; Fragile X, p.468. Amenorrhoea can also be produced by extreme prolonged stress or near-total separation from society or family[428]. Other causes include hyper- and hypothyroidism, pp.484,485; premature ovarian failure; chemotherapy; Turner's, p.570; Cushing's, p.449; Kallmann syndrome, p.495; galactosaemia, p.472 – and many others[580].

Non-menstrual disorders occasionally present with monthly timing (p.62). For milestones of menarche see p.411. For details of history taking, examination, menorrhagia, and unusual cycle-lengths see[698]). See also relation to fasting, p.465.

Psychological and behavioural aspects
Pelvic pain and/or irritability occur in many women in the few days before periods start. There are often mood changes (p.309), emotional lability (p.70) and migraines (p.141). Severe but rare complications include psychosis[403] and catamenial epilepsy, which occur perimenstrually, probably due to the effects of progesterone and progesterone-derived neurosteroids on GABA function[163].

All these neurological/psychological symptoms can appear years before menarche (p.411), when oestradiol cycling begins[216,1476]. This can be quite irregular. After menarche, the cycling gradually becomes regular. Crying is also very common in postnatal blues.

Extra issues in ID include premenstrual self-harm or stereotypies, and education including normalisation. Most teens who can toilet independently can learn to manage pads[1290].

Mental fatigue: p.323.
Mental Retardation: see *Intellectual Disability*.
Mercury: p.330.
Metabolism: crises, p.381; major pathways, p.382; disorders, p.381.

Microcephaly: this means a head circumference (p.409) 2 sd below the mean for age and sex. Severe microcephaly is 3 sd below the mean. Among congenital cases there are many genetic and chromosomal causes, as well as many maternal diseases, and stroke or infection in the foetus (see[67]).

Microcephaly of postnatal onset has numerous causes, some of them partially treatable, including amino acidopathies, Rett, p.541; ataxia telangiectasia, p.454, head injury, p.477; stroke, p.556; meningitis and encephalitis, p.461; HIV encephalopathy, p.479; lead poisoning, p.330; chronic renal failure, hypothyroidism, p.485; anaemia, p.421; malnutrition, p.504; and congenital heart disease (see[67]).

Microsleeps: p.72.
Middle child syndrome: see *Birth order*.
Midline stereotypies: p.64.
Migraine: p.141.
Milestones: p.55.

Mimicry: copying someone for social communication (such as mockery, or wanting to annoy, or wanting to be like someone, or perhaps wanting to communicate but not knowing what to say). This is different from echolalia and echopraxia which are usually done without awareness of the fact that they are copied, and with much less social understanding (p.459). Mimicry often has exaggerated diction, and eye contact during or afterwards.

Minuchin, Salvador: influential family therapist, p.213.

Mirror movements: inadvertently moving both sides of the body together. A subtype of *synkinesis*, p.560; and of *bilateral movements*, p.431; and a soft sign of neurological immaturity[907]. Test by showing the child how to touch his left thumb to each of his left fingers in turn; look for right hand movement (which is normal in infancy but unusual after age 10). Other examples include: (a) In infancy, both limbs tend to move together, preventing, e.g., tying shoelaces. (b) In Klippel-Feil syndrome [1693] there are neck and spine abnormalities, and usually mirror movements: While grasping something with one hand, they cannot let go with the other (so cannot climb a ladder). Contrast *mirror system*, below.

Mirror system: hypothetical neural system that underlies our copying other people's body posture, facial expressions and behaviour (such as yawning, laughing, sniffing and scratching); feeling what we imagine they are feeling; and priming of their goals and their cognitive and social judgments[103]. See Möbius syndrome, p.178; *facial expressions (using)*, p.464; *utilisation behaviours*, p.572; *overflow*, p.520.

Miscarriages: loss of a pregnancy between conception and 24 weeks gestation. About half of all women have at least one miscarriage, though very early miscarriages often occur undetected. Single gene mutations do not usually cause miscarriages, but major chromosomal defects are found in about half of all miscarriages[1296]. Recurrent (three or more) miscarriages are often caused by aneuploidy (which increases with maternal age), uterine abnormalities, antiphospholipid syndrome, or thrombophilia[1296].

Misery: in children, p.313; in mothers, p.174.

Mitochondrial disorders: this is usually a shorthand for primary disorders of mitochondrial metabolism affecting oxidative phosphorylation (oxphos). This is the most common group of inborn errors of metabolism (1/7000)[1041,1605]. Consider this in any progressive disorder; or developmental problems accompanied by abnormality in any other system. It is also an uncommon cause of hallucinations; chronic fatigue, migraine, depression[860] and medication-resistant psychiatric disorders[44]. Defects are often passed in the female line[1789], but new mutations are more common.

Aspects of mitochondrial function linked to disease
 (a) Coenzyme-Q10 (ubiquinone) is most needed in tissues with a high metabolic rate, so metabolic defects of CoQ10 primarily affect muscle, brain and nerves. CoQ10 deficiency causes ID with spasticity, axial hypotonia and failure to thrive. There are diverse and partial forms. Look for elevated plasma lactate; cerebellar atrophy; CoQ10 in muscle (not plasma). (b) *Leigh syndrome* is a devastating neurodegenerative disorder resulting from any of a wide range of mutations in mitochondria; however *Leigh-like syndrome* covers the entire spectrum from severe disorder to normality, with onset at any age[500]. Some cases of Leigh syndrome are caused by CoQ10 deficiency. (c) Fatty acid oxidation occurs in mitochondria. Inherited disorders of fatty acid metabolism affect about 1 in 9000 and can cause exercise intolerance, hypotonia, and/or ID[568]; the best-known example is MCADD, p.418. (d) There are numerous other mitochondrial conditions affecting development of infants and children; but the presenting problem is not often behavioural.

Screening tests
Because lactate is broken down in mitochondria, serum lactate is elevated in many mitochondrial disorders. Also test pyruvate, ketone bodies, plasma acylcarnitines, urinary organic acids, and ammonia.

MMORPG: massively multiplayer online role-playing games, p.573.

MMR: (a) A mixture of three attenuated viruses, used to immunise against measles, mumps and rubella (see *viruses*, p.573). This often causes a mild viral illness lasting up to three weeks. Because MMR is given in the same developmental period when some autistic children regress, MMR was incorrectly blamed for autism. However, changing from MMR to individual immunisations (as was done in Japan) did not decrease rate of diagnosis of autism[712].

(b) Mild Mental Retardation (see *Intellectual disability*, p.491).

MMSE: Mini-Mental State Examination, p.400.
Möbius syndrome: p.178.

MLD: *Moderate* Learning Difficulty (similar to *Mild* Learning Disability, see p.497).

Monotropism: this has two meanings. (1) Bowlby's suggestion of the unique importance of the mother (see p.195); (2) the idea that the core problem in autism is excessive focus on something, also called "attention tunnelling" [1125] (but see p.183).

Mood: p.461.

Mood stabilisers: medications used mainly in epilepsy, bipolar affective disorder, and violence. See also *ideographs*, p.487.

Mosaicism: two (or more) distinct genotypes within one individual[1478]. Subtypes include:

> *Postzygotic mutation*: an anomaly occurs in one cell in a very early embryo, then propagates to form a significant part of the child. This accounts for some of the milder forms of, e.g., Down's syndrome, p.455, Turner syndrome, p.570 and pyruvate carboxylase deficiency[1710]. Gonadal mosaicism in a parent can result in transmission of an autosomal dominant condition to more than one child, even when both parents are unaffected[1478].

> *Lyonisation*: Because the X-chromosome can function singly, as in XY males, one of the X's in XX females is inactivated. This effectively reduces the severity of some genetic diseases in females[1710], e.g. in Rett's, p.541; Fabry's disease, p.464.

Mothers: see parents, p.525; parenting☼, p.189; attachment☼, p.195; mother's heartbeat, p.61; social skills first used with mother, p.169.

> *Special difficulties facing some mothers*
> Single mothers, p.213; maternal mental health including depression, pp.173, 193–194; stress in pregnancy, p.300; mothers with ID, p.212; trapped wives, p.212; risks of young motherhood, p.268; mothers in prison, p.535; assisted conception, p.424; foetal alcohol syndrome, p.467; foetal valproate, p.572; mothers with PKU, p.529.

> *Problematic relationships with mother*
> See poor relationship with mother☼, p.193; daughter grooming mother, p.225; over-dependence on mother, p.43; child working to keep mother happy, p.112; Munchausen by proxy, p.206; mother obsequious to son, p.212; fear of losing mother, p.313; overprotection or infantilising, p.214.

> *Maternal role in specific problems of child*
> Mother's role in chronic fatigue, p.323; role in anorexia, p.334; role in parental alienation, p.187; role in difficulty separating, p.197; mother's relation to early menarche, p.411.

> *Other mothering issues*
> Oversociability of child to mother-figures, p.173; child's behaviour being worst with mother, p.201; misguided criticisms of mothering, p.271; ways of assessing parenting, pp.365, 556; monotropism, p.509; child staying off school to help mother, p.215; transition objects, p.567.

Motivation: *intrinsic* motivations are the "end purposes" of behaviour, as distinct from the countless *extrinsic* purposes of behaviours[1328]. For a general list of motivations see p.395. However most of the lists in this book contain some motives for behaviours. The distinction from some senses of *drives* is now outdated (see p.456).

> Motivational interviewing, p.355; Motivational Assessment Scale, p.365; loss of motivation in depression, p.313; amotivational state

with cannabis use, p.258; Yerkes-Dodson law and optimal level of anxiety/motivation, p.40; motivational orientation, p.534.

Mouthing: p.56.
MRI: magnetic resonance imaging (e.g. of the brain), p.374.
MSLT: Multiple Sleep Latency Test. See narcolepsy, p.72.
MSU: mid-stream urine.

Multiple personality: also called Dissociative Identity Disorder. This is a highly contentious topic: proponents identify cases frequently, and opponents claim this is because they ask leading questions and reward positive answers. The observation that families of people with DID have generally not seen any specific signs before contact with professionals suggests that most cases learn a behaviour akin to self-hypnosis, that becomes increasingly florid during sessions with a clinician who repeatedly raises the possibility[1257]. It is rare in children, and below puberty it can be difficult to distinguish non-florid cases from imaginary friends, pseudo-regression, acting, normal forgetting and "contextually determined sense of identity" (see examples in[717]). The causes and comorbidities are very similar to those of other dissociative symptoms[717] (see *dissociation*, p.453); and it is important to consider the possibility of psychosis[511].

Multiple sclerosis: acquired demyelination causing plaques in the white matter of the brain, with episodic exacerbations and very variable timecourse. Varied neurologic problems are seen, especially weakness, regression and transient visual deficits[988]. Risk is increased by multiple genotypes; family history of autoimmune disease; and exposure to Epstein Barr virus (p.478) and mononucleosis[65]. Half of all under-18 patients are depressed or anxious, and lists of their main concerns have been published which can aid in assessment and treament[1732]. See also *temperature-sensitivity*, p.562; *myelin*, p.510.

Multiple Sleep Latency Test: see narcolepsy, p.72.

Munchausen's syndrome: p.362; Munchausen by proxy (medical child abuse), p.206.

Muscular dystrophy: a large group of hereditary disorders causing progressive weakness. Intelligence is generally stable, and distributed about 1 sd below that of the unaffected population, i.e. mild ID is common [1061].

Duchenne MD is the best known, affecting 1 in 3500 males. It causes proximal muscle weakness (p.87). The first sign usually appears at age 3-4 and is often clumsiness (p.89, especially of running in games) or difficulty climbing stairs. Duchenne is usually fatal by age 30. Diagnosis of specific genetic subtypes is important as specific treatments are becoming available.

Mutism: p.153. Pseudo-mutism, p.151.
Myalgic encephalomyelitis: p.323.

Myasthenia: rapid tiring of muscles (both eyelids or mouth droops after 20 minutes). Seen in myasthenia gravis which is an autoimmune attack (p.427) on acetylcholine receptors. Also in congenital myasthenic syndromes, which are more diverse and severe.

Myelin: fatty sheath on axons that makes them conduct signals much faster, both in the central nervous system (see *white matter*, p.574) and in peripheral nerves.

Leukodystrophies (p.498) affect myelin development. See also acute and chronic inflammatory demyelinating polyneuropathies (AIDP/CIDP) such as Guillain-Barré, p.87; peripheral demyelination in Charcot-Marie-Tooth, p.87; central pontine myelinolysis, p.436; sphingomyelin, p.552.

Myoclonus: shock-like jerks not voluntarily reproducible. They can be regular, oscillatory or single. Common examples are hiccups; when falling asleep (hypnic jerks, p.200); and in startles, p.552 (see hyperekplexia, p.483). Also seen in epilepsy and many neurological disorders, in which they have been described as fragments of epilepsy. They can originate in the cortex or subcortically, and the pattern of the jerk (e.g. unilateral or bilateral, synchronous or progressive, ascending or descending) can suggest where, though neurophysiological investigation is far more precise[630]. See other twitches, p.101; movements, p.85; tardive myoclonus, p.561, jaw myoclonus, p.52.

Nail-biting: this occurs most when bored, alone and/or frustrated. Surprisingly, it does not seem to be increased by anxiety[432]. Nail-biting usually starts well before puberty and inproves thereafter, whereas anxiety disorders tend to start and worsen *post*pubertally. Furthermore, severe nail-biters are seen without any psychiatric problem (see cases in[1206]). See *behavioural addictions*, p.260.

One can measure the free length of nails, or the amount of impingement on the nailbed. One rating system is: *mild*: free edge of nail is irregular but reasonably intact; *moderate*: the free edge of the nail is absent; *severe*: the fingernail is bitten beyond the free edge so the nail margin is below the soft tissue border. Moderate or worse biting declines from 50% at age 10 to 15% at age 18[999]. Most children who bite their nails bite all ten fingers severely. The fingernails are usually bitten in a sequence, with the ring finger left till last because it is most awkward to bite.

Names and name-changing: p.239.

Narcissism: this means excessive preoccupation with one's physical or mental endowments. It can be grandiose/exhibitionistic or vulnerable/sensitive (there are many variations of these terms[246]). Many narcissistic children become aggressive when they are shamed[1600]. See Narcissistic Personality Disorder, p.241.

Narcolepsy: p.72.

Naughtiness: knowing one shouldn't do something, and doing it anyway (p.249). Anger (p.287), aggressive behaviour (p.289), oppositionality (p.253) and many other symptoms in this book are often considered to be naughtiness. Some naughtiness is developmentally useful. Healthy naughtiness (exploration of boundaries to see what happens) should happen regularly, e.g. once or twice per day from age 3 to 6, e.g. hitting a smaller sibling to see the reaction. Normally after age 8 this is occasional, mild and covert. *By itself*, naughtiness does not cause dysfunction in family, peer group or school. However, the term implies moral blame, and most professionals avoid it because blame damages the child's self-esteem and relationships. Rather than simply blaming, it is more useful to look for specific causes, many of which have effective remedies.

Navigation skills: these should be assessed directly and on history, using practical tests as well as maps and drawings. Several distinct contexts should be assessed, e.g. home, finding her way to school or in school, finding the waiting room in the clinic, knowing whether she has been in this room before (in severe cases she will not know the answer even when shown a closet or storage room). For detailed assessment methods see[229,230].

These skills are limited in several circumstances: mental age under 5; with preoccupation or performance anxiety; with memory consolidation or recall problems; damage to right parietal cortex, p.512; agenesis of the corpus callosum, p.445. Bumping into doorways or overhanging tree branches can arise from excess haste (p.79), clumsiness (p.89), reading a book, visual problems (p.133) or spatial neglect (p.512). If damage to the parietal lobes is the cause, there may be coexisting apraxia (p.89). There are distinct cortical systems for locations near oneself, for objective maps, and for perspective views[1156].

NEET: "not in employment, education or training." A term used since about 2000. NEETs are sometimes caricatured as inactive, workshy or unemployable; but the group is heterogeneous, including as it does school-leavers who are young mothers, disabled, chronically sick, doing voluntary work, studying at home, resting, caring for relatives, or travelling the world. The group therefore includes both highly privileged and able young people, and those who are having difficulty taking the next step. The number of young people who are NEET quadruples to 30% in the summer months, but being NEET for six months is a strong predictor of long-term NEET[531]. See also *unemployment*, p.570.

Negative expressed emotion: refers to parents (and other relatives, teachers, etc.) who when talking about or to a child, use terms that are hostile or critical, or who are emotionally over-involved, e.g. blaming themselves for a child's problems. Reducing EE in a family reduces the risk of a relapse of schizophrenia, mood disorder, or eating disorder[243]. Criticism by parents increases teenagers' self-harm, especially in teenagers who are critical of themselves[1728]. The effect of expressed emotion in ADHD is more complex, and may interact with lack of maternal warmth to increase the risk of later conduct problems[1516]. Compare "double-bind" (p.356).

Neglect: this has two meanings: (a) a type of child abuse, p.274; and (b) acting as if part of space did not exist. This can affect peripersonal space, personal space, perceptual space (including imagination), motor function (e.g. motor neglect, p.96), or any combination of these[244]. Drawing of half-clocks[444], and clapping to the midline[1199], are simple signs. Underlying causes are much broader than the classically recognised parietal damage (p.513), and include unilateral migraine[465], deficits in spatial working memory[1223], and possibly the writing direction of the local language. For practical tests see[625]. *Artefactual* neglect occurs if a child stops a cancelling test at a fold or shadow on the page.

Neocortex: a ventral *what* path converges on the temporal pole (damage to which causes visual agnosia in *Klüver-Bucy*, p.496); and a more dorsal *where* path converges to the parietal and then the frontal cortex[670].

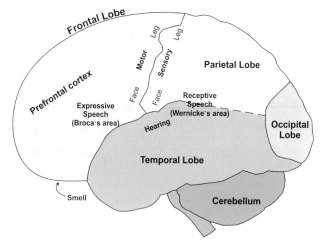

Figure 32. Principal lobes of the brain.

- Frontal lobe: areas include motor, oculomotor, dorsolateral, lateral orbitofrontal, and anterior cingulate (see frontal signs, p.469). Each area has a distinct function, so several frontal syndromes are recognised, as follows[349]. Dorsolateral damage causes reduced verbal fluency, poor constructional strategies, and difficulty in maintaining or shifting set (see[1178]). Orbitofrontal lesions cause irritability, tactlessness, and sometimes excessive imitation and utilisation behaviours (p.572). The anterior cingulate cortex (ACC) detects inconsistency (i.e. conflict between sources of information)[654]. Damage to the ACC can cause akinetic mutism, p.97.
- Parietal lobe: this processes spatial information including navigation (p.512), judging of objects' size or weight[952]; and numbers (with a number line[385]; see *dyscalculia*, p.457). See spatial neglect, p.512; motor neglect, p.96; and simultanagnosia, p.122. The right parietal cortex may have a role in the misjudgment of body size in anorexia nervosa[1157].
- Occipital lobe: this performs visual processing and visual imagery, which is driven both visually and via association tracts.
- Temporal lobe: this includes the auditory cortex, p.512; hippocampus, p.478; and amygdala, p.421. Problems include auditory hallucinations, p.344; temporal lobe epilepsy, p.562; *Klüver-Bucy*, p.496; olfactory hallucinations, p.344.
- Insula: this is cortex in the depths of the lateral fissure. It has roles in homeostasis, taste, and pain processing, p.136.

See also epilepsy, p.73; migraine, p.141; corpus callosum, p.445; *compartmentalization*, p.443; *connectivity*, p.444.

Neural tube defects: these include spina bifida (p.551), cranium bifidum / encephalocoele, anencephaly, hydranencephaly, porencephaly. These are increased in foetal valproate syndrome, p.572; and folate deficiency, p.467.

Nerves (peripheral): see Eaton-Lambert syndrome, p.459; congenital analgesia, p.136; Fabry's disease, p.464; Guillain-Barré, p.87; neurofibromatosis, p.514.

NES: Neurological Evaluation Scale, p.58.

NESS: Neurological Examination for Subtle Signs, p.58.

Neuroacanthocytosis: a broad family of disorders, causing movement disorders and spiky (Gk "acantha", a thorn) red blood cells. Neuroacanthocytoses are degenerative conditions often first appearing in adolescence, with a wide range of neurological abnormalities including dystonia, chorea (p.439), odd gait, continuous belching (p.430), eye movement problems, epilepsy and often eventually hypokinesis.

> One subgroup occurs due to abnormalities in lipid metabolism (e.g. abetalipoproteinaemia, p.417). Degeneration of the basal ganglia, with tongue- and lip-biting, is seen in chorea-acanthocytosis[1704]. For suggested investigations see [1703,1704]. Despite the name, acanthocytes are not always found[121].

Neurofibromatosis (von Recklinghausen disease): an autosomal dominant condition occurring in 1 in 2500 births[1776]. It is a neurophakomatosis (p.514).

> *Diagnostic signs*. The most visible signs are café-au-lait spots and axillary freckling. Cutaneous neurofibromata may be palpable, sometimes within associated lipomas. Neurofibromata often increase at puberty. NIH criteria are any two of: six or more café-au-lait spots (>0.5 cm prepubertally or >1.5 cm postpubertally); axillary freckling; two or more neurofibromas; two or more iris hamartomas (Lisch nodules); a distinctive bone lesion; or a first-degree relative diagnosed using the same criteria.

> *Genetic testing* is for mutations in the NF1 gene, and SPRED1 testing for NF1-like-syndrome should also be considered[1065].

> *Effects*. NF is a highly variable syndrome, and a few patients are disfigured. Nearly half are mildly learning disabled, and visuospatial skills may be particularly affected. About a third have ADHD, and there is an increased prevalence of autism and mood problems (see[1120]). Regular paediatric checks are needed to detect and treat cardiovascular, renal, visual, and endocrine problems.

Neurofilaments and neurotubules: relevant to SSPE, p.557; Lyme disease, p.501; neuroacanthocytosis, p.514; tuberous sclerosis, p.569; Alzheimer's.

Neuroleptic malignant syndrome (NMS): muscle rigidity (can be just head and neck), high fever, tachycardia, hypertension, tachypnea, autonomic instability (p.428), clouding of consciousness. This is an idiosyncratic reaction to normal doses of neuroleptics (typical and atypical neuroleptics, as well as some other psychotropic medicines). It needs emergency medical attention due to the risk of renal damage. Relevant tests include creatine phosphokinase, p.446; and iron, which is often low. For distinction from serotonin syndrome see p.548. The balance between ACh and dopamine seems to determine NMS[1544] as well as parkinsonism.

Neurological signs, hard and soft: p.58

Neuropathic pain: p.136

Neurophakomatoses: developmental disorders including benign tumours (hamartomas) of skin and neural tissue. Examples include *neurofibromatosis*, p.514; *tuberous sclerosis*, p.569; *Von Hippel-Lindau* disease (retinal changes, cerebellar ataxia); and Sturge-

Weber syndrome (with port wine haemangiomas in the skin and brain). *Ataxia telangiectasia*, p.454, is sometimes included.

Neurosteroids: see p.506.
Neurotransmitters: p.398.
Nightmares: see p.456.
Night terror: p.200.

NMDA: a subtype of glutamate receptor (N-methyl-D-aspartate). See glutamate, p.474; anti-NMDA, p.422.

NMS: neuroleptic malignant syndrome, p.514.

Nomenclature: in adult psychiatry a distinction has traditionally been made between the *form* of symptoms and their *content*[1123]. Behavioural nomenclature is less systematic, with the most common patterns named after a single characteristic aspect:

Aspect	Common examples
motivation	*gratification* phenomena (usually used as a euphemism for masturbation)
motivation at first glance	anorexia, challenging behaviour, school refusal
delay until symptoms	*tardive* dyskinesia (implies it is the result of long-term antipsychotic treatment)
trigger	*startle* syndromes are triggered by unexpected stimuli
duration	*tics* are usually rapid
content	*echolalia* (implies automaticity or interest only in the sound); *coprolalia* (implies that this is a tic)
location	*midline* stereotypies; *hand*-regard
repetitiveness	*stereotypies*
what they are not	*pseudo*-hallucination (ambiguous: implies brief, partial, or faked)
mechanism	*pseudo*-fit (implies faked)

The examples in the right column constitute a conventional shorthand for common behaviours. When describing less common forms, common terms can be combined (tardive tics, pseudo-echolalia) or they can be described at a lower, more detailed, "phenomenological" level. See also *ideographs*, p.487.

Non-behaviours: this entry describes children who apparently voluntarily refrain from activities (as distinct from non-conscious processes, p.570). Assessing what children don't do, and the way they don't do it, can be difficult.

The simplest cases are easy: the proposed activity is simply not enjoyable (e.g. homework) so the child does something else. However for children to come to professional attention, non-behaviours generally have to be more disabling than most referred *behaviours* are (because behaviours usually bother adults more than non-behaviours). Their being prolonged and rather invisible and invariant makes it much more difficult to work out the causes. This is all the more true if the non-behaviour precludes interaction with professionals.

An operant explanation can be (and usually is) produced for most non-behaviours. Refusing to follow mum (p.557) is often a simple example, as is a child's failure to participate in normal activities when he is preoccupied by imaginary friends (p.231). However, many non-behaviours are not operants at all, but are produced by an innate response to anxiety[204,1021] which has been described as the "refusal-withdrawal-regression spectrum"[768] (see p.296). Frozen watchfulness (p.470), selective mutism (p.153) and pervasive refusal (p.527) often combine the innate response and the operant mechanism. In other situations the gain is rather amorphous, such as keeping the predictability of the environment at a manageable level (see p.126).

Inflexibility (p.234), as a trait and/or increased by anxiety, is often a characteristic of these children and their relatives. For discussion of some common aspects of the dynamics of causation and investigation, see *chronic fatigue*, p.323.

not attending school: p.217	*learned helplessness*: p.96
fight-flight-freeze: p.296	*panic*: p.301
party refusal: p.125	*avoidance*: p.429
Pervasive Refusal: p.527	*refusals*: p.540
food refusal: p.332	*not opening presents*: p.312
not eating: p.331	simple and complex effects
anorexia nervosa: p.332	of anxiety: p.296
Chronic fatigue: p.323	*behavioural inhibition*: p.296
Selective mutism and	*perverse effects*: p.528
related avoidant	*dissociation*: p.453
behaviours: p.153	*unwanted nonbehaviour*:
sensory intolerance: p.125	p.353
sulking: p.557	*oppositionality*: p.253.
refusing to follow: p.557	

Non-declarative memory: p.37.
Non-ketotic hyperglycinaemia: p.350.

Non-stimulant: word used to refer to atomoxetine, a treatment for ADHD that has very similar actions to *Stimulants*, p.555. See also *ideographs*, p.487.

Non-verbal Learning Disability (NVLD): p.28.

Non-verbal children: preverbal developmental stage, p.143; Not speaking much, p.151; Regression, p.41.

Testing non-verbal children
Cognitive: When a child's language abilities are impaired, or no translator is available, his other abilities can be assessed using a non-verbal method such as the Leiter International Performance Scale or Raven's Matrices.
Social: Social interest can be assessed non-verbally, using observation of free play; non-verbal elements of the ADOS such as eye-contact; and games (such as chess, playing with balls, tapping or drawing for them to copy, crawling fingers toward them, or give-me-five, p.378). For social interactions by blind and sighted babies see p.134.
Flexibility: Assess his enthusiasm for changes initiated by himself or others (using games as above; more details on p.234).

Noonan syndrome: genetic syndrome that is surprisingly common (perhaps 1 in 1000, with variable expression). Heart defects, short stature, wide-spaced eyes, webbed neck and low-set ears with thick rims, generally normal IQ or mild ID. Caused by multiple single gene defects, some of which can be tested for.

Noradrenaline (also called norepinephrine): a transmitter that regulates behaviour[70] and enhances learning[726]. It increases anxiety, and in extremis it also signals fight-or-flight (p.466).

Levels are increased by stimulants (p.555) or opiate withdrawal, and reduced by clonidine (p.441) or opiates[71]. It is mainly released by the locus coeruleus, but it is also produced by some rare phaeochromocytoma tumours, p.529. Sudden drop in noradrenaline is a core mechanism in cataplexy, p.436. Deficiency is one of the causes of ✠ADHD[60], p.79

NOS: Means "not otherwise specified". See *Atypical disorders*, p.426.

Nose-picking: Practically all people pick their noses, many of them more than 20 times a day[42]. The main reasons are to unclog the nose, to relieve discomfort, and for cosmetic purposes. 17% of teenagers think they have a serious nose-picking problem, but their nose-picking is no different from the other 83%[42].

Not doing something: see *non-behaviours*, p.515.
Not listening: p.129.

Novelty: this produces unexpected uncertainty (an example of *expected* uncertainty is the weather being different each day)[1813]. People differ in the amount of novelty they crave. Novelty, stimulants, and reward briefly reduce children's activity level (see *dopamine appetite*, p.322).

Nutrients: p.327.
NVLD: see *Non-verbal Learning Disability*, p.28.
Obesity: p.335.

Object persistence: the important physical principle, learned in infancy, that an object cannot spontaneously appear or disappear (continuity, or object permanence), occupy the same space as another object (solidity), break apart (cohesion), fuse with another object (boundedness) or change size, shape or colour[88]. Infants learn that self-propelled (or animate) objects are able to violate some but not all of these rules[88]. They also learn that after an object's disappearance, the best way to bring it back is by calling if it is animate, and by reaching if it is inanimate[926]. For intelligence testing methods in infancy, see p.59.

Object relations: a framework describing how an infant creates (and later uses) internal models in his mind, representing people and aspects of people. Object relations is usually seen as a branch of psychoanalysis, separate from classical psychoanalysis which focuses on the discharge of impulses[643]. From an object relations point of view an infant is always in a relationship with his mother and with himself; whereas from a classical point of view he becomes attached to mother only because she satisfies his oral drive. See splitting, p.552; projective identification, p.535; transition object, p.567; Melanie Klein, p.495. Compare *object persistence*, above.

Obsession: the common meaning of this term is any repetitive behaviour (pp.61, 63) or dominating interest (p.229). The psychiatric meaning, used in this book, is of recurrent fears that are experienced as the person's own thoughts, but are unwelcome and often lead to attempts (compulsions) to inactivate them [1487], contributing to a diagnosis of Obsessive Compulsive Disorder (OCD, p.65).

Conundrum 15: Obsession or psychosis

A conventional rule is that the effort to resist these ideas distinguishes obsessions from psychosis or simple preference. However this rule is unreliable in adults, and even more so in children. Contrary to the usual assumption that ideas cause behaviour, in many children who are developing OCD, the compulsions start months or years before the child can describe any obsession (and sometimes even in the absence of vague fears).

Obsessive Compulsive Disorder (OCD), p.65; obsessive compulsive behaviour (OCB), p.63

Obsessive slowness: p.95

Obstructive sleep apnoea: this happens mainly in the obese but can also be caused by large tonsils. Whereas in adults, daytime sleepiness is the most common effect, in children hyperactivity is a more common effect. OSA may be more common in orientals, in whom it may make a substantial contribution to daytime inattention [728] or daytime sleepiness, p.321.

OCB: obsessive compulsive behaviours, p.63.
OCD: Obsessive Compulsive Disorder, p.65.
Occipital Horn syndrome: p.32.
OCP: see *oral contraceptive pill*.
Oculogyric crisis: p.93.
ODD: Oppositional Defiant Disorder, p.519.
Odd ideas: p.348.
Odour: see *body odour*.
Offending: see *criminality*, p.446.

Only child: child without siblings. In most environments, the benefits of greater access to parents and resources seem to outweigh the disadvantage of no access to siblings [1263], perhaps because only children often play with neighbours or cousins. However only children are often stereotyped [1118] as selfish (pp.179, 179), unfriendly (p.181), inflexible (p.234), and overconfident (p.244). The impression that only children are different may arise from their being an obvious subgroup of small families, who are indeed different from large families (see *siblings*, p.548). First-borns with no siblings yet (some of whom will continue as only children) are more likely until age 5 to be taken to the doctor, perhaps because their parents are less experienced or have more time [1338].

"On the spectrum": usually means having Autistic Spectrum Disorder (p.427). The graph at the right shows one of the "spectra" related to autism in the population[314]. Working out where on this continuum should be considered impaired (p.17) is subjective.

The phrase is misleading as (a) everyone is on a spectrum; and (b) it implies that there is only one spectrum, indicating a common aetiology for all three areas of difficulty, whereas there is also a spectrum for each area[1371], and in addition many non-autism-related spectra that contribute to referral and diagnosis (e.g. see figures on pp.60 and 83).

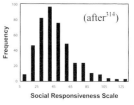

(after[314])

Figure 33. Population distribution of sociability.

Operationalized Psychodynamic Diagnostics (OPD-2): One of the most successful attempts to specify in detail (i.e. to operationalise) the signs of psychodynamic processes[1194,1438]. It is far more detailed than DSM (p.385) regarding what patients say, and especially how they describe their feelings. It is not yet as well developed as DSM;it requires considerably more subjective interpretation than DSM; and unfortunately there is minimal consideration of children, adolescents, or people with ID. See *axes*, p.16; *personality*, p.241.

Opiates and opioids: these terms are often used interchangeably, but formally *opiates* are chemicals derived from the opium poppy (morphine, codeine and synthetic variants of them such as heroin) whereas *opioids* are chemicals with different structures that work on the same receptors (e.g. methadone and endogenous peptide ligands such as enkephalins and endorphins)[227]. They are released from the hypothalamus during severe exercise, pain, excitement, and orgasm. There are many subtypes of opioid receptor, and opioids differ in which ones they act on. Antagonists include naltrexone and naloxone.

Opiates and opioids sedate, relieve pain, and can produce euphoria, leading them to be major drugs of abuse. See heroin abuse and withdrawal, p.258; overwhelming states, p.69; toxic substances in pregnancy, p.566.

Individual variation
There is great inter-individual variability in the amount of pain relief obtained with opiates, and some of the genes underlying this have been identified[249]. A few long-term self-harmers may be addicted to the pleasant effects of endogenous opioids (p.317). See also *anorexia nervosa*, p.334.

Opisthotonus: p.93.
Oppositional: ☂ habitually acting against others, p.253.

Oppositional Defiant Disorder: ☂ includes traits related to oppositionality, p.253. ODD may be separable into irritability (with outbursts, anger and easily annoyed), headstrong (argumentative, non-compliant, rule-breaking), and hurtful traits (spitefulness and vindictiveness)[1558]. About half of children with a diagnosis of ODD go on in adolescence to receive a diagnosis of Conduct

Disorder (p.249), and in turn about half of those with a diagnosis of CD go on in adulthood to receive a diagnosis of Antisocial Personality Disorder (p.242)[1096]. See *disruptive behaviour.*

Oral contraceptive pill: steroid medication that occasionally causes depression or anxiety. It can also be used to reduce "perimenstrual" symptoms, which can start years before menarche (p.506).

Orexin: see *Hypocretin*, p.485.

Organelles: cell components separated by a membrane. These include mitochondria, p.508; lysosomes, p.501; peroxisomes, p.526.

Orgasm: p.71. See also masturbation, p.115.
OSA: obstructive sleep apnoea, p.518.
OT: Occupational Therapist.
OTC: ornithine transcarbamylase, p.571.
Overactivity: see hyperactivity, p.79.

Overexcited: this is a state of positive emotional arousal, leading to ill-judged, repetitive, noisy giggling or shouting, as in parties. Contributors include long-term temperament (see *hyperthymia*, p.264) and short-term stimulation (e.g. other people's laughter, funny faces, or even eye contact). It sometimes happens in rough play when tickles or wrestling cause giggling and requests for more, i.e. a positive feedback cycle. A similar effect can be produced by rewards in ADHD (see *perverse effects*, p.528). After excess stimulation is removed, overexcitement generally fades within a few minutes.

Overflow: spread of activation to apparently unconnected behaviours, in a more or less uncontrolled way. Synkinesis is sometimes due to overflow but that term is usually used to describe fairly precise movement patterns, p.560.

During REM sleep, some impulses leak past the paralysis of sleep, so producing observable movements. Similarly many people move defensively when watching a violent film or playing a violent computer game (see mirror system, p.507). See also overflow of annoyance to things that did not cause it, p.292.

Speech increases the excitability of the hand area in motor cortex, and it has been suggested that this "overflow" of activation may account for the prevalence of hand gestures accompanying speech[1058]. Similarly, excitement-induced flapping is usually confined to the arms but in extreme excitement can overflow to the legs (p.105).

An example of overflow in *time* is perseveration, p.527; a less cognitive example is the *selfish goal principle*[102]: According to this, multiple goals act simultaneously, and continue to influence behaviour even after the person is thinking about other things. This is similar to the better-known effect of sensory, cognitive, and emotional inputs of which we are unaware *priming* both perception and behaviour.

One example of sensory overflow is synaesthesia, p.559. The generalisation of classical conditioning produces associational overflow, p.440. People monitor their own body movements less than their facial expressions, so when they try to deceive, behavioural signs of deception are more likely to *leak* to the body than to the face[1763].

See also overflow of liquid faeces, p.341.

Over-generosity: see *sharing*, p.179.

Overgrowth: [1142] (a) large birth weight, or neonatal macrosomia, typically defined as weight over 4.5 kg. This is usually caused by maternal hyperglycaemia or obesity. Large babies increase the risk of birth trauma to baby and mother, and prenatal hyperglycaemia increases the risk of postnatal hypoglycaemia. Rare causes include Sotos, p.551; Beckwith-Wiedemann, p.429; and many other syndromes[1142]; (b) secondary overgrowth, e.g. in overeating, p.335; (c) focal overgrowth, i.e. one part of the body growing faster than others, is seen in Beckwith-Wiedemann, p.429; isolated hemihyperplasia, Proteus and CLOVE syndromes[1092]; and of the tongue and feet in acromegaly.

Oversociability: p.173.

Overvalued idea: This term is often used in adult psychiatry: "an acceptable, comprehensible idea pursued by the patient beyond the bounds of reason … The patient's whole life comes to resolve around this one idea … similar to a passionate political, religious, or ethical conviction." [1487]. Unlike obsessions (p.517), overvalued ideas are welcome. They are characteristic of anorexia nervosa and hypochondriasis. In children the terms preoccupation and dominating interest (p.229) are more common ☂. Closely related ideas include:

▶ inflexibility (p.234)

▶ overvalued beliefs/lessons. With mental age under about 5, some common lessons (e.g. to keep hands clean) can be followed too strictly: the remedy is to teach the more complicated lesson of *when* to clean hands. Other examples include excessive fears about noise-induced deafness (p.131) or the importance of tidiness.

Overweight: p.335.

Overwork: this means working more than one can endure. It is sometimes used to mean exceeding one's recuperative capacity – which is common in children, many of whom become increasingly tired as Friday approaches, and also during the course of each term. Individuals differ in their capacity for work, and repeated minor illness is one of the signs that this has been exceeded. Ask the child about a typical week, including Kumon, therapies, tutors, clubs, homework (p.481), chores and jobs, and ensure he has adequate sleep and some free time most days, particularly at weekends. Severe overwork is unusual[22] but important in a small minority. Parental overwork can also be problematic, mainly if it affects both parents.

Oxytocin: traditionally viewed as the hormone that stimulates milk let-down in lactation, this is now realised to have more general emotional and/or social functions. It is probably involved in attachment and in sexual behaviour, as well as in reduction of fear and aggression[250]. In normal adults, oxytocin increases the amount of time spent looking at people's eyes (and to a lesser extent their mouths)[628].

As expected, therefore, oxytocin ameliorates some of the social symptoms of ☂ autism. Surprisingly, initial data suggest it helps people who are socially inappropriate more than those who are socially disinterested[36]. In addition, alterations in the oxytocin receptor gene may be associated with just the social symptoms of autism[1738].

P-levels: a way of indicating the attainment level of people with learning disabilities (as opposed to the ability to learn, for which the best indicator is IQ, p.59). P-levels are used in UK schools to track the progress of children with ID, and in the definitions of degrees of *learning difficulty*, p.497. For example, the following is a brief overview of the mathematics P-levels:

P1   Child sometimes reacts or appears alert.
P2   Child is proactive and shows preferences.
P3   Child indicates choices by gestures.
P4   Child shows object permanence (p.517), and matches similar objects.
P5   Child can identify which is the bigger or smaller object.
P6   Child puts shapes in a shape-sorter, and obeys a request to put one object on or inside another.
P7   Child understands forward and backwards. Child uses words for shapes and physical concepts (heavy, more, enough).
P8   Child knows something about time and days of the week.

Pacing: p.114.
Pain: p.135.

Palate, high arched: the appearance of a dark narrow chasm behind the teeth (pictures available online). It is found in many named syndromes, most famously Marfan's, p.505, and Ehlers-Danlos, p.460; but it can also be a mild variant of cleft lip/palate, p.440.

Palilalia: p.62.

PANDAS (paediatric autoimmune neurological disorders associated with streptococcus):

PANDAS is a cause of episodic neurological problems including tics, hyperactivity, Sydenham's chorea; encephalitis lethargica (see below); and obsessionality[358,1575]. However, note that it is not always caused by streptococcus: vaccines and non-strep infections can sometimes trigger or re-start it (an anamnestic response). PANDAS occurs mainly in developing countries, where it is often accompanied by other signs of autoimmune disorder (rheumatic fever, i.e. arthritis, erythema marginatum, damage to heart valves).

Look for an episodic problem *physically distant from the site of infection*. Local irritation often contributes to tics, so non-local sequelae are needed to argue a systemic mechanism such as PANDAS. For example, throat-clearing without other behavioural symptoms cannot be reliably attributed to PANDAS.

Classical signs (not very common)
- choreo-athetoid movements (p.439)
- milkmaid's grip: while gripping your hand tightly, the strength fluctuates (as if milking a cow)
- myoclonic jerks (p.511)
- encephalitis lethargica[357]. This includes sleep disturbance, lethargy, parkinsonism, dyskinesias and neuropsychiatric symptoms. Although the 1918 epidemic coincided with an influenza pandemic, the flu did not directly cause the EL[357].

To confirm the association

- Repeated exacerbation by sore throats
- Repeated relief by antibiotic.

Immunology

ASOT and anti-DNAase B indicate distant or more recent infection, respectively (but they don't prove this is the cause). Anti-basal-ganglia antibodies, and in the acute phase anti-Group A β-haemolytic streptococcus IgM, all contribute to the diagnosis. Elevated anti-basal ganglia antibodies are found in over half of children referred to specialist clinics with washing, repeating, or counting rituals [359].

Panics: p.301.

Paradoxes: When we see something that seems incongruous or seems to contradict itself the cause is usually that our understanding of the child, or the diagnosis, or the medication, was wrong. Such paradoxes should not be glossed over as they are often the key to working out what is causing a behaviour.

See paradoxical disinhibition with benzodiazepines, p.430 (there are similar effects with antiepileptics); the paradox of unselfishness, p.167; paradox of good-enough parenting needing to be imperfect, p.190; paradoxical increase in speech following brain damage, p.556; perverse effects of training, p.528; paradoxical response to praise or punishment in autism, p.528; counterproductive effect of criticism (see *negative expressed emotion*, p.512).

Paradoxes of ADHD

The term *paradox* has been applied to ADHD in many senses, one of which is that these children *appear* to be faster but actually have slower response times [942]. More commonly the term refers to the complexities of stimulant effects, some of which are listed here.

- Stimulants should *stimulate*, i.e. increase behaviours, but instead at therapeutic doses they reduce activity level. This is because they make children focus more (of course, usually on stationary objects such as books), so they move around less.
- Even though there are many causes of hyperactivity, impuslvity, and inattention, stimulants help most of them (p.79).
- Low doses make children concentrate better, but high doses make them too still, or mindlessly repetitive, called the zombie effect (p.310). This is because the anti-hyperactive effects of ADHD have an inverted-U relationship with dose, as do the cognitive benefits, which peak earlier[476,1585].
- Methylphenidate can produce a moderate high, but probably only at high doses and in a minority of adults[1686]. The paradox is that these medicines, when given in children with a diagnosis of ADHD, probably *reduce* the long-term risk that children will become addicts[1762].
- For decades many have thought that stimulant-induced behavioural improvement was a characteristic of ADHD not shared with control children[e.g. 977]. This is probably wrong as a generalisation[1306,1307,1685] (but see[533]). (However, a relatively minor quantitative difference has not been excluded[1760] and even large differences cannot be excluded for small subgroups. These discrepancies are due to differences in MPH response caused by combinations of ☂ ADHD-related alleles[1541], which would be found in children both with and without a diagnosis of ADHD, rather than by ADHD.)

- In normal adults and presumably in adolescents, methylphenidate in therapeutic doses may increase *subjective* restlessness, apparently the reverse of its effect in children[1686] but this is a much smaller effect than the useful effects seen in children.

Paranoia: The *common* meaning is the feeling of being in danger, or thinking that everyone is against them, or everyone is looking at them. The term has had many other meanings in the past century (see references in[522]), including oversensitive, suspicious, mistrustful, and even schizophrenic. Like *psychotic*, it has also been used as a term indicating clinical severity – but about a third of the general public regularly have self-referential thoughts that are either odd or persecutory[523] (related statistics for children are on p.347).

The *psychiatric* meaning is "excessively self-referential", of which a mild example would be often thinking peers were talking about you. Of self-referential ideas only some are persecutory: a mild example would be the brief suspicion that a stranger crossed the road to avoid you, and a severe example would be delusional (p.348) certainty that Secret Service agents on every street corner are looking for you. Alternatively, self-referential ideas can be very pleasant, e.g. the delusion that you have won the lottery. Simple questioning can clarify whether self-referentiality is accompanied by feelings of persecution (see checklist in[608]). *Paranoid schizophrenia* is defined as schizophrenia (p.543) with auditory hallucinations or delusions (because most of both tend to be self-referential).

Special factors in children: (a) Most children are very egocentric (p.180) until well after school entry. Things interest them to the extent that they affect them, and they assume anyone they meet is interested in them. This is different from clinical paranoia in which events experienced as self-referential are interesting or puzzling or frightening. (b) Children are obviously smaller, and have less control over their surroundings, than grown-ups; for many children a feeling of being at risk is often appropriate. Some children have learned that they often misunderstand other people, or that other people tease them. Both of these views are common in children who have been bullied/teased (p.219). (c) Bizarre comments may result from cognitive errors such as concrete thinking about social intentions; failure to question magical ideas (p.502); or cognitive dissonance (p.355). One child responded to any questions from professionals with "you're going to trick me" which sounded paranoid but was actually an effective technique he had learned to avoid being tricked by peers.

Links: when we feel we are being looked at, this results mainly from visual or auditory clues, but many patients would concur with the few scientists who think we use other senses (e.g.[1468]). It is important not to overlook the possibility of drug abuse (especially cannabis, p.257), depression, p.313; schizophrenia ☂ or schizophrenic prodrome, p.543.

Paraneoplastic conditions: disorders caused by the remote effects of cancer[604,1098]. These are rare in children but important to detect. Eaton-Lambert syndrome, p.459; Stiff Person syndrome, p.555.

Parasomnia: p.200.
Parasuicide: p.317.
Parasympathetic Nervous System: see *autonomic nervous system*, p.428.

Parathyroid: small endocrine glands next to the thyroid gland in the neck. They produce parathyroid hormone (parathormone), which elevates blood calcium, p.435 and lowers phosphate. *Primary* hyperparathyroidism is rare in children and usually caused by an easily treatable parathyroid adenoma[555]. It causes hypercalcaemia, p.483, and primary hypofunction causes hypocalcaemia, p.485. *Secondary* parathyroid disorders are attempts by the gland to compensate for other disorders, so results on blood testing can be the opposite of these.

See also velocardiofacial syndrome, p.572.

Parents: see family, p.465; mothers, p.509; fathers, p.465; parents who have other difficulties, p.191.

Common patterns of family dynamics, p.211; necessary aspects of parenting, p.189; good-enough parenting, p.190; parents' ideas about what is wrong, p.13; acceptability of explanations to parents, p.19; explaining complex formulations to parents, p.19; parental alienation, p.187.

Child arguing with parents, p.162; parents sensitised to a particular behaviour, p.205; parent wary of child, p.107; parents complaining about normal behaviour, p.205; behaviour better with dad than with mum, p.201; parents' role in school non-attendance, p.217.

Attachment, p.195; difficulty separating, p.197; sharing a bed with parents, p.198; abuse, p.271ff.

Parkinsonism: this is the triad of rigidity, tremor, and reduced movements (for slow or reduced movements see p.95; for other causes of tremor see p.61). The tremor is characteristically 4–6 Hz in the hands (called *pill-rolling*). The combination of rigidity and tremor is often detectable as cogwheel rigidity at the elbow. The *festinant gait* has short rapid steps without arm-swing, sometimes while leaning forward. The face is mask-like. It is often accompanied by depression. Anosmia or hyposmia is usually present[1071], which can help to establish the diagnosis.

The only common cause in young people is side-effects of medication, including antipsychotics, p.422; SSRIs, p.552; tetrabenazine, pethidine, sedatives, anti-emetics, calcium channel blockers, and isoniazid. Other causes of basal ganglia damage that can cause parkinsonism include infection or autoimmunity (see encephalitis lethargica, p.522), heavy metals, carbon monoxide, stroke, p.556; and many rare genetic syndromes (e.g. juvenile parkinsonism, with a diurnal or perimenstrual fluctuation[1806]). See also *dystonia*, p.458; *basal ganglia*, p.429.

Paroxysm: sudden unpredictable symptoms, usually severe.

Passive-Aggressive: this is a common term for people who avoid confrontation (especially to authority, by speaking cryptically, sulking or being sullen, being late, or agreeing to do work they know they won't have time for). One difficulty with the *idea* is that it is sometimes perfectly sensible to avoid an argument, or to avoid unnecessary work. A problem with the *term* is that it implies aggression is the cause, even though that is obviously not always the case (i.e. it is an *ideograph*, p.487). The place of Passive Aggressive Personality Disorder in DSM is only provisional, partly because most of the symptoms are also attributable to other PDs or to other individual characteristics such as oppositionality (p.253), argumentativeness (p.162) and/or a belief that life is unfair[1380].

Passivity: p.95.

Pathognomonic signs: these are single signs that establish a diagnosis. Because children experiment with every behaviour they can imagine, highly repeated behaviours are more likely to be pathognomonic. Among the most reliable are hard neurological signs, p.58; specific *behavioural phenotypes*, p.430; frozen watchfulness, p.470; dilated or pinpoint pupil, p.258; and immature behaviours that should have already disappeared, p.56.

Pat phrase: p.158.
Pathological Demand Avoidance: see *Pervasive Refusal*, p.527.
PD: personality disorder, p.241.
PDA: Pathological Demand Avoidance (above).
PDD: Pervasive Developmental Disorder. This is the DSM term for autism-related conditions, p.183. See also *pervasive*, p.527.
PDD-NOS: Pervasive Developmental Disorder, not otherwise specified. See pp.426, 183.
Pedantry: p.163.
Peer relationships: p.171.
PEG: percutaneous endoscopic gastrostomy. See tube feeding, p.333.

Peroxisomal disorders: peroxisomes are organelles found in most cells. They contain enzymes for metabolism of very long chain fatty acids, and for detoxification. Disorders of peroxisomes include Refsum's disease, p.499; adrenoleukodystrophy, p.498 and several β-oxidation disorders. There is also a separate group of disordered perixisome production, which causes severe multiorgan disease in infancy. Several of the peroxisomal disorders primarily affect white matter, i.e. are leukodystrophies, p.498. Tests for these include[1659]: MRI; VLCFA, phytanic acid; and plasmalogens for adrenoleukodystrophy, Zellweger syndrome, single enzyme peroxisomal defects.

Perpetuating factors: aspects of the child or the world that make a problem persist once it has started. They are generally not able to start the problem on their own. Perpetuating and protective factors are often more amenable to treatment than predisposing or precipitating factors.
    i) Pleasant and unpleasant effects from the environment (including from people) become learned, and so affect behaviour. This is sometimes called *feedback*, though the more precise term is *reinforcement*, and can be used to calibrate a child's behaviour to his environment. For example, most children will learn to regulate their noisiness and activity to different environments. Negative feedback from teachers can add to positive reinforcement from antisocial peers, to perpetuate disengagement and further naughtiness (see "conduct disorder", p.249). For a more complex example see figure on p.355.
    ii) *Amplifying feedback loops* produce effects that grow. These can be useful or harmful (called vicious cycles). Examples include achieving recognition in a peer group (whether antisocial, school marks, etc.) in which one has to repeatedly try to outdo past performances and peers (e.g. in *gangs*, p.472); children who become increasingly excited by the continuing response of others to their excitement (p.520); the effect of social status on mood (p.172); self-fulfilling prophecies in general (e.g. p.323); and the itch-scratch cycle (p.110).
    iii) Perpetuation by triggering a new process. Examples include transient eye problems precipitating a long-lasting blink tic

(p.108); habitual throat-clearing precipitated by an infection; and some autoimmune responses (p.522).

Persecuted: see *paranoid*.

Perseveration: an effect of short-term memories influencing behaviour after the memories are no longer relevant. The term excludes long-term memory or interests. For distinction from *stereotypy*, see p.554.

An influential system of classification[1425] is:

- o Continuous perseveration = abnormal continuation of a current behaviour (e.g. perseverative automatism, p.427)
- o Stuck-in-set perseveration: continuous and inappropriate maintenance of the current framework in which one is working (i.e. the set)
- o Recurrent perseveration: when a stimulus recurs, all or part of the previous response (or stimulus) intrudes again, even though attention was apparently shifted to something new.

Other classification systems include sensory perseveration; emotional perseveration[1519]; high-level perseveration (area of interest) v low level (sounds); and object perseveration: see *Klüver-Bucy*, p.496. For various theories of perseveration, and ways of classifying them, see[1425].

Persona: p.237.

Personal space (or interpersonal space): the volume around a person within which movements of strangers are uncomfortable. This forms the basis of multiple defensive behaviours[607]. Avoidant people keep a larger interpersonal space[803], as do people who are listening through headphones[970].

Personality and *Personality Disorder*: p.241.

Personality clash: this should mean what it says: a fundamental incompatibility between two people's personalities. That is rare, and the term is usually used in an intentionally vague way, to mean friction between two specific people, i.e. "these people don't get on and there's no point in discussing why that is." However in practice it is often useful to find a reason, and many are listed for *pair friction*, p.172; *hatred*, p.187; and *bullying*, p.219.

Bullying is often wrongly described as a personality clash; it can appear to affect only the single known victim just because everyone else has put up with it. Personality clashes can appear in any relationship; bullying requires a hierarchical one (p.219).

Pervasive: term applied to behaviours or disorders, meaning that they permeate all aspects of a child's life, i.e. they cannot be circumvented simply by avoiding problematic situations. For the contrast between the pervasiveness of autism, and the non-pervasiveness of selective mutism, see p.156. Pervasiveness is also characteristic of severe emotional states, e.g. exercising pervasively, p.65; pervasive mutism, p.151; histrionics, p.479. The degree of pervasiveness is a key part of the assessment of poor communication, p.166; feeding problems, p.331; and hallucinations, p.343. Emotional abuse is also usually pervasive, p.277. See also Pervasive Refusal syndrome, below.

Pervasive Refusal syndrome: refusal of several of: food, school, mobilisation, speech, and self-care; when very severe it is sometimes called "total refusal syndrome". Like chronic fatigue (p.323) it typically starts with a clear organic illness, followed by a downward spiral of reducing activity, and can last a year or more. Unlike chronic fatigue, the person strongly, physically, and sometimes angrily, resists activities associated with recovery, such as being taken in a wheelchair to a school on the ward. The reason for this may be that rehabilitation, in common with premorbid pressures to high achievement, is experienced as coercive[913]. During physical examination, one boy tensed his quadriceps to prevent a sore knee being flexed – and then after the thigh was raised on a pillow kept the leg rigidly off the bed for five exhausting yet mute minutes. Consider sexual or physical abuse (pp.273–275), severe cognitive dissonance, p.355; depression, p.309; physical causes (pp.321, 87, 527); catatonia, p.98; and other *non-behaviours*, p.515. This diagnostic category, and the related Pathological Demand Avoidance, have not caught on widely[547], because the children are usually treated using more common diagnoses (see *rigidity*, p.233). Other related behaviours are discussed in[913] and[1147].

Perverse (or paradoxical) effects of training: this means training that changes behaviour but in an unwanted way. (This is not the same as *deviant behaviour*, p.49, or training that doesn't change behaviour.)

Of rewards: as in politics, performance targets will lead the children to find any way of meeting the target, even if their way is useless and not what the parent had in mind. If children are rewarded every time they produce something in the toilet, they will produce smaller amounts more frequently. In hyperactive children, use of rewards alone can reduce performance, if the children become overexcited[501], p.520. Praise can be shocking and unpleasant for some autistic children, especially if it involves physical contact, close approach, eye-to-eye contact and speech being louder than usual.

Of punishments: most children deprived of a trip to the park (e.g. as a punishment for being rowdy) will just become more rowdy. Children being pushed to do homework they find difficult become increasingly upset, sometimes preventing the calm thought needed to find the answer. If a child doesn't want to be in the car or shop, a noisy tantrum may get him out (thereby reinforcing the bad behaviour) and eventually may prevent mum from taking him in the car ever, or shopping when she doesn't have a babysitter, neither of which results is in the child's long-term interests. An exaggerated version of this scenario is seen in some children with autism who prefer time away from other people, so time-out even in a boring place will become a target to be worked for, by misbehaving. A few children with autism or profound ID even enjoy being threatened or snarled at by parents. See also punishments that increase the original incentive for misbehaviour, p.250; misbehaviour to avoid punishment, pp.256, 341; punishment causing violence, p.291; relation to fire-setting, p.466; other adverse aspects of punishments, p.538.

Of boundaries: if boundaries are too strict (i.e. prohibitions), and other motivators (such as role models and family warmth) are insufficient, children may rebel, and fail to learn skills of self-regulation, persuasion and compromise. For example, if totally prohibited from drinking alcohol, a teen will not learn how to drink socially (which is, of course, desirable in some cultures).

Perverse (or paradoxical) effects of defence mechanisms and coping strategies: avoiding situations that provoke anxiety can prevent a child learning how to cope with them. Avoiding school can cause much greater problems in the long run.

PET scans: p.374.

PFC: Prefrontal cortex, see p.513.

Phaeochromocytoma: rare tumours, half of which are genetically determined. The most common presentations in children are sustained anxiety and hypertension[177]. Also characteristic are episodes with sudden onset, then tailing off over seconds to hours, classically with the triad of headaches (p.139), pallor/sweating (p.558) and hypertension. Palpitation, tremor, weight loss and nausea are common, but symptoms depend on the specific combination of catecholamines being produced by the tumour[667]. Vision can become blurry, snowy, or have black spots or pulsatile scotomata during episodes[1602].

Phenomenology: the usual scientific sense is of studies that relate empirical observations to each other rather than to underlying theories. In psychology, the term refers to the careful analysis of subjective experiences.

Phenylketonuria (PKU): the first successfully treated genetic cause of severe ID (p.32). It is managed in most of the world by a heel-prick test at birth, followed when detected by a low phenylalanine diet and other measures. Unresolved issues include mothers with PKU who don't keep their strict diet during pregnancy (including mothers with unrecognised PKU who are about 1/10 000 in some studies); detection in immigrants (p.488, and the unknown effectiveness of such delayed treatment); relaxation of diet in childhood, p.482; and "mild PKU" which is often not treated but which apparently causes IQ 10 points lower than controls[646]. Consider this especially in fair-haired children with blue eyes, in dark-haired families.

Photophobia: fear of light. It can result from photalgia (eye pain caused by light), headache, painful tear production, conditioned fear of skin photosensitivity, or aversion to arousal. It is crucial to consider eye disease as some cases need emergency management !!. Ophthalmological causes include corneal inflammation, cataract, p.436; glaucoma, p.474; exotropia, ocular albinism, and retinal degenerative disease[1517]. Photophobia is also seen in chronic fatigue, p.323; migraine, p.128; dilated pupils; *scotopic sensitivity* or Meares-Irlen syndrome, p.52; central dazzle, p.66.

Children with autism have increased rates of photophobia. Some shield their eyes in unusual ways, e.g. using a curtain of thick hair and sitting away from windows (see migraine in ID, p.142). Some dislike artificial lights, especially flickering fluorescent lights. They are prone to restrictive eating which in severe cases depletes vitamin A (p.328) sufficiently to cause photophobia and severe optic atrophy[1031].

Photosensitivity: adversely affected by light (see also *photophobia*, p.529).

(a) Photosensitive epileptic discharges can be trivial, or can interfere briefly with brain function, or can trigger grand mal fits; there are diverse molecular causes[1143]. Visually evoked epilepsy is not a distinct form of epilepsy; rather, visual stimuli are one way of provoking epileptiform discharges (p.73). They are in fact the most common external triggers for seizures, and depend on the wavelength, the intensity, and the size of the stimulus[1221]. Televisions, disco lights, and flickering sunlight are the commonest causes of this effect.

(b) Photosensitive skin rashes. The most common in children is the polymorphous light eruption occurring at the start of the sunny season, often with raised 2–5 mm spots. Other causes include[747] drug-sensitivity (e.g. ibuprofen, chlorpromazine); pellagra, p.329; and lupus, p.560. Genetic causes include albinism; porphyria, p.532; Hartnup disease, p.477; phenylketonuria, p.529; and xeroderma pigmentosum, p.454.

Piaget: Psychologist who described the typical stages of a child's cognitive development:

Name of stage	age	description
Sensorimotor	0–2	interacting with the environment
Pre-operational	2–7	starting to use symbols
Concrete operations	7–12	using rules such as conservation of volume when pouring.
Formal operations	12–adult	abstract thought.

Piaget based these on observation of his own relatives, and less able children obviously progress more slowly (see graphs in[1465]). The *formal operations* stage is probably reached by only a minority of adults. Some of the criticisms of Piagettian staging are that children only gradually learn to use the more advanced thinking for more and more subject areas, and they can move backward temporarily if they are anxious, tired, or ill.

Pica: p.336.
Pink, love of: p.247.

Pituitary gland: an endocrine gland at the base of the brain, beneath and controlled by the hypothalamus (p.485).

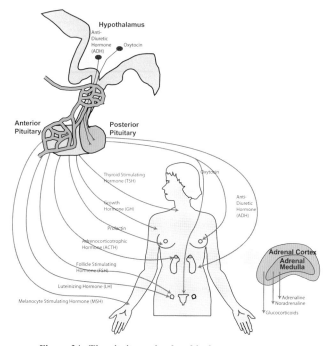

Figure 34. The pituitary gland and its hormones.

PKU: phenylketonuria, p.529.

Placenta: histological, biochemical and pathological examination of the child's placenta, or the placenta from a subsequent pregnancy, can shed light on a child's developmental problems, e.g. revealing some treatable inborn errors of metabolism. Ultrasound examination provides related information, but in far less detail.

Placental insufficiency has many causes, including pre-eclampsia, p.535; cocaine abuse, and antiphospholipid syndrome. Depending on timing and severity, it can cause general growth retardation or fairly specific delay in gastrointestinal maturation[1619].

Play: p.221.
PNET: primitive neuroectodermal tumour, rare and mainly below age 10.
Pointing: p.170.
Poisoning: see *toxic substances*, p.566.

Polycystic ovaries: amultifactorial endocrine disorder affecting about 7% of women[1170], which increases testosterone levels (p.554), causing numerous effects including acne, increased hair growth, irregular periods, often obesity, and possibly a reduction in verbal fluency[1434]. Depression is a common complication in adolescence. PCO is more common in women with epilepsy, and is also increased by valproate (p.572).

Polydipsia: drinking too much, p.338.

POMC: pro-opiomelanocortin, the precursor molecule of ACTH, melanocyte stimulating hormone, endorphins and lipotropins. See *hair*, p.475; intake-regulating hormones, p.491.

Porphyrias: a family of rare inherited metabolic disorders, of which some cause neuropsychiatric symptoms[336]. Symptoms can include neuropathy, acute confusion, psychosis, anxiety, hypomania, autonomic instability (p.428), abdominal pain and severe rashes. Symptoms are chronic or episodic (especially premenstrual), and can be precipitated by starvation, infection, alcohol, or by porphyrinogenic medications such as erythromycin, steroids, anti-epileptics and benzodiazepines (a detailed list is in the *British National Formulary*). Urine is characteristically purple; but it is possible to have mild porphyria without the colour being obviously abnormal. Test for urine porphobilinogen during an attack. Negative blood porphyrin/porphobilinogen results are unreliable, and positive results may be chance associations rather than causal[336,732].

Post-concussive syndrome: see *head injury*, p.477.

Post-ictal: after a seizure. See post-ictal tests, p.74; post-ictal confusion, p.75; post-ictal coma, p.97; post-ictal psychosis, below; sleep following breath-holding spells, p.434.

Post-ictal psychosis: psychosis following a seizure or cluster of seizures[1672], usually occurring after a lucid interval of up to 72 hours and lasting days to weeks[1622]. See also interictal psychosis, p.449; and other causes of *cycloid psychosis*, p.449.

Post-traumatic feeding disorder: see choking phobia, p.333.

Post-traumatic Stress Disorder (PTSD): For DSM criteria, see p.389. Intrusive thoughts, images and dreams follow the same time course, appearing within a few weeks after trauma (occasionally appearing months or even years after the trauma[1010]) and gradually fading over a year or more[1132]. A handicapping unfocused anxiety persists in the absence of any stimulus. All symptoms are strongly related to the degree of exposure[1132]. Related cognitions and dysfunctional strategies are often found[448]. PTSD is unlikely in infancy, although there may be secondary effects of the carers' response to trauma (p.567).

Diagnoses of PTSD are unconvincing unless people talk about or draw or enact intrusive experiences; or there is a clear onset of anxious avoidance (p.429) of stimuli closely related to the trauma – but not of other stimuli (so this diagnosis can be difficult in ID[1067]).

Fundamental questions about this diagnosis remain uncertain, including whether it is distinct from other diagnoses, whether it is reasonable to include the causation in the definition, and diagnostic thresholds[e.g. 1742]. Some traumas cause many problems as well as, or instead of, PTSD (e.g. rape[1674]). Some traumas cause generalised anxiety (p.297); others cause simple phobias (p.307), i.e. with avoidance but without the other symptoms of PTSD[1010].

For pseudo-PTSD, see[859]. See also *trauma*, p.567; *intrusions*, p.493; classical conditioning, p.440. For help with diagnostic difficulties, see[758]. For the relationship to conditioned arousal, see p.127.

Posturing: p.93.

Pouting (of lips): see baby talk, p.43; and if combined with a frown, sulking, p.557. See also frontal signs such as snout reflex and visual rooting, p.469; masturbation, p.115.

Poverty: absolute poverty is defined internationally as access to less than about a dollar a day (for other definitions see[203]). There are more poor people in middle-income countries than in poor countries[25]. Poverty affects children mainly through malnutrition (p.504), exposure to infections (p.490), and inadequate schooling. There is a much increased rate of ID in poor countries[142], though overall population intelligence is probably similar (see discussion of IQ tests, p.59). Physical illness has a far greater social and educational impact on the poor than on the rich[1388].

Relative poverty is a concept applied to developed countries, and to the developed (usually urban) areas of poorer countries. It is defined in various ways such as having less than half the average income, or not having access to specific goods (e.g. a telephone or an indoor toilet). Relative poverty reduces lifespan, and increases many health risks[1768]. It increases the risk of conduct problems, but not the risk of anxiety or depression in children[322]. Many mediating factors have been suggested, in the parents and their parenting[1590], in the children, and in the environment[802]. These include parents' IQ, education, and mental health; social support, children's temperament, exposure to crime, status, sense of control, social exclusion, and the amount of adult time available for supervision. *Inequality* per se seems to be at most a minor factor[983].

Absolute and relative poverty are sometimes called *old* and *new* poverty. See also poverty as an effect of prison, p.535; of parental drug abuse, p.257; as a risk factor for physical abuse, p.273; assessment in home visit, p.365; clothing, p.441.

Prader-Willi syndrome: children are dysmorphic, and grossly overweight by age 2. Individuals differ in severity and precise symptoms depending on the precise location and size of the deletion (Type 2 is milder and has a smaller deletion than Type 1; mUPD type has no deletion but more social impairment[1084]). Multiple hypothalamic functions become dysregulated. Usually underactive, with daytime sleepiness[248] and mild to moderate ID (with relative strengths in LTM and jigsaw puzzles). From middle childhood most have points on their skin of severe skin-picking (p.549) or plucking continuing despite bleeding, as well as severe nose picking, palate picking and rectal digging[1436,1761], possibly caused by a reduced sensitivity to pain[1280] necessitating intense local damage merely to scratch an itch.

From adolescence, the mUPD subtype has a high risk of psychotic bipolar disorder[1514,1671] which is atypical in the extent of confusion and its resolution within days; so better called *cycloid psychosis* (p.449). The deletion subtype has increased risk of non-psychotic depression.

Age at assessment	Features sufficient to prompt DNA testing for PWS (after [633])
Birth to 2 years	1. Profound hypotonia with poor suck necessitating tube feeding (this sign may not be present in partial forms of PWS[383])
2–6 years	1. Hypotonia with history as above 2. Global developmental delay
6–12 years	1. History of hypotonia as above 2. Global developmental delay 3. Excessive eating (hyperphagia; preoccupation with food) with central obesity if uncontrolled
13 years through adulthood	1. Cognitive impairment; usually mild mental retardation 2. Excessive eating (hyperphagia; preoccupation with food) with central obesity if uncontrolled 3. Hypothalamic hypogonadism and/or typical behaviour problems (including temper tantrums and obsessive-compulsive features).

Pragmatics: p.144.

Precipitating factors: factors that trigger a problem (compare *perpetuating factors*).

A special type of precipitant works via *escalation*. If this feeds back to increase the problems (i.e. if this forms a vicious cycle) it is very likely to become a major problem soon. Escalation can be physiological (bedrest in chronic fatigue reduces strength); emotional (e.g. overbreathing in panic is interpreted as a sign of further danger); focusing on or ignoring problems; misattribution (p.426); catastrophising; social reinforcement or social contagion; health carer responses; or cultural norms[850].

Predictable irrationality: also called cognitive biases or meta-heuristics or cognitive illusions[852]:

- If a child expects a food to taste bad (or good), it is much more likely to do so[Chapter 9 of 57].
- Arbitrary coherence, i.e. comparing an object with recent *anchor objects*, even if they are irrelevant, or relative to a similar object even when dissimilar objects could be more relevant to the task[Chapter 2 of 57].
- Children who have worked hard to achieve something will value it more[Chapter 7 of 57].
- People will work to avoid losing options, even when they know those options are useless[Chapter 8 of 57].
- Motivational orientation: even if children are doing something because they enjoy it, rewarding the behaviour can alter their motivation, so they no longer do it if rewards are not available[1713].
- Being overimpressed by inadequate cases – and by heresy; liking extraordinary or positive findings.
- Looking for confirmatory evidence rather than disproof (see *bubble bursting*, p.435).
- Motivated or wishful thinking (with secondary gain, p.471); e.g. for simplicity, immediate gratification, consolation, moral meaning[1472].
- A need for control and simplicity.
- A reluctance to change views (which increases with IQ because of ability to defend position).
- Overutilising cognitive heuristics[801]. For examples in diagnosis, see p.18.
- Mistaking unexplained for inexplicable, indisproveable for true, and association for causation (p.553).

- Failing to weight adequately all the other ideas that would have to be overturned for a new one to be true.
- Deductive errors such as circular reasoning and inappropriate *reductio ad absurdam*[569].
- inconsistency of behaviour, e.g. pp.77-79.
- *memory distortions*, p.40.

Pre-eclampsia: this is the most common serious complication of pregnancy. It consists of severe maternal hypertension, proteinuria, and visual symptoms which if untreated progress to maternal seizures (when it is called eclampsia). Emergency delivery is often necessary. Many mothers recall that they were diagnosed with pre-eclampsia, when actually they had full eclampsia. Following either pre-eclampsia or eclampsia, long-term effects are mainly due to low birth weight (p.432) and prematurity (p.432)[1801].

Prefrontal cortex: p.513.
Prematurity: p.432.
Premenstrual symptoms: p.506.
Pre-pulse inhibition: p.462.

Pressure of speech: an increase in the amount of spontaneous speech, which is also difficult to interrupt. The speaker is usually loud, emphatic and insistent socially, though he may also talk when no one is listening. Some sentences are interrupted in the rush to get on to the next idea. The rate is over 150 words per minute, though medicines can reduce the speed while leaving the other aspects unchanged[43].

Prison: there are many difficulties for children with parents in prison, including the separation; the disorganisation of their lives; the impact on the free parent who is now coping alone; unpleasant visits to prison; poverty; the trauma of the arrest and any crimes they witnessed; the many underlying difficulties that led to arrest in the first place; genetic effects; and the parent as a role model[1126]. Problems are usually greatest when it is the mother who is in prison[360].

For some children, parental imprisonment provides respite from abuse and domestic violence. Such children are often preoccupied by thoughts of what will happen after dad is discharged (or escapes): will he attack mum, or will he kidnap the child he was closest to? In these cases the approaching release date brings increasing anxiety.

Note that in American usage, *prison* is for substantial sentences, whereas *jail* is for brief sentences or pre-trial detention.

Procrastination: delaying doing something. Causes include disliking the task; other interests or distractions (e.g. drug misuse), lack of energy (pp.323, 322, 309), poor confidence that they will succeed, perfectionism, depression, impulsivity (p.79); attention from parents during the procrastination; lack of immediate reward for task completion; poor judgment of the passage of time; failure to allocate priorities appropriately. It has been suggested that even saccades, which take a fraction of a second, may include a "process of procrastination" that allows slowly-acting higher centres the chance to influence rapid reflexes[1319].

Projective identification (p.i.): there are many different definitions of this. The essence is that emotions observed in one person actually were initiated in another person – and that the transfer was not explicit. More specifically, people make prophecies about themselves, which become self-fulfilling because of the signals (verbal and non-verbal) they send to other people. The following table shows some types of p.i.[798]

Level	Name	Description
Minimal p.i (some would say not p.i.)	Projection (of an aspect of myself)	experiencing a person's actions as though they were due to my assumption, even though I have no interaction with them. The term p.i. could not be used for projection of something that wasn't part of myself, e.g. a standard stereotype.
Incomplete p.i.	Projection (of an aspect of myself) *onto*	acting toward a person based on my assumption
Full p.i.	Projection (of an aspect of myself) *into*	acting in such a way that the person changes his behaviour in accord with my assumption (the result depends on how the recipient changes). If he does not change at all, full p.i. didn't happen.

Projective identification is thought to be an essential part of the mother-child relationship, in at least two main ways[957]. First, a mother can want her baby to feel her love, so she tries to express her love in ways he can recognise (she knows she has succeeded when he makes similar expressions). Second, a child when terrified may want his mother to feel this, so that she will do something about it: a good mother interrupts this by calming him and demonstrating a mature assessment of the situation. Parents can "project" their own views of individual children *onto* those children, some of whom will conform, and this can have helpful or damaging effects.

The term *p.i.* is most used by psychoanalysts, denoting specific underlying mechanisms of object relations (p.517); but in practice it is often impossible to know whether such mechanisms have acted[439] (examples in[583]; see also[1407,1548]). It is usually more rigorous to use simpler alternative descriptions for the behaviours described as examples of p.i. For example, re-enactment of familiar roles can often produce the same observable behaviours as p.i. Similar confusion can arise from oppositionality (p.253) or expressed emotion (p.512)[1072]. Mirror neurons (p.507) may form part of the mechanism of some apparent p.i.[1057] (see also *self-identity*, p.237).

Prolactin: hormone that promotes milk production. It is physiological in lactating mothers, but when it occurs in other people is abnormal (called galactorrhoea). Raised levels can suppress sexual interest in both sexes[864], and the menstrual cycle in women.

Prolactin is often increased by some antipsychotics, up to five times the upper limit of normal[296]. However the level can return nearly to normal within a year of continued treatment[779]. Risperidone causes dose-dependent menstrual irregularity in a third of women, and galactorrhoea in a small proportion[779]. Levels over five times the upper limit of normal, or persistence of symptoms after stopping antipsychotics may indicate prolactinoma and generally need investigation[296].

Prolactin levels are somewhat higher in black people than in whites. Elevation after seizures (p.73) can be helpful in distinguishing them from pseudoseizures.

Prosody: p.148.
Pseudo-acquisition of a skill: p.44.
Pseudo-behaviours: p.363.
Pseudo-experiences: p.364.
Pseudo-sociability: p.167.

Pseudobulbar palsy: labile affect (sometimes called pseudobulbar affect, p.70) combined with dysarthria and *dysphagia*. This indicates damage to upper motor neurons that project to brainstem nuclei controlling speech and eating. See p.70.

Pseudologia fantastica: p.256.
Pseudoscience: a body of knowledge that is internally consistent but does not make risky disproveable predictions about the world outside the theory. The most commonly cited example is Freud's interpretations of psychopathology[1552]. DSM-style psychiatric disorders (p.385) have similar difficulty in that they are essentially a categorisation system, yet the large number of studies papers on each category are often taken as proof that each category has a distinct physical existence[1426].

Pseudoscience also refers broadly to poor scientific thinking. For example, many writers on specific conditions (including website authors, parents and professionals) assume that *associated* symptoms are actually part of a condition (e.g. oppositionality being thought to be part of ADHD), or are as permanent as the rest of the condition, so mistakenly do not seek help for them. NICE guidelines claim that the best-evidenced treatment for depression is CBT, but social interventions such as stopping child abuse and bullying are so obviously effective that randomised trials would be unethical.

Psychomotor retardation: this has a paediatric sense (developmental delay or ID, especially in infancy) and a psychiatric sense (the reduction in number and speed of movements and utterances, often seen in depression). Both senses cause confusion and are best avoided. For the psychiatric sense, the term "psychomotor slowing" is less likely to cause upset or confusion (p.95).

Psychopathy: p.280.

Psychosis: loss of contact with reality. Insight (p.491) can be present, absent or partial; but the unreality is usually only partial. Symptoms include hallucinations, p.343; delusions, p.347; thought disorder, p.563; catatonia, p.98. Paranoid psychosis usually refers to paranoid ideas (p.524) that have reached delusional strength (discussed on p.348). *Primary* psychosis usually refers to schizophrenia. *Functional* psychosis is a broader term meaning psychosis resulting from a mental illness (e.g. schizophrenia, p.543; depression, p.309; mania, p.261). Like *paranoid*, the word *psychotic* is sometimes used very loosely[1502], e.g. to refer to imaginative ideas, impairing ideas, or dangerous ideas. Historically the term *child psychosis* included both autism and childhood onset schizophrenia (COS) [1398]. See also causes, pp.343–347; investigations, p.349; antipsychotics, p.422; interictal and cycloid psychosis, p.449.

‼ Acute psychosis needs urgent management due to (a) the fact that treatment reduces relapse and functional decline; (b) the possibility of finding a treatable progressive biological cause; (c) social risks.

DSM's "Brief Psychotic Disorder" lasts from 24 hours to one month, usually precipitated by a major social stressor in a predisposed individual. DSM's "Acute Stress Disorder" has similar causes but refers to dramatically odd behaviour and ideas lasting a few days after trauma, when this seems more dissociative (p.453) than psychotic.

Conundrum 16: Autism or psychosis

This is not really a forced choice, as other explanations need to be considered as well (pp.345, 347), and occasional children have both conditions. The proportion of children with autism-related disorders who develop psychosis is much higher than expected for the general population. There is some genetic overlap between autism and schizophrenia[234], and cognitively autism has some similarity with the negative symptoms of schizophrenia[327].

Talking to oneself can appear in either condition, but in autism it is usually echolalia or the repetition of stereotyped phrases in a fixed tone of voice. In contrast, an otherwise normal child's response to hallucinated voices contains a normal degree of emotion and variability.

Laughing out of the blue (p.111) is quite common in both conditions. An autistic child would be less likely to make eye contact or other non-verbal communication during this.

There are quite separate age peaks, with autism almost always apparent before age 4, and COS exceedingly rare below age 7 (see figure in[1398]). Unlike autism, characteristic features of COS include delusions, hallucinations, incongruous affect, perplexity and loosening of associations[869]. COS is much rarer than autism, and seems to occur mainly in children with language delay and other symptoms of autism – but there is occasionally difficulty distinguishing between them[424,1305,1536].

Unusual cases can sometimes be clarified by other features, such as whether other family members were affected. Another aid is that, compared with COS, autism is much more commonly associated with ID. Autism tends to be stable above age 5 (improving gradually over many years[521]), whereas functional psychosis tends to get worse (worsening over weeks to months). General distrust of others should make one consider child abuse (p.271) or other trauma (p.567), or paranoia (p.524); all of these are more likely if another family member is affected. When high or low mood causes delusions or hallucinations, the content is mood-congruent.

PTSD: see *post-traumatic stress disorder*, p.532.
Puberphonia: p.147.
Puberty: p.411.

Punishment: this is either something the child doesn't like, or (more usefully) something that reduces inappropriate behaviours (contrast *reinforcement*, p.540).

Rewards are usually more useful than punishments because they keep a child engaged in a task. However, if a child is fully engaged in a task, the combination of appropriate rewards and punishments is more effective in encouraging his learning than using just rewards or just punishments[206].

The most common cause of punishments not working is that they are delivered erratically, are not actually punishments, or are outweighed by a reward delivered at the same time (e.g. mum's voice and attention). This doesn't usually necessitate bigger or different punishments (or rewards) – just that they become more reliable, more immediate or closer together.

Time-out (sometimes called *time-out from positive reinforcement* to suggest that it is not a punishment) is for most children a definite punishment, which is non-violent and effective for modifying behaviour[477,1354]. Many children enjoy time-outs that take place in their bedroom with TV and computer, so these will not reduce problem behaviours. Probably more important than the details of the time-out location, is that the child should enjoy it less than where he was before[1511].

Physical (corporal) punishment is widely deprecated yet widely used[911]. It has good immediate effect, but can damage the parent-child relationship, especially if used severely. It carries a risk of escalation. It is associated with many adverse long-term outcomes but whether this effect is causative is not yet clear[456].

See also excessive punishments, pp.209, 210; punishment as aspect of abuse, p.273; self-punishment, pp.117, 317; perverse effects of punishments, p.528.

Pyromania: a misleading term; see *Fire*, p.466.
Querulousness: p.162.
Quibbling: p.162.
Rabbits, love of: p.246.

Race: There are many ways of grouping people (p.251) or oneself (see self-identity, p.237), or singling out others (see bullying, p.220), but race may have a special capacity to inflame – visible, unchangeable, familial, historical, political; cultural (p.448). For a detailed discussion of the impact of race on psychiatry see[162].

Ramadan: p.465.
Rage: p.71.

Rasmussen's encephalitis/syndrome: progressive neurological decline with multiple seizure types and cerebral hemi-atrophy. One symptom is epilepsia partialis continua (p.461).

Rating scales: see *Checklist diagnosis*, p.24.
RBMT: Rivermead Behavioural Memory Test, p.38.
Reaction formation: p.305.
Reading: p.51.

Recklessness: taking inadequate care of safety. In general useage *reckless* means the same as *impulsive*: performing actions without adequately considering the benefits of waiting.

A commonplace example is a child (or adult) being careless when crossing the road. A more extreme example, both because it is more dangerous and because it was thought about for longer, is climbing on to a table to perform the first back-flip of one's life.

Evaluations of risk by children
A child's awareness of risk is indicated by flinching, p.107; frozen watchfulness, p.470; staying at a distance; and signs of anxiety (p.296). Children overestimate risk when they are anxious; and in

OCD, p.65; and in paranoia, p.524. Conversely, many children underestimate risk. The most common cause is ID; for example it is quite common for children with ID to underestimate the risk of climbing out of windows. People with amygdala damage do not feel sufficient fear in some situations (see *Klüver-Bucy*, p.496); nor do some psychopaths, p.280; nor those with congenital analgesia, p.136.

Response of children to risks they recognise
There are many reasons for one child to be more reckless than another (p.79).

There are also many factors other than the child that contribute to accidents: see causes of accidents, p.417. See also *risk*, p.542.

Reconsolidation: there is a great deal of evidence that even after memories have been consolidated (made permanent) they can be altered. This makes a lot of sense: a parent knows what his child looks like, and thinks this is unforgettable, yet the knowledge is continually updated as the child grows. Reconsolidation may provide the mechanism for the creation of false memories[650] (p.465).

Reference: see *Ideas of reference*.
Refsum's disease: p.499.

Refuge: women at risk of domestic violence are sometimes offered emergency accommodation, usually with their children at a secret address, away from their usual home area so they are unlikely to be seen by people who would inform the partner. This can make it impossible for them to receive appointment letters, etc. A sudden change of school is often needed.

A large proportion of the children involved have witnessed the domestic violence or have been abused themselves. The women seek refuge after an average of 28 assaults[1722]. A substantial number return home to stay with the original perpetrator.

Refugees: one percent of the world's population have left home to seek safety, roughly half of these outside their home country. Over half of these are children[488]. Many have been malnourished, p.504, or chronically infected, p.490. After arrival they often suffer a prolonged stay in a reception centre with minimal psychosocial care. Following this, they usually have to go to school without knowing the local language; and many live in serial temporary accommodations with parents who may themselves be traumatised and unemployed, p.570. See also *immigrants*, p.488.

A special subgroup of refugees is those who arrive unaccompanied, with or without family contacts. About 1000 arrive in Belgium annually, of whom 95% are aged 11 or above[401]. They suffer very high rates of anxiety, depression and post-traumatic symptoms[402] (see p.567).

Refusal: this is often used imprecisely to refer to things that children don't do, regardless of whether they are actually refusing, or unable (especially important in school refusal), or just preferring something else. See the broader concept of *non-behaviours*, p.515.

Regression: p.41.

Reinforcement: this word has a useful, precise meaning from the field of operant conditioning, i.e. stimuli that increase the likelihood of an

Glossary and Index

organism doing something. This is distinct from *reward*, which is the subjective pleasure experienced (p.353).

With children, most voluntary behaviours start through *experimentation* (p.463), soon become used to satisfy particular *drives* (p.456) and later become *habits*, that is learned automatic behaviours that continue to be used even when the drive is not active.

Commonly reinforced behaviours in children include drawing, p.56; tantrums, p.286; repetitive behaviours in autism, p.64. See *functional analysis*, p.365.

Religion: religion can function as a practice, belief, affiliation, or an identity[1321]. Ethnic groups differ greatly in the extent to which adolescents participate in religious practice[1498]. In most cultures, girls participate more than boys. People who participate regularly in religious activities tend to be more regular in other aspects of their lives (sleeping, eating, exercising) and to engage in less risk-taking behaviour[1321], especially less drug-taking[406]. Some of the benefits to children in religious families arise from the support their parents obtain. Teenagers can rebel by becoming much less[431] or much more religious than their parents, or by religious conversion. In general religion is a protective factor, but ceases to be so if it leads to interpersonal or intrapersonal conflict (e.g. p.355). Warning signs of this include dramatic religious change and unconventional religious beliefs. Occasionally, discussion with a religious leader can clarify the situation (see [861]). See also Ramadan, p.465; traditional cultural practices, p.448; religious rituals as superstimuli, p.558; distinguishing religious from psychotic experiences, p.347.

REM: rapid eye movement (phase of sleep).

Repetitive behaviours: pp.61, 63; repetitive speech, p.157.

Resilience: protective factors (p.394). A child is protected not only by factors in himself, but also in his strongest relationship; in his immediate family; his extended family; and his neighbourhood. An example within himself is that children with certain alleles of the serotonin transporter (p.547) are protected against long-term emotional sequelae of abuse and other negative life events (p.499). See protective factors in domestic violence, p.454; trauma, p.567; discussions of perpetuating factors, p.526, and of *religion*, p.541.

Resistance: opposing a force, especially not wanting to change. See treatment resistance, p.567; waxy flexibility and gegenhalten, p.98; resistance to comforting, p.390; "psychological insulin resistance", p.451. See also resistance to urges in OCD, p.65, 101; in psychosis, p.65; and in tics, p.101.

Restless legs syndrome: p.200.

Reticular formation: a collective term for the parts of the brainstem lacking in obvious structure. Historically the reticular formation was thought to control alertness. More recently some have suggested it controls what "mode" an animal is in. In apparent contrast to this idea, the small chunks in which it is studied tend to have functions closely related to nearby motor and sensory nuclei.

Rett syndrome: onset is typically about age 1–2, but can occur as late as age 4. Most lose hand skills and all language, over several months to years. The child becomes increasingly self-preoccupied but gaze is preserved; a few partially recover.

The loss of active grasping, loss of pincer grip, and onset of severe apraxia affecting all activities clearly differentiate Rett from autism; hyperventilation (p.484) is also more common in Rett. The degree of slowing of head growth usefully predicts severity. Ninety per cent have bursts of seizures lasting a few days, followed by a seizure-free week or more.

The standard description is of replacement of useful hand movements by midline stereotypies (p.64) such as hand-wringing and hand-rubbing, but in fact *using joined hands to do many activities* is a better description (see[1596] for photos). The hands may be stabilising each other in the face of tremor and ataxia. However this does not always appear even in MECP2-confirmed cases, and many other stereotypies appear as well[1596]. The stereotypies become simpler and slower as the disease progresses.

Great variability
Boys with this gene die soon after birth (see[469] for details of the whole MECP2 spectrum). Severity in girls is very variable due to X-inactivation and distinct point-mutations; some live to middle age[469,637]. A similar phenotype does rarely follow encephalitis.

Reye syndrome: p.99.
RIBA: repetitive interests, behaviours and activities[1001].
Rigidity: p.234.

Risk: predictions of unexpected negative events. For evaluations *by children* of risks they face, and their responses to these evaluations, see *recklessness*, p.539.

Evaluations by staff of all risks following from a known fact
Risk posed by sexual behaviour, p.267; by headbanging, p.119; by fire-setting, p.466; by sleeping in parents' bed, p.198; by running away, p.210; by toxic substances, p.566; by obesity, p.335; by time on the internet, p.492; by poverty, p.533.

ID increases some risks while reducing others. Wandering off (p.209) is both more common and more risky in ID and autism. Children with epilepsy have high risk of falls. In some areas teens with mild ID are at high risk of carrying guns or becoming involved in drug-related crimes[1208]. However the greater degree of supervision (at home and in a special school) can reduce the risk of drug abuse, alcohol use, gang membership, or sexual activity below that of other teens[1208].

Evaluations by staff of likelihood of specific negative events
Risk that child is being abused, p.271; risk that child will harm self, p.319 or others, pp.283, 245 or will kill, p.282; risk of suicide, p.320; risk that this symptom is being fabricated, induced or exaggerated, p.359; risk of maternal depression, p.174.

Other aspects of risk
Key role of risk in assessment of child, p.15; importance of collecting full information to minimise risk, p.22; inadequacy of intuition in assessing risk, p.18; At Risk register, p.272; risk of psychiatric disorder, pp.334, 394; importance of risky predictions in science, p.537. See also *statistics*, p.553.

Ritual. this term is used in two different ways: (a) *sequences* of behaviours (p.547) such as bedtime rituals and (b) behaviours that are performed to neutralise underlying fears (see OCD, p.65).

Role-play: p.222.
Rudeness: p.161.

Rumination: (a) Depressive ruminations are repeated negative thoughts. Similar repetitivity can be seen in OCD and autism. Terms for normal rumination include contemplation, reflection, pondering and reconsidering. The term is not used for primarily sensory mental repetitions, such as imaginary worlds, imagery, and imagining a tune.

(b) Repeated regurgitation starting within 30 minutes after meals. It is started by use of tongue/throat muscles or by fingers in mouth, usually triggering an adapted belch or a learned relaxation of the lower oesophageal sphincter. Anatomical abnormalities such as hiatal hermia can contribute. The child lies contentedly and may also have other self-entertaining activities (p.545).

In infancy it is fairly common, and the food remains in the mouth. It sometimes continues longer, causing tooth erosion similar to that in bulimia. If the behaviour persists for years, e.g. in ID or autism, it can evolve into more complicated behaviours such as putting the food on the floor and smearing or re-eating it.

The parents may describe this as vomiting, and in rare cases half-digested food may be spat out or dribbled. However it is a separate mechanism, which does not cause nausea or the sympathetic signs of vomiting (p.337) and is relatively effortless.

Running away: p.210.
Running off: p.209.

Saccades: rapid eye movements, taking the eye from one fixation point to another, lasting about 1/20 second. These are driven by both visual and task information[674,927] and can be extremely complex, e.g. in reading[1324].

Scanpaths are sequences of saccades used to explore a visual scene. *Antisaccades* are movements *away* from a visual stimulus, which can be performed voluntarily if desired. See also other types of eye movement, p.52; blinks with saccades, p.121; cerebellum, p.437; procrastination of reflex, p.535; slowed saccades, p.552.

SAD: Separation Anxiety Disorder, p.391; Seasonal affective disorder, p.314.
Safety: see *recklessness*, p.539; *risk*, p.542.
Sanfilippo disease: p.502.
SCAN: Schedules for Clinical Assessment in Neuropsychiatry[1796].

Schistosomiasis (or bilharzia): infection with schistosoma, acquired by playing or walking in infected non-salty water in the tropics. Chronic infection can cause anaemia, p.421; fatigue, p.323; growth stunting, and impaired cognitive development[844]. See also worms, p.576.

Schizophrenia: a diverse group of causes of psychosis (p.537). Schizophrenia typically has florid episodes of Schneiderian symptoms (p.544), lasting weeks to months, superimposed on chronic functional decline. Look for family history, paranoia (p.524), soft neurological signs (p.58).

By definition, *childhood onset schizophrenia (COS)* also called *very early onset schizophrenia (VEOS)* starts below age 13, and *early onset schizophrenia* starts below age 18. COS is rare, and an unlikely diagnosis unless other family members are affected.

Caveats: The notion of schizophrenia as a single disorder, or even as a coherent group of disorders, is strongly questioned[1426]. In common with other psychiatrically recognised "syndromes" such as catatonia (p.98) or chronic fatigue (p.323), comprehensive medical assessment is necessary (p.349). Diagnosis based purely on DSM criteria does not reliably predict outcome[1536] and should usually be deferred until at least two episodes have occurred. Because antipsychotics help many problems (p.422), the diagnosis is not strongly supported by positive response to an antipsychotic. Similarly, incongruous affect and signs of puzzlement (such as broad smiles) are increased in schizophrenia but not sufficiently to help much with diagnosis[786].

Schizophrenic prodrome: several months of declining function preceding frank pychotic symptoms. In such a situation there is a very high risk of schizophrenia developing, if there is family history [see p.379 of 1747]. It is unlikely if the child has good friendships and is progressing normally at school. Prodrome is suggested by self-isolation, school-avoidance, an astonishingly messy room, personality change, gradual worsening of mood (including low mood and delusional mood, a feeling that something odd is going on, or academic difficulties over months (school essays can be useful to assess whether thought processes are deteriorating). Ask: "Are there thoughts that are too difficult to put into words?" Apparent prodromes can have neurological causes[727] (see *regression*, p.41).

Relapse: relapse can be detected earlier by being alert for symptoms from previous episodes (for excellent suggestions on how to do this see[171]). People with ID have the same signs, plus vaguer symptoms such as elation, fear, swearing, challenging behaviour, and even not doing as they are told (which is only noticeable in very obedient children).

Relationship to other disorders: rediagnosis of childhood schizophrenia as bipolar affective disorder (p.264) is common. Relationship to autism, p.538; to mutism, p.151; to pre-pulse inhibition, p.462. Immaturity, ID and autism are far more common than schizophrenia but can cause schizophrenia-like symptoms[424] (for more details see pp.343–347.). For a clear genetic and neuroanatomical exposition see[1069].

Schneiderian (first-rank) symptoms: these occur in schizophrenia and in organic disorders[1012]. They include audible thoughts, hallucinated voices of two or more people conversing, hallucinated voices commenting on the person's actions, thought broadcasting / withdrawal / insertion, somatic passivity (p.95), delusional perception. For discussion see[1487].

School: p.215.
Scoliosis: p.93.
Scratching: p.110.

Scream: a very loud simple non-verbal utterance. This is different from shouting (or screaming *at*) which has verbal content. *Crying* (p.315) includes sobs and lasts longer than screams, but screams can be superimposed on longer-term crying, for example when a source of cuddles enters the room, or when an abdominal pain is exacerbated.

Causes

Screams can be in fright (p.296), rage (p.71), pain (p.135), excitement, or laughter; and they can be reinforced by attention or demand avoidance, as in tantrums (p.286). It can be difficult to exclude physical causation in people who cannot localise pains, e.g. infants and those with ID (see p.135). Screams in sleep are most often due to night terrors (p.200) or seeking attention or reassurance. Children eventually learn not to scream in migraine, as it worsens the headache, but they often scream with ear pain.

A few people with ID and/or autism scream because they like the sound or find it relaxing – in which case it is prolonged and there is no accompanying communication. Rare causes include hallucinations (p.343), hypoglycaemia (p.82), fits[1566], recurrent vertigo (p.454), and mucopolysaccharidoses (p.501).

Social aspects
Chimpanzees can distinguish between tantrum screams, aggressor screams, mild victim screams, and severe victim screams[1495,1496]; human parents usually can too.

Some infants scream when others would whimper or cry, as an aspect of their temperament (p.561). Some children (mainly young girls), react to surprises with high-pitched squeals or screams, accompanied by freezing (p.296) or flap-like movements (p.105). This may be an evolved response to danger[1021], possibly signalling unwanted submission by social subordinates, as it seems to do in monkeys[1457].

Scurvy: p.329.
Seasonal Affective Disorder (SAD): p.314.
Secondary gain: p.471.
Secrecy: consider drug abuse, p.257; OCD, p.65.
Segawa syndrome: see *dystonia*, p.458.
Selective mutism: p.153.
Self-consciousness: see social anxiety, p.298.

Self-entertainment: usually refers to simple experimental or exploratory activities done by oneself for fun, as the simplest form of play (p.221).

The most common usage of the term is for the waving of limbs, squealing, babbling, and shaking of rattles, under a mental age of 2 or so. Similar behaviours at later ages include tapping pencils, humming, running around, and provoking people. By rights the term could include hobbies such as drawing, reading, TV, computer games, and indeed all *interests* (p.229). Music can be related, an "auditory cheesecake, an exquisite confection crafted to tickle the sensitive spots of… our mental faculties." [1256] Some forms of dissociation (p.453) such as daydreaming (p.450) are not simply calming, so could be described as self-entertainment.

Characteristic signs are looking at what is done, and, for the simpler movements, speed (compare *spinning*, p.104). Children first learn self-entertainment skills that work in the environments where they are bored – so boredom (p.322) and upset will be seen in environments that lack the equipment children have learned to use for self-entertainment. This is universal, but can be worse in ID or inflexible children. Most children are very pleased to have activities suggested by adults: it is not easy for them to initiate activities that they have not seen or been taught.

Contrast *gratification phenomena*, p.474, which are done repetitively because they feel good; and *self-soothing* behaviours, p.61. A table linking all these is on p.124.

Self-harm: pp.319, 317.
Self-identity: p.237.
Selfishness: p.179.
Self-injury: usually refers to violent behaviours that leave a mark, p.317.
Self-soothing: p.61.
Semantics: p.144.

Semantic Pragmatic Disorder: affectionate but socially and linguistically odd. In conversation, often gives too little or too much information (p.163), or unusual content (p.229). Not a standard term, and usually included under the broad umbrella of Autistic Spectrum Disorder ☝. See *Semantics*, *Pragmatics*.

Sensation-seeking (includes seeking arousal, and seeking a specific sensation): p.123.

Sensitisation means becoming more aware of a sensation. Sensitisation can be accompanied by anxiety, fear, avoidance – and eventually in some circumstances increased acuity. Sensitisation is generally arousing, and rather nonspecific, whereas habituation (the decrement in function with repeated presentations of a stimulus) affects only the activated paths[1011].

A localised painful stimulus causes, over the next few minutes to days, an increase in the pain elicited by the same stimulus (hyperalgesia), and over a broader area of skin, the perception of pain elicited by normally innocuous stimuli (allodynia, p.136)[707]. In chronic painful conditions, hypervigilance (an attentional or arousal phenomenon) causes not only increased pain-sensitivity but also increased intolerance to strong stimuli in other modalities.

See *parents sensitised to a particular behaviour*, p.205; sensitisation to environment in session, p.77; sensitisation to direct gaze in Fragile X, p.176; in addiction, p.259; conditioned arousal or sensory amplification, p.127; sensitisation and failure of habituation in tinnitus, p.565. See also *desensitisation*, p.451.

Sensitive period: discussed with *critical period*, p.447

Sensitivity has four meanings: intolerance (p.125), upsettability, acuity, and empathy. The word *sensitivity* is most often used in lay talk to describe people who are **easily upset**, often due to low self-esteem or self-confidence (pp.151,295,309). The term is sometimes used in the engineering sense of elevated sensory function or **acuity**.

The common therapeutic sense of *sensitivity* is elevated **empathy** (experiencing another person's situation). In principle, such *experiencing* can be divided into understanding (i.e. Theory of Mind, p.563), doing, and feeling[181]. In practice, it is difficult to work out whether a child empathises with another's pain (see p.170). He may help someone because he gets credit for demonstrating a caring role; conversely he may turn his back because he finds the other's suffering overwhelming.

Relationship between empathy and acuity
Whether empathy has any association with enhanced acuity is unclear, though the idea has some plausibility as anxious people are more able to detect things that are concordant with their own feelings and less good at perceiving discordant feelings[524];

similarly, people who congenitally cannot feel pain are less likely to perceive pain in others [367]. However, even though rare highly empathic people *may* have heightened sensory or emotional function, the vast majority of people with sensory intolerance have no special empathy. They also have no enhanced acuity [e.g. 1392]. This is a useful reminder that clinicians' *empathy* can clarify a patient's problems, to a modest degree, but cannot reliably "understand and make meaningful"[1123].

Sensory defensiveness: p.125.
Sensory Integration, sensory processing deficits: p.125.
Sensory intolerance: p.125.
Sensory sensitivity: see *Sensitivity*.
Sensory tic: p.231.
Separation anxiety: p.197

Septo-Optic Dysplasia: A group of rare congenital conditions of greatly varying severity, with various combinations of pituitary hormone abnormalities (p.531), optic nerve hypoplasia, and midline brain defects (such as agenesis of the septum pellucidum or corpus callosum). Common characteristics are small stature (growth hormone deficiency), ID and visual impairment (which may be anything from strabismus or nystagmus to blindness)[1723]. Other associations include obesity, anosmia and deafness.

Sequence: several actions that are done in order. (a) Many people have invariant sequences (e.g. checking their hair then their collar and glasses, or checking websites in a particular order) that reduce their anxiety, or are simple habits. Sometimes there is an underlying obsession (p.517) that allows a diagnosis of OCD. Autistic people's sequences are often more frequent, more unusual, and less concealed than other people's. (b) Behavioural sequences under automatic, subcortical control are attributed to *central pattern generators* in the spinal cord and brainstem[413]. Such sequences include walking, crawling, breathing, swallowing and utilisation behaviours, p.572. Difficulty in performing sequential movements is a *frontal sign*, p.469.

Serotonin: neuromodulatory transmitter involved in anxiety, impulsivity, sleep, eating, libido and learning. Inherited abnormalities in 5HTT-LPR (serotonin linked polymorphism region) may lead to some children being more prone than others, to mood disorders following abuse ([269] but for debate see[1348] and[1146,1403]) or following maternal anxiety during pregnancy[1260]. Other inherited serotonin abnormalities have a smaller effect, increasing impulsivity/hyperactivity[481]. Serotonin neurons in the dorsal raphe fire while an animal withholds planned responses[1094], which may explain why suicide victims have reduced serotonin activity[1286]. See *SSRI*, p.552; *serotonin syndrome*, below.

There are many serotonin receptors[1152]:

- Gq/11-coupled receptors: 5HT-2A (LSD), 2B (non-neural), 2C (SSRI, weight)
- Gs-coupled receptors: 5HT-4 (learning in hippocampus), 6 (enhances memory),7 (mood and sleep)
- Gi/o-coupled receptors: 5HT-1A (buspirone anxiolytic), 1B (aggression, impulsivity, SSRI), 1D (antimigraine drugs), 1E (unknown function), 1F (new antimigraine drugs), 5A (little known)
- Ion-channel receptor: 5HT-3 (ondansetron anti-nausea).

'Serotonin syndrome': SSRI toxicity. The most severe effects of toxicity are generalised involuntary muscle activity with hyperthermia, which can be fatal[753]. Such severe cases usually result from the use of an SSRI (p.552) with an MAO inhibitor. Milder signs include confusion, hypomania (p.263), agitation, shivering; sweating (p.558); diarrhoea; hyper-reflexia; *myoclonus*, p.511. It is distinguished from neuroleptic malignant syndrome (p.514) because it includes hyper-reflexia and clonus, whereas NMS has normal reflexes with lead pipe or cogwheel rigidity.

Sex: see Sexual abuse, p.275; sexual and sexualised behaviour, p.269; disinhibition, p.261; masturbation, p.115; inserting things in penis, p.118; sexual maturation in anorexia, p.334; homosexuality, p.481; gender roles: pp.247, 248, 243; obsessions in OCD, p.65; effect on eye contact, p.175; sex as a social drive, p.168; relationship to attachment, p.195; co-sleeping, p.198; possible relationship to hobbies, p.223, 246, 248; bipolar affective disorder, p.264; age norms, p.269; puberty, p.411. For patterns of sexual relationships in a school, see[123].

Sex chromosome disorder: abnormal structure or number of the X or Y chromosome. The most common are:

XO	Turner's	p.570	1/2500 females
XXY	Klinefelter's	p.496	1/1000 males
XXX	Triple X	p.568	1/1000 females
XYY	(not a syndrome)	usually normal	1/1000 males

It is worth considering whether the parents have the misunderstanding that sex-chromosome abnormalities would cause sexualised or otherwise disinhibited behaviour (there is generally no such connection).

Sharing: p.179; sharing a bed with parents, p.198; professional information sharing, p.414.

Shoplifting: p.250.

Showing off: can result from simple immaturity, competition with peers, attention-seeking, following a role model or cultural norm, trying to be respected, or trying to build up his own self-esteem. Most children proudly show their drawings to parents, and this is often up to ten times an hour. Many children boast of what their parents do or how big their house is.

Shuddering attacks: p.71.
Shyness: p.181.
SIADH: syndrome of inappropriate anti-diuretic hormone, p.338.

Siblings: see *family*, p.465; *sibling rivalry*, p.213; *only child*, p.518; effect of birth order on child labour in poorer countries, p.575.

Many studies have attempted to relate birth order to the child's personality, sexuality or intelligence. The effect sizes are small, necessitating vast studies, and the results are disputed. The clearest results to date are that children's IQ is lower in larger families, and that the later children's IQs are also slightly lower[134] (by about one point of IQ for each step in family size or birth rank[1564]). There has been no detailed study of a suggested "middle child syndrome".

Mechanisms implicated in making siblings different from one another include greater parental investment in the first and last children; dominance by elder children; children adopting behavioural niches in the family; each sibling trying to be an individual; and cultural stereotypes[1564].

First children probably identify more with parents and authority, and are more conformist than later children[1565]. This seems to be because later children usually can't match the eldest in terms of conformity (as he is older), so they find other ways to compete for parental attention.

Sick role: p.487.

Sickle cell: a hemoglobin variant that when homozygous causes red blood cells to clump up especially when dehydrated, infected or hypoxic, leading to excruciatingly painful vaso-occlusive crises. The homozygous form is called sickle *disease*; sickle *trait* is heterozygous and much milder. Children with sickle disease have a somewhat increased rate of psychiatric symptoms, but IQ is unaffected[746]. The relationship to night-time wetting is multifactorial: see discussion in[496].

Side-effects of treatments: p.568.

Skin-picking: almost everyone does this sometimes, mainly picking at pimples and scabs to remove them. It often starts in adolescence, and 4% of college students say it is a severe problem for them[1764]. When it is strenuous or involves healthy skin it is important to look for causes, such as anxiety, self-loathing, emotional dyscontrol (p.69) or congenital anaesthesia (p.136), as well as sequelae such as disfigurement or feeling helpless. Like hair-pulling and nail-biting (p.511), skin-picking is done mainly when the person is sitting thinking about something else. In contrast people harming themselves intentionally (p.317) are often deeply interested in the picking. Simulants (p.555) can increase skin-picking, presumably by increasing the focus on small irregularities in the skin.

SLD: severe learning difficulty, p.497.
SLE: systemic lupus erythematosus, p.560.
Sleep: pp.199, 200. For age norms and daytime sleepiness see p.321.
Slowness: p.95.
SLT: speech and language therapy.
SM: selective mutism, p.153 or sadomasochism (see sadism, p.281).
Smearing: p.342.
Smell: see p.122 and *body odour*.

Smiles: The earliest smiles are nonsocial responses to pleasure, but these have an important role in helping carers bond. They can appear from the first day of life. Social smiles, which are reciprocal responses to faces or smiles, appear in 90% by 3 months. Smiling at himself in the mirror starts at 4–8 months. Smiles are not unitary phenomena, but can be shaped and mixed with other emotional signs[452]. Fixed grins that appear only in the consultation may be an attempt to minimise problems, or to be polite in some cultures. More permanent fixed grins (i.e. not directed at people) are seen quite often in autism, in some dementias, in advanced Wilson's disease (p.575), tetanus (p.490) and other dystonias. Relationship to laughter: p.111; faces that are naturally smiley: p.178; inability to smile: p.178; smiles out of the blue when in love: p.309; sign of hallucination: p.343; in headbanging: p.119; relationship to vision: p.133; role in conversation, p.144.

Smith-Magenis syndrome: a defect in the RAI1 gene, found once in 15000 births[621]. This causes a variable degree of ID, a very communicative personality, hyperactivity, self-injury, stereotypies (esp. with mouth), and a small maxilla and philtrum that can give the impression of a large jaw[202]. Facial features gradually become coarser in adolescence. Characteristic behaviours include self-hugging, nail-yanking, insertion of objects into body orifices (p.118), and hand-licking before page-flicking. Reversed melatonin secretion (highest in the daytime, see graphs in[621] and[202]) is in some way associated with reduced night-time sleep (p.199) and increased daytime sleepiness and naps. 75% have a non-progressive peripheral neuropathy with reduced sensitivity to pain and a characteristic appearance of the leg muscles.

Sniffing: p.109.
Sociability: p.519.
Social anxiety: p.298.
Social care services: see Social Services Department, p.550.

Social constructionism: many individual characteristics can be depicted as a normal distribution in the population (figures on pp.83, 519) yet most societies recognise only problems at one end of such distributions (e.g. high impulsivity, or low sociability). Thus definitions of disorders reflect not only objective variation between people, but group decisions regarding what should be viewed as pathological. Societies also determine disorder thresholds (i.e. the level of symptoms or impairment that will admit the child to a diagnosis or sick role (p.487).

Changes in prevailing beliefs influence which conditions are given a medical label. For example, homosexuality was in DSM until 1973; and most damaging social relationships still are not.

See also *ideograph*, p.487.

Social / observational learning: a key process, learning from the behaviours and reactions of parents, peers and teachers. The following can be problematic: learned violence[100], p.291; specific fears[1086,1124], p.307; folie imposee, p.347; culturally determined disorders, p.448; learned pedantry, p.163; social behaviour, p.162; eating habits. For many culturally determined examples of body language see [1114]. See also *personal space*, p.527. The term *observational learning* is more appropriate for skills that could be equally well learned from machines (e.g.[714]).

Social Services Department. This has legal, practical and financial roles. Typically it is subdivided into child (child protection, also called child welfare; adoption and fostering; emergencies; young offenders; ID and physical disabilities), adult (mental health; domestic violence; ID and physical disabilities; post-hospital recovery; and elderly). In some countries it includes aspects of housing, education and benefits.

Social worker: see Social Services Department, above.

Sociogram: a diagram of social relationships. A sociogram can include many kinds of information such as strength of friendship or animosity, sexual relationships[123], power structures, family rifts and groupings. This information can be usefully added on top of the genetic information in a genogram, p.203. Using a simple questionnaire completed by each child in a class, a sociogram can be constructed to show bullies, high-status children (p.172) and bystanders (this is called a *sociometric survey* and is useful in predicting social risks and planning interventions. Free software can be downloaded.)

Soft neurological signs: p.58.
Soiling: vague term, can mean any type of faecal misplacement, p.341.
Solvent abuse: p.258.
Somatising/Somatoform: p.359.

Sotos syndrome: cerebral gigantism, with large head, hypotonia and mild ID[1142]. Many have dysgenesis of the corpus callosum, p.445. See *overgrowth*, p.521.

Specific Learning Disabilities: disabilities previously thought to be unrelated to overall cognitive function. The most commonly described are *dyslexia*, p.51; dyspraxia, p.89; writing difficulty, p.53; and dyscalculia, p.457. Callosal agenesis (p.445) can cause major navigational difficulty even in the presence of fully normal IQ results. Some would also include problems revealed in a subscale of an IQ test, such as NVLD, p.28; and language problems, p.145. For other kinds of discrepancy on testing, see p.33. For distinct meanings of *learning disability* see p.498.

SPECT: single photon emission CT, see p.374.

Spectrum: describes purportedly unitary clinical conditions that are manifest differently in different children. The word implies that the manifestations could differ quantitatively or qualitatively; whereas *continuum* implies that they only differ quantitatively. See "On the spectrum", p.519, which refers to autistic spectrum disorders. Others include OCD spectrum, schizophrenia spectrum, "Tourettes Plus". In all these cases it is likely that the impression of such simple variation in a population is created by the amalgamation of numerous traits that are rare or have small effects [1770].

Speech problems: p.147. See also *Language problems*, p.145.

Spinal cord: see *posturing*, p.93; *spina bifida*, below; *spinal muscular atrophy*, p.551. Spinal reflexes include the stretch reflex; startle, p.552; erection, p.462. For central pattern generators see *sequence*, p.547.

Spina bifida: a neural tube defect (p.513). Its severity ranges from unnoticeable, to incompatible with life.

The mildest form, spina bifida occulta, is remarkably common, affecting 20% of normal people, in a few of whom it is associated with urodynamic abnormalities. It may be revealed by a trivial tuft of sacral hair, epidermal cysts, or X-ray[494].

If the skin is open it is generally repaired soon after birth. Ten per cent of these go on to have minimal or no disability[733].

Severe forms have a high-level lesion (with the lowest pin-prick-unimpaired dermatome at L2 or above), and sometimes hydrocephalus. These people often have problems with urinary and faecal continence and sexual function, and orthopaedic problems in the back, legs and feet[1668]. IQ is lowered in those with hydrocephalus. Even higher sensory levels (i.e. thoracic) are associated with renal abnormalities.

Spinal muscular atrophy: an autosomal recessive condition causing partial degeneration of motor units (spinal motor neurons and their muscle fibres). Infants with Type I have difficulty within the first 6 months of life and usually die by 4 years. Children with Type II show weakness by 18 months, and will always need support to stand. Patients with Type III develop variable degrees of weakness, with onset between 18 months and 30 years of age. Type IV has onset after age 30. Severity is epigenetically regulated[664].

Spinning: p.104.

Sphingomyelin: a lipid occurring in myelin (p.510) and in red blood cell membranes. Sphingomyelin accumulates in Niemann-Pick disease, Type A causing severe brain damage and early death in infants; and Type B affecting the liver and spleen but not the brain, and occurring in later childhood.

Niemann-Pick type C[1708] causes psychosis *years before* ataxia, slowed saccades, hepatosplenomegaly. Test LFT, fibroblast enzymes.

Splitting: this has a straightforward meaning (thinking of people in all-good or all-bad, black-or-white terms) and a subtler psychoanalytic meaning (a defence mechanism, p.303, or an infantile stage of development in which good things and bad things have to be separate from one another in the mind: see *object relations*, p.517). Splitting has direct effects on social dynamics. Splitting is common when several other people are involved, as in a family (p.187), or when outpatient or inpatient care brings a patient into contact with multiple professionals[532]. For example, patients are often over-enthusiastic about their current favourite therapist, while condemning all previous therapists.   It is important to bear in mind that most such situations have many possible causes other than splitting: e.g. politeness, optimism, simple concrete thinking, conformity with groups of people who have aligned themselves together (or who seem to have done so), or the current therapist actually being better or more amenable (which is quite likely if the patient has been referred on to someone more likely to help).

SSADH: see *GABA*, p.470.
SSD: Social Services Department, p.550.
SSPE: subacute sclerosing panencephalitis, p.557.

SSRI: selective serotonin reuptake inhibitor. a class of medications used in treating depression, anxiety, obsessionality and, occasionally, repetitive behaviours. Uncommon side-effects include dry mouth, GI upset and serotonin syndrome (p.548).

A common and important side-effect is mood elevation (also called "behavioural activation") causing troublesome disinhibition (p.261).   The effect increases with dose and duration, and in ID. It occurs with all SSRIs, but can sometimes be avoided by using ultra-low doses, and is less severe with sertraline than with fluoxetine. Such disinhibition probably accounts for adolescents on SSRIs having an increased rate of non-fatal suicidal-like behaviour despite a decreased rate of suicide[1610].

SST: Strange Situation Test, p.556.

Stammer: see *Stutter* which is the more common term (*stammer* more used in UK and clinically).

Startle syndromes: A startle is a fast reflex response to unexpected threat, consisting of lowered eyebrows, eyes closed, lips horizontally stretched and neck taut (all these are the opposite of the much slower expression of surprise[453]). Physiologically, startling is increased in anxious states (also called fear-potentiated startle, as in PTSD, p.389). Some anxious people also startle to innocuous cues[1320], and have other enhanced reflexes too; in neonates this is called jitteriness. There are three categories of abnormal startles[93]. These are (a) hyperekplexia, p.483 (b) slower, learned culture-specific syndromes (p.448) such as Jumping Frenchmen of Maine, in which sufferers can jump, swear, repeat phrases, hit or fall over when startled; and (c) stimulus-induced disorders. Syncope (p.74) is sometimes caused this way. Startle epilepsy is another example, initiated by an unexpected stimulus, but a tonic/clonic seizure ensues. Contrast sleep-starts, p.200; breath-holding spells, p.434; pre-pulse inhibition of startle, p.462.

Starvation: Severe malnutrition (for less severe malnutrition see p.504). Starvation can be of sudden onset (see e.g. *fasting*, p.465; *diabetes*, p.451) or long-term protein-calorie malnutrition, which is categorised as marasmus or kwashiorkor.

Classically, kwashiorkor results from protein deficiency, and marasmus from deficiency in both energy and protein (for formal classification see p.504). The child with kwashiorkor is lethargic yet severely irritable, with diarrhoea and patchy red skin, whereas the marasmic child is very thin but has a normal mental state. Kwashiorkor is mainly seen in poor countries, and in rich countries it is an easily missed diagnosis that can result from restricted diet (whether caused by child or parent[1609]).

Starvation can cause severe repetitiveness (p.63) and cognitive inflexibility[837] (p.234). See also anorexia nervosa, p.334; neglect, p.274; metabolic crises, p.381.

Statistics: problem of multiple tests, pp.373,532. Distinction between population risk and risk in individual, p.24. Distinguishing association from causation, pp.195,411,432,490,539,571. Attribution, p.426; Flynn effect, p.59; Occam's razor, p.14. Risk, p.542; *a posteriori* versus *a priori* risk, p.21. IQs that "cannot be calculated", p.33.

Status: one's position in a social hierarchy. See *Status among peers*, p.172; status of first-borns or sons, p.214; legal status, p.495; socioeconomic status (*poverty*, p.533). The medical, non-hierarchical use of *status* emphasises persistence in time, e.g. status epilepticus lasts over 20 minutes, cf. pseudoseizure status, p.74.

Stealing: p.250.

Stereotyped: actions with no obvious or normal purpose, with repetitions that are unnecessarily similar to one another, p.85. *Also* interests always pursued in the same way. Stereotyped *interests* are unnecessarily constrained (p.227).

Stereotypy: a movement that is repeated unnecessarily uniformly and unusually frequently, generally for months or years. The uniformity may arise because they are innate subcortical behaviours (e.g. flaps, p.105) or, more ominously, because the child learns to pursue a particular sensation (monotropism, p.509). Purposelessness and involuntariness are sometimes included in definitions but they are debatable or variable: many stereotypies are performed to relieve or achieve sensations (see stimming, p.64; headbanging, p.119). Mannerisms (p.505) and normal repetitions (pp.61, 63, 156) should

be excluded. Even though stereotypies are abnormal, they can
appear in otherwise normal children, in which case they started in
the first 3 years[1078], are not of interest to the child, are easily
suppressed, do not impair function, and happen mainly when
stressed or excited and not asleep[993]. Midline stereotypies, p.64.
Parents *stereotyping* the child, p.214.

Conundrum 17: Stereotypy or perseveration

Stereotypies can be recognised over at least a few days, because
they persist through sleep, whereas perseverations continue
whatever attention was focused on in the last few seconds or
minutes. Stereotypies have "higher rates of activity but in a
decreasing number of response categories"[985], as if the motivation
were arising repeatedly, uncalled for, whereas perseverations are
"repetitive but not excessive"[1344] as though recent memories
continue to influence the expression of later, unrelated,
understandable motivations.

Sterile interests: interests that are circumscribed (i.e. have few
associations), with little social relevance, that would not interest
most people (p.227). Examples include tube lines, stones (p.226);
hair (p.225); earlobes, drapery and other hanging objects; part-
objects (perhaps related to autistic skill in block design subtests,
p.36). Reduction of sterility with maturation, p.229.

Steroids: the main groups of steroid hormones are the sex hormones
(testosterone; oestrogens, p.506, progesterone); mineralocorticoids
which regulate electrolytes; and glucocorticoids. See also cerebrotendinous xanthomatosis, p.32; neurosteroids, p.506.

Testosterone and related chemicals are also called androgenic-
anabolic steroids. They build muscle bulk and masculinise.

Testosterone increases at puberty in boys, and is often blamed for
violence in adolescence. Across the population the effect seems to
be small[196] as should perhaps be expected from the high frequency
of violence committed by testosterone-free small children.
However about 10% of men exposed to 4x normal levels do
become aggressive or manic[1266], so an effect of normal levels may
also be confined to a minority. Trait dominance is directly related
to baseline testosterone levels, and the level of aggression produced
by a losing situation is proportional to changes in testosterone
level[260]. It is not clear whether testosterone is the cause or whether
it is raised by such situations – for example it is raised in the winner
after a game of chess[1030].

Both sexes are also exposed to low levels of testosterone from their
mother's adrenal glands while in utero, and this apparently
produces a dose-related reduction in eye contact and vocabulary[74],
and an increased interest in balls and toys, over social videos[23] (the
effect is about a tenth that of male karyotype)[75,1006]. Half of female
twins are also exposed to testosterone from their co-twins, and this
contributes to a reduction in anorexia nervosa (p.334). In
comparison with these situations, the levels of androgens present in
foetuses with congenital adrenal hyperplasia are much higher and
do somewhat increase the rate of gender identity disorder and
homosexuality, but only in females[701]. In adult women,
testosterone reversibly reduces verbal fluency[1434].

Males have a longer fourth finger : second finger ratio which seems
to be caused by testosterone, possibly due to the simple fact that

males are bigger[882]. See also the relation of testosterone to personality, p.241; stealing and other antisocial behaviour, p.250; puberphonia, p.147; steroid abuse, p.258; polycystic ovaries, p.531.

Glucocorticoids are so called because they raise blood sugar and are released by the adrenal cortex (under control of ACTH, see figure on p.531). They are increased by stress (p.125) and are useful as medicines to reduce inflammation, e.g. in asthma (p.424, including some inhalers). However in the brain they can in certain circumstances increase inflammation[1518].

When released in stress, glucocorticoids can strengthen fear memories (in conjunction with noradrenaline[1372]) while limiting formation of other memories (p.478). Excess can cause Cushing's, p.449; disinhibition, p.261; anxiety, p.299; depression, p.311; and psychosis, p.537. Severe deficiency can cause Addison's disease, p.419.

Abusive treatment in childhood appears to increase children's proneness to depression in adulthood[208], and their life-long cortisol response to stress[1633]; both of these outcomes are confined to the 25% of the population with one genotype of the CRH receptor (see *imprinting*, p.489). See also *hippocampus*, p.478.

Stiff man syndrome: see *Stiff person syndrome.*

Stiff person syndrome: Stiffness in the trunk and/or limbs, of variable severity. In mild form it can be taken for primary anxiety, as patients are characteristically afraid of falling, and their stiffness is exacerbated by emotional or sensory stimulation. It is somewhat similar to tetanus (p.490), and caused by autoimmunity (p.427) to GAD65[471]. The following are frequently associated: diabetes, p.451; epilepsy, ataxia, extrapyramidal signs[1258]. Consider also anxiety, p.295; startle conditions, p.552; catatonia, p.98; postures, p.93; gait, p.471.

Stimming: p.64.

Stimulants: medicines that increase arousal, including methylphenidate, dexamfetamine, cocaine, and theophylline (some would include caffeine, nicotine, and *non-stimulants*, p.516). They are very useful in treating ADHD and narcolepsy. Like sedatives, they usually reduce activity levels, but completely unlike sedatives, they increase precision and attention. The most common side-effects are reduction in appetite (p.331) and, if given too close to bedtime, sleep onset difficulty (p.199). The zombie effect, p.310, indicates excess dose. See also *paradoxes of ADHD*, p.523.

STM: short-term memory. In adults, this holds about 6–7 items, each of which can be a "chunk" of considerable complexity[82,1077]. Clinically it is tested using digit span (p.452) or Corsi block-tapping (p.399). For other clinical signs see pp.149, 157, 357. STM is specially weak in some conditions, such as Fragile X, p.468. In Down's syndrome, verbal STM is weaker than visuospatial, whereas the reverse is true in Williams syndrome[1711]. Contrast *working memory*, p.575.

Stones: (for collecting stones, see p.226). Kidney stones are uncommon in children. Children experience far less pain with urinary stones than do adolescents and adults. When present they can occasionally assist in diagnosing inborn errors of metabolism that contribute to behavioural symptoms[301]. This is especially likely if parents are consanguinous or or relatives also have the combination of stones and developmental problems. Investigation of the urine is almost always more revealing than the composition of the stones[683]; but a stone history is easier to obtain from distant relations.

- Urinary infection often causes stones.
- Oxalate: stones are most likely to be caused by intestinal problems or increased dietary load. The rare genetic conditions of primary hyperoxaluria types 1 and 2 also cause stones in children, but not neurological or psychiatric problems.
- Calcium phosphate: follows immobilisation
- Silica: following excess silica ingestion (e.g. in diet supplements)
- Amino acids
  - Cystinuria (2%): renal stones even in heterozygotes for cystinuria[464]
- Purines
  - Urate:
    - In complete or partial HGPRT deficiency (see Lesch-Nyhan, p.318)
    - PRPP overactivity also causes gout, deafness, and neurodevelopmental problems[301].
    - von Gierke (Type 1 glycogen storage disease)[301].
  - Xanthine: In xanthine oxidase deficiency type 1, with myopathy; in type 2: epilepsy and severe ID[194].
  - Adenine: APRT deficiency (no neurological problem).

Storage disorders: intracellular accumulation of a specific chemical causes insidious neurological decline. Some are treatable (e.g. p.498 and [299,1461]). A few of the leukodystrophies (p.498) are storage disorders. See:
  - i)   lysosomes: p.501
  - ii)   peroxisomes: p.526
  - iii)   lipidoses[1573]
  - iv)   xanthomas (contain lipid): cerebro-tendinous xanthomatosis, p.32
  - v)   glycogen storage diseases (11 types)
  - vi)   iron: Friedreich's ataxia, p.92.

Strange Situation Test: this is a way of assessing an attachment (p.195) relationship in young children, by taking mother out of the clinic room for a minute or so, and observing how the child copes. It can be used formally for research (for which it has some limitations [1399]) and informally in the clinic to obtain pragmatic information on how mother and child manage the departure and return, and how well the child continues to explore (e.g. trying new toys) in mother's absence. The Modified SST is useful when the child has neurodevelopmental problems[1365,1366], see also p.196. Naturalistic observation is less stressful to the child and may produce more meaningful results (useful behavioural signs for the Attachment Q-Sort are listed in[1716]).

Stress response: the physical and psychological response to threats. The immediate response is mediated by the sympathetic nervous system, p.428, releasing noradrenaline, p.516 and adrenaline, p.420. These increase the heart rate, tense the muscles, and reduce blood flow to the skin. The longer term response is mediated by glucocorticoids, p.555. See also fight-flight-or-freeze, p.296.

Stroke: the most common meaning is loss of effective blood supply to a *part* of the brain. This can be caused by inadequate oxygen supply through an artery (infarction) or rupture of an artery (haemorrhage). The results of a stroke last more than a day, whereas a *transient ischaemic attack* (TIA, p.72) typically lasts less than an hour.

There are very many underlying causes of which a likely one can be identified in about two-thirds of paediatric cases[1345]. Birth is a very high-risk time for strokes, probably more because of the hypercoagulable state than due to trauma (for causes see[1140] and vitamin K, p.328).

Stroke can be followed by focal neurological deficits, long-term emotional incontinence, (p.70), and paradoxically an *increase* in speech due to disinhibition (though not in young children)[118].

Watershed infarcts do not result from a single artery blockage, instead affecting the brain areas far from main arteries. They have many causes in children[968], including sepsis, encephalitis, congenital heart disease, sickle (p.549), hypotensive episodes, and vasculitis. Hypoxic-ischaemic encephalopathy (p.486) can cause multiple watershed infarcts. *Cortical* watershed infarcts affect strips of cerebral cortex, whereas *internal* watershed infarcts affect cerebral white matter[1099].

Stupor: p.97.
Sturge-Weber syndrome: p.514.

Stutter (or stammer): frequent involuntary interruption. This most often refers to speech (p.157), but there are also stammering nod (common in ASD) and stammering gait.

Subacute sclerosing panencephalitis (SSPE): Fatal complication of measles seen mainly in developing countries, in the unimmunised. Decline can take several years, including myoclonus (p.511), seizures, intellectual decline, and sometimes visual hallucinations. Diagnosis requires characteristic EEG findings and antimeasles antibody in CSF. It is easily confused with catatonia, depression, functional disorder or simple epilepsy[1277].

Subjective experiences: these are self-evidently important and are too often ignored[1172]. They are important as motivators in their own right (e.g. of imaginary play, p.231), and sometimes also as indicators of underlying social or biological problems. The radical behaviourist notion that these are mere "hypothetical constructs" is thoroughly outdated now. When a child cannot describe his subjective experiences (or gives an unreliable account), there are still many fairly direct ways to obtain the information, such as his facial expressions, linear analogue or picture scales, play (p.221), drawings, physical examination, temperature, and even response to antacids (p.374).

See hallucinations, p.343; subjective experience of dread, p.296; delusional mood, p.544; self-esteem, pp.313, 261; love, p.501; hatred, p.187; cognitive dissonance, p.355; subjective experiences out of the blue in epilepsy, p.76.

Sublimation: p.305.
Substance abuse: p.267.
Suicide and suicidal ideas: p.317.

Sulking: being silent or withdrawn, as an expression of anger or resentment (whereas an *active/externalising* expression of these feelings is a tantrum or rage or violence, pp.286, 71, 289). Sulks can be overt (e.g. with a scowl and a pout, and sometimes foot-stamping or refusing to follow or running off, p.209); or sulks can be private to varying degrees. A child pressurised to do impossible homework may just sit there, in which case fuming and sulking and misery can usually be distinguished; possible underlying factors include learned helplessness (p.96; consider depression) and cognitive dissonance, p.355. A child sulking about being in clinic is not his usual self, and this can cause professionals to make mistakes in assessments, especially of his social skills. Compare *passive-aggressive*, p.525; *non-behaviours*, p.515.

Superstimuli, supernormal stimuli: animals obviously evolve responses to stimuli. When the stimuli are used for communication between organisms, they can become tightly constrained and remarkably effective, so in some cases the stimulus seems to force the recipient to respond, even when this is damaging to them[1612]. Humans don't usually have such overpowering responses to single stimuli, but certain situations in human cultures press several buttons at the same time, making responses very likely indeed, even when this is damaging to the person. These could be called *amalgam superstimuli* (compare amalgam fears, p.307; see also gratification phenomena, p.474; self-entertainment, p.545). (The mechanism taking place over evolutionary time may be analogous to superstitious learning within a lifetime: the Baldwin effect[95]; see also[1530]).

Real things	...subverted by these superstimuli
acquisitiveness	many people can't stop collecting books, stamps, jewellery....
bright things	Jewels and flowers attract humans (and magpies). Lights attract moths, city lights attract sea turtles.
ingestion • sugar • pleasant aromas • feeling of water (cold+smooth)	sweets for kids (with sweetness, colour, and flavour), double cheeseburgers, milk shakes
emotions • feeling rewarded/high • relaxation	licit and illicit drugs
mating signals: • waist-hip ratios • healthy skin • smiles, teeth • large pupils	subverted by skirts, padded shoulders, low neckline, makeup, erotic films, some fetishes, Australian jewel beetles mating with beer-bottles[668], sexual pictures on internet (p.115)
nurturing the young: • gapes of nestling birds • large eyes • a baby's cry	birds sitting on enormous eggs placed in their nests[1611]. Similarly, parental feeding subverted by the larger gape of cuckoo chicks.
multiple drives	refined cultural composites: good cooking, music, art, beauty, religion[384]. Computer games (p.573)

Superstition: superstitious learning, e.g. because a cough was followed by thunder, believing that it will work again.

SW: Social worker. See Social Services, p.550.
Swallowing difficulty: see oromotor apraxia, p.90; choking phobia, p.333.
Swearing: p.161.

Sweating: eccrine sweat glands, found all over the body but especially on the palms and soles, secrete odourless salty water which has a mainly thermoregulatory role. Apocrine sweat glands, found in the armpits and genital area, secrete a thicker, more smelly sweat.

Here excess sweating is discussed (for inadequate sweating or anhydrosis see[290]). Some people sweat much more than is needed to regulate their temperature. In severe cases the sweat runs down the face, drips off the hands, and penetrates through thick jackets. Underarm sweating can be socially embarrassing, especially in females. Facial sweat is the most difficult to hide.

Generalised sweating. The most common causes are heat and exercise, and sympathetic drive (p.428) – especially due to anxiety, pain or drug withdrawal. Rarer causes[290,1547] include SSRIs, pp.548,552; hyperthyroidism, p.484, diabetes, p.451; hypoglycaemia, p.82; phaeochromocytoma, p.529; disease of the hypothalamus or pituitary, p.531; lymphoma; and hereditary autonomic neuropathies (p.136). Night-time sweating can be a sign of nocturnal seizures, p.76; tuberculosis, p.569; lymphoma; endocarditis; acromegaly; and Prinzmetal (episodic) angina[290].

Localised sweating. When severe this is called congenital hyperhidrosis; it is not qualitatively different from normal sweating but is an exaggerated sweat response. Localised sweating usually disappears in sleep.

Palms and soles are the most common sites, and underarms are often also affected. Whereas most of the body's sweating is controlled by temperature, these areas are more responsive to anxiety[290,1625]. Damp hands can make it difficult to hold a pen, and can smear the ink on written work: 4% of adolescents have hands sufficiently sweaty to drench a handkerchief, and about 0.2% have spontaneous dripping from the hands[1625]. When present, damp palms are a useful sign of anxiety, as they can be detected on initial handshake – but most anxious people do not have damp palms. Eating very spicy food causes many people to sweat symmetrically on their scalp, whereas one-sided gustatory sweating merits investigation. Rare causes of localised sweating include Frey's syndrome (the cheek becomes red and sweaty when the person salivates).

For cold damp hands see p.129. See also Reflex sympathetic dystrophy, p.136; body odour, p.433; Fabry's disease, p.464.

Symbol: one thing that represents another, by association, resemblance or convention. For general discussion see p.14. See also symbols in pre-operational stage, p.530; symbolism by lego, p.500; symbolic play, p.221 (and its place in diagnosis of autism, p.388); symbolic pains, p.135; penile symbol, p.228; private symbols, p.145; symbolic triggers of PTSD symptoms, p.389.

See also symbolic causes of cleaning, p.112; of pulling one's hair, p.117; of intolerances, p.128; of special interests, p.232; of loving rabbits, p.246; of loving horses, p.248; of stealing, p.250; of self-harm, p.318; of fabricated symptoms, pp.361–362.

Sympathetic nervous system: see *autonomic nervous system,* p.428.
Sympathomimetics: see *autonomic nervous system,* p.428.

Synaesthesia: sensation in one modality eliciting perception in that modality plus a second sensory modality. This occurs in about 4% of the general population, or considerably more if a broader definition is used[1481]. It is well described in children, for example digits having colours associated with them[610]. Synaesthesia has been divided into high and low level based on the level of information processing at which the crossover occurs[1298]. It appears to be due to aberrant connections between cortical areas[1386]. It has inspired much artistic creativity.

Syncope: p.74.
Syndromes: p.383.

Synkinesis: two movements that occur together, when the patient only thought of one of them. This is often useful, e.g. swinging our arrms when walking, or bracing our trunk when lifting something. Most people can suppress such arm-swinging (*avoidable synkinesis*), but not the trunk-bracing (*obligatory synkinesis*).

Examples of synkinesis: Fogs' sign (hands turn in when walking on inside edges of feet, described by Fog and Fog) – normal until age 9 in girls and 10 in boys[1578,1586]. From age 3, most children can tiptoe, but their associated arm movements only gradually disappear until they are gone by age 8. Mirror movements (p.507) are a subtype of synkinesis. Synkinesis is the basis of Hoover's test for pseudo-paralysis (p.87). For other examples of synkinesis see[907].

Systemic Lupus Erythematosus (SLE): autoimmune condition mainly seen in young women. Signs include a butterfly rash on the face (i.e. with relative sparing of nasolabial creases), joint pains, fatigue, fever, headache (p.139), Raynaud's phenomenon (p.562), and neurolupus[792]. Neurolupus can include cognitive impairment, psychiatric symptoms (depression, anxiety and occasionally psychosis[727]), and movement disorders (e.g. tremor, chorea, p.439; myoclonus, p.511). The first-line test is ANA; other relevant tests include: CRP, Complement (C3,C4), ENA, dsDNA[117]. Rarely, anti-dsDNA gives a true positive even when ESR, CRP and ANA are all normal[117].

Systemising: this means searching for precise, reliable, consistent or lawful patterns or structure in data[109]. Baron-Cohen has suggested that autistic people have a strong systematising trait and a weak empathising trait[109]. Systemising can also be driven by obsessionality, poor long-term memory, or the demands of academia.

The great systemisers of science do not just collect facts but find simple overarching principles: Darwin for species, Freud for dreams, Marx for ideologies, Levi-Strauss for cultures, Jimmy Carr for jokes[258]. They do not seem to have been autistic.

Life-long collectors of facts (who may look for patterns but rarely find overarching principles) are sometimes unsociable but there are many exceptions: Samuel Johnson of the dictionary, Victor McKusick who created the OMIM genetic database[822], and Richard Fortey for trilobites, who describes serious collectors as "obdurate people, odd people, admirable people"[513,1774]. See also *taxonomy*.

Tag: personal graffito, like a signature, sometimes used to assert personal or gang territory (see *gangs*, p.472).

Talking to himself: the content will indicate whether the child is just thinking out loud, or rehearsing a conversation or favourite DVD. Repetitive speech has many causes, p.157. If a name comes up repeatedly it may be an imaginary friend, p.231. Consider also auditory hallucinations, p.343. Rarely, the content will indicate odd ideas, p.347.

Tantrum: p.286.

Tardive movements: refers to repetitive movements appearing usually after using antipsychotics for many years. The most common is tardive dyskinesia (p.62) but tardive myoclonus, dystonia, akathisia (p.114) and other symptoms have been described[493].

Taste: oral, p.122; aesthetic, p.128.

Tattoos: being a culturally determined behaviour (p.448), the significance of this depends on the time and the place. In American adolescents, tattoos are a marker of risk-taking behaviour that includes at least double the rate of drug taking and sexual behaviour.

Taxonomy: the science of working out which categories exist; or conversely deciding that objects exist on a continuum. Calling a grouping of objects a category, or a taxon, implies that there are discrete boundaries and there is a notable paucity of intermediate forms. A taxonomist has to use personal judgment to decide which groupings of problems are most appropriate[1814], and in some cases practical characteristics of the groupings, such as treatability or acceptability may be more important than their innate characteristics such as visible symptoms, age of appearance, or chronicity.

For psychiatric examples see p.487; for non-psychiatric examples see[1010,1568]. An example of improper taxonomy is in an ancient Chinese encyclopaedia that divides the animal kingdom into many overprecise, vague, transient, irrelevant or overlapping categories, including: those that belong to the emperor, embalmed ones, ones that are trained, suckling pigs, those that tremble as if they were mad, those drawn with a very fine camel's hair brush, those that have just broken a flower vase, and those that resemble flies from a distance[200].

Tay-Sachs: p.502.
Teachers: see *school*, p.215.
Tearfulness: p.108.
Teddy bear: see *Transition object*.

Teeth: unusual teeth are found in many syndromes – reach for Smith[787] after the child's parents are out of the room. See bruxism, p.200; holoprosencephaly, p.480; cleft lip, p.440; eroded teeth in anorexia nervosa, p.334 and in rumination, p.543.

Temperament: predispositions found first in infancy[581]. One system that is quite easy to relate to specific disorders often diagnosed at later ages is EASI: Emotionality, Activity, Sociability, and Impulsivity[241]. A more detailed parcellation[1601] includes:

- Activity level (p.79)
- Regularity (of sleeping, eating, and elimination: this makes the infant much easier to manage)
- Initial reaction (withdrawal or approach: *behavioural inhibition*, p.296 versus *exuberance*, p.464). Some infants push a new toy away, spit out new food, or reject a new playgroup.
- Adaptability (versus *rigidity*, p.234). Some infants adapt their initial reactions and others do not.

- Intensity (screaming rather than whimpering; jumping for joy rather than smiling. This can be utterly exhausting for caregivers)
- Mood (p.313). See *hyperthymia*, p.264; *dysthymia*, p.314.
- Distractibility (p.453)
- Persistence and attention span (p.79)
- Sensitivity (p.546).

Based on these, 40% of babies are "easy" , 10% are "difficult" and 15% are "slow to warm up"[1601].

Elements of this have been incorporated into other systems, e.g. personality disorders, p.241; personality, p.241. See also *novelty*, p.517; *warmth*, p.574. *Exuberance*, p.464, includes several of the above factors.

Temperature of body: (see also temperature sensation, p.122). Antipsychotics (p.422) impair temperature-regulation allowing people to become too hot or cold. Cold hands sometimes indicate excessive doses of antipsychotics, in which case they are usually accompanied by some signs of parkinsonism, p.525.

Causes of raised temperature
The most common causes are infection, p.490; and exercise in hot weather. Obese people overheat faster and are more prone to suffer from exertional heat increase[541]. Consider also hyperthyroidism, p.484; phaeochromocytoma, p.529; salicylate intoxication, p.99; stimulants, p.555; status epilepticus; dehydration, p.450; neuroleptic malignant syndrome, p.514; injury; and encephalitis (for more causes see[1482]).

Effects of external heat
Gentle heat has a soporific effect. This may be one of the modes of action of benzodiazepines (p.430), which raise the temperature of the limbs substantially[561]. However, people in England are more likely to commit suicide on hotter days[1211]; in other climates other patterns may be seen (see[1404]). Symptoms of multiple sclerosis (p.510) may first appear in a hot bath, or may be exacerbated by a hot bath or by an unrelated fever.

Effects of external cold
Raynaud's phenomenon is reversible colour change in fingers (or other extremities). Contributory factors include smoking, β-blockers, vibration, connective tissue disease, underweight or anorexia nervosa, and exposure to cold. The majority of cases are benign but further investigation is justified if there are abnormal nailfold capillaries or antinuclear antibodies[1162]. In hand-arm vibration syndrome (vibration white finger) sensory loss and reduced tendon reflexes are found, confined to the limbs that have been exposed to excess vibration.

Temporal lobe: p.513.

Temporal lobe epilepsy (TLE): traditionally, temporal lobe epilepsy (TLE) has been believed to be the epilepsy most likely to cause psychiatric symptoms, but it now seems that other focal epilepsies are just as likely to do so[9]. See *temporal lobe*, p.513; *epilepsy*, p.73; *blinking*, p.108.

Testosterone: p.554.
Tetanus: p.490.
TFT: thyroid function tests. See *thyroid*, below.

Thalassaemia: disease of haemoglobin synthesis. It is transmitted in autosomal recessive fashion, and in some tropical regions 10–20% of the population are carriers. Its severe homozygous form (thalassaemia major) causes severe anaemia which necessitates regular transfusions and medication. Especially in poor countries it has profound effects on the social, emotional and economic life of the child and his or her family, and shortens life expectancy, typically to 20–30 years[1388].

Theory of Mind, ToM: knowing that other people have different beliefs from us, and being able to predict them. One of the most influential theories of autism is that sufferers have a deficiency in ToM[110].

There are several problems with this theory. It is non-explanatory in that it exists at the same level of complexity as autism; and it does not account for the separability of the three disordered domains of autism (p.183). It does not account for deficits associated with autism that seem quite separate from ToM[1580], such as stereotypies and deficits in face recognition or empathy; or that precede any substantial ToM, such as gaze abnormalities occurring in the first year of life in relatives of autistic children[459]. It does not explain why some children with severe ID have, whereas others don't have, social separateness and excess stereotypies (p.185); and it doesn't account for clever autistic people who learn to pass ToM tests.

There are several ways to assess ToM:

In the Sally-Anne game one doll (Sally) hides chocolate in a basket and goes out of the room; then another doll (Anne) steals the chocolate. When Sally re-enters the room, the child is asked where Sally will look for the chocolate. If the child is consistently right, he has a developmental age of 4 or above, *and* good linguistic skills, *and* a ToM[185]. Failure in the task can be caused by problems in any of these areas (e.g. immaturity, language deficit, or autism).

More advanced *second order* ToM involves reasoning about other people's lies, white lies, misunderstandings, sarcasm, pretending, jokes, figures of speech, double bluffs, and forgetting (for the Happé test and age norms see[1177]).

Thought disorder: disorganisation of thinking. This is a graded phenomenon, but the term is usually reserved for severely abnormal cases, and then it is one of the categories of behaviour described as psychotic (p.537). It is most apparent in speech, especially if an unusual sequence of sentences is written down or recorded and the person (over a mental age of about 10) is given a chance to explain the sequence of his thoughts. If he can explain the sequence he is not thought disordered; but failure to do this can be due to ID, language disorder, p.145; unusual ideas, or thought disorder (in this approximate order of likelihood).

Some subtypes of thought disorder[1487] are flight of ideas (with connections made so fast they are difficult to follow); circumstantial thinking (in which the person repeatedly explains unnecessary details, i.e. fails to distinguish figure from ground, but eventually does answer the question); tangential thinking (in which one thought leads to another and the determining tendency is lost); and derailment (sudden switches to an unrelated topic, also called knight's move thinking). Some would also include illogicality, agramaticism, slowed thinking or speech devoid of ideas, perseveration (p.527), broadening of category boundaries, fantasy thinking or habitually thinking imaginatively about the future.

It is important to realise that many of these patterns are heard in normal immature speech. Such speech often includes loose associations and magical thinking, p.502. In addition, children only gradually acquire an awareness of the listener's needs[254]. Hence, identification of characteristic "thought disorder" patterns in children even up to age 16 cannot be taken as evidence of psychosis or schizophrenia[52].

Like psychosis, thought disorder is a broad umbrella term. It is usually used in describing people with severe mental illness such as mania, drug intoxication or schizophrenia, but similar speech patterns can also be heard in many other situations. These include immaturity (above); abnormal grammar in people following the rules of another language; the consistent following of idiosyncratic thought sequences in autism; abrupt changes of focus in partial seizures; specific language impairment; brain injury; and the "speaking in tongues" in some churches.

Thought disorder can be elicited in children by reading a standard story and asking open-ended questions about it.

Absurd questions ('Did the slithy 27 green?') can sometimes elicit a thought-disordered reply in people who are vulnerable to it, even if they are perfectly able to answer straightforward questions. This is not ethical if you already know the person is intermittently psychotic and he is upset by the question; but it may be useful in demonstrating lack of symptoms if no others can be found.

Throwing: p.103.

Thyroid: relevance to mental health problems in childhood is rare. Can contribute to ADHD ☂. Check heart rate (p.478) and consider blood test in fatigue, underachievement, slow growth. Goitre can accompany both hypo- and hyper-thyroidism. Benign transient abnormalities in thyroid hormones can be ruled out by repeating the blood test after 3–6 months[916]. See *hypothyroidism*, p.485; *hyperthyroidism*, p.484.

Thumb-sucking: a majority of children develop a non-nutritive sucking habit, which can be of thumb, finger or dummy. It is one of the self-soothing behaviours (p.61). Dummy-sucking usually finishes by nursery, and thumb-sucking by age 10. There can be slight effects on dental and face morphology. In regression: p.41. In autism: p.261. As a gratification phenomenon: p.115.

TIA (Transient ischaemic attacks): p.72.

Tic: p.101; distinguishing from compulsions, p.101; distinction from pseudo-tics, p.102; sensory tics, p.231; tics creating inattention, p.81.

Timecourse: the progression of a problem, typically over weeks to years. It has several aspects including age of onset, duration and fluctuations (which are typically altered by treatments). Monitoring the timecourse can be difficult but crucial: for example it can establish the cause of a problem and the effectiveness of treatment (p.365).

Standard words are used to describe phases of disease. Problems *progress* and eventually cross the impairment threshold (p.17).

They can *remit* either spontaneously or as a *response* to therapy. *Relapse* occurs after partial or brief improvement. *Recurrence* describes a new episode occuring well after the end of a previous episode, usually with an intervening gap of months or more.

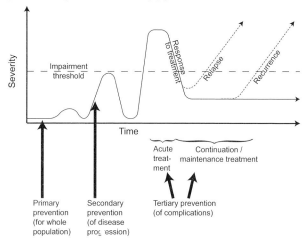

Figure 35. Terminology for timecourse of disease.

For various conditions with a wide range of timecourses: see pp.61–63; for various timecourses of intolerance see p.125; for multiple sclerosis, p.510. For shorter timecourses, i.e. minutes to days, see *crescendos*, p.77; experimental persona, p.240. For the interaction of long and short timecourses: in hyperactivity see p.79; in mood changes see p.306. For disorders that have characteristic ages of onset see p.43.

For figures depicting timecourse: for headaches see p.139; for symptoms in general see p.13.

Tinnitus: this is the perception of sound in the ears with no external source. Thirty per cent of healthy children hear it, up to twice a day[1082]. These children have heard the noises as long as they can remember, and so can't remember when it started. They assume that it is normal, and few are bothered by it.

It is usually impossible to know whether a non-verbal child has tinnitus, unless he makes the sound of a bee or indicates a bee via Makaton (p.502). At least half of children with other ear problems report tinnitus. See also *basilar migraine*, p.142; *hallucinations*, p.344.

Tinnitus is most often heard in quiet surroundings. It tends to be more of a problem if children have difficulty paying attention to their work anyway, or if they are miserable or feeling anxious about the significance of the tinnitus[41]. Like chronic pain, tinnitus grows through sensitisation (p.546) and/or fails to habituate properly[1707]. Patients affected with either have a greatly increased rate of depression, anxiety and hypochondriasis[752], some of which presumably predates the pain or the tinnitus.

TLE: temporal lobe epilepsy, p.562.
Toe-walking: see *Gait*, p.471.

Toilet: toilet-training, pp.339–340; fear/avoidance of toilets, pp.341, 153, 308; perverse effects of training, p.528; prolonged sitting on the toilet or going too often, p.340.

Tomboy: a girl who acts like a boy. The term is mainly used before puberty. Girls described as tomboys are generally somewhere between girls and boys in their playmate preference, choice of toys, and appearance; but they are judged to be just as attractive as other girls[87]. See *clothing*, p.441; frequency at various ages, p.267; effects of prenatal testosterone in girls, p.554. Distinguish from *Gender Identity Disorder*, p.267.

TORCH: see *infections*, p.490.
Touching: p.132.
Tourette syndrome: p.102.

Toxic substances: this includes all substances that are harmful to the body (the term *toxin* means such substances that are produced biologically). Many nutrients can become toxic if taken in excess (list on p.327). Medicines can be toxic due to overdose, interaction with other medicines, or idiosyncratic metabolism (see e.g. serotonin syndrome, p.548; neuroleptic malignant syndrome, p.514; cytochromes, p.450; insulin overdose, p.451). See alcohol and illicit drugs, p.257; heavy metals, p.330; traditional remedies, p.448; water intoxication, p.338. Occasionally pica is toxic, p.336.

The reason for ingestion can be deliberate self-harm (p.317), accident (greatest from age 1 to 3, p.331: consider poor supervision, p.274 or lack of safe storage / childproof containers), deliberate poisoning by others (pp.282, 206), or risk-taking (p.539) as when a group of teenagers share a bottle of vodka.

The most common substances causing death in children under 6 are analgesics (especially paracetamol/acetaminophen), cleaning products, iron tablets, oil or paint thinner, antidepressants, insecticides, anticonvulsants and cocaine[1460].

Intoxication usually means a temporary change in mental state caused by ingestion, especially of alcohol or illicit drugs.

Toxic substances in pregnancy
Cigarette smoking is correlated with slightly lower birth weight – but most such children's difficulties are not due to the cigarettes themselves but to other factors in the mother's life such as background disadvantage and a less positive attitude to child-rearing[1045]. Prenatal maternal smoking is usually followed by postnatal smoking (by mother and/or father), which increases the risk of respiratory tract infections, asthma and ear infections[411]. See also foetal alcohol syndrome, p.467; foetal valproate syndrome, p.572; oxidative stress[1148].

At least 10% of pregnant women take illicit substances during pregnancy. This does not cause any significant increase in malformations[1652], but use of cocaine causes low birth weight and preterm delivery; and use of opiates during pregnancy probably reduces birth weight slightly and can cause transient withdrawal symptoms after delivery[1435]. Smoking, drinking of alcohol, and illicit drug use in pregnancy tend to co-occur and all are much more common in women who are experiencing domestic violence[1042] or not attending prenatal checks.

TPN: total parenteral nutrition. See tube feeding, p.333.
Transient ischaemic attacks (TIAs): p.72.

Transition[al] object: at least half of infants become specially fond of one (or a few) toys in infancy, and many find this comforts them when lonely or sad right through adolescence (see self-soothing, p.61). Most often it is a teddy, doll, blanket, or pillow, but in teenage boys it is just as likely to be another (non-fluffy) object[468] such as a gift or phone. The first such "non-me" possession in toddlerhood may help the child to imagine that mother is present, and help him to create an internal working model of her.

Transmitters: p.398.

Trauma: there are many kinds of trauma, including abuse, p.271; bereavement, p.430; birth trauma, p.437; head injury, p.477; parental separation, illness, natural disaster and financial problems. Distinctive, salient, brief events are usually recalled exceptionally clearly. Children exposed to longer-lasting or more numerous trauma may be more likely to develop memory deficits (see *hippocampus*, p.478) but findings in this area are inconsistent[1644] and in some cases differences may have preceded the trauma. Although most children have surprisingly few long-term adverse effects following trauma[1546], effects in a low-resilience minority are severe[269] (see p.541). See also *Post-Traumatic Stress Disorder*, p.532; *amnesia*, p.421; *false memory*, p.465.

Traumatic brain injury: see *Head injury*, p.477.

Treatments: treatments are largely excluded from this book, but they do of course have close connections with assessment.

Overlap between assessment and treatment
Obviously, most treatments are based on a view of the underlying cause(s) of the problem. The view can be scientifically based, as is the emphasis of this book; or culturally based: see *religion*, p.541; *nutrition*, p.327.

Treatment planning is often a part of assessment. For example, an assessor often focuses on problem areas that are most treatable. Treatment decisions such as whether it is safe for the child to go home, are based in part on assessments of risk. The system of diagnosis called OPD-2 (p.519) includes aspects of treatment suitability as part of the assessment.

A good assessment can itself be therapeutic, in several ways. It can organise thinking, put things in context, either normalise or provide a label; make the patient aware that there are treatments available; and make the patient feel supported and understood[1362]. A confident conclusion to the assessment probably contributes to treatment efficacy[1603]. The effect of a new diagnosis on self-identity is often positive (p.237); and it can bring a feeling of understanding, and access to information, social support, and sometimes funds.

Treatment failure / treatment resistance
Knowing that good treatments have failed is an important contribution to assessment. It may indicate an inadequate assessment; treating symptoms rather than causes; addressing predisposing or precipitating rather than perpetuating or protective factors (pp.394, 526); inadequate treatment; use of medicines that lose some effectiveness (such as benzodiazepines, p.430; and sometimes antipsychotics, p.422); comorbidity; poor adherence to the treatment; medicine interactions; abnormal metabolism (see cytochromes, p.450); a transition to pseudo-symptoms (p.359) or

other disorder; secondary gain (p.471: even a need to rebel); or that there is a undetected physical disease underlying the mental state[898].

Side-effects of treatments
In clinical practice one frequently meets patients who have undergone treatments, especially expensive private treatments, with neither the seller nor the parents able to judge the evidence properly.

It has been suggested, controversially, that side-effects of talking therapies should be considered as carefully as side-effects of medication[1174]. Parallels between medicines and talking therapies include non-specific therapeutic effects; dependence; "withdrawal effects" at the end of talking therapies; and temporary worsening of symptoms during exposure therapies.

Some treatments affect life-long *traits*. The effects are usually small and temporary (there are more likely to be large positive effects if a substantial disorder is effectively treated). It is not usually practical to measure these traits both on and off medication (for methods see p.33). Hence the choice of whether to administer tests on or off medicines depends on whether one wants to discover the child's potential or his underlying need. (a) The clearest example is the temporary effect of many medicines on IQ. For example, IQ scores are typically elevated a few points by stimulants (e.g.[567,1288], especially on coding tasks and especially in non-anxious children[186]; improving visuospatial function more than verbal function[570]; and different subtests have different optimal doses[1237]) as well as perhaps by other "cognitive enhancers"[573]; and lowered a few points by medicines that reduce attention, such as antipsychotics and antihypertensives[872,1513]. (b) Similarly, clinical experience suggests that scores on tests of sociability (ADOS, p.183) are improved by medicines that improve mood, and can be worsened by stimulants.

For some side-effects of medications, see SSRI, p.552; antiepileptics, p.422; antipsychotics, p.422; stimulants, p.555. For trials of medication as a part of assessment, see p.374. For difficulties in the mapping from diagnosis to treatment, see *ideograph*, p.487; epilepsy, p.73. See also *iatrogenic*, p.486.

Tremor: p.61.

Triplet repeat inherited disorders: some of these appear at earlier ages (and more severely) in children than in their parents:
    iv)   Huntington's chorea, p.482
    v)   myotonic dystrophy (type 2 can come to attention any time in childhood or adulthood, with muscle pain, stiffness, fatigue, or lower limb weakness)[380]
    vi)   hereditary ataxias, e.g. Friedreich's ataxia, p.92
    vii) Fragile X[974] (p.468).

Triple X syndrome: One of the sex chromosome disorders (p.548). It usually remains undiagnosed because it is mild, often with long legs, problems with language or auditory development, and some difficulty in long-term relationships[1201]. IQs are somewhat below the general population, averaging 81[138].

Truant: p.217.

TS: Tourette syndrome, p.101; Turner syndrome, p.570; tuberous sclerosis, p.569; or trans-sexual.

TSH: thyroid stimulating hormone. See thyroid, p.564; diagram, p.531.
Tube-feeding: p.333.

Tuberculosis (TB): infection with *Mycobacterium tuberculosis*. This can affect behaviour through systemic effects of infection (such as malaise); by local effects on any body system (such as lungs or joints); or if it has reached within the CNS, by direct effects on CNS function (the brain or spinal cord becomes involved in 1% of cases; this is especially common in small children). Symptoms are very varied, but the commonest symptoms are failure to thrive, loss of weight, poor appetite, headache and abdominal pain, neck stiffness, seizures, cranial nerve palsies, hemiplegia, confusion and coma. An exposure history is essential: Two thirds have had recent contact with someone known to be infected with TB. Many tests exist, none of them reliable in children, and can be considered depending on urgency and available resources: chest X-ray, sputum microscopy, CSF microscopy, tuberculin skin test (TST). Detection is difficult and diagnostic algorithms are available[1607].

Tuberous Sclerosis: A genetic disorder affecting 1 in 6000: 90% develop epilepsy, and many other developmental problems are common, including ID, autism, and various neurological symptoms. External signs include angiofibromas in a butterfly-shaped distribution on the nose and cheeks, fingernail fibromas (p.466), hypopigmented macules, and shagreen patches (thick dimpled skin usually on the back) [338]. Regular paediatric review is needed because of the risk of developing internal tubers, the monitoring of epilepsy, and the possibility of medication developments[472].

Tumours: many parents worry that regressions may have been caused by a tumour. Symptoms of an actual tumour can be focal or diffuse[1637]. Diffuse symptoms include headache (especially postural or changing, see pp.139); seizures (p.73 and see[1637]); early morning nausea and vomiting; lethargy, deteriorating performance in school, mood change, irritability and, in infants, increased head circumference and bulging fontanelle. Focal signs include ataxia, nystagmus, cranial nerve palsies, focal peripheral weakness or sensory changes, visual field defects, Parinaud syndrome (failure of upgaze with other signs[1637]), aphasia, growth slowing, and paraneoplastic symptoms (p.524). Tumours usually cause steady progression of symptoms. See also paraneoplastic effects, p.524; hydrocephalus, p.482; craniopharyngioma, p.446.

Malignancy and cancer mean tumours with the ability to jump to other body areas. When children are diagnosed with cancer, the mother's coping depends on her social supports and her problem-solving ability[421]. Malignant cancers with rate per million children under 14[635]:

- Leukaemia: 41
- CNS: 29 (astroglia 17, PNET 6, ependymoma 2)
- Other: neuroblastoma 9, non-Hodgkin's lymphoma 8, Wilm's 8, Hodgkin's lymphoma 6, rhabdomyosarcoma 5, embryonal rhabdomyosarcoma 3, germ cell 4, retinoblastoma 4, osteosarcoma 4, Ewing's sarcoma 4.

When parents have cancer, the main effects on the children occur through parental depression or poor family communication[1718]; see also *bereavement*, p.430. Inherited disorders with cancer predisposition include polyposis; neurophakomatoses, p.514; DNA repair defects, p.454; overgrowth syndromes such as Beckwith-

Wiedemann, p.429; Multiple Endocrine Neoplasia, and many others[1554]. Children of families with these conditions need detailed specialist follow-up (e.g.[1145]).

Especially in the tropics, some intracranial growths are infections.

Turner syndrome: 45,XO phenotype: females with short stature, webbed neck, gonadal dysgenesis, and hearing loss. IQs are somewhat below the general population, averaging 85[138]. About a third are mosaics (p.509).

Turn-taking: a skill generally acquired between ages 3 and 6, and seen in queuing and in games. Poor turn-taking is listed in DSM as a symptom of impulsivity (pp.489, 387). The ability to wait in a particular queue depends on knowledge of social norms and sanctions; plus the balance of self-entertainment skills, desire to be with someone in the queue, desire to conform, desire to run around or explore, and desire to get the thing being queued for (e.g. if hungry may jump to the front of a food queue, but if not hungry will leave the queue).

Twitching: p.101.
UECr: urea, electrolytes and creatinine (kidney function tests).
Unaccompanied minors: see *refugees*, p.540.

Unconscious: this has several meanings (some of which are listed below). See also dissociation, p.453; unconscious triggers, p.63; difficulties of classification, p.359; defence mechanisms, p.305.
- Lack of responding (as in coma, p.97; or sleep, p.200). These can also be partial, i.e. *semiconscious*.
- Non-conscious: immediate unintentional processes that do not usually reach awareness. Examples include breathing; regulation of hormone levels (p.531); and the mirror system (p.507).
- Non-declarative, i.e. non-recallable learning (p.37)
- Information that has been explicitly available but he is not currently aware of. Such information influences responses without being explicitly recallable (see repression, p.421). This is important in priming of recall, and in attitudes (p.425) that influence behaviour even though the person is apparently unaware of them.
- Some therapists take the view that we each have a "dynamic unconscious", that is constantly active and processing information[150]. A version of this posits that *all* processing is performed by an "unconscious mind", and what we call consciousness is just a mechanism for revealing a small portion of this. However, while there is no doubt that there are nonconscious processes and influences, there is no evidence that they are sufficiently integrated, continuous, independent, cognitive, symbolic, or aware to deserve the term *mind*, nor indeed sufficiently "striving" to justify the term *dynamic*[438]. The stronger versions contradict current understanding, e.g. of the gradual fading of most traumatic memories that are not brought to consciousness ([210,For further discussion see 807]).
- The dynamics of a group, especially if the individual is not aware of why interactions are proceeding as they are.

Unemployment: this can affect parents or teenagers.

Parental unemployment lowers the mood of single parents, often leading to more frequent punishments and some depression in children[1051]. Among the adolescents with financial concerns, there is increased anxiety and lower self-esteem.

For the relationship between post-school teenage unemployment and criminal behaviour, see p.446. See also work, p.575; NEET, p.512.

Unlearning: this has several closely related meanings: replacing an obsolete fact with a new one; reducing the size or certainty of a prediction (e.g. learning that something that was important is less so now); or a subtype of extinction (p.463) that acts when the memory has not yet been consolidated[843]. Contrast forgeting, p.468.

A specific deficit in unlearning aversive stimuli may cause some PTSD (see conditioned aversion, p.127). Unlearning can also be prevented by cognitive dissonance, or by a sense of duty (e.g. "It would be very naughty to disbelieve my teacher"; "If mother could lie to me once should I ever believe her? who could I trust?").

Autistic people often seem especially slow to unlearn. For example, an autistic boy learned to say "six" when asked his age, and never managed to change this to seven, eight, etc. Formal testing of autistic children shows no deficit in motor learning or unlearning[560], so the apparent fixity presumably results from their having practised their old skills so much more than the new ones; or because they actually like them more than any available reward for changing.

Unsociability: p.181.
Unwanted behaviours: p.353.

"Unwanted child": pregnancies that are either mistimed, or unwanted at conception, are *associated with* prenatal and postnatal maternal behaviours that adversely affect the child's development – but the unwantedness itself does not cause these problems[794].

Urea-cycle disorders: a group of several genetic disorders. They typically appear in the first few months of life, but the *late onset urea cycle disorders* can also present later in childhood with chronic symptoms suggesting ADHD, autism, ID, language disorder, psychomotor retardation, agitation, psychosis, or confusion[1137,1455]. These are important to recognise as they respond better to dietary than to pharmacological treatment. The diagnosis is more likely if there are also digestive problems, nausea or meat refusal. There is often an identifiable trigger such as starvation (p.553), dehydration, or variation in protein supply either externally (weaning or varying the diet) or internally (infections, surgery, or chemotherapy) [661,1137], or the introduction of valproate[408]. Look for previous recurrent neurological "accidents" wrongly attributed to other causes; extreme metabolic upset perimenstrually[189]; but not for kidney stones. Measure the blood ammonia, liver enzymes and clotting. Specific disorders[1137]:

- OTC (ornithine transcarbamylase) deficiency[1347] is the commonest urea-cycle defect. It is X-linked and the partial form seen in girls can be as severe as that in boys[464,1137]. Even the common heterozygotes for OTC deficiency can reduce their risk of hyperammonaemic crises by limiting their protein intake[464].
- ASS (arginosuccinate synthetase) deficiency
- ASL (arginosuccinate lyase) deficiency

- Very rare: arginase deficiency, NAGS (N-acetylglutamate synthase) deficiency, CPS (carbamoylphosphatase synthetase) deficiency.

URTI: Upper respiratory tract infection.
UTI: Urinary tract infection.

Utilisation behaviour: simple automatic behaviours such as grasping or handling objects, apparently triggered by aspects of the environment, and occurring without high-level control[53]. They are object-appropriate but not context-appropriate. These occur more in ADHD[1159], where they are probably the basis of some fidgeting; and also in frontal dementias[947] (see *frontal signs*, p.469). Some imitation movements triggered by the *mirror system* (p.507) may be similar to utilisation behaviours except for having social triggers[947].

Vacuolated lymphocytes: this is a cheap (but labour-intensive) first-line screening test when metabolic disease is suspected[38]. Abnormal accumulations of metabolic byproducts appear as vacuoles, or holes, of varying size, colour, and distribution within cells. This can be conveniently seen in white blood cells.

This forms a screen for mucopolysaccharidoses (p.501), Niemann-Pick disease (p.552), glycogen storage disorders (p.556) and various other rare metabolic disorders[38]. In most centres it is being replaced by a white cell enzymes screening battery.

Valproate: a medication used to treat epilepsy, bipolar disorder and migraines. It can induce polycystic ovary syndrome (p.531) in a small proportion of women[779].

Foetal valproate syndrome: a wide range of major developmental anomalies is seen in babies of mothers who used the anti-epileptic medication valproate during pregnancy[846]. The rate of 14% of exposed mothers is several times the rate seen in controls or with the other anti-epileptics[847]. Effects are dose-related, and can include spina bifida (p.551), cardiac and skeletal abnormalities. This may be due to valproate's anti-folate action[1197], as folate deficiency can cause neural tube defects (p.513). However the effect is not always avoidable by folate supplementation; and some of the neurodevelopmental problems in these children are inherited from their epileptic mothers.

Vandalism: damaging property. About 30% of 12-year-olds report having done this, rising to 50% by age 21[1037], though the severity varies enormously. It is often an expression of contempt or envy or protest, but it can also be an incidental result of childish experimentation or competition ("who can break the highest window in that building?").

Vanishing white matter disease: see *leukodystrophies*, p.498.
VCFS: see *Velocardiofacial syndrome*.

Vegan diet: a diet without any animal products, i.e. without meat, poultry, fish, eggs and dairy products[836]. The health of vegans is usually comparable to that of omnivores and vegetarians, but there is increased risk of B_{12} deficiency, p.329; and hypocalcaemia, p.485. See *micronutrient deficiencies*, p.327; *diet*, p.452.

VEOS: very early onset schizophrenia. See *schizophrenia*, p.543.

Velocardiofacial syndrome (also called diGeorge syndrome, VCFS): the most common microdeletion syndrome and the most common known genetic risk factor for schizophrenia (apart from having an affected identical twin or two schizophrenic parents). Its most common manifestations are heart defects (mild or severe), nasal speech (caused by cleft palate, p.440), mild ID, autism[1692], and seizures (caused by hypocalcaemia). Prepubertally there is increased ADHD and anxiety[613]; postpubertally there is increase in depression and psychotic symptoms[596,1670]. Affected people need to be screened for heart defects and hypoparathyroidism (p.525).

VEP: visual evoked potential, p.462.

Video games: highly efficient instruments for uninterrupted play (and potentially teaching), because they include variety, extrinsic as well as intrinsic rewards (e.g. magic cloaks and a sense of mastery), instant feedback, repetition, and rapidly adjusting difficulty levels[553]. Massively multiplayer online games (MMOGs) are more often damagingly attractive than games on a home computer, because of the social interaction, competition with real people, and the *persistent world* where events continue to occur even while the player is offline. Massively multiplayer online role-playing games (MMORPGs) are the most popular of all, perhaps because of the escapism (enhanced by avatars). This array of attractive characteristics creates irresistible superstimuli (p.558) though there is also a cumulation which can reasonably be called behavioural addiction (p.260).

See also indicators of severity, p.260; altruism, p.420; violence, p.289; internet, p.492.

Vineland tests: p.419.
Violence: p.289.

Viruses: here are some of the most important (see also *infections*, p.490; *MMR*, p.508).
   i)   Measles can cause encephalomyelitis or, months to years later, SSPE, p.557. Immunisable.
   ii) Mumps causes tender swelling of the parotid glands and sometimes the testes. Occasionally causes meningitis or encephalitis[1259] (p.461). Immunisable.
   iii) Rubella, see TORCH, p.490. Especially if infected in the first trimester of pregnancy, there is increased risk of miscarriage, stillbirth, and defects in heart, eyes, ears and brain. Immunisable.
   iv) Polio, a virus that kills motor neurons. It can cause weakness, death, or lifelong asymmetrical paralysis, most commonly of the legs. Immunisable.
   v)   HIV, p.479.
   vi) Herpes virus family, p.478.

Visual problems: p.133.
Vitamins: see *nutrients*, p.327.
VLCFA: very long chain fatty acids, see p.526.
VLDL: very low density lipoprotein (see abetalipoproteinaemia, p.417)

VMA: vanillyl mandelic acid, a metabolite of catecholamines (dopamine, epinephrine and norepinephrine). It is usually measured in 24-hour urine samples.

Voice: see *speech problems*, p.147.
Von Hippel-Lindau disease: p.514.
VP shunt: ventriculoperitoneal shunt (a treatment for hydrocephalus).

VP discrepancy: p.28.
WAIS: Wechsler Adult Intelligence Scale, p.59.
Wandering off: p.209.

Warmth: an aspect of

- temperament, p.561. In some children the impression of warmth can be misleading, and if excessive can lead to exploitation, e.g. in Williams syndrome[1018].
- relationships, and as one example of this it is a necessary aspect of parenting (p.189). Physical warmth has a soothing effect, and infants seek it[653]. See also *love*, p.501.
- individual social exchanges, e.g. smiling, speaking gently, praising, nodding, agreeing. Lack of warmth, e.g. in negative expressed emotion (p.512) adversely affects children and adolescents, especially those with other difficulties as well.

Washing machines: p.104.
WASI: Wechsler Abbreviated Scale of Intelligence, p.59.
Weakness: p.87.
Weapons, interest in: p.245.

Wernicke: (a) Wernicke's area of cerebral cortex, p.145; figure, p.513; and in disconnection syndromes, p.444.

(b) !! Wernicke-Korsakoff syndrome results from prolonged dietary deficiency of vitamin B1 (p.328), *when followed by* unaccustomed carbohydrates. It is rare in children but can follow starvation (p.553), anorexia[1249], or highly restricted diets (as in autism, exclusive rice-eating, or defective infant food / parenteral nutrition). The syndrome consists of Wernicke's encephalopathy (confusion, ataxia and nystagmus) and subsequently Korsakoff psychosis (anterograde and retrograde amnesia with confabulation, p.443). MRI is necessary to confirm[1826].

Wetting: night-time, p.339; daytime, p.340.
Wheels: p.104.
Whining: p.315.
White cell enzymes: p.572.

White matter: areas of the brain filled with axons connecting the cellular, grey, areas. The white colour comes from myelin, p.510.

Myelination of individual regions occurs at very different ages: motor roots during gestation; sensory roots until 6 months postnatally; cerebellar peduncles until 4 years; the reticular formation and cerebral association areas into adolescence.[1805] The left arcuate fasciculus, connecting temporal and frontal cortex, develops steadily until at least age 15, presumably contributing to the maturation of speech[1232]. In contrast, the development of the internal capsule, carrying motor fibres among others, is largely complete by age 6, reflecting early motor maturation.

Though individual white matter disorders are rare, their overall prevalence is about 1 in 6000. The white matter of the brain can develop incorrectly, as in leukodystrophies, p.498; or agenesis of the corpus callosum, p.445, or can be damaged later, as in multiple sclerosis, p.510; B_{12} deficiency, p.329; biotinidase deficiency; and in autoimmune thyroid disease (for other causes see[1659]). See also *connectivity*, p.444; *stroke*, p.556; *ciliopathies*, p.440.

WIAT: Wechsler Individual Achievement Test, p.51.
Williams syndrome: p.177.

Wilson's disease: genetic disease of excess copper, also called hepatolenticular degeneration. Symptoms include tiredness, confusion, catatonia, psychosis, depression, bleeding, tremors. Signs include dystonia / parkinsonism, myoclonus/spasticity, Kayser-Fleischer ring on iris (may not be visible without slit-lamp), liver inflammation. Tests: LFT, plasma copper and caeruloplasmin (or 24-hour urinary copper).

Winnicott, Donald: introduced the ideas of good-enough parenting, p.190; transition object, p.567; and the Squiggle Game, p.378.

WISC: Wechsler Intelligence Scale for Children, p.59.

Withdrawn: consider autism, p.183; abuse, p.271; depression, p.309; sulking, p.557; masturbation, p.115.

WMS: Wechsler Memory Scale, p.38.

Wolfram syndrome: also called DIDMOAD as an acronym for diabetes insipidus, p.338; diabetes mellitus, p.451; optic atrophy, and low-frequency deafness. It can also cause ID, peripheral neuropathy, and ataxia. Heterozygotes have increased risk of psychiatric disorders.

WORD: Wechsler Objective Reading Dimensions, p.51.
Word-finding difficulty: p.149.

Work: this term can be used in a very broad sense of activities that produce obvious benefit for the family; or can be restricted to regular paid employment outside the family (see also unemployment, p.570.) The problem of working children "is better described as a normal part of the life of the relatively poor in all societies"[1745]. Child labour is most likely to impair a child's health and development if it prevents the child going to school, or if the child is not protected from physical hardship[1745].

In poorer countries, parental unemployment substantially increases the likelihood of adolescents leaving school to take jobs to support the family[435]. The younger children in a family are typically spared from this because they cannot earn as much as their older siblings[463].

Child labour laws regulate the types of work a child may do, and specify a maximum number of hours per day, which typically differs between school days and holidays. The laws typically say nothing regarding household work. In the Netherlands, and presumably in most other countries, the majority of teenagers at some time work for money in ways that contravene child labour laws – usually by choice in order to earn money for themselves[1745].

Working memory (WM): this is defined to include not only storage but also the ability to *manipulate* information in memory, i.e. it is not a subset or type of memory. The standard view of WM incorporates a visuospatial sketchpad, a phonological loop, and a central executive[83]. See the WM subscale of IQ tests, p.36; brief tests of WM, p.399; WM deficits giving the impression of inattention, p.82; role of cerebellum, p.437; spatial WM, p.512.

Formally, short-term memory (STM, p.555) is different in that STM does not do any processing[83] – but in practice the terms are used interchangeably. See also *memory*, p.37.

Worms: see pinworm, p.82; whipworm, p.47; schistosomiasis, p.543; eating worms, p.336. Children in endemic areas are often infected from the age of weaning, and remain affected with several types of worm simultaneously[427,844].

Writing: p.53. See also use of written interviews for shy children, p.23; handwriting or not writing as a form of redaction, p.415.

Worster-Drought syndrome: p.90.
W-posture: p.483
WPPSI: Wechsler Preschool and Primary Scale of Intelligence, p.59.
Writer's cramp: see *Dystonia*, p.458.
Xeroderma pigmentosum: p.454.
XO: Turner syndrome, p.570 or xanthine oxidase, p.555.
Yerkes-Dodson law: p.40.
Young offenders: see *Criminality*, p.446.
Zombie effect: p.310.
Zoning out: p.75.
Zoophilia: p.268.

References

1. Abell, S. C., Wood, W. & Liebman, S. J. Children's Human Figure Drawings as measures of intelligence: The comparative validity of three scoring systems. *J. Psychoeduc. Assess.* **19**, 204-215 (2001).
2. Abikoff, H., Courtney, M. E., Szeibel, P. J. & Koplewicz, H. S. The effects of auditory stimulation on the arithmetic performance of children with ADHD and nondisabled children. *J. Learn. Disabil.* **29**, 238-246 (1996).
3. Abrams, D., Wetherell, M., Cochrane, S., Hogg, M. A. & Turner, J. C. Knowing what to think by knowing who you are: self-categorization and the nature of norm formation, conformity and group polarization. *Br. J Soc. Psychol* **29 (Pt 2)**, 97-119 (1990).
4. Accardo, P., Caul, J. & Whitman, B. Excessive water drinking. A marker of caretaker interaction disturbance. *Clin. Pediatr. (Phila)* **28**, 416-418 (1989).
5. Achenbach, T. *Manual for the CBCL/4-18 and 1991 Profile.* University of Vermont, Dept of Psychiatry, Burlington, VT (1991).
6. Achenbach, T. M. & Edelbrock, C. S. The classification of child psychopathology: a review and analysis of empirical efforts. *Psychol Bull.* **85**, 1275-1301 (1978).
7. Ackil, J. K. & Zaragoza, M. S. Memorial consequences of forced confabulation: Age differences in susceptibility to false memories. *Developmental Psychology* **34**, 1358-1372 (1998).
8. Adams, M., Kutcher, S., Antoniw, E. & Bird, D. Diagnostic utility of endocrine and neuroimaging screening tests in first-onset adolescent psychosis. *J Am Acad. Child Adolesc. Psychiatry* **35**, 67-73 (1996).
9. Adams, S. J. *et al.* Neuropsychiatric morbidity in focal epilepsy. *Br. J. Psychiatry* **192**, 464-469 (2008).
10. Addolorato, G. *et al.* Affective and psychiatric disorders in celiac disease. *Dig. Dis* **26**, 140-148 (2008).
11. Adelson, P. D. & Kochanek, P. M. Head injury in children. *J Child Neurol* **13**, 2-15 (1998).
12. Adler, L. E. *et al.* Schizophrenia, sensory gating, and nicotinic receptors. *Schizophr. Bull.* **24**, 189-202 (1998).
13. Adler, R. H. *et al.* How not to miss a somatic needle in the haystack of chronic pain. *J. Psychosom. Res* **42**, 499-505 (1997).
14. Adolph, K. E., Joh, A. S., Franchak, J. M., Ishak, S. & Gill, S. V. Flexibility in the development of action in Morsella, E., Bargh, J. A. & Gollwitzer, P. M. (eds.), *Oxford Handbook of Human Action.*pp. 399-426 (Oxford University Press, New York,2008).
15. Ahmed, A. O., Green, B. A., McCloskey, M. S. & Berman, M. E. Latent structure of intermittent explosive disorder in an epidemiological sample. *J. Psychiatr. Res.* **44**, 663-672 (2010).
16. Ahmed, F. Vitamin A deficiency in Bangladesh: a review and recommendations for improvement. *Public Health Nutrition* **2**, 1-14 (1998).
17. Aicardi, J. *Diseases of the Nervous System in Childhood.* Cambridge University Press, Cambridge (1998).
18. Akcam, T. *et al.* Voice changes after androgen therapy for hypogonadotrophic hypogonadism. *The Laryngoscope* **114**, 1587-1591 (2004).
19. Akiskal, H. S. Classification, diagnosis and boundaries of bipolar disorders: a review in Maj, M., Akiskal, H. S., Lopez-Ibor, J. J. & Sartorius, N. (eds.), *Bipolar Disorder.*pp. 1-52 (John Wiley & Sons,2002).
20. Alaggia, R. An ecological analysis of child sexual abuse disclosure: considerations for child and adolescent mental health. *J Can. Acad. Child Adolesc. Psychiatry* **19**, 32-39 (2010).
21. Albanese, A. & Lalli, S. Is this dystonia? *Movement Dis.* **24**, 1725-1731 (2009).
22. Aldgate, J. & McIntosh, M. *Time well spent: a study of well-being and children's daily activities.* Social Work Inspection Agency, Edinburgh (2006).
23. Alexander, G. M., Wilcox, T. & Farmer, M. E. Hormone-behavior associations in early infancy. *Horm. Behav* **56**, 498-502 (2009).
24. Ali-Khan, S. E., Daar, A. S., Shuman, C., Ray, P. N. & Scherer, S. W. Whole genome scanning: resolving clinical diagnosis and management amidst complex data. *Pediatr. Res* **66**, 357-363 (2009).
25. Alkire, S. & Santos, M. E. *Acute multidimensional poverty: A new index for developing countries.* Oxford Poverty and Human Development Initiative, Oxford (2010).
26. Allen, L. H. The nutrition CRSP: what is marginal malnutrition, and does it affect human function? *Nutr Rev,* **51**, 255-267 (1993).
27. Allen, P. M., Gilchrist, J. M. & Hollis, J. Use of visual search in the assessment of pattern-related visual stress (PRVS) and its alleviation by colored filters. *Invest Ophthalmol. Vis. Sci.* **49**, 4210-4218 (2008).
28. Alloway, T. P., Gathercole, S. E., Kirkwood, H. & Elliott, J. The cognitive and behavioral characteristics of children with low working memory. *Child Dev.* **80**, 606-621 (2009).
29. Alloy, L. B., Just, N. & Panzarella, C. Attributional style, daily life events, and hopelessness depression: Subtype validation by prospective variability and specificity of symptoms. *Cog. Ther. Res.* **21**, 321-344 (1997).
30. Almond, D. & Mazumder, B. *Health Capital and the Prenatal Environment: The Effect of Maternal Fasting During Pregnancy.* National Bureau of Economic Research, Cambridge,MA (2008).
31. Amador, X. F. & David, A. S. *Insight and psychosis: Awareness of illness in schizophrenia and related disorders.* Oxford University Press, Oxford (2004).
32. Ambelas, A. Life events and mania. A special relationship? *Br. J. Psychiatry* **150**, 235-240 (1987).
33. American Psychiatric Association *Diagnostic and statistical manual of mental disorders, 4th edn, Text Revision (DSM-IV-TR).* American Psychiatric Press Inc., Arlington (2000).
34. Amiri, K., Hagerman, R. J. & Hagerman, P. J. Fragile X Associated Tremor/Ataxia Syndrome: An Aging Face of the Fragile X Gene. *Arch. Neurol.* **65**, 19-25 (2008).
35. Amsel, A. Frustration theory--many years later. *Psychol. Bull.* **112**, 396-399 (1992).
36. Andari, E. *et al.* Promoting social behavior with oxytocin in high-functioning autism spectrum disorders. *Proc. Natl. Acad. Sci. U. S. A* **107**, 4389-4394 (2010).
37. Anderson, C. A. Temperature and aggression: effects on quarterly, yearly, and city rates of violent and nonviolent crime. *J. Pers. Soc. Psychol* **52**, 1161-1173 (1987).
38. Anderson, G., Smith, V. V., Malone, M. & Sebire, N. J. Blood film examination for vacuolated lymphocytes in the diagnosis of metabolic disorders; retrospective experience of more than 2,500 cases from a single centre. *J Clin Pathol* **58**, 1305-1310 (2005).
39. Anderson, G. M. Conceptualizing autism: the role for emergence. *J. Am. Acad. Child Adolesc. Psychiatry* **48**, 688-691 (2009).
40. Anderson, K. L. Perpetrator or victim? Relationships between intimate partner violence and well-being. *J. Marriage and Family* **64**, 851-863 (2002).
41. Andersson, G. & McKenna, L. The role of cognition in tinnitus. *Acta Otolaryngol. (Stockh).* **126**, 39-43 (2006).

42. Andrade, C. & Srihari, B. S. A preliminary survey of rhinotillexomania in an adolescent sample. *J. Clin. Psychiatry* **62**, 426-431 (2001).

43. Andreasen, N. C. *Scale for the assessment of positive symptoms*. University of Iowa, Iowa City (1984).

44. Anglin, R. E., Rosebush, P. I. & Mazurek, M. F. Treating Psychiatric Illness in Patients With Mitochondrial Disorders. *Psychosomatics* **51**, 179 (2010).

45. Angold, A., Costello, E. J., Farmer, E. M., Burns, B. J. & Erkanli, A. Impaired but undiagnosed. *J. Am. Acad. Child Adolesc. Psychiatry* **38**, 129-137 (1999).

46. Annett, M. Patterns of hand preference for pairs of actions and the classification of handedness. *Br. J. Psychol.* **100**, 491-500 (2009).

47. Anon. Obsessional slowness. *Br. Med. J* **5921**, 685-686 (1974).

48. Antrop, I., Roeyers, H., Van Oost, P. & Buysse, A. Stimulation seeking and hyperactivity in children with ADHD. *J. Child Psychol. Psychiatry* **41**, 225-231 (2000).

49. Apgar, V. The newborn (Apgar) scoring system. *Pediatr Clin North Am* **13**, 645-650 (1966).

50. Applebaum, J., Cohen, H., Matar, M., Rabia, Y. A. & Kaplan, Z. Symptoms of posttraumatic stress disorder after ritual female genital surgery among Bedouin in Israel: Myth or Reality? *Primary Care Companion to J. Clin. Psychiatry* **10**, 453-456 (2008).

51. Arbib, M. A. From grasp to language: embodied concepts and the challenge of abstraction. *J Physiol Paris* **102**, 4-20 (2008).

52. Arboleda, C. & Holzman, P. S. Thought disorder in children at risk for psychosis. *Arch Gen. Psychiatry* **42**, 1004-1013 (1985).

53. Archibald, S. J., Mateer, C. A. & Kerns, K. A. Utilization behavior: clinical manifestations and neurological mechanisms. *Neuropsychol. Rev.* **11**, 117-130 (2001).

54. Ardila, A. & Rosselli, M. Acalculia and dyscalculia. *Neuropsychol. Rev.* **12**, 179-231 (2002).

55. Arendt, M. *et al*. Testing the self-medication hypothesis of depression and aggression in cannabis-dependent subjects. *Psychol Med.* **37**, 935-945 (2007).

56. Argyle, M. & Dean, J. Eye-contact, distance and affiliation. *Sociometry* **28**, 289-304 (1965).

57. Ariely, D. *Predictably irrational*. HarperCollins, London (2008).

58. Ariely, D., Bracha, A. & Meier, S. Doing good or doing well? Image motivation and monetary incentives in behaving prosocially. *Am. Econ. Rev.* (2009).

59. Arnold, G. L., Griebel, M. L., Porterfield, M. & Brewster, M. Pyruvate carboxylase deficiency: Report of a case and additional evidence for the "Mild" phenotype. *Clin. Pediatrics* **40**, 519-521 (2001).

60. Arnsten, A. F. Genetics of childhood disorders: XVIII. ADHD, Part. 2: Norepinephrine has a critical modulatory influence on prefrontal cortical function. *J. Am. Acad. Child Adolesc. Psychiatry* **39**, 1201-1203 (2000).

61. Arnulf, I. *et al*. Kleine-Levin syndrome: A systematic study of 108 patients. *Ann. Neurol.* **63**, 482-493 (2008).

62. Aruffo, R. N., Ibarro, S. & Strupp, K. R. Encopresis and anal masturbation. *J. Am. Psychoanal. Assoc.* **48**, 1327-1354 (2000).

63. Asbring, P. Chronic illness - a disruption in life: identity-transformation among women with chronic fatigue syndrome and fibromyalgia. *J. Adv. Nurs.* **34**, 312-319 (2001).

64. Asch, S. E. Effects of group pressure upon the modifications and distortions of judgements in Guetzkow, H. (ed.), *Groups, Leadership, and Men*. (Carnegie, Pittsburgh,1951).

65. Ascherio, A. & Munger, K. Epidemiology of multiple sclerosis: from risk factors to prevention. *Semin. Neurol* **28**, 17-28 (2008).

66. Asher, S. R. & Parker, J. G. Significance of peer relationship problems in childhood in Schneider, B. H., Attili, G., Nadel, J. & Weissberg, R. P. (eds.), *Social competence in developmental perspective*.pp. 5-23 (Kluwer, Dordrecht,1989).

67. Ashwal, S. Practice Parameter: Evaluation of the child with microcephaly (an evidence-based review). *Neurology* **73**, 887-897 (2009).

68. Aslin, R. N. & Fiser, J. Methodological challenges for understanding cognitive development in infants. *Trends Cogn Sci.* **9**, 92-98 (2005).

69. Asquith, S. & Cutting, E. Murder by children: Principles for a preventive strategy in Tunstill, J. (ed.), *Children and the state, whose problem?*pp. 141-160 (Cassell, London,1999).

70. Aston-Jones, G. & Cohen, J. An integrative theory of locus coeruleus-norepinephrine function: adaptive gain and optimal performance. *Annu. Rev. Neurosci* **28**, 403-450 (2005).

71. Aston-Jones, G. & Kalivas, P. W. Brain norepinephrine rediscovered in addiction research. *Biol. Psychiatry* **63**, 1005-1006 (2008).

72. Atlantis, E., Barnes, E. H. & Singh, M. A. F. Efficacy of exercise for treating overweight in children and adolescents: a systematic review. *Int. J. Obes.* **30**, 1027-1040 (2006).

73. Austin, J. K. *et al*. Behavior problems in children before first recognized seizures. *Pediatrics* **107**, 115-122 (2001).

74. Auyeung, B. *et al*. Fetal testosterone and autistic traits. *Br J Psychol* **100**, 1-22 (2009).

75. Auyeung, B. *et al*. Fetal testosterone predicts sexually differentiated childhood behavior in girls and in boys. *Psychol. Science* **20**, 144-148 (2009).

76. Avan, B., Richter, L. M., Ramchandani, P. G., Norris, S. A. & Stein, A. Maternal postnatal depression and children's growth and behaviour during the early years of life: exploring the interaction between physical and mental health. *Arch. Dis. Child.* **95**, 690-695 (2010).

77. Avramidis, E., Bayliss, P. & Burden, R. A survey into mainstream teachers' attitudes towards the inclusion of children with special educational needs in the ordinary school in one local education authority. *Educat. Psychol.* **20**, 191-212 (2000).

78. Axelrod, F. B., Chelimsky, G. G. & Weese-Mayer, D. E. Pediatric autonomic disorders. *Pediatrics* **118**, 309-321 (2006).

79. Ayala, R., Shu, T. & Tsai, L. H. Trekking across the brain: the journey of neuronal migration. *Cell* **128**, 29-43 (2007).

80. Azmanov, D. N. *et al*. Further evidence for allelic heterogeneity in Hartnup disorder. *Hum. Mutat.* **29**, 1217-1221 (2008).

81. Baas, J. M., Milstein, J., Donlevy, M. & Grillon, C. Brainstem correlates of defensive states in humans. *Biol Psychiatry* **59**, 588-593 (2006).

82. Baddeley, A. The magical number seven: still magic after all these years? *Psychol Rev.* **101**, 353-356 (1994).

83. Baddeley, A. Working memory: Looking back and looking forward. *Nat. Rev. Neurosci.* **4**, 829-839 (2003).

84. Bagheri, M. M., Kerbeshian, J. & Burd, L. Recognition and management of Tourette's syndrome and tic disorders. *Am Fam Physician* **59**, 2263-2274 (1999).

85. Baguley, D. M. Hyperacusis. *JRSM* **96**, 582-585 (2003).

86. Baier, P. C. *et al*. Olfactory dysfunction in patients with narcolepsy with cataplexy is restored by intranasal Orexin A (Hypocretin-1). *Brain* **131**, 2734-2741 (2008).

87. Bailey, J. M., Bechtold, K. T. & Berenbaum, S. A. Who are tomboys and why should we study them? *Arch. Sex. Behav.* **31**, 333-341 (2002).

88. Baillargeon, R., Li, J., Gertner, Y. & Wu, D. How Do Infants Reason About Physical Events? in Goswami, U. (ed.), *Wiley-Blackwell Handbook of Childhood Cognitive Development*.pp. 11-48 (Blackwell Publishing Ltd, Oxford,2011).

89. Baird, G. & Gringras, P. Physical examination and medical investigation in Rutter, M. *et al.* (eds.), *Rutter's Child and Adolescent Psychiatry*.pp. 317-335 (Blackwell, Oxford,2008).

90. Baker, K. & Beales, P. L. Making sense of cilia in disease: The human ciliopathies. *Am. J. Med. Genetics Part C* **151**, 281-295 (2009).

91. Baker, P. J. Chronic Lyme disease: in defense of the scientific enterprise. *FASEB J.* **24**, 4175-4177 (2010).

92. Bakker, E. & Wyndaele, J. J. Changes in the toilet training of children during the last 60 years: the cause of an increase in lower urinary tract dysfunction? *BJU Int.* **86**, 248-252 (2000).

93. Bakker, M. J., van Dijk, J. G., van den Maagdenberg, A. M. & Tijssen, M. A. Startle syndromes. *Lancet Neurol.* **5**, 513-524 (2006).

94. Baldwin Jr, D. C., Daugherty, S. R., Rowley, B. D. & Schwarz, M. D. Cheating in medical school: a survey of second-year students at 31 schools. *Acad. Med.* **71**, 267-273 (1996).

95. Baldwin, J. M. A new factor in evolution. *Am. Naturalist* **30**, 441-451 (1896).

96. Ball, T., Bush, A. & Emerson, E. *Psychological interventions for severely challenging behaviours shown by people with learning disabilities*. British Psychological Society, Leicester (2004).

97. Ballas, N., Lioy, D. T., Grunseich, C. & Mandel, G. Non-cell autonomous influence of MeCP2-deficient glia on neuronal dendritic morphology. *Nat. Neurosci.* **12**, 311-317 (2009).

98. Bambauer, K. Z. & Connor, D. F. Characteristics of aggression in clinically referred children. *CNS Spectr* **10**, 709-718 (2005).

99. Bancroft, J. & Vukadinovic, Z. Sexual addiction, sexual compulsivity, sexual impulsivity, or what? Toward a theoretical model. *J. Sex Res* **41**, 225-234 (2004).

100. Bandura, A., Ross, D. & Ross, S. A. Transmission of aggression through imitation of aggressive models. *J Abnorm. Soc. Psychol* **63**, 575-582 (1961).

101. Banken, J. A. Clinical utility of considering digits forward and digits backward as separate components of the Wechsler Adult Intelligence Scale-Revised. *J. Clin. Psychol.* **41**, 686-691 (1985).

102. Bargh, J. A., Green, M. & Fitzsimons, G. The Selfish Goal: Unintended Consequences of Intended Goal Pursuits. *Soc. Cogn* **26**, 534-554 (2008).

103. Bargh, J. A. & Williams, L. E. The nonconscious regulation of emotion in Gross, J. J. (ed.), *Handbook of emotion regulation*.pp. 429-445 (Guilford Press, New York,2007).

104. Bariaud, F. Age differences in children's humor in McGhee, P. E. (ed.), *Humour and children's development*.pp. 15-45 (Haworth Press, London,1989).

105. Barnerias, C. *et al.* Pyruvate dehydrogenase complex deficiency: four neurological phenotypes with differing pathogenesis. *Dev Med Child Neurol* **52**, e1-e9 (2010).

106. Barnes, S. Is sport better than sex? *The Times* **14 Nov**, 92 (2008).

107. Baron, I. S. *Neuropsychological evaluation of the child*. Oxford University Press, New York (2004).

108. Baron, R., Binder, A. & Wasner, G. Neuropathic pain: diagnosis, pathophysiological mechanisms, and treatment. *Lancet Neurol* **9**, 807-819 (2010).

109. Baron-Cohen, S. Autism, hypersystemizing, and truth. *Q. J Exp. Psychol (Colchester.)* **61**, 64-75 (2008).

110. Baron-Cohen, S. The autistic child's theory of mind: a case of specific developmental delay. *J. Child Psychol. Psychiatry* **30**, 285-297 (1989).

111. Barsky, A. J. *et al.* Hypochondriacal patients' appraisal of health and physical risks. *Am. J. Psychiatry* **158**, 783-787 (2001).

112. Bartels, A. & Zeki, S. The neural basis of romantic love. *Neuroreport* **11**, 3829-3834 (2000).

113. Bartlett, M. S. *et al.* Towards automatic recognition of spontaneous facial actions in Ekman, P. & Rosenberg, E. L. (eds.), *What the face reveals*. (Oxford University Press, New York,2005).

114. Bartley, G. B. The differential diagnosis and classification of eyelid retraction. *Trans. Am. Ophthalmol. Soc.* **93**, 371-387 (1995).

115. Bassell, G. J. & Gross, C. Reducing glutamate signaling pays off in fragile X. *Nat. Med.* **14**, 249-250 (2008).

116. Basti, S. & Greenwald, M. J. Principles and paradigms of pediatric cataract management. *Indian J Ophthalmol.* **43**, 159-176 (1995).

117. Basu, A. P. *et al.* Spotting the wolf in sheep's clothing (SLE). *Arch. Dis. Child-Education & practice edition* **95**, 105-111 (2010).

118. Bates, E. *et al.* Differential effects of unilateral lesions on language production in children and adults. *Brain Lang.* **79**, 223-265 (2001).

119. Bateson, G., Jackson, D. D., Haley, J. & Weakland, J. Toward a theory of schizophrenia. *Behav. Sci.* **1**, 251-264 (1956).

120. Bauer, M. S. & Mitchner, L. What is a "mood stabilizer"? An evidence-based response. *Am. J Psychiatry* **161**, 3-18 (2004).

121. Bayreuther, C., Borg, M., Ferrero-Vacher, C., Chaussenot, A. & Lebrun, C. Chorea-acanthocytosis without acanthocytes. *Rev. Neurol. (Paris).* **(in press)**, (2009).

122. Beaman, A. L., Klentz, B., Diener, E. & Svanum, S. Self-awareness and transgression in children: two field studies. *J. Pers. Soc. Psychol.* **37**, 1835-1846 (1979).

123. Bearman, P. S., Moody, J., Stovel, K. & Thalji, L. Social and sexual networks: The national longitudinal study of adolescent health in Morris, M. (ed.), *Network Epidemiology*.pp. 201-220 (Oxford University Press, Oxford,2004).

124. Beaudet, A. L. Which way for genetic-test regulation? Leave test interpretation to specialists. *Nature* **466**, 816-817 (2010).

125. Beaulieu-Prevost, D. & Zadra, A. Dream recall frequency and attitude towards dreams. *Personality & Individ Differences* **38**, 919-927 (2005).

126. Beaumont, S. L. Conversational styles of mothers and their preadolescent and middle adolescent daughters. *Merrill-Palmer Q. J. Devel. Psychol* **46**, 119-139 (2000).

127. Beaven, D. W. & Brooks, S. E. *Color atlas of the nail in clinical diagnosis*. Wolfe Medical, London (1984).

128. Bebbington, A. & Miles, J. The supply of foster families for children in care. *Br. J. Social Work* **20**, 283-307 (1990).

129. Beck, A. T., Brown, G., Berchick, R. J., Stewart, B. L. & Steer, R. A. Relationship between hopelessness and ultimate suicide: a replication with psychiatric outpatients. *Am. J. Psychiatry* **147**, 190-195 (1990).

130. Beck, A. T., Weissman, A., Lester, D. & Trexler, L. The measurement of pessimism: the hopelessness scale. *J. Consult. Clin. Psychol.* **42**, 861-865 (1974).

131. Becker, D. V., Kenrick, D. T., Neuberg, S. L., Blackwell, K. C. & Smith, D. M. The confounded nature of angry men and happy women. *J. Pers. Soc. Psychol* **92**, 179-190 (2007).

132. Belelli, D. *et al.* Extrasynaptic GABAA receptors: form, pharmacology, and function. *J Neurosci* **29**, 12757-12763 (2009).

133. Beligere, N. & Rao, R. Neurodevelopmental outcome of infants with meconium aspiration syndrome: report of a study and literature review. *J. Perinatol.* **28**, S93-S101 (2008).

134. Belmont, L. & Marolla, F. A. Birth order, family size, and intelligence. *Science* **182**, 1096-1101 (1973).

135. Belsky, J. *et al.* Family rearing antecedents of pubertal timing. *Child Dev* **78**, 1302-1321 (2007).

136. Benazzi, F., Koukopoulos, A. & Akiskal, H. S. Toward a validation of a new definition of agitated depression as a bipolar mixed state (mixed depression). *European Psychiatry* **19**, 85-90 (2004).

137. Benbadis, S. The differential diagnosis of epilepsy: a critical review. *Epilepsy Behav* **15**, 15-21 (2009).

138. Bender, B. G., Harmon, R. J., Linden, M. G., Bucher-Bartelson, B. & Robinson, A. Psychosocial competence of unselected young adults with sex chromosome abnormalities. *Am. J. Med. Genet. (Neuropsych. Genetics)* **88**, 200-206 (1999).

139. Benjamin, B. *Endolaryngeal surgery*. Martin Dunitz, London (1998).

140. Benjet, C., Thompson, R. J. & Gotlib, I. H. 5-HTTLPR moderates the effect of relational peer victimization on depressive symptoms in adolescent girls. *J Child Psychol Psychiatry* **51**, 173-179 (2010).

141. Bent, S., Bertoglio, K. & Hendren, R. L. Omega-3 fatty acids for autistic spectrum disorder: a systematic review. *J Autism Dev Disord.* **39**, 1145-1154 (2009).

142. Bergen, D. C. Effects of poverty on cognitive function: a hidden neurologic epidemic. *Neurology* **71**, 447-451 (2008).

143. Bergen, S. E., Gardner, C. O. & Kendler, K. S. Age-related changes in heritability of behavioral phenotypes over adolescence and young adulthood: a meta-analysis. *Twin. Res Hum. Genet* **10**, 423-433 (2007).

144. Berger, L. M., McDaniel, M. & Paxson, C. Assessing parenting behaviors across racial groups: Implications for the child welfare system. *Soc. Serv. Rev.* **79**, 653-688 (2005).

145. Berger, L. R. The Winnicott Squiggle Game: a vehicle for communicating with the school-aged child. *Pediatrics* **66**, 921-924 (1980).

146. Bergeron, M. J., Simonin, A., Burzle, M. & Hediger, M. A. Inherited epithelial transporter disorders-an overview. *J Inherit. Metab Dis* **31**, 178-187 (2008).

147. Berginer, V. M. *et al.* Chronic diarrhea and juvenile cataracts: think cerebrotendinous xanthomatosis and treat. *Pediatrics* **123**, 143-146 (2009).

148. Berk, R. A. Verbal-performance IQ discrepancy score: a comment on reliability, abnormality, and validity. *J Clin Psychol* **38**, 638-641 (1982).

149. Berkson, J. Limitations of the application of the fourfold table analysis to hospital data. *Biometrics* **2**, 47-53 (1946).

150. Berlin, H. A. The Neural Basis of the Dynamic Unconscious. *Neuropsychoanalysis* **13**, 5-31 (2011).

151. Berlingeri, M. *et al.* Nouns and verbs in the brain: Grammatical class and task specific effects as revealed by fMRI. *Cognitive neuropsychology* **25**, 528-558 (2008).

152. Berlyne, D. E. Novelty and curiosity as determinants of exploratory behavior. *Br. J. Psychol* **41**, 68-80 (1950).

153. Bermanzohn, P. C. *et al.* Hierarchy, reductionism, and 'comorbidity' in the diagnosis of schizophrenia in Hwang, M. Y. & Bermanzohn, P. C. (eds.), *Schizophrenia and comorbid conditions*.pp. 1-30 (American Psychiatric Publishing, Arlington,2001).

154. Bernabei, P., Cerquiglini, A., Cortesi, F. & D'Ardia, C. Regression versus no regression in the autistic disorder: developmental trajectories. *J Autism Dev Disord.* **37**, 580-588 (2007).

155. Bernard, S. & Turk, J. *Developing mental health services for children and adolescents with learning disabilities*. Royal College of Psychiatrists, London (2009).

156. Bernard, S. H. Parents with learning disabilities - the assessment of parenting ability. *Adv. Mental Health & Learn. Dis* **1**, 14-18 (2007).

157. Berne, E. *Games people play: The psychology of human relationships*. Grove Press, (1964).

158. Berrios, G. E. Stupor: a conceptual history. *Psychol Med* **11**, 677-688 (1981).

159. Berry, G. T. Galactosemia and amenorrhea in the adolescent. *Ann. N. Y. Acad. Sci.* **1135**, 112-117 (2008).

160. Besag, F. M. Childhood epilepsy in relation to mental handicap and behavioural disorders. *J. Child Psychol. Psychiatry* **43**, 103-131 (2002).

161. Besag, F. M. C. A child with Attention-Deficit Disorder, autistic features and frequent epileptiform discharges in Schmidt, D. & Schachter, S. C. (eds.), *Puzzling Cases of Epilepsy, Second Edition*.pp. 296-298 (Academic Press, New York,2010).

162. Bhugra, D. & Bhui, K. Racism in psychiatry: paradigm lost--paradigm regained. *Int. Rev. Psychiatry* **11**, 236-243 (1999).

163. Biagini, G., Panuccio, G. & Avoli, M. Neurosteroids and epilepsy. *Curr. Opin. Neurol* **23**, 170-176 (2010).

164. Biddle, L., Donovan, J., Hawton, K., Kapur, N. & Gunnell, D. Suicide and the internet. *Br. Med. J.* **336**, 800-802 (2008).

165. Biederman, J. *et al.* Further evidence of association between behavioral inhibition and social anxiety in children. *Am. J. Psychiatry* **158**, 1673-1679 (2001).

166. Bills, A. G. Blocking: A new principle of mental fatigue. *Am. J. Psychol.* **43**, 230-245 (1931).

167. Bindu, P. S., Shehanaz, K. E., Christopher, R., Pal, P. K. & Ravishankar, S. Intermediate maple syrup urine disease: Neuroimaging observations in 3 patients from South India. *J. Child Neurol.* **22**, 911-913 (2007).

168. Binnie, C. D. Cognitive impairment during epileptiform discharges: is it ever justifiable to treat the EEG? *Lancet Neurol* **2**, 725-730 (2003).

169. Birbaumer, N. *et al.* Deficient fear conditioning in psychopathy: a functional magnetic resonance imaging study. *Arch. Gen. Psychiatry* **62**, 799-805 (2005).

170. Bircan, I. Genetics of obesity. *J. Clin. Res. Ped. Endo* **2009**, 54-57 (2009).

171. Birchwood, M., Spencer, E. & McGovern, D. Schizophrenia: early warning signs. *Adv. Psychiat. Treat.* **6**, 93-101 (2000).

172. Bird, E. K. R. The case for bilingualism in children with Down Syndrome in Paul, R. (ed.), *Language disorders from a developmental perspective: essays in honor of Robin S.Chapman*.pp. 249-275 (Lawrence Erlbaum, Mahwah,NJ,2007).

173. Bird, T. D., Carlson, C. B. & Hall, J. G. Familial essential (" benign") chorea. *Br. Med. J.* **13**, 357-362 (1976).

174. Biro, F. M. *et al.* Pubertal Assessment Method and Baseline Characteristics in a Mixed Longitudinal Study of Girls. *Pediatrics* **126**, e583-e590 (2010).

175. Bishop, G. H. The skin as an organ of senses with special reference to the itching sensation. *J Invest Dermatol.* **11**, 143-154 (1948).

176. Bishop, L. *et al.* Severe methylenetetrahydrofolate reductase (MTHFR) deficiency: A case report of nonclassical homocystinuria. *J. Child Neurol.* **23**, 823-828 (2008).

177. Bissada, N. K. *et al.* Pheochromocytoma in children and adolescents: a clinical spectrum. *J Pediatr. Surg.* **43**, 540-543 (2008).

178. Black, B. & Uhde, T. W. Elective mutism as a variant of social phobia. *J. Am. Acad. Child Adolesc. Psychiatry* **31**, 1090-1094 (1992).

179. Black, M. M. Zinc deficiency and child development. *Am. J. Clin. Nutr.* **68**, 464S-469S (1998).

180. Blackwood, N. J., Howard, R. J., Bentall, R. P. & Murray, R. M. Cognitive neuropsychiatric models of persecutory delusions. *Am. J. Psychiatry* **158**, 527-539 (2001).

181. Blair, R. J. R. Responding to the emotions of others: Dissociating forms of empathy through the study of typical and psychiatric populations. *Conscious. Cogn.* **14**, 698-718 (2005).

182. Blank, M. J. Adoption nightmares prompt judicial recognition of the tort of wrongful adoption: Will New York follow suit. *Cardozo Law Rev.* **15**, 1687-1744 (1993).

183. Blaskewitz, N., Merten, T. & Kathmann, N. Performance of children on symptom validity tests: TOMM, MSVT, and FIT. *Arch. Clin. Neuropsychol.* **23**, 379-391 (2008).

184. Block, J. J. Issues for DSM-V: internet addiction. *Am. J Psychiatry* **165**, 306-307 (2008).

185. Bloom, P. & German, T. P. Two reasons to abandon the false belief task as a test of theory of mind. *Cognition* **77**, B25-B31 (2000).

186. Blouin, B., Maddeaux, C., Firestone, J. S. & van, S. J. Predicting response of ADHD symptoms to methylphenidate treatment based on comorbid anxiety. *J. Atten. Disord.* (2009).

187. Bocchetta, A. Psychotic mania in glucose-6-phosphate-dehydrogenase-deficient subjects. *Ann. Gen. Hosp. Psychiatry* **2**, 6 (2003).

188. Bokan, J. A., Ries, R. K. & Katon, W. J. Tertiary gain and chronic pain. *Pain* **10**, 331-335 (1981).

189. Boles, R. G. & Stone, M. L. A patient with arginase deficiency and episodic hyperammonemia successfully treated with menses cessation. *Mol. Genet. Metab.* **89**, 390-391 (2006).

190. Bolton, D., Dearsley, P., Madronal-Luque, R. & Baron-Cohen, S. Magical thinking in childhood and adolescence: Development and relation to obsessive compulsion. *Br. J. Dev. Psychol.* **20**, 479-494 (2002).

191. Bolton, D. *et al.* Normative childhood repetitive routines and obsessive compulsive symptomatology in 6-year-old twins. *J. Child Psychol Psychiatry* (2009).

192. Bolton, J. M., Robinson, J. & Sareen, J. Self-medication of mood disorders with alcohol and drugs in the National Epidemiologic Survey on Alcohol and Related Conditions. *J. Affect. Disord.* **115**, 367-375 (2009).

193. Bolton, P. F., Pickles, A., Murphy, M. & Rutter, M. Autism, affective and other psychiatric disorders: patterns of familial aggregation. *Psychol. Med.* **28**, 385-395 (1998).

194. Bonioli, E. *et al.* Combined deficiency of xanthine oxidase and sulphite oxidase due to a deficiency of molybdenum cofactor. *J. Inherit. Metab. Dis.* **19**, 700-701 (1996).

195. Bonnet, M., Decety, J., Jeannerod, M. & Requin, J. Mental simulation of an action modulates the excitability of spinal reflex pathways in man. *Brain Res Cogn Brain Res* **5**, 221-228 (1997).

196. Book, A. S. & Quinsey, V. L. Re-examining the issues: A response to Archer et al. *Aggression and Violent Behavior* **10**, 637-646 (2005).

197. Boreham, R. & Shaw, A. *Drug use, smoking and drinking among young people in England in 2001.* Department of Health, Norwich (2002).

198. Born, L., Koren, G., Lin, E. & Steiner, M. A new, female-specific irritability rating scale. *J. Psychiatry Neurosci.* **33**, 344-354 (2008).

199. Borowsky, I. W., Hogan, M. & Ireland, M. Adolescent sexual aggression: risk and protective factors. *Pediatrics* **100**, E7 (1997).

200. Borthwick, C. Mental Retardation, Dementia, and the Age of Majority. *Disability & Society* **9**, 519-531 (1994).

201. Bottoms, B. L., Shaver, P. R., Goodman, G. S. & Qin, J. In the name of God: A profile of religion-related child abuse. *J. Social Issues* **51**, 85-112 (1995).

202. Boudreau, E. A. *et al.* Review of disrupted sleep patterns in Smith-Magenis syndrome and normal melatonin secretion in a patient with an atypical interstitial 17p11.2 deletion. *Am. J Med Genet. A* **149A**, 1382-1391 (2009).

203. Bourguignon, F. & Chakravarty, S. R. The measurement of multidimensional poverty. *J. Econ. Inequality* **1**, 25-49 (2003).

204. Bracha, H. F. & Maser, J. D. Anxiety and posttraumatic stress disorder in the context of human brain evolution: a role for theory in DSM-V? *Clin. Psychol* **15**, 91-97 (2008).

205. Bracha, H. S. Freeze, flight, fight, fright, faint: adaptationist perspectives on the acute stress response spectrum. *CNS. Spectr.* **9**, 679-685 (2004).

206. Brackbill, Y. & O'hara, J. The relative effectiveness of reward and punishment for discrimination learning in children. *J. Comp. Physiol. Psychol.* **51**, 747-751 (1958).

207. Bradford, H. F. Glutamate, GABA and epilepsy. *Prog. Neurobiol.* **47**, 477-511 (1995).

208. Bradley, R. G. *et al.* Influence of child abuse on adult depression: moderation by the corticotropin-releasing hormone receptor gene. *Arch Gen. Psychiatry* **65**, 190-200 (2008).

209. Braff, D. L., Geyer, M. A. & Swerdlow, N. R. Human studies of prepulse inhibition of startle: normal subjects, patient groups, and pharmacological studies. *Psychopharmacology (Berl)* **156**, 234-258 (2001).

210. Brandon, S. *et al.* Reported recovered memories of child sexual abuse. *Psychiatr. Bull.* **21**, 663-665 (1997).

211. Brandt, J. & Van Gorp, W. G. Functional ("psychogenic") amnesia. *Semin. Neurol.* **26**, 331-340 (2006).

212. Breakefield, X. O. *et al.* The pathophysiological basis of dystonias. *Nat Rev. Neurosci* **9**, 222-234 (2008).

213. Bredenoord, A. J. & Smout, A. J. P. M. Physiologic and pathologic belching. *Clin. Gastroenterol. Hepatol* **5**, 772-775 (2007).

214. Brent, D. A. & Maalouf, F. T. Pediatric depression: Is there evidence to improve evidence-based treatments? *J. Child Psychol Psychiatry* **50**, 143-152 (2009).

214a. Breslau, N. & Rasmussen, B. K. The impact of migraine: Epidemiology, risk factors, and co-morbidities. Neurology 56, S4–-12 (2001).

215. Brim, D., Townsend, D. B., DeQuinzio, J. A. & Poulson, C. L. Analysis of social referencing skills among children with autism. *Res. Autism Spectrum Dis* **3**, 942-958 (2009).

216. Brockington, I. F. Monthly psychosis starting before the menarche. *Arch. Women Ment. Health* **12**, 121-122 (2009).

217. Brod, M., Kongso, J. H., Lessard, S. & Christensen, T. L. Psychological insulin resistance: patient beliefs and implications for diabetes management. *Qual. Life Res.* **18**, 23-32 (2009).

218. Broer, S. *et al.* Iminoglycinuria and hyperglycinuria are discrete human phenotypes resulting from complex mutations in proline and glycine transporters. *J Clin Invest* **118**, 3881-3892 (2008).

219. Bromley, S. M. Smell and taste disorders: a primary care approach. *Am. Fam. Physician* **61**, 427-440 (2000).

220. Brooks, R. M. & Mott, A. M. Domestic violence: what should paediatricians do? *Arch. Dis. Child.* **93**, 558-560 (2008).

221. Broom, L., Beem, H. P. & Harris, V. Characteristics of 1,107 petitioners for change of name. *Am. Sociol. Rev.* **20**, 33-39 (1955).

222. Brotman, M. A. *et al.* Prevalence, clinical correlates, and longitudinal course of severe mood dysregulation in children. *Biol. Psychiatry* **60**, 991-997 (2006).

223. Brown, G. W. & Harris, T. O. Aetiology of anxiety and depressive disorders in an inner-city population. 1. Early adversity. *Psychol Med* **23**, 143-154 (1993).

224. Brown, J. B. & Lloyd, H. A controlled study of children not speaking at school. *J. Assoc. Workers Maladjusted Child* **3**, 49-63 (1975).

225. Brown, R. J. Psychological mechanisms of medically unexplained symptoms: an integrative conceptual model. *Psychol Bull.* **130**, 793-812 (2004).

226. Browne, K. D. & Hamilton-Giachritsis, C. The influence of violent media on children and adolescents:a public-health approach. *Lancet* **365**, 702-710 (2005).

227. Brownstein, M. J. A brief history of opiates, opioid peptides, and opioid receptors. *Proc. Natl. Acad. Sci. U. S. A.* **90**, 5391-5393 (1993).

228. Bruno, M. A. *et al.* Locked-In Syndrome in Children: Report of Five Cases and Review of the Literature. *Pediatr. Neurol.* **41**, 237-246 (2009).

229. Brunsdon, R., Nickels, L. & Coltheart, M. Topographical disorientation: towards an integrated framework for assessment. *Neuropsychological Rehab* **17**, 34-52 (2007).

230. Brunsdon, R., Nickels, L., Coltheart, M. & Joy, P. Assessment and treatment of childhood topographical disorientation: A case study. *Neuropsychological Rehab* **17**, 53-94 (2007).

231. Bryon, M. Interventions with children who are tube-fed in Southall, A. & Schwartz, A. (eds.), *Feeding problems in children: a practical guide.* (Radcliffe Medical Press, Abingdon,2000).

232. Buchanan, R. W. & Heinrichs, D. W. The Neurological Evaluation Scale (NES): a structured instrument for the assessment of neurological signs in schizophrenia. *Psychiatry Res* **27**, 335-350 (1989).

233. Bundak, R. *et al.* Analysis of puberty and pubertal growth in healthy boys. *Eur. J. Pediatr.* **166**, 595-600 (2007).

234. Burbach, J. P. H. & van der Zwaag, B. Contact in the genetics of autism and schizophrenia. *Trends Neurosci.* **32**, 69-72 (2009).

235. Burgess, P. W. & McNeil, J. E. Content-specific confabulation. *Cortex* **35**, 163-182 (1999).

236. Burgess, P. W. & Shallice, T. Response suppression, initiation and strategy use following frontal lobe lesions. *Neuropsychologia* **34**, 263-272 (1996).

237. Burgos-Vargas, R. A case of childhood-onset ankylosing spondylitis: diagnosis and treatment. *Nat. Clin. Pract. Rheumatol.* **5**, 52-57 (2009).

238. Busby, K. & Pivik, R. T. Failure of high intensity auditory stimuli to affect behavioral arousal in children during the first sleep cycle. *Pediatr. Res* **17**, 802-805 (1983).

239. Busby, K. A., Mercier, L. & Pivik, R. T. Ontogenetic variations in auditory arousal threshold during sleep. *Psychophysiology* **31**, 182-188 (1994).

240. Busch, F. N., Milrod, B. L. & Shear, M. K. Psychodynamic Concepts of Anxiety in Stein, D. J., Hollander, E. & Rothbaum, B. O. (eds.), *Textbook of Anxiety Disorders.*pp. 117-128 (Amer Psychiatric Pub Inc, Arlington,2009).

241. Buss, A. H. & Plomin, R. *Temperament: Early developing personality traits.* Lawrence Erlbaum, Mahwah, NJ (1984).

242. Butcher, L. M. & Plomin, R. The nature of nurture: A genomewide association scan for family chaos. *Behav. Genet.* **38**, 361-371 (2008).

243. Butzlaff, R. L. & Hooley, J. M. Expressed emotion and psychiatric relapse: a meta-analysis. *Arch. Gen. Psychiatry* **55**, 547-552 (1998).

244. Buxbaum, L. J. *et al.* Hemispatial neglect: Subtypes, neuroanatomy, and disability. *Neurology* **62**, 749-756 (2004).

245. Buzzard, A. & Nicholson, S. Deaf parents of deaf children. *Sites: a journal of social anthropology and cultural studies* **3**, 126-142 (2006).

246. Cain, N. M., Pincus, A. L. & Ansell, E. B. Narcissism at the crossroads: Phenotypic description of pathological narcissism across clinical theory, social/personality psychology, and psychiatric diagnosis. *Clin. Psychol. Rev.* **28**, 638-656 (2008).

247. Camden ACPC *Child Protection Guidelines from the Area Child Protection Committee.* (1993).

248. Camfferman, D., McEvoy, R. D., O'Donoghue, F. & Lushington, K. Prader Willi Syndrome and excessive daytime sleepiness. *Sleep Med. Rev.* **12**, 65-75 (2008).

249. Campa, D., Gioia, A., Tomei, A., Poli, P. & Barale, R. Association of ABCB1/MDR1 and OPRM1 gene polymorphisms with morphine pain relief. *Clin. Pharmacol. Ther.* **83**, 559-566 (2007).

250. Campbell, A. Oxytocin and Human Social Behavior. *Personality and Social Psychology Review* **14**, 281-295 (2010).

251. Campo, J., Hardy, S., Merckelbach, H., Nijman, H. & Zwets, A. The urge to change appearance in different psychopathological categories. *Acta Neuropsychiatrica* **19**, 104-108 (2007).

252. Cantwell, D. P. & Baker, L. Differential diagnosis of hyperactivity. *J. Dev. Behav. Pediatr.* **8**, 159-170 (1987).

253. Capitani, E. *et al.* Posterior cerebral artery infarcts and semantic category dissociations: a study of 28 patients. *Brain* **132**, 965-981 (2009).

254. Caplan, R., Guthrie, D., Fish, B., Tanguay, P. E. & David-Lando, G. The Kiddie Formal Thought Disorder Rating Scale: clinical assessment, reliability, and validity. *J Am Acad. Child Adolesc. Psychiatry* **28**, 408-416 (1989).

255. Capute, A. J. & Accardo, P. J. Linguistic and auditory milestones during the first two years of life: a language inventory for the practitioner. *Clin. Pediatr. (Phila)* **17**, 847-853 (1978).

256. Carlson, G. A. The challenge of diagnosing depression in childhood and adolescence. *J Affect. Disord.* **61**, 3-8 (2000).

257. Caron, C. & Rutter, M. Comorbidity in child psychopathology: concepts, issues and research strategies. *J. Child Psychol. Psychiatry* **32**, 1063-1080 (1991).

258. Carr, J. & Greeves, L. *The naked jape.* Penguin Books, London (2007).

259. Carr, M. & Gill, D. Polyuria, polydipsia, polypopsia:" Mummy I want a drink". *Arch. Dis. Child.* **92**, e139-e143 (2007).

260. Carre, J. M., Putnam, S. K. & McCormick, C. M. Testosterone responses to competition predict future aggressive behaviour at a cost to reward in men. *Psychoneuroendocrinology* **34**, 561-570 (2009).

261. Carter, A. S., Davis, N. O., Klin, A. & Volkmar, F. R. Social development in autism in Volkmar, F. R., Paul, R., Klin, A. & Cohen, D. J. (eds.), *Handbook of autism and pervasive developmental disorders.*pp. 312-334 (John Wiley and Sons, Hoboken,2005).

262. Carter, C. J. Schizophrenia Susceptibility Genes Directly Implicated in the Life Cycles of Pathogens: Cytomegalovirus, Influenza, Herpes simplex, Rubella, and Toxoplasma gondii. *Schizophr. Bull.* (2008).

263. Caruso, E. M., Rahnev, D. A. & Banaji, M. R. Using conjoint analysis to detect discrimination. *Social Cognition* **27**, 128-137 (2009).

264. Casasanto, D., Willems, R. & Hagoort, P. Body-specific representations of action verbs: Evidence from fMRI in right-and left-handers. Proceedings of the 31st Annual Conference of the Cognitive Science Society , 875-880. 2009.
Ref Type: Conference Proceeding

265. Casby, M. W. The development of play in infants, toddlers, and young children. *Comm. Dis. Q* **24**, 163-174 (2003).

266. Case, A., Lin, I. F. & McLanahan, S. How hungry is the selfish gene? *Econ. J.* **110**, 781-804 (2000).

267. Cashdan, E. A sensitive period for learning about food. *Human Nature* **5**, 279-291 (1994).

268. Caspi, A., Roberts, B. W. & Shiner, R. L. Personality development: stability and change. *Annu. Rev. Psychol* **56**, 453-484 (2005).

269. Caspi, A. *et al.* Influence of life stress on depression: moderation by a polymorphism in the 5-HTT gene. *Science* **301**, 386-389 (2003).

270. Cass, H. Visual impairment and autism: current questions and future research. *Autism* **2**, 117-138 (1998).

271. Cassano, G. B. *et al.* The bipolar spectrum: a clinical reality in search of diagnostic criteria and an assessment methodology. *J. Affect. Disord.* **54**, 319-328 (1999).

272. Castellanos, F. X., Sonuga-Barke, E. J., Milham, M. P. & Tannock, R. Characterizing cognition in ADHD: beyond executive dysfunction. *Trends Cogn Sci.* **10**, 117-123 (2006).

273. Castellanos, F. X. & Tannock, R. Neuroscience of attention-deficit/hyperactivity disorder: the search for endophenotypes. *Nat. Rev. Neurosci.* **3**, 617-628 (2002).

274. Catani, M. & ffytche, D. H. The rises and falls of disconnection syndromes. *Brain* **128**, 2224-2239 (2005).

275. Cerel, J., Fristad, M. A., Verducci, J., Weller, R. A. & Weller, E. B. Childhood bereavement: Psychopathology in the 2 years postparental death. *J. Am. Acad. Child Adolesc. Psychiatry* **45**, 681-690 (2006).

276. Cermolacce, M., Sass, L. & Parnas, J. What is Bizarre in Bizarre Delusions? A Critical Review. *Schizophr. Bull.* **(in press)**, (2010).

277. Chadwick, O., Rutter, M., Brown, G., Shaffer, D. & Traub, M. U. A prospective study of children with head injuries: II. Cognitive sequelae. *Psychol. Med.* **11**, 49 (1981).

278. Chalder, T. *et al.* Development of a fatigue scale. *J. Psychosom. Res.* **37**, 147-153 (1993).

279. Chamberlain, S. R. *et al.* A neuropsychological comparison of obsessive-compulsive disorder and trichotillomania. *Neuropsychologia* **45**, 654-662 (2007).

280. Chamberlain, S. R., Fineberg, N. A., Blackwell, A. D., Robbins, T. W. & Sahakian, B. J. Motor inhibition and cognitive flexibility in obsessive-compulsive disorder and trichotillomania. *Am. J. Psychiatry* **163**, 1282-1284 (2006).

281. Chan, D. W. Giftedness of Chinese students in Hong Kong. *Gifted Child Q* **52**, 40-54 (2008).

282. Chandran, M., Tharyan, P., Muliyil, J. & Abraham, S. Post-partum depression in a cohort of women from a rural area of Tamil Nadu, India. Incidence and risk factors. *Br. J Psychiatry* **181**, 499-504 (2002).

283. Changizi, M. A. & He, D. Four correlates of complex behavioral networks: differentiation, behavior, connectivity, and compartmentalization. *Complexity* **10**, 13-40 (2005).

284. Chapman, W. P. & Jones, C. M. Variations in cutaneous and visceral pain sensitivity in normal subjects. *J. Clin. Invest* **23**, 81-91 (1944).

285. Charman, T. & Baird, G. Practitioner review: Diagnosis of autism spectrum disorder in 2- and 3-year-old children. *J. Child Psychol. Psychiatry* **43**, 289-305 (2002).

286. Chatoor, I., Ganiban, J., Harrison, J. & Hirsch, R. Observation of feeding in the diagnosis of posttraumatic feeding disorder of infancy. *J Am. Acad. Child Adolesc. Psychiatry* **40**, 595-602 (2001).

287. Chatoor, I. & Khushlani, D. Eating disorders in Luby, J. L. (ed.), *Handbook of preschool mental health.* (Guilford Press, New York,2006).

288. Cheng, Y., Chou, K. H. & Chen, I. Atypical development of white matter microstructure in adolescents with autism spectrum disorders. *Neuroimage* **50**, 873-882 (2010).

289. Chervin, R. D., Dillon, J. E., Archbold, K. H. & Ruzicka, D. L. Conduct problems and symptoms of sleep disorders in children. *J. Am. Acad. Child Adolesc. Psychiatry* **42**, 201-208 (2003).

290. Cheshire, W. P. & Freeman, R. Disorders of sweating. *Semin. Neurol.* **23**, 399-406 (2003).

291. Cho, H. J., Menezes, P. R., Hotopf, M., Bhugra, D. & Wessely, S. Comparative epidemiology of chronic fatigue syndrome in Brazilian and British primary care: prevalence and recognition. *Br. J Psychiatry* **194**, 117-122 (2009).

292. Choudhry, N. K., Fletcher, R. H. & Soumerai, S. B. Systematic review: The relationship between clinical experience and quality of health care. *Ann. Intern. Med.* **142**, 260-273 (2005).

293. Christie, D. Introduction to IQ testing in Skuse, D. (ed.), *Child psychology and psychiatry: An introduction.*pp. 29-32 (Medicine Publishing, Abingdon,2003).

294. Cieraad, I. Gender at play: Decor differences between boys' and girls' bedrooms in Casey, E. & Martens, L. (eds.), *Gender and consumption.*pp. 197-218 (Ashgate Publishing, Ltd, Aldershot,2007).

295. Cipolotti, L. *et al.* Recollection and familiarity in dense hippocampal amnesia: A case study. *Neuropsychologia* **44**, 489-506 (2006).

296. Citrome, L. Current guidelines and their recommendations for prolactin monitoring in psychosis. *J. Psychopharmacol. (Oxf).* **22**, 90-97 (2008).

297. Clarke, A. R., Barry, R. J., Irving, A. M., McCarthy, R. & Selikowitz, M. Children with attention-deficit/hyperactivity disorder and autistic features: EEG evidence for comorbid disorders. *Psychiatry Res* **(in press)**, (2010).

298. Clarke, D. J., Littlejohns, C. S., Corbett, J. A. & Joseph, S. Pervasive developmental disorders and psychoses in adult life. *Br. J. Psychiatry* **155**, 692-699 (1989).

299. Clarke, L. A. The mucopolysaccharidoses: a success of molecular medicine. *Expert Reviews in Mol. Medicine* **10**, 1-17 (2008).

300. Coats, D. K., Paysse, E. A. & Kim, D. S. Excessive blinking in childhood: a prospective evaluation of 99 children. *Ophthalmology* **108**, 1556-1561 (2001).

301. Cochat, P. *et al.* Nephrolithiasis related to inborn metabolic diseases. *Pediatr. Nephrol.* **25**, 415-424 (2010).

302. Cochen, V. *et al.* Vivid dreams, hallucinations, psychosis and REM sleep in Guillain-Barre syndrome. *Brain* **128**, 2535-2545 (2005).

303. Cockerell, O. C., Rothwell, J., Thompson, P. D., Marsden, C. D. & Shorvon, S. D. Clinical and physiological features of epilepsia partialis continua. Cases ascertained in the UK. *Brain* **119 (Pt 2)**, 393-407 (1996).

304. Coddington, R. D. The significance of life events as etiologic factors in the diseases of children. II. A study of a normal population. *J Psychosom. Res* **16**, 205-213 (1972).

305. Cohen, D. & MacKeith, S. A. *The development of imagination: The private worlds of childhood.* Routledge, London (1991).

306. Cohen, D. *et al.* Absence of cognitive impairment at long-term follow-up in adolescents treated with ECT for severe mood disorder. *Am. J. Psychiatry* **157**, 460-462 (2000).

307. Cole, P. M. & Deater-Deckard, K. Emotion regulation, risk and psychopathology. *J. Child Psychol Psychiatry* **50**, 1327-1330 (2009).

308. Cole, T. J., Bellizzi, M. C., Flegal, K. M. & Dietz, W. H. Establishing a standard definition for child overweight and obesity worldwide: international survey. *Br. Med. J* **320**, 1240-1243 (2000).

309. Coles, M. E. & Heimberg, R. G. Memory biases in the anxiety disorders: current status. *Clin. Psychol. Rev.* **22**, 587-627 (2002).

310. Coll, C. G., Kagan, J. & Reznick, S. Behavioral inhibition in young children. *Child Dev.* **55**, 1005-1019 (1984).

311. Colville, G. A. & Mok, Q. Psychological management of two cases of self injury on the paediatric intensive care unit. *Arch. Dis. Child* **88**, 335-336 (2003).

312. Conicella, E. *et al.* The child with headache in a pediatric emergency department. *Headache: J. Head Face Pain* **48**, 1005-1011 (2008).

313. Connellan, J., Baron-Cohen, S., Wheelwright, S., Batki, A. & Ahluwalia, J. Sex differences in human neonatal social perception. *Inf. Behav. Devel* **23**, 113-118 (2000).

314. Constantino, J. N., Hudziak, J. J. & Todd, R. D. Deficits in reciprocal social behavior in male twins: evidence for a genetically independent domain of psychopathology. *J. Am. Acad. Child Adolesc. Psychiatry* **42**, 458-467 (2003).

315. Cooper, H., Nye, B., Charlton, K., Lindsay, J. & Greathouse, S. Effects of summer vacation on achievement test scores. *Rev. Educ. Res* **66**, 227-268 (1996).

316. Corballis, M. C., Hattie, J. & Fletcher, R. Handedness and intellectual achievement: An even-handed look. *Neuropsychologia* **46**, 374-378 (2008).

317. Corbett, B. A., Mendoza, S., Abdullah, M., Wegelin, J. A. & Levine, S. Cortisol circadian rhythms and response to stress in children with autism. *Psychoneuroendocrinology* **31**, 59-68 (2006).

318. Corbett, J. Development, disintegration and dementia. *J. Ment. Defic. Res* **31 (Pt 4)**, 349-356 (1987).

319. Corrigan, N., Stewart, M., Scott, M. & Fee, F. Predictive value of preschool surveillance in detecting learning difficulties. *Arch. Dis. Child* **74**, 517-521 (1996).

320. Corsica, J. A. & Spring, B. J. Carbohydrate craving: a double-blind, placebo-controlled test of the self-medication hypothesis. *Eat. Behav* **9**, 447-454 (2008).

321. Costello, D. J., Eichler, A. F. & Eichler, F. S. Leukodystrophies: Classification, diagnosis, and treatment. *Neurologist* **15**, 319-328 (2009).

322. Costello, E. J., Compton, S. N., Keeler, G. & Angold, A. Relationships between poverty and psychopathology: A natural experiment. *JAMA* **290**, 2023-2029 (2003).

323. Costello, E. J., Worthman, C., Erkanli, A. & Angold, A. Prediction from low birth weight to female adolescent depression: a test of competing hypotheses. *Arch. Gen. Psychiatry* **64**, 338-344 (2007).

324. Costigan, M., Scholz, J. & Woolf, C. J. Neuropathic pain: A maladaptive response of the nervous system to damage. *Ann. Rev. Neurosci.* **32**, 1-32 (2011).

325. Cotton, R. G. H. *et al.* The human variome project. *Science* **322**, 861-862 (2008).

326. Courchesne, E. & Pierce, K. Why the frontal cortex in autism might be talking only to itself: local over-connectivity but long-distance disconnection. *Curr. Opin. Neurobiol.* **15**, 225-230 (2005).

327. Couture, S. M. *et al.* Comparison of social cognitive functioning in schizophrenia and high functioning autism: more convergence than divergence. *Psychol Med.* **(in press)**, 1-11 (2009).

328. Covanis, A. Eyelid myoclonia and absence in Delgado-Escueta, A. V. *et al.* (eds.), *Adv.Neurol., vol.95: Myoclonic Epilepsies.*pp. 185-196 (Lippincott Williams & Wilkins, Philadelphia,2005).

329. Cowling, V. *Children of parents with mental illness 2: Personal and clinical perspectives.* Acer Press, Melbourne (2004).

330. Cox, A. D. Maternal depression and impact on children's development. *Arch Dis Child* **63**, 90-95 (1988).

331. Cox, M. V. *Children's drawings of the human figure.* Lawrence Erlbaum Associates, Hove, East Sussex (1993).

332. Craig, M. C. *et al.* Altered connections on the road to psychopathy. *Mol. Psychiatry* **14**, 946-953 (2009).

333. Cramer, P. *Protecting the self: defense mechanisms in action.* Guilford Press, New York (2006).

334. Cramer, P. Longitudinal study of defense mechanisms: late childhood to late adolescence. *J. Pers.* **75**, 1-24 (2007).

335. Crawford, T. N. *et al.* Self-reported attachment, interpersonal aggression, and personality disorder in a prospective community sample of adolescents and adults. *J Pers. Disord.* **20**, 331-351 (2006).

336. Crimlisk, H. L. The little imitator--porphyria: a neuropsychiatric disorder. *J Neurol Neurosurg Psychiatry* **62**, 319-328 (1997).

337. Crimlisk, H. L. *et al.* Slater revisited: 6 year follow up study of patients with medically unexplained motor symptoms. *Br. Med. J.* **316**, 582-586 (1998).

338. Crino, P. B., Nathanson, K. L. & Henske, E. P. The tuberous sclerosis complex. *N. Engl. J. Med.* **355**, 1345-1356 (2006).

339. Critchley, E. Hearing children of deaf parents. *J. Laryngol. Otol.* **81**, 51-62 (1967).

340. Critchley, M. The clinical significance of dysprosody. *Psychol Med.* **11**, 9-10 (1981).

341. Critchley, M. D. & Hoffman, H. L. The syndrome of periodic somnolence and morbid hunger (Kleine-Levin syndrome). *Br. Med. J.* **1**, 137-139 (1942).

342. Crockenberg, S. C., Leerkes, E. M. & Lekka, S. K. Pathways from marital aggression to infant emotion regulation: the development of withdrawal in infancy. *Infant Behav Dev* **30**, 97-113 (2007).

343. Crompton, D. E. & Berkovic, S. F. The borderland of epilepsy: clinical and molecular features of phenomena that mimic epileptic seizures. *Lancet Neurol.* **8**, 370-381 (2009).

344. Croskerry, P. Achieving quality in clinical decision making: cognitive strategies and detection of bias. *Acad. Emerg. Med.* **9**, 1184-1204 (2002).

345. Crowson, R. L. The home schooling movement: a few concluding observations. *Peabody J. Educ.* **75**, 294-300 (2000).

346. Cuesta, M. J., Peralta, V. & de Leon, J. Neurological frontal signs and neuropsychological deficits in schizophrenic patients. *Schizophr. Res.* **20**, 15-20 (1996).

347. Cuesta, M. J., Peralta, V. & Juan, J. A. Abnormal subjective experiences in schizophrenia: Its relationships with neuropsychological disturbances and frontal signs. *Eur. Arch. Psychiatry Clin. Neurosci.* **246**, 101-105 (1996).

348. Culbert, K. M., Breedlove, S. M., Burt, S. A. & Klump, K. L. Prenatal hormone exposure and risk for eating disorders: a comparison of opposite-sex and same-sex twins. *Arch. Gen. Psychiatry* **65**, 329-336 (2008).

349. Cummings, J. L. Frontal-subcortical circuits and human behavior. *Arch. Neurol.* **50**, 873-880 (1993).

350. Cunningham, W. A. & Zelazo, P. D. Attitudes and evaluations: A social cognitive neuroscience perspective. *Trends Cog. Sci.* **11**, 97-104 (2007).

351. Cuttler, C. & Graf, P. Checking-in on the memory deficit and meta-memory deficit theories of compulsive checking. *Clin. Psychol Rev.* **29**, 393-409 (2009).

352. d'Augelli, A. R. Mental health problems among lesbian, gay, and bisexual youths ages 14 to 21. *Clin. Child Psychol. Psychiatry* **7**, 433-456 (2002).

353. Dadds, M. R., El, M. Y., Wimalaweera, S. & Guastella, A. J. Reduced eye gaze explains "fear blindness" in childhood psychopathic traits. *J Am Acad. Child Adolesc. Psychiatry* **47**, 455-463 (2008).

354. Dadds, M. R. & Fraser, J. A. Fire interest, fire setting and psychopathology in Australian children: a normative study. *Aust. N. Z. J Psychiatry* **40**, 581-586 (2006).

355. Dadds, M. R. *et al.* Attention to the eyes and fear-recognition deficits in child psychopathy. *Br. J. Psychiatry* **189**, 280-281 (2006).

356. Dahmen, J. C. & King, A. J. Learning to hear: plasticity of auditory cortical processing. *Curr. Opin. Neurobiol.* **17**, 456-464 (2007).

357. Dale, R. C. *et al.* Encephalitis lethargica syndrome: 20 new cases and evidence of basal ganglia autoimmunity. *Brain* **127**, 21-33 (2004).

358. Dale, R. C. & Heyman, I. Post-streptococcal autoimmune psychiatric and movement disorders in children. *Br. J. Psychiatry* **181**, 188-190 (2002).

359. Dale, R. C., Heyman, I., Giovannoni, G. & Church, A. W. Incidence of anti-brain antibodies in children with obsessive-compulsive disorder. *Br. J. Psychiatry* **187**, 314-319 (2005).

360. Dallaire, D. H. Children with incarcerated mothers: Developmental outcomes, special challenges and recommendations. *J. Appl. Dev. Psychol* **28**, 15-24 (2007).

361. Dally, A. The rise and fall of pink disease. *Social History of Medicine* **10**, 291-304 (1997).

362. Dalton, K. & Dalton, M. J. Characteristics of pyridoxine overdose neuropathy syndrome. *Acta Neurol Scand* **76**, 8-11 (1987).

363. Daly, D. A. & Burnett, M. L. Cluttering: assessment, treatment planning, and case study illustration. *J. Fluency Dis.* **21**, 239-248 (1996).

364. Daly, M. & Wilson, M. An assessment of some proposed exceptions to the phenomenon of nepotistic discrimination against stepchildren. *Annales Zoologici Fennici* **38**, 287-296 (2001).

365. Dansak, D. A. On the tertiary gain of illness. *Compr. Psychiatry* **14**, 523-534 (1973).

366. Dantzer, R., O'Connor, J. C., Freund, G. G., Johnson, R. W. & Kelley, K. W. From inflammation to sickness and depression: when the immune system subjugates the brain. *Nat Rev. Neurosci* **9**, 46-56 (2008).

367. Danziger, N., Prkachin, K. M. & Willer, J. C. Is pain the price of empathy? The perception of others' pain in patients with congenital insensitivity to pain. *Brain* **129**, 2494-2507 (2006).

368. Dapretto, M. *et al.* Understanding emotions in others: mirror neuron dysfunction in children with autism spectrum disorders. *Nat. Neurosci.* **9**, 28-30 (2006).

369. Dauvilliers, Y., Arnulf, I. & Mignot, E. Narcolepsy with cataplexy. *Lancet* **369**, 499-511 (2007).

370. David, C. N. *et al.* Child onset schizophrenia: High rate of visual hallucinations. *J. Am. Acad. Child Adolesc. Psychiat* **50**, 681-686 (2011).

371. David, T. J. *Symptoms of disease in childhood.* Wiley-Blackwell, Oxford (1995).

372. David, T. J. The overworked or fraudulent diagnosis of food allergy and food intolerance in children. *J. R. Soc. Med.* **78**, 21-31 (1985).

373. Davidsson, J., Collin, A., Olsson, M. E., Lundgren, J. & Soller, M. Deletion of the SCN gene cluster on 2q24.4 is associated with severe epilepsy: an array-based genotype-phenotype correlation and a comprehensive review of previously published cases. *Epilepsy Res* **81**, 69-79 (2008).

374. Davies, S. & Crawley, E. Chronic fatigue syndrome in children aged 11 years old and younger. *Arch Dis Child* **93**, 419-421 (2008).

375. Davis, C. & Carter, J. C. Compulsive overeating as an addiction disorder. A review of theory and evidence. *Appetite* **53**, 1-8 (2009).

376. Davis, M., Walker, D. L., Miles, L. & Grillon, C. Phasic vs sustained fear in rats and humans: role of the extended amygdala in fear vs anxiety. *Neuropsychopharmacology Rev* **35**, 105-135 (2010).

377. Davison, S. E. The management of violence in general psychiatry. *Adv. Psychiat. Treat.* **11**, 362-370 (2005).

378. Dawes, R. *House of Cards.* Free Press, New York (1994).

379. Dawson, N. V. Cognitive limitations and methods for improving judgments: Implications for establishing medically relevant performance goals. *Frontiers in Laboratory Practice Research* **1995**, 354-363 (1995).

380. Day, J. W. *et al.* Myotonic dystrophy type 2: molecular, diagnostic and clinical spectrum. *Neurology* **60**, 657-664 (2003).

381. de Buys Roessingh, A. S., Loriot, M. H., Wiesenauer, C. & Lallier, M. Lambert-Eaton myasthenic syndrome revealing an abdominal neuroblastoma. *J Pediatr. Surg.* **44**, E5-E7 (2009).

382. De Ribaupierre, S., Rilliet, B., Cotting, J. & Regli, L. A 10-year experience in paediatric spontaneous cerebral haemorrhage: which children with headache need more than a clinical examination? *Swiss Medical Weekly* **138**, 59-69 (2008).

383. De Smith, A. J. *et al.* A deletion of the HBII-85 class of small nucleolar RNAs (snoRNAs) is associated with hyperphagia, obesity and hypogonadism. *Hum. Mol. Genet.* **18**, 3257-3265 (2009).

384. Deeley, P. Q. The religious brain. *Anthropology & Medicine* **11**, 245-267 (2004).

385. Dehaene, S., Piazza, M., Pinel, P. & Cohen, L. Three parietal circuits for number processing. *Cog. neuropsychol* **20**, 487-506 (2003).

386. Delaney, K. R. Top 10 milieu interventions for inpatient child/adolescent treatment. *J Child Adolesc. Psychiatr. Nurs.* **19**, 203-214 (2006).

387. Delange, F. Iodine requirements during pregnancy, lactation and the neonatal period and indicators of optimal iodine nutrition. *Public Health Nutr.* **10**, 1571-1580 (2007).

388. Delanty, N., Vaughan, C. J. & French, J. A. Medical causes of seizures. *Lancet* **352**, 383-390 (1998).

389. DeMaio-Feldman, D. Somatosensory processing abilities of very-low-birth weight infants at school age. *Am. J. Occup. Ther* **48**, 639-645 (1994).

390. DeMeyer, W. Megalencephaly in children. Clinical syndromes, genetic patterns, and differential diagnosis from other causes of megalocephaly. *Neurology* **22**, 634-643 (1972).

391. Demirkaya, M., Sevinir, B., Ozdemir, O., Nazlioglu, H. O. & Okan, M. Lymphoma of the Cavernous Sinus Mimicking Tolosa-Hunt Syndrome in a Child. *Pediatr. Neurol.* **42**, 351-354 (2010).

392. Denckla, M. B. Revised neurological examination for subtle signs. *Psychopharmacol. Bull.* **21(4)**, 773-800 (1985).

393. Denecke, J. Biomarkers and diagnosis of congenital disorders of glycosylation. *Expert Opinion on Medical Diagnostics* **3**, 395-409 (2009).

394. Denisoff, R. S. & Romanowski, W. Katzman's "Rock Around the Clock": A pseudo event? *The Journal of Popular Culture* **24**, 65-78 (1990).

395. Denny, K. & Sullivan, V. O. The economic consequences of being left-handed: Some sinister results. *J. Hum. Resour.* **42**, 353 (2007).

396. Denson, T. F. Displaced Aggression in Children and Adolescents in Bhave, S. Y. & Saini, S. (eds.), *The AHA syndrome and cardiovascular diseases.*pp. 43-54 (Anshan Ltd, New Delhi,2008).

397. Denson, T. F., Pedersen, W. C. & Miller, N. The displaced aggression questionnaire. *J. Pers. Soc. Psychol.* **90**, 1032-1051 (2006).

398. Denton, W. H. Issues for DSM-V: relational diagnosis: an essential component of biopsychosocial assessment. *Am. J. Psychiatry* **164**, 1146-1147 (2007).

399. Department of Health *Women's mental health: Into the mainstream.* Department of Health, London (2002).

400. Depienne, C. *et al.* Spectrum of SCN1A gene mutations associated with Dravet syndrome: analysis of 333 patients. *J Med Genet.* **46**, 183-191 (2009).

401. Derluyn, I. & Broekaert, E. Unaccompanied refugee children and adolescents: the glaring contrast between a legal and a psychological perspective. *Int. J Law Psychiatry* **31**, 319-330 (2008).

402. Derluyn, I., Broekaert, E. & Schuyten, G. Emotional and behavioural problems in migrant adolescents in Belgium. *Eur. Child Adolesc. Psychiatry* **17**, 54-62 (2008).

403. Deuchar, N. & Brockington, I. Puerperal and menstrual psychoses: the proposal of a unitary etiological hypothesis. *J. Psychosom. Obstet. Gynaecol.* **19**, 104-110 (1998).

404. Devlin, L. & Morrison, P. J. Accuracy of the clinical diagnosis of Down syndrome. *Ulster Med. J.* **73**, 4-12 (2004).

405. deVries, M. W. & deVries, M. R. Cultural relativity of toilet training readiness: A perspective from East Africa. *Pediatrics* **60**, 170 (1977).

406. Dew, R. E. *et al.* Religion/Spirituality and adolescent psychiatric symptoms: a review. *Child Psychiatry Hum. Dev.* **39**, 381-398 (2008).

407. Diaz, B., Baus, C., Escera, C., Costa, A. & Sebastian-Galles, N. Brain potentials to native phoneme discrimination reveal the origin of individual differences in learning the sounds of a second language. *Proc. Natl. Acad. Sci. U. S. A* **105**, 16083-16088 (2008).

408. DiCarlo, J. Metabolic Encephalopathies in Children in McCandless, D. W. (ed.), *Metabolic Encephalopathy.*pp. 137-148 (Springer,2009).

409. Dickson, A., Toft, A. & O'Carroll, R. E. Neuropsychological functioning, illness perception, mood and quality of life in chronic fatigue syndrome, autoimmune thyroid disease and healthy participants. *Psychol Med.* **39**, 1567-1576 (2009).

410. Diener, E., Lucas, R. E. & Scollon, C. N. Beyond the hedonic treadmill: revising the adaptation theory of well-being. *Am Psychol* **61**, 305-314 (2006).

411. DiFranza, J. R., Aligne, C. A. & Weitzman, M. Prenatal and postnatal environmental tobacco smoke exposure and children's health. *Pediatrics* **113**, 1007-1015 (2004).

412. DiMario, F. J., Jr. Paroxysmal nonepileptic events of childhood. *Semin. Pediatr. Neurol.* **13**, 208-221 (2006).

413. Dimitrijevic, M. R., Gerasimenko, Y. & Pinter, M. M. Evidence for a spinal central pattern generator in humans. *Annals- NY Acad. Sciences* **860**, 360-376 (1998).

414. Dinklage, D. Asperger's Disorder and Nonverbal Learning Disabilities: How are these two disorders related to each other? *Asperger's Association of New England* (2001).

415. Dishion, T. J., Veronneau, M. H. & Myers, M. W. Cascading peer dynamics underlying the progression from problem behavior to violence in early to late adolescence. *Dev. Psychopathol.* **22**, 603-619 (2010).

416. Dittmar, H. Are you what you have? *Psychologist* **17**, 206-210 (2004).

417. Djukic, A. Folate-responsive neurologic diseases. *Pediatr. Neurol* **37**, 387-397 (2007).

418. Dmitruk, V. M. "Experimental neurosis" in cats: fact or artifact? *J. Abnorm. Psychol* **83**, 97-105 (1974).

419. Dodds, L., Fell, D. B., Joseph, K. S., Allen, V. M. & Butler, B. Outcomes of pregnancies complicated by hyperemesis gravidarum. *Obstet. Gynecol.* **107**, 285-292 (2006).

420. Dogangun, B. *et al.* The treatment of psychogenic polydipsia with risperidone in two children diagnosed with schizophrenia. *J Child Adolesc. Psychopharmacol.* **16**, 492-495 (2006).

421. Dolgin, M. J. *et al.* Trajectories of adjustment in mothers of children with newly diagnosed cancer: a natural history investigation. *J Pediatr. Psychol* **32**, 771-782 (2007).

422. Donsante, A. *et al.* Differences in ATP7A gene expression underlie intrafamilial variability in Menkes disease/occipital horn syndrome. *J. Med. Genetics* **44**, 492-497 (2007).

423. Doss, A. J. Evidence-based diagnosis: incorporating diagnostic instruments into clinical practice. *J. Am. Acad. Child Adolesc. Psychiatry* **44**, 947-952 (2005).

424. Dossetor, D. R. 'All that glitters is not gold': misdiagnosis of psychosis in pervasive developmental disorders--a case series. *Clin Child Psychol Psychiatry* **12**, 537-548 (2007).

425. Doty, R. L., Shah, M. & Bromley, S. M. Drug-induced taste disorders. *Drug Saf.* **31**, 199-215 (2008).

426. Dowdney, L. & Skuse, D. Parenting provided by adults with mental retardation. *J Child Psychol Psychiatry* **34**, 25-47 (1993).

427. Drake, L. J. & Bundy, D. A. P. Multiple helminth infections in children: impact and control. *Parasitology* **122**, 73-81 (2001).

428. Drew, L. & Stifel, E. N. Secondary amenorrhea among young women entering religious life. *Obstet. Gynecol.* **32**, 47-51 (1968).

429. Drummond, C. R., Ahmad, S. A. & Rourke, B. P. Rules for the classification of younger children with nonverbal learning disabilities and basic phonological processing disabilities. *Arch. Clin. Neuropsychol.* **20**, 171-182 (2005).

430. Drummond, K. D., Bradley, S. J., Peterson-Badali, M. & Zucker, K. J. A follow-up study of girls with gender identity disorder. *Dev. Psychol.* **44**, 34-45 (2008).

431. Dudley, R. L. Alienation from religion in adolescents from fundamentalist religious homes. *J. Sci. Study Religion* **17**, 389-398 (1978).

432. Dufrene, B. A., Watson, T. S. & Kazmerski, J. S. Functional Analysis and Treatment of Nail Biting. *Behav. Modif.* **32**, 913-927 (2008).

433. Dulcan, M. K. & Martini, D. R. *Concise guide to child and adolescent psychiatry.* American Psychiatric Press, Washington, DC (2005).

434. Dummit, E. S., III *et al.* Systematic assessment of 50 children with selective mutism. *J. Am. Acad. Child Adolesc. Psychiatry* **36**, 653-660 (1997).

435. Duryea, S., Lam, D. & Levison, D. Effects of economic shocks on children's employment and schooling in Brazil. *J. Develop. Econ.* **84**, 188-214 (2007).

436. Dutton, D. G. The complexities of domestic violence. *Am. Psychol* **62**, 708-709 (2007).

437. Dwyer, P., Stokes, H., Tyler, D. & Holdsworth, R. *Negotiating staying and returning.* University of Melbourne, Melbourne (1998).

438. Eagle, M. N. Psychological Processes and Neural Correlates. *Neuropsychoanalysis* **13**, 37-42 (2011).

439. Eagle, M. N. A critical evaluation of current conceptions of transference and countertransference. *Psychoanal. Psychol.* **17**, 24-37 (2000).

440. Eaves, L., Silberg, J. & Erkanli. A. Resolving multiple epigenetic pathways to adolescent depression. *J. Child Psychol Psychiatry* **44**, 1006-1014 (2003).

441. Ebert, R. S. & Long, J. S. Mental Retardation and the Criminal Justice System: Forensic Issues in Hall, H. V. (ed.), *Forensic psychology and neuropsychology for criminal and civil cases.* pp. 375-392 (Taylor & Francis, Boca Raton, 2008).

442. Ecker, C. *et al.* Investigating the predictive value of whole-brain structural MR scans in autism: a pattern classification approach. *Neuroimage* **49**, 44-56 (2010).

443. Edelstyn, N. M. J., Baker, S. R., Ellis, S. J. & Jenkinson, P. A cognitive neuropsychological and psychophysiological investigation of a patient who exhibited an acute exacerbated behavioural response during innocuous somatosensory stimulation and movement. *Behav. Neurol.* **15**, 15-22 (2004).

444. Eden, G. F., Wood, F. B. & Stein, J. F. Clock drawing in developmental dyslexia. *J. Learn. Disabil.* **36**, 216-228 (2003).

445. Egger, H. L. & Angold, A. Common emotional and behavioral disorders in preschool children: presentation, nosology, and epidemiology. *J. Child Psychol Psychiatry* **47**, 313-337 (2006).

446. Eggermann, T. Silver-Russell and Beckwith-Wiedemann syndromes: opposite (epi)mutations in 11p15 result in opposite clinical pictures. *Horm. Res* **71**, 30-35 (2009).

447. Egliston, K. A., McMahon, C. & Austin, M. P. Stress in pregnancy and infant HPA axis function: conceptual and methodological issues relating to the use of salivary cortisol as an outcome measure. *Psychoneuroendocrinology* **32**, 1-13 (2007).

448. Ehlers, A. & Clark, D. M. A cognitive model of posttraumatic stress disorder. *Behav. Res. Ther.* **38**, 319-345 (2000).

449. Eigsti, I. M. & Bennetto, L. Grammaticality judgments in autism: Deviance or delay. *J. Child Lang.* **36**, 999-1021 (2009).

450. Ekbom, K. & Ulfberg, J. Restless legs syndrome. *J. Internal Medicine* **266**, 419-431 (2009).

451. Ekman, P. An argument for basic emotions. *Cognition & Emotion* **6**, 169-200 (1992).

452. Ekman, P., Friesen, W. V. & O'Sullivan, M. Smiles when lying in Ekman, P. & Rosenberg, E. (eds.), *What the face reveals.* pp. 201-216 (Oxford University Press, New York, 1997).

453. Ekman, P., Friesen, W. V. & Simons, R. C. Is the startle reaction an emotion? in Ekman, P. & Rosenberg, E. (eds.), *What the face reveals.* pp. 21-39 (Oxford University Press, New York, 1997).

454. Eley, T. C. & Stevenson, J. Specific life events and chronic experiences differentially associated with depression and anxiety in young twins. *J. Abnorm. Child Psychol.* **28**, 383-394 (2000).

455. Ellenbogen, J. M., Payne, J. D. & Stickgold, R. The role of sleep in declarative memory consolidation: passive, permissive, active or none? *Curr. Opin. Neurobiol.* **16**, 716-722 (2006).

456. Elliman, D. & Lynch, M. The physical punishment of children. *Arch. Dis. Child.* **83**, 196-198 (2000).

457. Ellis, A. An operational reformulation of some of the basic principles of psychoanalysis. *Psychoanal. Rev.* **43**, 163-180 (1956).

458. Ellis, R. J., Calero, P. & Stockin, M. D. HIV infection and the central nervous system: a primer. *Neuropsychol. Rev.* **19**, 144-151 (2009).

459. Elsabbagh, M. *et al.* Neural correlates of eye gaze processing in the infant broader autism phenotype. *Biol. Psychiatry* **65**, 31-38 (2009).

460. Embirucu, E. K., Martyn, M. L., Schlesinger, D. & Kok, F. Autosomal recessive ataxias: 20 types, and counting. *Arq Neuropsiquiatr.* **67**, 1143-1156 (2009).

461. Emck, C., Bosscher, R., Beek, P. & Doreleijers, T. Gross motor performance and self-perceived motor competence in children with emotional, behavioural, and pervasive developmental disorders: a review. *Dev. Med. Child Neurol* **51**, 501-517 (2009).

462. Emerson, J. & Babtie, P. *The dyscalculia assessment*. Continuum Publishing Corp, London (2010).

463. Emerson, P. M. & Souza, A. P. Birth order, child labor, and school attendance in Brazil. *World Devel.* **36**, 1647-1664 (2008).

464. Endres, W. Inherited metabolic diseases affecting the carrier. *J. Inher. Metab. Dis.* **20**, 9-20 (1997).

465. Enoki, H., Takeda, S., Hirose, E., Matsubayashi, R. & Matsubayashi, T. Unilateral spatial neglect in a child with hemiplegic migraine. *Cephalalgia* **26**, 1165-1167 (2006).

466. Eppig, C., Fincher, C. L. & Thornhill, R. Parasite prevalence and the worldwide distribution of cognitive ability. *Proceedings of the Royal Society B: Biological Sciences* **(in press)**, (2010).

467. Epstein, A. W. Recurrent dreams; their relationship to temporal lobe seizures. *Arch Gen. Psychiatry* **10**, 25-30 (1964).

468. Erkolahti, R. & Nystrom, M. The prevalence of transitional object use in adolescence: is there a connection between the existence of a transitional object and depressive symptoms? *Eur. Child Adolesc. Psychiatry* **18**, 400-406 (2009).

469. Erlandson, A. & Hagberg, B. MECP2 abnormality phenotypes: clinicopathologic area with broad variability. *J. Child Neurol.* **20**, 727-732 (2005).

470. Ermer, E. & Kiehl, K. A. Psychopaths are impaired in social exchange and precautionary reasoning. *Psychol. Science* **21**, 1399-1405 (2010).

471. Espay, A. J. & Chen, R. Rigidity and spasms from autoimmune encephalomyelopathies: stiff-person syndrome. *Muscle Nerve* **34**, 677-690 (2006).

472. Ess, K. C. Tuberous sclerosis complex: a brave new world? *Curr. Opin. Neurol* **23**, 189-193 (2010).

473. Evans, D. W. *et al.* Ritual, habit, and perfectionism: the prevalence and development of compulsive-like behavior in normal young children. *Child Dev.* **68**, 58-68 (1997).

474. Evans, J. L. *What about the children? How to help children survive separation and divorce*. Bantam Press, (2009).

475. Evans, S. E., Davies, C. & DiLillo, D. Exposure to domestic violence: A meta-analysis of child and adolescent outcomes. *Aggression and Violent Behavior* **13**, 131-140 (2008).

476. Evans, S. W. *et al.* Dose-response effects of methylphenidate on ecologically valid measures of academic performance and classroom behavior in adolescents with ADHD. *Exp. Clin. Psychopharmacol.* **9**, 163-175 (2001).

477. Fabiano, G. A. *et al.* An evaluation of three time-out procedures for children with attention-deficit/hyperactivity disorder. *Behavior Therapy* **35**, 449-469 (2004).

478. Fair, D. A. *et al.* Development of distinct control networks through segregation and integration. *Proc. Natl. Acad. Sci. U. S. A* **104**, 13507-13512 (2007).

479. Fairburn, C. G. & Harrison, P. J. Eating disorders. *Lancet* **361**, 407-416 (2003).

480. Fancher, T. L., Kamboj, A. & Onate, J. Interpreting liver function tests. *Curr. Psychiat.* **6**, 61-68 (2007).

481. Faraone, S. V. *et al.* Molecular genetics of attention-deficit/hyperactivity disorder. *Biol. Psychiatry* **57**, 1313-1323 (2005).

482. Farmer, T. W. The social dynamics of aggressive and disruptive behavior in school: Implications for behavior consultation. *J. Educ. Psychol. Consult.* **11**, 299-321 (2000).

483. Farrington, D. P., Gallagher, B., Morley, L., St Ledger, R. J. & West, D. J. Unemployment, school leaving, and crime. *Br. J. Criminology* **26**, 335-356 (1986).

484. Farrington, D. P., Jolliffe, D., Loeber, R., Stouthamer-Loeber, M. & Kalb, L. M. The concentration of offenders in families, and family criminality in the prediction of boys' delinquency. *J. Adolesc.* **24**, 579-596 (2001).

485. Farzin, F. *et al.* Autism spectrum disorders and attention-deficit/hyperactivity disorder in boys with the fragile X premutation. *J. Dev. Behav. Pediatr.* **27**, S137-S144 (2006).

486. Fava, M. *et al.* Difference in treatment outcome in outpatients with anxious versus nonanxious depression: a STAR* D report. *Am. J. Psychiatry* **165**, 342-351 (2008).

487. Favazza, A. R. The coming of age of self-mutilation. *J. Nerv. Ment. Dis.* **186**, 259-268 (1998).

488. Fazel, M. & Stein, A. The mental health of refugee children. *Arch. Dis. Child.* **87**, 366-370 (2002).

489. Feely, M. P., O'Hare, J., Veale, D. & Callaghan, N. Episodes of acute confusion or psychosis in familial hemiplegic migraine. *Acta Neurol Scand* **65**, 369-375 (1982).

490. Feinstein, C. & Singh, S. Social phenotypes in neurogenetic syndromes. *Child Adolesc. Psychiatr. Clin. N. Am.* **16**, 631-647 (2007).

491. Ferguson, C. J. *et al.* Violent video games and aggression: causal relationship or byproduct of family violence and intrinsic violence motivation? *Crim. Justice & Behav* **35**, 311-332 (2008).

492. Ferguson, T. *The young delinquent in his social setting*. Oxford University Press, London (1952).

493. Fernandez, H. H. & Friedman, J. H. Classification and treatment of tardive syndromes. *Neurologist.* **9**, 16-27 (2003).

494. Fidas, A. *et al.* Prevalence and patterns of spina bifida occulta in 2707 normal adults. *Clin. Radiol.* **38**, 537-542 (1987).

495. Field, A. P. & Schorah, H. The verbal information pathway to fear and heart rate changes in children. *J Child Psychol Psychiatry* **48**, 1088-1093 (2007).

496. Field, J. J., Austin, P. F., An, P., Yan, Y. & DeBaun, M. R. Enuresis is a common and persistent problem among children and young adults with sickle cell anemia. *Urology* **72**, 81-84 (2008).

497. Fink, M. & Taylor, M. A. The catatonia syndrome: forgotten but not gone. *Arch Gen. Psychiatry* **66**, 1173-1177 (2009).

498. Finkelhor, D. Sex among siblings: a survey on prevalence, variety, and effects. *Arch Sex Behav* **9**, 171-194 (1980).

499. Finlay-Jones, R. & Brown, G. W. Types of stressful life event and the onset of anxiety and depressive disorders. *Psychol. Med.* **11**, 803-815 (1981).

500. Finsterer, J. Leigh and Leigh-like syndrome in children and adults. *Pediatr. Neurol.* **39**, 223-235 (2008).

501. Firestone, P. & Douglas, V. The effects of reward and punishment on reaction times and autonomic activity in hyperactive and normal children. *J. Abnorm. Child Psychol.* **3**, 201-216 (1975).

502. First, M. B., Frances, A. & Pincus, H. A. *DSM-IV-TR Handbook of differential diagnosis*. American Psychiatric Publishing, Inc., Arlington (2002).

503. Fishbain, D. A., Cutler, R. B., Rosomoff, H. L. & Rosomoff, R. S. Is there a relationship between nonorganic physical findings (Waddell signs) and secondary gain/malingering? *Clin. J. Pain* **20**, 399-408 (2004).

504. Fishell, G. & Rudy, B. Mechanisms of inhibition within the telencephalon: "where the wild things are". *Annu. Rev Neurosci* **34**, 535-567 (2011).

505. Fisher, J. R. W., Hammarberg, K. & Baker, G. H. W. Antenatal mood and fetal attachment after assisted conception. *Fertil. Steril.* **89**, 1103-1112 (2008).

506. Flaschker, N. *et al.* Description of the mutations in 15 subjects with variant forms of maple syrup urine disease. *J. Inherit. Metab. Dis.* **30**, 903-909 (2007).

507. Florance, N. R. *et al.* Anti-N-methyl-D-aspartate receptor (NMDAR) encephalitis in children and adolescents. *Ann. Neurol* **66**, 11-18 (2009).

508. Fohrman, D. A. & Stein, M. T. Psychosis: 6 steps rule out medical causes in kids. *J. Fam. Prac.* **5**, (2006).

509. Foley, D. C. & McCutcheon, H. Detecting pain in people with an intellectual disability. *Accid. Emerg. Nurs.* **12**, 196-200 (2004).
510. Folstein, M. F., Folstein, S. E. & McHugh, P. R. Mini-mental state. A practical method for grading the cognitive state of patients for the clinician. *J. Psychiatr. Res.* **12**, 189-198 (1975).
511. Foote, B. & Park, J. Dissociative identity disorder and schizophrenia: differential diagnosis and theoretical issues. *Curr. Psychiat. Rep.* **10**, 217-222 (2008).
512. Forsyth, R. J. Neurological and cognitive decline in adolescence. *J Neurol Neurosurg Psychiatry* **74**, i9-i16 (2003).
513. Fortey, R. *Dry Store Room No.1: The secret life of the Natural History Museum.* Harper Press, London (2008).
514. Fowler, H. W. *A Dictionary of Modern English Usage.* Oxford University Press, Oxford (1946).
515. Fox, N. A., Henderson, H. A., Marshall, P. J., Nichols, K. E. & Ghera, M. M. Behavioral inhibition: linking biology and behavior within a developmental framework. *Annu. Rev. Psychol* **56**, 235-262 (2005).
516. Fox, N. A., Henderson, H. A., Rubin, K. H., Calkins, S. D. & Schmidt, L. A. Continuity and discontinuity of behavioral inhibition and exuberance: Psychophysiological and behavioral influences across the first four years of life. *Child Dev.* **72**, 1-21 (2001).
517. Foy, E. Parental grieving of childhood disability: a rural perspective. *Australian Social Work* **50**, 39-44 (1997).
518. Franic, S., Middeldorp, C. M., Dolan, C. V., Ligthart, L. & Boomsma, D. I. Childhood and adolescent anxiety and depression: Beyond heritability. *J. Am. Acad. Child Adolesc. Psychiat* **49**, 820-829 (2010).
519. Frankfurt, H. On Truth, Lies, and Bullshit in Martin, C. (ed.), *The Philosophy of Deception*.pp. 37-48 (Oxford University Press, USA, New York,2009).
520. Fredrickson, B. L. The broaden-and-build theory of positive emotions. *Philosophical Transactions of the Royal Society B: Biological Sciences* **359**, 1367-1377 (2004).
521. Freeman, B. J., Del'Homme, M., Guthrie, D. & Zhang, F. Vineland Adaptive Behavior Scale scores as a function of age and initial IQ in 210 autistic children. *J. Autism Dev. Disord.* **29**, 379-384 (1999).
522. Freeman, D. The experience of paranoia deserves centre stage. *Br. J. Psychiatry* **193**, 81-82 (1998).
523. Freeman, D. *et al.* Psychological investigation of the structure of paranoia in a non-clinical population. *Br. J. Psychiatry* **186**, 427-435 (2005).
524. Frenkel, T. I., Lamy, D., Algom, D. & Bar-Haim, Y. Individual differences in perceptual sensitivity and response bias in anxiety: evidence from emotional faces. *Cognition & Emotion* (2008).
525. Fridlund, A. J. & Loftis, J. M. Relations between tickling and humorous laughter: preliminary support for the Darwin-Hecker hypothesis. *Biol Psychol* **30**, 141-150 (1990).
526. Fried, I., Wilson, C. L., MacDonald, K. A. & Behnke, E. J. Electric current stimulates laughter. *Nature* **391**, 650 (1998).
527. Friedrich, W. N. *et al.* Child Sexual Behavior Inventory: normative, psychiatric, and sexual abuse comparisons. *Child Maltreat.* **6**, 37-49 (2001).
528. Frith, C. Is autism a disconnection disorder? *Lancet Neurol* **3**, 577 (2004).
529. Fujiwara, J., Nakahara, S., Enomoto, T., Nakata, Y. & Takita, H. The effectiveness of O2 administration for transient ischemic attacks in moyamoya disease in children. *Childs Nerv. Syst.* **12**, 69-75 (1996).
530. Fuller, G. N., Marshall, A., Flint, J., Lewis, S. & Wise, R. J. Migraine madness: recurrent psychosis after migraine. *Br. Med. J.* **56**, 416-418 (1993).
531. Furlong, A. Not a very NEET solution: Representing problematic labour market transitions among early school-leavers. *Work, Employment & Society* **20**, 553-569 (2006).
532. Gabbard, G. O. Splitting in hospital treatment. *Am. J. Psychiatry* **146**, 444-451 (1989).
533. Gainetdinov, R. R., Wetsel, W. C. & Caron, M. G. Serotonin and the therapeutic effects of Ritalin (Response). *Science* **288**, 11a-11b (2000).
534. Galanopoulou, A. S. GABA-A Receptors in Normal Development and Seizures: Friends or Foes? *Current Neuropharmacology* **6**, 1-20 (2008).
535. Gall, J. " Binkie Flutter," an Apparently Voluntary Behavior of Infants, Possibly Related to Vibratory Jaw Movements in Dogs: Report of 4 Cases. *Pediatrics* **115**, e367-e369 (2005).
536. Gallagher, S., Phillips, A. C., Oliver, C. & Carroll, D. Predictors of psychological morbidity in parents of children with intellectual disabilities. *J Pediatr. Psychol* **33**, 1129-1136 (2008).
537. Garber, J., Zeman, J. & Walker, L. S. Recurrent abdominal pain in children: psychiatric diagnoses and parental psychopathology. *J. Am. Acad. Child Adolesc. Psychiatry* **29**, 648-656 (1990).
538. Garcia, A. M. *et al.* Phenomenology of early childhood onset Obsessive Compulsive Disorder. *J. Psychopathol. Behav. Assessment* **31**, 104-111 (2009).
539. Garcia-Cazorla, A. *et al.* Mental retardation and inborn errors of metabolism. *J Inherit. Metab Dis* **32**, 597-608 (2009).
540. Gard, M. G. & Kring, A. M. Sex differences in the time course of emotion. *Emotion* **7**, 429-437 (2007).
541. Gardner, J. W. *et al.* Risk factors predicting exertional heat illness in male Marine Corps recruits. *Med & Science in Sports & Exercise* **28**, 939-944 (1996).
542. Gardner, M. & Steinberg, L. Peer influence on risk taking, risk preference, and risky decision making in adolescence and adulthood: an experimental study. *Dev. Psychol.* **41**, 625-635 (2005).
543. Gardner, R. M. & Brown, D. L. Body image assessment: A review of figural drawing scales. *Personality & Individ Differences* **48**, 107-111 (2010).
544. Gardner, W. N. The pathophysiology of hyperventilation disorders. *Chest* **109**, 516-534 (1996).
545. Gargus, J. J. & Tournay, A. Novel mutation confirms seizure locus SCN1A is also familial hemiplegic migraine locus FHM3. *Pediatr. Neurol* **37**, 407-410 (2007).
546. Garralda, E. M. & Chalder, T. Practitioner review: chronic fatigue syndrome in childhood. *J. Child Psychol. Psychiatry* **46**, 1143-1151 (2005).
547. Garralda, M. E. Pathological demand avoidance syndrome or psychiatric disorder? *Arch Dis. Child* **(electronic letter, 22.7.2003)**, (2003).
548. Garralda, M. E. Somatisation in children. *J. Child Psychol. Psychiatry* **37**, 13-33 (1996).
549. Gathercole, S. E., Pickering, S. J., Ambridge, B. & Wearing, H. The structure of working memory from 4 to 15 years of age. *Dev Psychol* **40**, 177-190 (2004).
550. Gauchat, A., Zadra, A., Tremblay, R. E., Zelazo, P. D. & Seguin, J. R. Recurrent dreams and psychosocial adjustment in preteenaged children. *Dreaming* **19**, 75-84 (2009).
551. Gellerman, D. M. & Suddath, R. Violent fantasy, dangerousness, and the duty to warn and protect. *J. Am. Acad. Psychiatry and the Law Online* **33**, 484-495 (2005).
552. Gentile, D. A. *et al.* The effects of prosocial video games on prosocial behaviors: international evidence from correlational, longitudinal, and experimental studies. *Pers. Soc. Psychol. Bull.* **35**, 752-763 (2009).
553. Gentile, D. A. & Gentile, J. R. Violent video games as exemplary teachers: a conceptual analysis. *J. Youth Adolesc.* **37**, 127-141 (2007).
554. Genuis, S. J. & Bouchard, T. P. Celiac disease presenting as autism. *J Child Neurol* **25**, 114-119 (2010).
555. George, J., Acharya, S. V., Bangar, T. R., Menon, P. S. & Shah, N. S. Primary hyperparathyroidism in children and adolescents. *Indian J. Pediatr.* **77**, 175-178 (2010).

556. Gerlach, A. L., Wilhelm, F. H., Gruber, K. & Roth, W. T. Blushing and physiological arousability in social phobia. *J Abnorm. Psychol* **110**, 247-258 (2001).

557. Ghaziuddin, M. *Mental health aspects of autism and Asperger syndrome*. Jessica Kingsley, Philadelphia (2005).

558. Ghaziuddin, M. & Gerstein, L. Pedantic speaking style differentiates Asperger syndrome from high-functioning autism. *J. Autism Dev. Disord.* **26**, 585-595 (1996).

559. Gibbs, J., Appleton, J. & Appleton, R. Dyspraxia or developmental coordination disorder? Unravelling the enigma. *Arch Dis Child* **92**, 534-539 (2007).

560. Gidley Larson, J. C., Bastian, A. J., Donchin, O., Shadmehr, R. & Mostofsky, S. H. Acquisition of internal models of motor tasks in children with autism. *Brain* **131**, 2894-2903 (2008).

561. Gilbert, S. S., Burgess, H. J., Kennaway, D. J. & Dawson, D. Attenuation of sleep propensity, core hypothermia, and peripheral heat loss after temazepam tolerance. *Am. J. Physiol- Regulatory, Integrative, Comp. Physiol.* **279**, 1980-1987 (2000).

562. Gilbert, W. M., Jacoby, B. N., Xing, G., Danielsen, B. & Smith, L. H. Adverse obstetric events are associated with significant risk of cerebral palsy. *Am. J. Obstet. Gynecol.* **(in press)**, (2010).

563. Gillberg, C. Practitioner review: physical investigations in mental retardation. *J Child Psychol Psychiatry* **38**, 889-897 (1997).

564. Gillberg, C. & Coleman, M. *The biology of the autistic syndromes*. MacKeith Press, London (2000).

565. Gillberg, C., Harrington, R. & Steinhausen, H.-C. *A clinician's handbook of child and adolescent psychiatry*. Cambridge University Press, Cambridge (2006).

566. Gillberg, C. & Kadesjo, B. Why bother about clumsiness? The implications of having developmental coordination disorder (DCD). *Neural Plast.* **10**, 59-68 (2003).

567. Gillberg, C. *et al.* Long-term stimulant treatment of children with attention-deficit hyperactivity disorder symptoms. A randomized, double-blind, placebo-controlled trial. *Arch Gen. Psychiatry* **54**, 857-864 (1997).

568. Gillingham, M. B. Nutrition Management of Patients with Inherited Disorders of Mitochondrial Fatty Acid Oxidation in Acosta, P. B. (ed.), *Nutrition Management of Patients With Inherited Metabolic Diseases*.pp. 369-403 (Jones & Bartlett Pub, Sudbury,MA,2010).

569. Gilovich, T. *How we know what isn't so: the fallibility of human reason in everyday life*. Free Press, New York (1993).

570. Gittelman-Klein, R. & Klein, D. F. Methylphenidate effects in learning disabilities: Psychometric changes. *Arch. Gen. Psychiatry* **33**, 655-664 (1976).

571. Glaser, D. Emotional abuse and neglect (psychological maltreatment): a conceptual framework. *Child Abuse Negl.* **26**, 697-714 (2002).

572. Glimcher, P. W. Indeterminacy in brain and behavior. *Annu. Rev. Psychol* **56**, 25-56 (2005).

573. Glue, P. & Patterson, T. Can drug treatments enhance learning in subjects with intellectual disability? *Aust. N. Z. J. Psychiatry* **43**, 899-904 (2009).

574. Godfrey, E. *et al.* Chronic fatigue syndrome in adolescents: do parental expectations of their child's intellectual ability match the child's ability? *J. Psychosom. Res* **67**, 165-168 (2009).

575. Goez, H. & Zelnik, N. Handedness in patients with developmental coordination disorder. *J. Child Neurol.* **23**, 151-154 (2008).

576. Goldacre, B. Pink, pink, pink, pink. Pink moan. Guardian . 25-8-2007.
      Ref Type: Newspaper

577. Goldacre, B. *Bad Science*. Harper Perennial, London (2008).

578. Goldberg, D. & Goodyer, I. *The origins and course of common mental disorders*. Taylor & Francis, London (2005).

579. Goldberg, R. J., Dubin, W. R. & Fogel, B. S. Behavioral Emergencies Assessment and Psychopharmacologic Management. *Clin. Neuropharmacol.* **12**, 233-248 (1989).

580. Golden, N. H. & Carlson, J. L. The pathophysiology of amenorrhea in the adolescent. *Ann. N. Y. Acad. Sci.* **1135**, 163-178 (2008).

581. Goldsmith, H. H. *et al.* Roundtable: What is temperament? Four approaches. *Child Dev.* **58**, 505-529 (1987).

582. Goldsmith, H. H., Van Hulle, C. A., Arneson, C. L., Schreiber, J. E. & Gernsbacher, M. A. A Population-Based Twin Study of Parentally Reported Tactile and Auditory Defensiveness in Young Children. *J. Abnorm. Child Psychol.* (2006).

583. Goldstein, W. N. Clarification of projective identification. *Am. J. Psychiatry* **148**, 153-161 (1991).

584. Gomez-Pinilla, F. Brain foods: the effects of nutrients on brain function. *Nat. Rev. Neurosci.* **9**, 568-578 (2008).

585. Gonzalez, G., Barros, G., Russi, M. E., Nu±ez, A. & Scavone, C. Acquired Neuromyotonia in childhood: case report and review. *Pediatric Neurology* **38**, 61-63 (2008).

586. Gonzalez-Alegre, P. & Afifi, A. K. Clinical characteristics of childhood-onset (juvenile) Huntington disease: report of 12 patients and review of the literature. *J. Child Neurol* **21**, 223-229 (2006).

587. Good, W. V. Behaviors of visually impaired children. *Semin. Ophthalmol.* **6**, 158-160 (1991).

588. Good, W. V. *et al.* Cortical visual impairment in children. *Surv. Ophthalmol.* **38**, 351-364 (1994).

589. Goodman, A. Neurobiology of addiction. An integrative review. *Biochem. Pharmacol.* **75**, 266-322 (2008).

590. Goodman, R. *Child and adolescent mental health services: Reasoned advice to commissioners and providers*. Maudsley (Discussion paper number 4), London (1997).

591. Goodman, R. Infantile autism: a syndrome of multiple primary deficits? *J. Autism Dev. Disord.* **19**, 409-424 (1989).

592. Goodman, R., Renfrew, D. & Mullick, M. Predicting type of psychiatric disorder from Strengths and Difficulties Questionnaire (SDQ) scores in child mental health clinics in London and Dhaka. *Eur. Child Adolesc. Psychiatry* **9**, 129-134 (2000).

593. Goodwin, G. M. & Malhi, G. S. What is a mood stabilizer? *Psychol. Med.* **37**, 609-614 (2007).

594. Goodyer, I. M. Recent undesirable life events: their influence on subsequent psychopathology. *Eur. Child Adolesc. Psychiatry* **5**, 33-37 (1996).

595. Gorelick, M. H., Shaw, K. N. & Murphy, K. O. Validity and reliability of clinical signs in the diagnosis of dehydration in children. *Pediatrics* **99**, e6 (1997).

596. Gothelf, D. *et al.* Risk factors for the emergence of psychiatric disorders in adolescents with 22q11.2 deletion syndrome. *Am. J. Psychiatry* **164**, 663-669 (2007).

597. Gouvier, W. D., Baumeister, A. & Ijaola, K. Neuropsychological disorders of children in Matson, J. L. (ed.), *Assessing childhood psychopathology and developmental disabilities*.pp. 151-182 (Springer, London,2009).

598. Graber, J. A., Lewinsohn, P. M., Seeley, J. R. & Brooks-Gunn, J. Is psychopathology associated with the timing of pubertal development? *J. Am. Acad. Child Adolesc. Psychiat.* **36**, 1768-1776 (1997).

599. Graham, P. Treatment interventions and findings from research: bridging the chasm in child psychiatry. *Br. J. Psychiatry* **176**, 414-419 (2000).

600. Graham, P., Turk, J. & Verhulst, F. *Child psychiatry: A developmental approach*. Oxford University Press, New York (1999).

601. Graham, S., Taylor, A. Z. & Hudley, C. Exploring achievement values among ethnic minority early adolescents. *J. Educ. Psychol.* **90**, 606-620 (1998).

602. Grahame, R. Joint hypermobility syndrome pain. *Curr. Pain Headache Rep.* **13**, 427-433 (2009).

603. Grammer, K. & Eibl-Eibesfeldt, I. The ritualisation of laughter in Koch, W. A. (ed.), *Naturlichkeit der Sprache und der Kultur*.pp. 192-214 (Bochum,1990).

604. Grant, R. & Graus, F. Paraneoplastic movement disorders. *Mov Disord.* **24**, 1715-1724 (2009).
605. Gray, K. & Wegner, D. M. The sting of intentional pain. *Psychol. Science* **19**, 1260-1262 (2008).
606. Gray, R. G. *et al.* Inborn errors of metabolism as a cause of neurological disease in adults: an approach to investigation. *J Neurol Neurosurg. Psychiatry* **69**, 5-12 (2000).
607. Graziano, M. S. & Cooke, D. F. Parieto-frontal interactions, personal space, and defensive behavior. *Neuropsychologia* **44**, 2621-2635 (2006).
608. Green, C. E. L. *et al.* Measuring ideas of persecution and social reference: the Green et al. Paranoid Thought Scales (GPTS). *Psychol. Med.* **38**, 101-111 (2007).
609. Green, H., James, R. A., Gilbert, J. D. & Byard, R. W. Medicolegal complications of pseudologia fantastica. *Leg. Med.* **1**, 254-256 (1999).
610. Green, J. A. K. & Goswami, U. Synesthesia and number cognition in children. *Cognition* **106**, 463-473 (2008).
611. Green, M. *Green & Richmond: Pediatric Diagnosis. Interpretation of Symptoms and Signs in Different Age Periods.* Saunders, Philadelphia (1980).
612. Green, S. M., Loeber, R. & Lahey, B. B. Child psychopathology and deviant family hierarchies. *J. Child Family Studies* **1**, 341-349 (1992).
613. Green, T. *et al.* Psychiatric disorders and intellectual functioning throughout development in velocardiofacial (22q11.2 deletion) syndrome. *J Am. Acad. Child Adolesc. Psychiatry* **48**, 1060-1068 (2009).
614. Greene, R. W., Abidin, R. R. & Kmetz, C. The Index of Teaching Stress: A measure of student-teacher compatibility. *J. School Psychology* **35**, 239-259 (1997).
615. Greenwald, A. G., McGhee, D. E. & Schwartz, J. L. Measuring individual differences in implicit cognition: the implicit association test. *J. Pers. Soc. Psychol* **74**, 1464-1480 (1998).
616. Greeves, L. G. *et al.* Effect of genotype on changes in intelligence quotient after dietary relaxation in phenylketonuria and hyperphenylalaninaemia. *Arch Dis. Child* **82**, 216-221 (2000).
617. Greitemeyer, T. Effects of songs with prosocial lyrics on prosocial thoughts, affect, and behavior. *J. Soc. Psychol.* **45**, 186-190 (2009).
618. Griffiths, T. D., Sigmundsson, T., Takei, N., Rowe, D. & Murray, R. M. Neurological abnormalities in familial and sporadic schizophrenia. *Brain* **121**, 191-203 (1998).
619. Grigorenko, E. L. Rethinking disorders of spoken and written language: generating workable hypotheses. *J. Dev. Behav. Pediatr.* **28**, 478-486 (2007).
620. Grillon, C., Baas, J. P., Lissek, S., Smith, K. & Milstein, J. Anxious responses to predictable and unpredictable aversive events. *Behav. Neurosci.* **118**, 916-924 (2004).
621. Gropman, A. L., Smith, A. C. M. & Duncan, W. Neurological aspects of the Smith-Magenis Syndrome in Nass, R. D. & Frank, Y. (eds.), *Cognitive and Behavioral Abnormalities of Pediatric Diseases.*pp. 231-243 (Oxford University Press, Oxford,2010).
622. Gross, J. J. The emerging field of emotion regulation: An integrative review. *Rev. Gen. Psychol.* **2**, 271-299 (1998).
623. Gross, J. J. & John, O. P. Individual differences in two emotion regulation processes: Implications for affect, relationships, and well-being. *J. Pers. Soc. Psychol.* **85**, 348-362 (2003).
624. Gross, T. F. The perception of four basic emotions in human and nonhuman faces by children with autism and other developmental disabilities. *J. Abnorm. Child Psychol* **32**, 469-480 (2004).
625. Grossi, D., LePore, M., Napolitano, A. & Trojano, L. On selective left neglect during walking in a child. *Brain Cogn* **47**, 539-544 (2001).
626. Gu, B. M. *et al.* Neural correlates of cognitive inflexibility during task-switching in obsessive-compulsive disorder. *Brain* **131**, 155-164 (2008).
627. Gu, F. *et al.* Erectile dysfunction in Fragile X patients. *Asian J Androl* **8**, 483-187 (2006).
628. Guastella, A. J., Mitchell, P. B. & Dadds, M. R. Oxytocin increases gaze to the eye region of human faces. *Biol. Psychiatry* **63**, 3-5 (2008).
629. Gude, T., Karterud, S., Pedersen, G. & Falkum, E. The quality of the DSM dependent personality disorder prototype. *Compr. Psychiatry* **47**, 456-462 (2006).
630. Guerrini, R., Bonanni, P., Parmeggiani, L., Hallett, M. & Oguni, H. Pathophysiology of myoclonic epilepsies in Delgado-Escueta, A. V. *et al.* (eds.), *Adv.Neurol., vol.95: Myoclonic Epilepsies.*pp. 23-46 (Lippincott Williams & Wilkins, Philadelphia,2005).
631. Guisinger, S. Competing paradigms for anorexia nervosa. *Am. Psychol* **63**, 199-200 (2008).
632. Gunay-Aygun, M., Cassidy, S. B. & Nicholls, R. D. Prader-Willi and other syndromes associated with obesity and mental retardation. *Behav. Genet.* **27**, 307-324 (1997).
633. Gunay-Aygun, M., Schwartz, S., Heeger, S., O'Riordan, M. A. & Cassidy, S. B. The changing purpose of Prader-Willi syndrome clinical diagnostic criteria and proposed revised criteria. *Pediatrics* **108**, E92 (2001).
634. Guntupalli, V. K., Kalinowski, J. & Saltuklaroglu, T. The need for self-report data in the assessment of stuttering therapy efficacy: repetitions and prolongations of speech. The stuttering syndrome. *Int. J Lang Commun. Disord.* **41**, 1-18 (2006).
635. Gurney, J. G. *et al.* Trends in cancer incidence among children in the US. *Cancer* **78**, 532-541 (1998).
636. Haas, H. L., Sergeeva, O. A. & Selbach, O. Histamine in the nervous system. *Physiol. Rev.* **88**, 1183-1241 (2008).
637. Hagberg, B. Rett syndrome: long-term clinical follow-up experiences over four decades. *J. Child Neurol.* **20**, 722-727 (2005).
638. Hagenah, J. M. *et al.* Distinguishing early-onset PD from dopa-responsive dystonia with transcranial sonography. *Neurology* **66**, 1951-1952 (2006).
639. Hagmann, P. *et al.* Mapping the structural core of human cerebral cortex. *PLoS Biol* **6**, 1479-1493 (2008).
640. Hall, D., Williams, J. & Elliman, D. *The child surveillance handbook.* Radcliffe Publishing, Oxford (2009).
641. Hallahan, B. *et al.* Brain morphometry volume in autistic spectrum disorder: a magnetic resonance imaging study of adults. *Psychol. Med.* **39**, 337-346 (2008).
642. Hamilton, L., Cheng, S. & Powell, B. Adoptive parents, adaptive parents: Evaluating the importance of biological ties for parental investment. *Am. Sociol. Rev.* **72**, 95-116 (2007).
643. Hamilton, N. G. A critical review of object relations theory. *Am. J. Psychiatry* **146**, 1552-1560 (1989).
644. Hamilton, W., Watson, J. & Round, A. Investigating fatigue in primary care. *Br. Med. J.* **341**, 502-504 (2010).
645. Hanks, J. W. & Venters, W. J. Nickel allergy from a bed-wetting alarm confused with herpes genitalis and child abuse. *Pediatrics* **90**, 458-460 (1992).
646. Hanley, W. B. Phenylketonuria: questioning the gospel. *Expert Rev. Endocrinol. Metab.* **2**, 809-816 (2007).
647. Hanoch, Y. & Vitouch, O. When Less is More. *Theory & Psychology* **14**, 427-452 (2004).
648. Happe, F., Ronald, A. & Plomin, R. Time to give up on a single explanation for autism. *Nat. Neurosci.* **9**, 1218-1220 (2006).
649. Haraldsson, E. Children who speak of past-life experiences: is there a psychological explanation? *Psychol Psychother.* **76**, 55-67 (2003).
650. Hardt, O., Einarsson, E. O. & Nader, K. A bridge over troubled water: reconsolidation as a link between cognitive and neuroscientific memory research traditions. *Annu. Rev. Psychol* **61**, 141-167 (2010).

651. Hardy, A. *et al.* Trauma and hallucinatory experience in psychosis. *J. Nerv. Ment. Dis.* **193**, 501-507 (2005).
652. Harlow, H. F. The nature of love. *Am. Psychol.* **13**, 673-685 (1958).
653. Harlow, H. F. Basic social capacity of primates. *Hum. Biol* **31**, 40-53 (1959).
654. Harmon-Jones, E. & Harmon-Jones, C. Action-based model of dissonance: a review of behavioral, anterior cingulate, and prefrontal cortical mechanisms *Social and Personality Psychology Compass* **2**, 1518-1538 (2008).
655. Harmony, T. Psychophysiological evaluation of neuropsychological disorders in children in Reynolds, C. R. & Fletcher-Janzen, E. (eds.), *Handbook of clinical child neuropsychology.*pp. 383-399 (Springer, New York,2009).
656. Harris, B. Whatever happened to little Albert. *Am. Psychol.* **34**, 151-160 (1979).
657. Harris, C. R. & Christenfeld, N. Humour, tickle, and the Darwin-Hecker hypothesis. *Cognition & Emotion* **11**, 103-110 (1997).
658. Harrison, A. G., Edwards, M. J. & Parker, K. C. H. Identifying students feigning dyslexia: preliminary findings and strategies for detection. *Dyslexia* **14**, 228-246 (2008).
659. Hartley, T. & Burgess, N. Complementary memory systems: competition, cooperation and compensation. *Trends Neurosci* **28**, 169-170 (2005).
660. Harvey, R. J. *et al.* A critical role for glycine transporters in hyperexcitability disorders. *Frontiers in Molecular Neuroscience* **1**, (2008).
661. Hasegawa, T. *et al.* Orthotopic liver transplantation for ornithine transcarbamylase deficiency with hyperammonemic encephalopathy. *J. Pediatr. Surg.* **30**, 863-865 (1995).
662. Hassett, A. L., Radvanski, D. C., Buyske, S., Savage, S. V. & Sigal, L. H. Psychiatric comorbidity and other psychological factors in patients with "Chronic Lyme Disease". *Am. J. Med.* **122**, 843-850 (2009).
663. Hatherill, S. & Flisher, A. Delirium in children with HIV/AIDS. *J Child Neurol* **24**, 879-883 (2009).
664. Hauke, J. *et al.* Survival motor neuron gene 2 silencing by DNA methylation correlates with spinal muscular atrophy disease severity and can be bypassed by histone deacetylase inhibition. *Hum. Mol. Genet.* **18**, 304-317 (2009).
665. Haut, S. Differentiating migraine from epilepsy. *Adv. Stud. Med.* **5**, S6-58-S6-65 (2005).
666. Haut, S. R., Bigal, M. E. & Lipton, R. B. Chronic disorders with episodic manifestations: focus on epilepsy and migraine. *Lancet Neurol.* **5**, 148-157 (2006).
667. Havekes, B., Romijn, J. A., Eisenhofer, G., Adams, K. & Pacak, K. Update on pediatric pheochromocytoma. *Pediatr. Nephrol.* **24**, 943-950 (2009).
668. Hawkeswood, T. J. Review of the biology and host-plants of the Australian jewel beetle Julodimorpha bakewelli (White, 1859)(Coleoptera: Buprestidae). *Calodema* **3**, 3-5 (2005).
669. Haworth, C. M. *et al.* Generalist genes and learning disabilities: a multivariate genetic analysis of low performance in reading, mathematics, language and general cognitive ability in a sample of 8000 12-year-old twins. *J Child Psychol Psychiatry* **50**, 1318-1325 (2009).
670. Haxby, J. V. *et al.* Dissociation of object and spatial visual processing pathways in human extrastriate cortex. *Proc. Natl. Acad. Sci. U. S. A* **88**, 1621-1625 (1991).
671. Hay, G. G. Feigned psychosis--a review of the simulation of mental illness. *Br. J. Psychiatry* **143**, 8-10 (1983).
672. Hayes, M. W., Graham, S., Heldorf, P., de, M. G. & Morris, J. G. A video review of the diagnosis of psychogenic gait: appendix and commentary. *Mov Disord.* **14**, 914-921 (1999).
673. Hayhoe, M. Vision using routines: A functional account of vision. *Visual Cognition* **7**, 43-64 (2000).
674. Hayhoe, M. & Ballard, D. Eye movements in natural behavior. *Trends Cogn Sci.* **9**, 188-194 (2005).
675. Haynie, D. L., Silver, E. & Teasdale, B. Neighborhood characteristics, peer networks, and adolescent violence. *Journal of Quantitative Criminology* **22**, 147-169 (2006).
676. Heap, G. A. & van Heel, D. A. Genetics and pathogenesis of coeliac disease. *Semin. Immunol.* **21**, 346-354 (2009).
677. Hebb, D. O. Drives and the CNS (Conceptual Nervous System). *Psychol. Rev.* **62**, 243-254 (1955).
678. Hegna, K. Coming out, coming into what? Identification and risks in the 'coming out' story of a Norwegian late adolescent gay man. *Sexualities* **10**, 582-602 (2007).
679. Heilman, K. M. Apraxia in Heilman, K. M. & Valenstein, E. (eds.), *Clinical Neuropsychology.*pp. 159-185 (Oxford University Press, New York,1993).
680. Heim, C. *et al.* Childhood trauma and risk for chronic fatigue syndrome: association with neuroendocrine dysfunction. *Arch. Gen. Psychiatry* **66**, 72-80 (2009).
681. Heiman, G. A. *et al.* Increased risk for recurrent major depression in DYT1 dystonia mutation carriers. *Neurology* **63**, 631-637 (2004).
682. Heinrich, L. M. & Gullone, E. The clinical significance of loneliness: A literature review. *Clin. Psychol. Rev.* **26**, 695-718 (2006).
683. Henderson, M. J. Renal stone disease-investigative aspects. *Arch. Dis. Child.* **68**, 160-162 (1993).
684. Heneghan, C. *et al.* Diagnostic strategies used in primary care. *Br. Med. J.* **338**, b946 (2009).
685. Hennequin, M., Morin, C. & Feine, J. S. Pain expression and stimulus localisation in individuals with Down's syndrome. *Lancet* **356**, 1882-1887 (2000).
686. Hennet, T. From glycosylation disorders back to glycosylation: What have we learned? *Biochimica et Biophysica Acta (BBA)-Molecular Basis of Disease* **1792**, 921-924 (2009).
687. Hensel, D. J., Fortenberry, J. D. & Orr, D. P. Factors associated with event level anal sex and condom use during anal sex among adolescent women. *J. Adolesc. Health* **(in press)**, (2009).
688. Hensley, C., Tallichet, S. E. & Singer, S. D. Exploring the possible link between childhood and adolescent bestiality and interpersonal violence. *J Interpers. Violence* **21**, 910-923 (2006).
689. Hepper, P. G., Wells, D. L. & Lynch, C. Prenatal thumb sucking is related to postnatal handedness. *Neuropsychologia* **43**, 313-315 (2005).
690. Herbert, M. *Behavioural Treatment of Children with Problems: A Practice Manual.* Academic Press, New York (1993).
691. Herman-Giddens, M. E. Vaginal foreign bodies and child sexual abuse. *Arch Pediatr. Adolesc. Med.* **148**, 195-200 (1994).
692. Hetherington, E. M. & Stanley-Hagan, M. The adjustment of children with divorced parents: a risk and resiliency perspective. *J Child Psychol Psychiatry* **40**, 129-140 (1999).
693. Hibbeln, J. R. Fish consumption and major depression. *Lancet* **351**, 1213 (1998).
694. Hill, C. M., Wheeler, R., Merredew, F. & Lucassen, A. Family history and adoption in the UK: conflicts of interest in medical disclosure. *Arch. Dis. Child.* **95**, 7-11 (2010).
695. Hill, P. Adjustment disorders in Rutter, M. & Taylor, E. (eds.), *Child and Adolescent Psychiatry.*pp. 510-519 (Blackwell, Oxford,2002).
696. Hill, P. Autism spectrum disorders and ADHD: diagnosis issues. *ADHD in Practice* **1**, 4-7 (2009).
697. Hill, W. F. Activity as an autonomous drive. *J Comp Physiol Psychol* **49**, 15-19 (1956).
698. Hillard, P. J. A. Menstruation in adolescents: what's normal, what's not. *Ann. N. Y. Acad. Sci.* **1135**, 29-35 (2008).
699. Hindley, P. Psychiatric aspects of hearing impairment. *J. Child Psychol Psychiatry* **38**, 101-117 (1997).
700. Hindley, P. & Salt, A. The hearing or visually impaired child in Martin, A. & Volkmar, F. R. (eds.), *Lewis's Child and Adolescent Psychiatry.*pp. 66-78 (Lippincott, Philadelphia,2007).

701. Hines, M., Brook, C. & Conway, G. S. Androgen and psychosexual development: core gender identity, sexual orientation and recalled childhood gender role behavior in women and men with congenital adrenal hyperplasia (CAH). *J Sex Res* **41**, 75-81 (2004).
702. Hiscock, M. The Flynn effect and its relevance to neuropsychology. *J Clin Exp Neuropsychol.* **29**, 514-529 (2007).
703. Hoffmann, G. F., Zschocke, J. & Nyhan, W. L. *Inherited metabolic diseases: a clinical approach.* Springer Verlag, Heidelberg (2010).
704. Hogan, D. P., Shandra, C. L. & Msall, M. E. Family developmental risk factors among adolescents with disabilities and children of parents with disabilities. *J. Adolesc.* **30**, 1001-1019 (2007).
705. Hoghughi, M. & Speight, A. N. Good enough parenting for all children--a strategy for a healthier society. *Arch Dis. Child* **78**, 293-296 (1998).
706. Holden, C. 'Behavioral' addictions: do they exist? *Science* **294**, 980-982 (2001).
707. Hollins, M. Somesthetic senses. *Annu. Rev. Psychol* **61**, 243-271 (2010).
708. Hollis, J., Allen, P. M., Fleischmann, D. & Aulak, R. Personality dimensions of people who suffer from visual stress. *Ophthalmic Physiol Opt.* **27**, 603-610 (2007).
709. Holmes, E. A. *et al.* Are there two qualitatively distinct forms of dissociation? A review and some clinical implications. *Clin Psychol Rev.* **25**, 1-23 (2005).
710. Holmes, G. The cerebellum of man. *Brain* **62**, 1-30 (1939).
711. Holsboer, F. & Ising, M. Stress hormone regulation: Biological role and translation into therapy. *Annu. Rev. Psychol* **61**, 81-109 (2010).
712. Honda, H., Shimizu, Y. & Rutter, M. No effect of MMR withdrawal on the incidence of autism: a total population study. *J Child Psychol Psychiatry* **46**, 572-579 (2005).
713. Hopkins, J. The dangers and deprivations of too-good mothering. *J. Child Psychotherapy* **22**, 407-422 (1996).
714. Hopper, L. M., Lambeth, S. P., Schapiro, S. J. & Whiten, A. Observational learning in chimpanzees and children studied through 'ghost' conditions. *Proc. Roy. Soc. B. Biol. Sci.* **275**, 835-840 (2008).
715. Hornor, G. Ano-genital herpes in children. *J. Pediatr. Health Care* **20**, 106-114 (2006).
716. Hornor, G. Sexual behavior in children: Normal or not? *J. Pediatr. Health Care* **18**, 57-64 (2004).
717. Hornstein, N. L. & Putnam, F. W. Clinical phenomenology of child and adolescent dissociative disorders. *J. Am. Acad. Child Adolesc. Psychiatry* **31**, 1077-1085 (1992).
718. Horowitz, M., Wilner, N. & Alvarez, W. Impact of Event Scale: a measure of subjective stress. *Psychosom. Med* **41**, 209-218 (1979).
719. Horton, A. M. The Halstead-Reitan neuropsychological test battery: Past, present, and future in Horton, A. M. & Wedding, D. (eds.), *The Neuropsychology Handbook, 3rd edition.*pp. 253-280 (Springer, New York,2008).
720. Horwood, J. *et al.* IQ and non-clinical psychotic symptoms in 12-year-olds: results from the ALSPAC birth cohort. *Br. J. Psychiatry* **193**, 185-191 (2008).
721. Hosser, D. & Bosold, C. A comparison of sexual and violent offenders in a German youth prison. *Howard J. Crim. Justice* **45**, 159-170 (2006).
722. Hotz, V. J., McElroy, S. W. & Sanders, S. G. Teenage childbearing and its life cycle consequences. *J. Hum. Resour.* **XL**, 683-715 (2005).
723. Howard, R. Linking extreme precocity and adult eminence: a study of eight prodigies at international chess. *High Ability Studies* **19**, 117-130 (2008).
724. Hoyme, H. E. *et al.* A practical clinical approach to diagnosis of fetal alcohol spectrum disorders: clarification of the 1996 institute of medicine criteria. *Pediatrics* **115**, 39-47 (2005).
725. Hsee, C. K. & Rottenstreich, Y. Music, pandas, and muggers: on the affective psychology of value. *J. Exp. Psychol. Gen.* **133**, 23-30 (2004).
726. Hu, H. *et al.* Emotion enhances learning via norepinephrine regulation of AMPA-receptor trafficking. *Cell* **131**, 160-173 (2007).
727. Huang, H.-C., Liu, C.-M. & Liu, C.-C. Psychiatric manifestations in systemic lupus erythematosus mimic psychotic prodrome. *Gen. Hosp. Psychiatry* (2009).
728. Huang, Y. S. *et al.* Attention-deficit/hyperactivity disorder with obstructive sleep apnea: a treatment outcome study. *Sleep Med.* **8**, 18-30 (2007).
729. Hudson, K. L. Prohibiting genetic discrimination. *New Engl. J. Med.* **356**, 2021-2023 (2007).
730. Hughes, D. L., Fey, M. E. & Long, S. H. Developmental sentence scoring: Still useful after all these years. *Topics in Language Disorders* **12**, 1-12 (1992).
731. Huibers, M. J. & Wessely, S. The act of diagnosis: pros and cons of labelling chronic fatigue syndrome. *Psychol Med* **36**, 895-900 (2006).
732. Hultdin, J., Schmauch, A., Wikberg, A., Dahlquist, G. & Andersson, C. Acute intermittent porphyria in childhood: a population-based study. *Acta Paediatr.* **92**, 562-568 (2003).
733. Hunt, G. M. Open spina bifida: outcome for a complete cohort treated unselectively and followed into adulthood. *Dev Med Child Neurol* **32**, 108-118 (1990).
734. Hunter, T. B. & Taljanovic, M. S. Foreign bodies. *Radiographics* **23**, 731-757 (2003).
735. Husain, K., Browne, T. & Chalder, T. A review of psychological models and interventions for medically unexplained somatic symptoms in children. *Child Adolesc. Mental Health* **12**, 2-7 (2007).
736. Hussain, K., Mundy, H., Aynsley-Green, A. & Champion, M. A child presenting with disordered consciousness, hallucinations, screaming episodes and abdominal pain. *Eur. J. Pediatr.* **161**, 127-129 (2002).
737. Huws, J. C. & Jones, R. S. P. Diagnosis, disclosure, and having autism: An interpretative phenomenological analysis of the perceptions of young people with autism. *J. Intellect. Develop. Disabil.* **33**, 99-107 (2008).
738. Hvidtjorn, D. *et al.* Cerebral palsy, autism spectrum disorders, and developmental delay in children born after assisted conception: a systematic review and meta-analysis. *Arch. Pediatr. Adolesc. Med.* **163**, 72-83 (2009).
739. Hyams, J. S. *et al.* Characterization of symptoms in children with recurrent abdominal pain: resemblance to irritable bowel syndrome. *J. Pediatr. Gastroenterol. Nutr.* **20**, 209-214 (1995).
740. Ichinose, H. *et al.* Hereditary progressive dystonia with marked diurnal fluctuation caused by mutations in the GTP cyclohydrolase I gene. *Nat. Genet.* **8**, 236-242 (1994).
741. Ihm, C. W. & Han, J. H. Diagnostic value of exclamation mark hairs. *Dermatology(Basel)* **186**, 99-102 (1993).
742. Ikoma, A., Steinhoff, M., Stander, S., Yosipovitch, G. & Schmelz, M. The neurobiology of itch. *Nat. Rev. Neurosci.* **7**, 535-547 (2006).
743. Illingworth, R. S. *Common symptoms of disease in children.* WileyBlackwell, Oxford (1988).
744. Illingworth, R. S & Lister, J. The critical or sensitive period, with special reference to certain feeding problems in infants and children. *J. Pediatrics* **65**, 839-848 (1964).
745. Illowsky, B. P. & Kirch, D. G. Polydipsia and hyponatremia in psychiatric patients. *Am. J. Psychiatry* **145**, 675-683 (1988).
746. Iloeje, S. O. Psychiatric morbidity among children with sickle-cell disease. *Dev Med Child Neurol* **33**, 1087-1094 (1991).
747. Inamadar, A. C. & Palit, A. Photosensitivity in children: An approach to diagnosis and management. *Indian J. Dermatol. Venereol. Leprol.* **71**, 73-79 (2005).
748. Innocenti, G. M. & Price, D. J. Exuberance in the development of cortical networks. *Nat Rev. Neurosci* **6**, 955-965 (2005).
749. Insel, T. R. Is social attachment an addictive disorder? *Physiol Behav.* **79**, 351-357 (2003).

750. Isaac, R. & Roesler, T. A. Medical Child Abuse in Giardino, A. P., Lyn, M. A. & Giardino, E. R. (eds.)pp. 291-305 (Springer, New York,2009).

751. Isaacs, E. B. *et al.* Hippocampal volume and everyday memory in children of very low birth weight. *Pediatr. Res* **47**, 713-720 (2000).

752. Isaacson, J. E., Moyer, M. T., Schuler, H. G. & Blackall, G. F. Clinical associations between tinnitus and chronic pain. *Otolaryngol. Head Neck Surg.* **128**, 706-710 (2003).

753. Isbister, G. K. & Buckley, N. A. The pathophysiology of serotonin toxicity in animals and humans: implications for diagnosis and treatment. *Clin. Neuropharmacol.* **28**, 205-304 (2005).

754. Isohanni, M. *et al.* Early developmental milestones in adult schizophrenia and other psychoses. A 31-year follow-up of the Northern Finland 1966 Birth Cohort. *Schizophr. Res* **52**, 1-19 (2001).

755. Itin, P. H. & Fistarol, S. K. Hair shaft abnormalities--clues to diagnosis and treatment. *Dermatology* **211**, 63-71 (2005).

756. Jacob, A. *et al.* Time course of anger and other emotions in women with borderline personality disorder: a preliminary study. *J. Behav Ther. Exp. Psychiatry* **39**, 391-402 (2008).

757. Jacob, R. G. & Furman, J. M. Psychiatric consequences of vestibular dysfunction. *Curr. Opin. Neurol.* **14**, 41-46 (2001).

758. Jacobs, W. J. & Dalenberg, C. Subtle presentations of post-traumatic stress disorder. Diagnostic issues. *Psychiatr. Clin. North Am.* **21**, 835-845 (1998).

759. Jaeken, J. & Matthijs, G. Congenital disorders of glycosylation: a rapidly expanding disease family. *Annu. Rev. Genomics Hum. Genet* **8**, 261-278 (2007).

760. Jakobovits, A. A. Fetal penile erection. *Ultrasound Obstet. Gynecol.* **18**, 405 (2001).

761. Jakobs, C., Jaeken, J. & Gibson, K. M. Inherited disorders of GABA metabolism. *J Inherit. Metab Dis* **16**, 704-715 (1993).

762. James, W. H. The sexual orientation of men who were brought up in gay or lesbian households. *J. Biosoc. Sci.* **36**, 371-374 (2004).

763. Jan, J. E., Groenveld, M. & Sykanda, A. M. Light-gazing by visually impaired children. *Develop. Med. Child. Neurol.* **32**, 755-759 (1989).

764. Janig, W. & Baron, R. Complex regional pain syndrome: mystery explained? *Lancet Neurol.* **2**, 687-697 (2003).

765. Jankovic, J. Tourette's syndrome. *N. Engl. J. Med.* **345**, 1184-1192 (2001).

766. Jankovic, J. & Kwak, C. Tics in other neurological disorders in Kurlan, R. (ed.), *Handbook of Tourette's syndrome and related tic and behavioral disorders.*2002).

767. Janosik, M. *et al.* Birth Prevalence of homocystinuria in Central Europe: Frequency and pathogenicity of mutation c. 1105C> T (p. R369C) in the cystathionine beta-synthase gene. *J. Pediatrics* **154**, 431-437 (2009).

768. Jaspers, T. *et al.* Pervasive refusal syndrome as part of the refusal-withdrawal-regression spectrum: critical review of the literature illustrated by a case report. *Eur. Child Adolesc. Psychiatry* **18**, 645-651 (2009).

769. Javitt, D. C. Glutamate as a therapeutic target in psychiatric disorders. *Mol. Psychiatry* **9**, 984-997 (2004).

770. Javitt, G. Assign regulation appropriate to the level of risk. *Nature* **466**, 817-818 (2010).

771. Jeejeebhoy, K. N. Benefits and risks of a fish diet--should we be eating more or less? *Nat Clin Pract. Gastroenterol. Hepatol.* **5**, 178-179 (2008).

772. Jelalian, E., Wember, Y. M., Bungeroth, H. & Birmaher, V. Practitioner review: bridging the gap between research and clinical practice in pediatric obesity. *J. Child Psychol Psychiatry* **48**, 115-127 (2007).

773. Jelicic, M. & Merckelbach, H. Traumatic stress, brain changes, and memory deficits: a critical note. *J Nerv Ment Dis* **192**, 548-553 (2004).

774. Jenny, C. Evaluating infants and young children with multiple fractures. *Pediatrics* **118**, 1299-1303 (2006).

775. Jensen, P. S. *et al.* Findings from the NIMH Multimodal Treatment Study of ADHD (MTA): implications and applications for primary care providers. *J. Dev. Behav. Pediatr.* **22**, 60-73 (2001).

776. Jha, S., Kumar, R., Kumar, M. & Kumar, R. Cerebral birth anoxia, seizures and Kluver-Bucy syndrome: some observations. *J. Pediatr. Neurol.* **3**, 227-232 (2005).

777. Ji, R. R., Kohno, T., Moore, K. A. & Woolf, C. J. Central sensitization and LTP: do pain and memory share similar mechanisms? *Trends Neurosci.* **26**, 696-705 (2003).

778. Jinnah, H. A. *et al.* Attenuated variants of Lesch-Nyhan disease. *Brain* **133**, 671 (2010).

779. Joffe, H. & Hayes, F. J. Menstrual cycle dysfunction associated with neurologic and psychiatric disorders: their treatment in adolescents. *Ann. N. Y. Acad. Sci.* **1135**, 219-229 (2008).

780. Johansson, T. & Fahlgren, H. Alexia without agraphia: lateral and medial infarction of left occipital lobe. *Neurology* **29**, 390-393 (1979).

781. Johnson, C. J. *et al.* Fourteen-year follow-up of children with and without speech/language impairments: Speech/language stability and outcomes. *J. Speech. Lang. Hear. Res.* **42**, 744-760 (1999).

782. Johnson, J. S. & Newport, E. L. Critical period effects in second language learning: the influence of maturational state on the acquisition of English as a second language. *Cogn Psychol* **21**, 60-99 (1989).

783. Johnson, M., Ostlund, S., Fransson, G., Kadesjo, B. & Gillberg, C. Omega-3/omega-6 fatty acids for attention deficit hyperactivity disorder: a randomized placebo-controlled trial in children and adolescents. *J Atten. Disord.* **12**, 394-401 (2009).

784. Johnson, M. K. & Raye, C. L. False memories and confabulation. *Trends Cog. Sci.* **2**, 137-145 (1998).

785. Johnston, J. R. Children of divorce who refuse visitation in Depner, C. E. & Bray, J. H. (eds.), *Nonresidential parenting.* (Sage Publications, London,1993).

786. Jones, I. H. & Pansa, M. Some nonverbal aspects of depression and schizophrenia occurring during the interview. *J Nerv Ment Dis* **167**, 402-409 (1979).

787. Jones, K. L. *Smith's Recognizable Patterns of Human Malformation.* Elsevier Saunders, Philadelphia (2006).

788. Jones, R. B. Impairment, disability and handicap--old fashioned concepts? *J. Med. Ethics* **27**, 377-379 (2001).

789. Jones, S. E. The Touch Log Record: A Behavioral Communication Measure in Manusov, V. (ed.), *The sourcebook of nonverbal measures: going beyond words.*pp. 67-82 (Lawrence Erlbaum Assoc Inc, Mahwah, NJ,2005).

790. Jones, S. E. & Yarbrough, A. E. A naturalistic study of the meanings of touch. *Communication Monographs* **52**, 19-56 (1985).

791. Jonides, J. *et al.* The mind and brain of short-term memory. *Annu. Rev. Psychol* **59**, 193-224 (2008).

792. Joseph, F. G. & Scolding, N. J. Neurolupus. *Pract. Neurol* **10**, 4-15 (2010).

793. Joseph, R. *Neuropsychology, neuropsychiatry, and behavioral neurology.* Plenum Press, New York (1990).

794. Joyce, T. J., Kaestner, R. & Korenman, S. The effect of pregnancy intention on child development. *Demography* **37**, 83-94 (2000).

795. Juberg, D. R., Alfano, K., Coughlin, R. J. & Thompson, K. M. An observational study of object mouthing behavior by young children. *Pediatrics* **107**, 135-142 (2001).

796. Julich, S. Stockholm syndrome and child sexual abuse. *J. Child Sex Abus.* **14**, 107-129 (2005).

797. Jurecka, A. *et al.* Hypoxanthine-guanine phosphoribosylotransferase deficiency-The spectrum of Polish mutations. *J. Inherit. Metab Dis* **JIMD Short Report #136 (2008) Online**, (2008).

798. Jureidini, J. Projective identification in general psychiatry. *Br. J. Psychiatry* **157**, 656-660 (1990).

799. Kachko, L., Efrat, R., Ami, S. B., Mukamel, M. & Katz, J. Complex regional pain syndromes in children and adolescents. *Pediatr. Int.* **50**, 523-527 (2008).

800. Kadosh, C. Virtual dyscalculia induced by parietal-lobe TMS impairs automatic magnitude processing. *Curr. Biol.* **17**, 689-693 (2007).

801. Kahneman, D. A perspective on judgment and choice: mapping bounded rationality. *Am. Psychol* **58**, 697-720 (2003).

802. Kaiser, A. P. & Delaney, E. M. The effects of poverty on parenting young children. *Peabody J. Educ.* **71**, 66-85 (1996).

803. Kaitz, M., Bar-Haim, Y., Lehrer, M. & Grossman, E. Adult attachment style and interpersonal distance. *Attach. Hum. Dev.* **6**, 285-304 (2004).

804. Kakooza-Mwesige, A., Wachtel, L. E. & Dhossche, D. M. Catatonia in autism: implications across the life span. *Eur. Child Adolesc. Psychiatry* **17**, 327-335 (2008).

805. Kalat, J. W. Speculations on similarities between autism and opiate addiction. *J. Autism Child Schizophr.* **8**, 477-479 (1978).

806. Kandel, E. R. Biology and the future of psychoanalysis: a new intellectual framework for psychiatry revisited. *Am. J. Psychiatry* **156**, 505-524 (1999).

807. Kandel, E. R. Biology and the future of psychoanalysis: a new intellectual framework for psychiatry revisited. *Am. J. Psychiatry* **156**, 505-524 (1999).

808. Kane, M. & Golovkina, T. Common Threads in Persistent Viral Infections. *J. Virol.* **(accepted for publication 2009)**, (2010).

809. Kanfer, F. H. & Duerfeldt, P. H. Age, class standing, and commitment as determinants of cheating in children. *Child Dev.* **39**, 545-557 (1968).

810. Kaplan, D. M. On stage fright. *The Drama Review: TDR* **14**, 60-83 (1969).

811. Kaplowitz, P. B. Subclinical hypothyroidism in children: normal variation or sign of a failing thyroid gland? *Int. J Pediatr. Endocrinol.* **(in press)**, (2010).

812. Kapoula, Z. *et al.* Free exploration of painting uncovers particularly loose yoking of saccades in dyslexics. *Dyslexia.* **15**, 243-259 (2009).

813. Kapp-Simon, K. A., Speltz, M. L., Cunningham, M. L., Patel, P. K. & Tomita, T. Neurodevelopment of children with single suture craniosynostosis: a review. *Child's Nervous System* **23**, 269-281 (2007).

814. Karlsgodt, K. H. *et al.* Developmental disruptions in neural connectivity in the pathophysiology of schizophrenia. *Dev. Psychopathol.* **20**, 1297-1327 (2008).

815. Kasese-Hara, M., Mayekiso, T., Modipa, O., Mzobe, N. & Mango, T. Depression, mothers' concerns and life-events experienced by HIV-positive, HIV-negative and mothers with unknown HIV status in Soweto. *S. A. J. Psychol.* **38**, 575-588 (2005).

816. Katusic, S. K., Colligan, R. C., Weaver, A. L. & Barbaresi, W. J. The forgotten learning disability: epidemiology of written-language disorder in a population-based birth cohort (1976-1982), Rochester, Minnesota. *Pediatrics* **123**, 1306-1313 (2009).

817. Kaufman, K. R., Endres, J. K. & Kaufman, N. D. Psychogenic Dyspnea and Therapeutic Chest Radiograph. *Death Stud.* **31**, 373-381 (2007).

818. Kaufman, L., Ayub, M. & Vincent, J. B. The genetic basis of non-syndromic intellectual disability: a review. *J. Neurodevel. Dis.* **2**, 182-209 (2010).

819. Kaufmann, R., Goldberg-Stern, H. & Shuper, A. Attention-deficit disorders and epilepsy in childhood: incidence, causative relations and treatment possibilities. *J. Child Neurol.* **24**, 727-733 (2009).

820. Kaukiainen, A. *et al.* Learning difficulties, social intelligence, and self-concept: connections to bully-victim problems. *Scand J Psychol* **43**, 269-278 (2002).

821. Kay, P. & Kolvin, I. Childhood psychoses and their borderlands. *Br. Med. Bull.* **43**, 570-586 (1987).

822. Kazazian, H. H. Remembering Victor McKusick. *Genomics* **92**, 185-186 (2008).

823. Kearney, C. A. Identifying the function of school refusal behavior: A revision of the School Refusal Assessment Scale. *J. Psychopathol. Behav. Assessment* **24**, 235-245 (2002).

824. Kearney, C. A. & Silverman, W. K. Family environment of youngsters with school refusal behavior. *Am. J. Family Therapy* **23**, 59-72 (1995).

825. Keel, P. K. & Klump, K. L. Are eating disorders culture-bound syndromes? Implications for conceptualizing their etiology. *Psychol. Bull.* **129**, 747-769 (2003).

826. Kelleher, A. Introduction, *On death and dying.* (Routledge, Abingdon,2009).

827. Kelley, H. H. & Michela, J. L. Attribution theory and research. *Annu. Rev. Psychol.* **31**, 457-501 (1980).

828. Kellner, M., Wiedemann, K. & Zihl, J. Illumination perception in photophobic patients suffering from panic disorder with agoraphobia. *Acta Psychiatr. Scand* **96**, 72-74 (1997).

829. Keltner, D. & Buswell, B. N. Embarrassment: Its distinct form and appeasement functions. *Psychol. Bull.* **122**, 250-270 (1997).

830. Kennedy, R. & McQueen, D. Bipolar affective disorder presenting as failure of parenting. *Aust. N. Z. J. Psychiatry* **44**, 392 (2010).

831. Kerbeshian, J., Burd, L. & Fisher, W. Lithium carbonate in the treatment of two patients with infantile autism and atypical bipolar symptomatology. *J. Clin. Psychopharmacol.* **7**, 401-405 (1987).

832. Kerbeshian, J., Burd, L., Randall, T., Martsolf, J. & Jalal, S. Autism, profound mental retardation and atypical bipolar disorder in a 33-year-old female with a deletion of 15q12. *J. Intellect. Disabil. Res.* **34**, 205-210 (1990).

833. Kerndt, P. R., Naughton, J. L., Driscoll, C. E. & Loxterkamp, D. A. Fasting: the history, pathophysiology and complications. *West. J. Med.* **137**, 379-399 (1982).

834. Kerrigan, J. F., Ng, Y., Chung, S. & Rekate, H. L. The hypothalamic hamartoma: a model of subcortical epileptogenesis and encephalopathy. *Semin. Pediatr. Neurol.* **12**, 119-131 (2005).

835. Kessler, R. C., Stein, M. B. & Berglund, P. Social phobia subtypes in the National Comorbidity Survey. *Am. J. Psychiatry* **155**, 613-619 (1998).

836. Key, T. J., Appleby, P. N. & Rosell, M. S. Health effects of vegetarian and vegan diets. *Proc. Nutr. Soc.* **65**, 35-41 (2006).

837. Keys, A., Brozek, J. & Henschel, A. *The biology of human starvation.* Univ.Minn.Press, Minneapolis (1950).

838. Kienhorst, C. W., De Wilde, E. J., Diekstra, R. F. & Wolters, W. H. Construction of an index for predicting suicide attempts in depressed adolescents. *Br. J. Psychiatry* **159**, 676-682 (1991).

839. Kihlstrom, J. F. Dissociative disorders. *Annu. Rev. Clin Psychol* **1**, 227-253 (2005).

840. Kikuchi, H. *et al.* Memory repression: Brain mechanisms underlying dissociative amnesia. *J. Cogn. Neurosci.* **22**, 602-613 (2010).

841. Kim, J. S. Post-stroke emotional incontinence after small lenticulocapsular stroke: correlation with lesion location. *J. Neurol.* **249**, 805-810 (2002).

842. Kimura, D. *Sex and cognition.* MIT Press, Boston (2000).

843. Kimura, R., Silva, A. J. & Ohno, M. Autophosphorylation of alphaCaMKII is differentially involved in new learning and unlearning mechanisms of memory extinction. *Learn. Mem.* **15**, 837-843 (2008).

844. King, C. H. & Dangerfield-Cha, M. The unacknowledged impact of chronic schistosomiasis. *Chronic. Illn.* **4**, 65-79 (2008).

845. King, N. J. & Bernstein, G. A. School refusal in children and adolescents: a review of the past 10 years. *J. Am. Acad. Child Adolesc. Psychiatry* **40**, 197-205 (2001).

846. Kini, U. Fetal valproate syndrome: a review. *Paediatr. Perinatal Drug Therapy* **7**, 123-130 (2006).

847. Kini, U., Adab, N., Vinten, J., Fryer, A. & Clayton-Smith, J. Dysmorphic features: an important clue to the diagnosis and severity of fetal anticonvulsant syndromes. *Arch Dis Child Fetal Neonatal Ed* **91**, F90-F95 (2006).

848. Kinket, B. & Verkuyten, M. Levels of ethnic self-identification and social context. *Soc. Psychol. Q.* **60**, 338-354 (1997).

849. Kirchheiner, J. & Rodriguez-Antona, C. Cytochrome P450 2D6 Genotyping: Potential Role in Improving Treatment Outcomes in Psychiatric Disorders. *CNS drugs* **23**, 181-191 (2009).

850. Kirmayer, L. J. & Sartorius, N. Cultural models and somatic syndromes in Dimsdale, J. E. *et al.* (eds.), *Somatic Presentations of Mental Disorders: Refining the Research Agenda for DSM-V.* pp. 19-38 (Am. Psychiatric Assoc, Arlington,2009).

851. Kirtley, D. D. & Sabo, K. T. Symbolism in the dreams of the blind. *Int. J. Rehabil. Res* **2**, 225-232 (1979).

852. Klaczynski, P. A. Motivated scientific reasoning biases, epistemological beliefs, and theory polarization: a two-process approach to adolescent cognition. *Child Dev.* **71**, 1347-1366 (2000).

853. Kleiner-Fisman, G. & Lang, A. E. Benign hereditary chorea revisited: A journey to understanding. *Mov. Disord.* **22**, 2297-2305 (2007).

854. Kleinknecht, R. A. The origins and remission of fear in a group of tarantula enthusiasts. *Behav. Res. Ther.* **20**, 437-443 (1982).

855. Klin, A., Lin, D. J., Gorrindo, P., Ramsay, G. & Jones, W. Two-year-olds with autism orient to non-social contingencies rather than biological motion. *Nature* **459**, 257-261 (2009).

856. Klonsky, E. D. & Moyer, A. Childhood sexual abuse and non-suicidal self-injury: meta-analysis. *Br. J. Psychiatry* **192**, 166-170 (2008).

857. Kluver, H. & Bucy, P. C. Preliminary analysis of functions of the temporal lobes in monkeys. *J. Neuropsychiatry Clin. Neurosci.* **9**, 606-620 (1938).

858. Knaapila, A. *et al.* Food neophobia shows heritable variation in humans. *Physiol Behav* **91**, 573-578 (2007).

859. Knoll, J. & Resnick, P. J. The detection of malingered post-traumatic stress disorder. *Psychiatr. Clin. North Am.* **29**, 629-647 (2006).

860. Koene, S. *et al.* Major depression in adolescent children consecutively diagnosed with mitochondrial disorder. *J Affect. Disord.* **114**, 327-332 (2009).

861. Koenig, H. G. Religion and mental health: what should psychiatrists do? *Psychiatr. Bull.* **32**, 201-203 (2008).

862. Koenigs, M., Baskin-Sommers, A., Zeier, J. & Newman, J. P. Investigating the neural correlates of psychopathy: a critical review. *Mol. Psychiatry* **(in press)**, (2010).

863. Koenigsknecht, R. A. & Lee, L. L. *The Assessment of Grammatical Development in Children and the Clinical Presentation of Grammatical Structure to Children with Language Problems. Final Report.* Northwestern Univ, (1974).

864. Kohen, D. & Wildgust, H. J. The evolution of hyperprolactinaemia as an entity in psychiatric patients. *J. Psychopharmacol. (Oxf)* **22**, 6-11 (2008).

865. Kohlschutter, A. *et al.* Leukodystrophies and other genetic metabolic leukoencephalopathies in children and adults. *Brain Dev.* **32**, 82-89 (2010).

866. Koht, J., Bjornara, K. A., Jorum, E. & Tallaksen, C. M. E. Ataxia with vitamin E deficiency in southeast Norway, case report. *Acta Neurol. Scand.* **120**, 42-45 (2009).

867. Kolker, S. *et al.* Guideline for the diagnosis and management of glutaryl-CoA dehydrogenase deficiency (glutaric aciduria type I). *J. Inherit. Metab. Dis.* **30**, 5-22 (2007).

868. Kolodny, E. H. & Pastores, G. M. Anderson-Fabry disease: extrarenal, neurologic manifestations. *J. Am. Soc. Nephrol.* **13**, S150-S153 (2002).

869. Kolvin, I., Ounsted, C., Humphrey, M. & McNay, A. Studies in the childhood psychoses. II. The phenomenology of childhood psychoses. *Br. J Psychiatry* **118**, 385-395 (1971).

870. Konofal, E. *et al.* Effects of iron supplementation on attention deficit hyperactivity disorder in children. *Pediatr. Neurol.* **38**, 20-26 (2008).

871. Kopp, S. & Gillberg, C. Selective mutism: a population-based study: a research note. *J. Child Psychol Psychiatry* **38**, 257-262 (1997).

872. Kornetsky, C., Vates, T. S. & Kessler, E. K. A comparison of hypnotic and residual psychological effects of single doses of chlorpromazine and secobarbital in man. *J. Pharmacol. Exp. Ther.* **127**, 51-54 (1959).

873. Kors, E. E. *et al.* Expanding the phenotypic spectrum of the CACNA1A gene T666M mutation: a description of 5 families with familial hemiplegic migraine. *Arch. Neurol.* **60**, 684-688 (2003).

874. Korzeniewski, S. J., Birbeck, G., DeLano, M. C., Potchen, M. J. & Paneth, N. A systematic review of neuroimaging for cerebral palsy. *J. Child Neurol.* **23**, 216-227 (2008).

875. Kosztolanyi, G. Does "ring syndrome" exist? An analysis of 207 case reports on patients with a ring autosome. *Hum. Genet.* **75**, 174-179 (1987).

876. Koutroumanidis, M. *et al.* The variants of reading epilepsy. A clinical and video-EEG study of 17 patients with reading-induced seizures. *Brain* **121 (Pt 8)**, 1409-1427 (1998).

877. Kozlowska, K. The developmental origins of conversion disorders. *Clin Child Psychol Psychiatry* **12**, 487-510 (2007).

878. Kraft, M. B. The face-hand test. *Dev Med Child Neurol* **10**, 214-219 (1968).

879. Kramer, J. M. & van, B. H. Genetic and epigenetic defects in mental retardation. *Int. J Biochem. Cell Biol.* **41**, 96-107 (2009).

880. Kramer, T. L., Robbins, J. M., Phillips, S. D., Miller, T. L. & Burns, B. J. Detection and outcomes of substance use disorders in adolescents seeking mental health treatment. *J. Am. Acad. Child Adolesc. Psychiatry* **42**, 1318-1326 (2003).

881. Kramer, U., de Roten, Y., Perry, J. C. & Despland, J. N. Specificities of defense mechanisms in bipolar affective disorder: Relations with symptoms and therapeutic alliance. *J. Nerv. Ment. Dis.* **197**, 675-681 (2009).

882. Kratochvil, L. & Flegr, J. Differences in the 2nd to 4th digit length ratio in humans reflect shifts along the common allometric line. *Biol. Lett.* **5**, 643-646 (2009).

883. Kubler-Ross, E., Wessler, S. & Avioli, L. V. On death and dying. *JAMA* **221**, 174-179 (1972).

884. Kuhn, T. S. *Structure of scientific revolutions.* Univ.Chicago Press, Chicago (1962).

885. Kulick, D. Gay and lesbian language. *Ann. Rev. Anthropology* **29**, 243-285 (2000).

886. Kullmann, D. M. & Hanna, M. G. Neurological disorders caused by inherited ion-channel mutations. *Lancet Neurol.* **1**, 157-166 (2002).

887. Kumar, R. & Lang, A. E. Tourette syndrome. Secondary tic disorders. *Neurol. Clin.* **15**, 309-331 (1997).

888. Kumari, V. & Postma, P. Nicotine use in schizophrenia: the self medication hypotheses. *Neurosci. Biobehav. Rev.* **29**, 1021-1034 (2005).

889. Kuppens, P., Allen, N. B. & Sheeber, L. B. Emotional inertia and psychological maladjustment. *Psychol. Science* **21**, 984 (2010).

890. Kutscher, M. L. *Kids in the Syndrome Mix.* Jessica Kingsley, London (2005).

891. Kwapil, T. R., Mann, M. C. & Raulin, M. L. Psychometric properties and concurrent validity of the schizotypal ambivalence scale. *J. Nerv. Ment. Dis.* **190**, 290-295 (2002).

892. Laberge, L., Tremblay, R. E., Vitaro, F. & Montplaisir, J. Development of parasomnias from childhood to early adolescence. *Pediatrics* **106**, 67-74 (2000).

893. Labov, T. Social structure and peer terminology in a black adolescent gang. *Language in Society* **11**, 391-411 (1982).
894. Lader, D., Singleton, N. & Meltzer, H. *Psychiatric comorbidity among young offenders in England and Wales.* Office for National Statistics, London (2000).
895. Lagerberg, D. Parents' observations of sexual behaviour in pre-school children. *Acta Paediatr.* **90**, 367-369 (2001).
896. Lahey, B. B., Pelham, W. E., Loney, J., Lee, S. S. & Willcutt, E. Instability of the DSM-IV Subtypes of ADHD From Preschool Through Elementary School. *Arch. Gen. Psychiatry* **62**, 896-902 (2005).
897. Lam, K. S., Bodfish, J. W. & Piven, J. Evidence for three subtypes of repetitive behavior in autism that differ in familiality and association with other symptoms. *J. Child Psychol Psychiatry* **49**, 1193-1200 (2008).
898. Lam, P. T. C. Treatment resistance in schizophrenia. *Hong Kong Medical Bulletin* **13**, 16-18 (2008).
899. Lambie, G. W. Motivational Enhancement Therapy: A Tool for Professional School Counselors Working With Adolescents. *Professional School Counseling* **7**, 268-276 (2004).
900. Lambrenos, K., Weindling, A. M., Calam, R. & Cox, A. D. The effect of a child's disability on mother's mental health. *Br. Med. J.* **74**, 115-120 (1996).
901. Lammer, C. & Weimann, E. Early onset of type I diabetes mellitus, Hashimoto's thyroiditis and celiac disease in a 7-yr-old boy with Down's syndrome. *Pediatric Diabetes* **9**, 423-425 (2008).
902. Lang, F., Floyd, M. R. & Beine, K. L. Clues to patients' explanations and concerns about their illnesses. A call for active listening. *Arch. Fam. Med.* **9**, 222-227 (2000).
903. Lanphear, B. P. The conquest of lead poisoning: a pyrrhic victory. *Environ. Health Perspect.* **115**, A484-A485 (2007).
904. Lanska, D. J. Functional weakness and sensory loss. *Semin. Neurol* **26**, 297-309 (2006).
905. Lanza, E. Can bilingual two-year-olds code-switch? *J Child Lang* **19**, 633-658 (1992).
906. Laplane, D. & Degos, J. D. Motor neglect. *Br. Med. J.* **46**, 152-158 (1983).
907. Larner, A. J. *A dictionary of neurological signs.* Springer, New York (2006).
908. Larsson, I. & Svedin, C. G. Sexual behaviour in Swedish preschool children, as observed by their parents. *Acta Paediatr.* **90**, 436-444 (2001).
909. Larsson, I. & Svedin, C. G. Teachers' and parents' reports on 3- to 6-year-old children's sexual behavior--a comparison. *Child Abuse Negl.* **26**, 247-266 (2002).
910. Larun, L., Nordheim, L. V., Ekeland, E., Hagen, K. B. & Heian, F. Exercise in prevention and treatment of anxiety and depression among children and young people. *Cochrane. Database. Syst. Rev.* **2009**, 1-52 (2006).
911. Larzelere, R. E. Disciplinary spanking: the scientific evidence. *J Dev. Behav Pediatr.* **29**, 334-335 (2008).
912. LaSalle, V. H. *et al.* Diagnostic interview assessed neuropsychiatric disorder comorbidity in 334 individuals with obsessive-compulsive disorder. *Depress. Anxiety* **19**, 163-173 (2004).
913. Lask, B. Pervasive refusal syndrome. *Adv. Psychiat. Treat.* **10**, 153-159 (2004).
914. Lauterbach, M. D., Stanislawski-Zygaj, A. L. & Benjamin, S. The differential diagnosis of childhood- and young adult-onset disorders that include psychosis. *J. Neuropsychiatry Clin. Neurosci.* **20**, 409-418 (2008).
915. Lavin, M. F. Ataxia-telangiectasia: from a rare disorder to a paradigm for cell signalling and cancer. *Nature Reviews Molecular Cell Biology* **9**, 759-769 (2008).
916. Lazar, I. *et al.* Natural history of thyroid function tests over 5 years in a large pediatric cohort. *J. Clin. Endocrinol. Metab.* **94**, 1678-1682 (2009).
917. Lazarus, R. S. A laboratory approach to the dynamics of psychological stress. *Adm. Sci. Q.* **8**, 192-213 (1963).
918. Le Couteur, A. *et al.* Autism Diagnostic Interview: a standardized investigator-based instrument. *J. Autism. Dev. Disord.* **19**, 363-387 (1989).
919. Leask, S. J., Done, D. J. & Crow, T. J. Adult psychosis, common childhood infections and neurological soft signs in a national birth cohort. *Br. J. Psychiatry* **181**, 387-392 (2002).
920. Lee, C. & Scherer, S. W. The clinical context of copy number variation in the human genome. *Expert Reviews in Mol. Medicine* **12**, e8 (2010).
921. Lee, H. P., Chae, P. K., Lee, H. S. & Kim, Y. K. The five-factor gambling motivation model. *Psychiatry Res* **150**, 21-32 (2007).
922. Lee, R. *et al.* A review of events that expose children to elemental mercury in the United States. *Ciencia & Sa\"de Coletiva* **15**, 585-598 (2010).
923. Lee, Z., Salekin, R. T. & Iselin, A. M. R. Psychopathic Traits in Youth: Is There Evidence for Primary and Secondary Subtypes? *J. Abnorm. Child Psychol.* **38**, 381-393 (2010).
924. Lees, A. J. Odd and unusual movement disorders. *J. Neurol. Neurosurg. Psychiatry* **72 Suppl 1**, I17-I21 (2002).
925. Leffler, D. A., Dennis, M., Edwards George, J. B. & Kelly, C. P. The interaction between eating disorders and celiac disease: an exploration of 10 cases. *Eur. J Gastroenterol. Hepatol.* **19**, 251-255 (2007).
926. Legerstee, M. A review of the animate inanimate distinction in infancy: Implications for models of social and cognitive knowing. *Early Development and Parenting* **1**, 59-67 (1992).
927. Leigh, R. J. & Kennard, C. Using saccades as a research tool in the clinical neurosciences. *Brain* **127**, 460-477 (2004).
928. Leitenberg, H., Detzer, M. J. & Srebnik, D. Gender differences in masturbation and the relation of masturbation experience in preadolescence and/or early adolescence to sexual behavior and sexual adjustment in young adulthood. *Arch. Sex Behav* **22**, 87-98 (1993).
929. Leitz, M. A. & Theriot, M. T. Adolescent Stalking. *J. Evidence-Based Social Work* **2**, 97-112 (2005).
930. Lempert, T., Brandt, T., Dieterich, M. & Huppert, D. How to identify psychogenic disorders of stance and gait. A video study in 37 patients. *J. Neurol.* **238**, 140-146 (1991).
931. Lempert, T., Dieterich, M., Huppert, D. & Brandt, T. Psychogenic disorders in neurology: frequency and clinical spectrum. *Acta Neurol. Scand.* **82**, 335-340 (1990).
932. Lempert, T. & Neuhauser, H. Migrainous vertigo. *Neurology Clinics* **23**, 715-730 (2005).
933. Lena, S. M. & Bijoor, S. Wrist cutting: a dare game among adolescents. *CMAJ.* **142**, 131-132 (1990).
934. Lenihan, F. Computer addiction - a sceptical view. *Adv. Psychiatric Treatment* **13**, 31-33 (2007).
935. Lenzenweger, M. F., Johnson, M. D. & Willett, J. B. Individual growth curve analysis illuminates stability and change in personality disorder features: the longitudinal study of personality disorders. *Arch. Gen. Psychiatry* **61**, 1015-1024 (2004).
936. Leslie, P., Carding, P. N. & Wilson, J. A. Investigation and management of chronic dysphagia. *Br. Med. J.* **326**, 433-436 (2003).
937. Leung, A. K. & Kao, C. P. Evaluation and management of the child with speech delay. *Am. Fam. Physician* **59**, 3121-3128 (1999).
938. Levin, I. & Bus, A. G. How is emergent writing based on drawing? Analyses of children's products and their sorting by children and mothers. *Dev. Psychol* **39**, 891-905 (2003).
939. Levin, K. H. Variants and mimics of Guillain Barre syndrome. *Neurologist* **10**, 61-74 (2004).
940. Levitt, S. D. & Dubner, S. J. *Super Freakonomics.* HarperCollins, New York (2009).
941. Levitt, S. D. & List, J. A. What do laboratory experiments measuring social preferences reveal about the real world? *J. Econ. Perspectives* **21**, 153-174 (2007).
942. Levy, F. & Swanson, J. M. Timing, space and ADHD: the dopamine theory revisited. *Aust. N. Z. J. Psychiatry* **35**, 504-511 (2001).

943. Levy, L. M. & Hallett, M. Impaired brain GABA in focal dystonia. *Ann. Neurol* **51**, 93-101 (2002).

944. Levy, Y. *et al.* Diagnostic clues for identification of nonorganic vs organic causes of food refusal and poor feeding. *J Pediatr. Gastroenterol. Nutr* **48**, 355-362 (2009).

945. Lewinsohn, P. M., Holm-Denoma, J. M., Small, J. W., Seeley, J. R. & Joiner, T. E. Separation anxiety disorder in childhood as a risk factor for future mental illness. *J. Am. Acad. Child Adolesc. Psychiatry* **47**, 548-555 (2008).

946. Lewis, C. M. *et al.* Genome-wide association study of major recurrent depression in the UK population. *Am. J. Psychiatry* **167**, 949-957 (2010).

947. Lhermitte, F., Pillon, B. & Serdaru, M. Human autonomy and the frontal lobes. Part I: Imitation and utilization behavior: A neuropsychological study of 75 patients. *Ann. Neurol.* **19**, 326-334 (1986).

948. Lheureux, P., Penaloza, A. & Gris, M. Pyridoxine in clinical toxicology: a review. *Eur. J Emerg. Med* **12**, 78-85 (2005).

949. Li, B. U. K., Murray, R. D., Heitlinger, L. A., Robbins, J. L. & Hayes, J. R. Heterogeneity of diagnoses presenting as cyclic vomiting. *Pediatrics* **102**, 583-587 (1998).

950. Li, C. S., Chen, S. H., Lin, W. H. & Yang, Y. Y. Attentional blink in adolescents with varying levels of impulsivity. *J. Psychiatr. Res.* **39**, 197-205 (2005).

951. Li, C.-Y., Mao, X. & Wei, L. Genes and (common) pathways underlying drug addiction. *PLoS Comput. Biol.* **4**, e2:1-6 (2008).

952. Li, Y., Randerath, J., Goldenberg, G. & Hermsdorfer, J. Grip forces isolated from knowledge about object properties following a left parietal lesion. *Neurosci. Lett.* **426**, 187-191 (2007).

953. Libow, J. A. Child and adolescent illness falsification. *Pediatrics* **105**, 336-342 (2000).

954. Lieberman, D. J. *Never be lied to again: How to get the truth in 5 minutes or less in any conversation or situation.* St Martin's Press, New York (1998).

955. Liese, J. G. *et al.* The burden of varicella complications before the introduction of routine varicella vaccination in Germany. *Pediatr. Infect. Dis. J.* **27**, 119-124 (2008).

956. Lifford, K. J., Harold, G. T. & Thapar, A. Parent-child hostility and child ADHD symptoms: a genetically sensitive and longitudinal analysis. *J. Child Psychol Psychiatry* (2009).

957. Likierman, M. Maternal love and positive projective identification. *J. Child Psychotherapy* **14**, 29-46 (1988).

958. Lima, D. & Zagalo-Cardoso, J. A. Kleine-Levin syndrome: clinical case and diagnosis difficulties. *Revista de Psiquiatria do Rio Grande do Sul* **29**, 328-332 (2007).

959. Lima, J. A. Laryngeal foreign bodies in children: a persistent, life-threatening problem. *Laryngoscope* **99**, 415-420 (1989).

960. Lin, J. & Staecker, H. Nonorganic hearing loss. *Semin. Neurol* **26**, 321-330 (2006).

961. Lin, P. T. & Hallett, M. The pathophysiology of focal hand dystonia. *J Hand Ther* **22**, 109-113 (2009).

962. Lin, P. Y. & Su, K. P. A meta-analytic review of double-blind, placebo-controlled trials of antidepressant efficacy of omega-3 fatty acids. *J. Clin. Psychiatry* **68**, 1056-1061 (2007).

963. Lindquist, B., Persson, E. K., Uvebrant, P. & Carlsson, G. Learning, memory and executive functions in children with hydrocephalus. *Acta Paediatr.* **97**, 596-601 (2008).

964. Lindstrom, L. H. Long-term clinical and social outcome studies in schizophrenia in relation to the cognitive and emotional side effects of antipsychotic drugs. *Acta Psychiatr. Scand Suppl* **380**, 74-76 (1994).

965. Link, B. G., Stueve, A. & Phelan, J. Psychotic symptoms and violent behaviors: probing the components of threat/control-override symptoms. *Soc. Psychiatry Psychiatr. Epidemiol.* **33**, 55-60 (1998).

966. Lintas, C. & Persico, A. M. Autistic phenotypes and genetic testing: state-of-the-art for the clinical geneticist. *J Med. Genet.* **46**, 1-8 (2009).

967. Lippman, C. W. Recurrent dreams in migraine: an aid to diagnosis. *J. Nerv. Ment. Dis.* **120**, 273-276 (1954).

968. Liu, A. Y., Zimmerman, R. A., Haselgrove, J. C., Bilaniuk, L. T. & Hunter, J. V. Diffusion-weighted imaging in the evaluation of watershed hypoxic-ischemic brain injury in pediatric patients. *Neuroradiology* **43**, 918-926 (2001).

969. Liu, Z. J., Ikeda, K., Harada, S., Kasahara, Y. & Ito, G. Functional properties of jaw and tongue muscles in rats fed a liquid diet after being weaned. *J Dent. Res* **77**, 366-376 (1998).

970. Lloyd, D. M., Coates, A., Knopp, J., Oram, S. & Rowbotham, S. Don't stand so close to me: the effect of auditory input on interpersonal space. *Perception* **38**, 617-620 (2009).

971. Lock, R. J., Virgo, P. F. & Unsworth, D. J. Pitfalls in the performance and interpretation of clinical immunology tests. *J Clin Pathol* **61**, 1236-1242 (2008).

972. Locker, D., Liddell, A., Dempster, L. & Shapiro, D. Age of onset of dental anxiety. *J. Dent. Res.* **78**, 790-796 (1999).

973. Loeber, R. Prevalence, Correlates, and Continuity of Serious Conduct Problems in Elementary School Children. *Criminology* **25**, 615-642 (1987).

974. Lombroso, P. J. & Ogren, M. P. Fragile X syndrome: keys to the molecular genetics of synaptic plasticity. *J Am. Acad. Child Adolesc. Psychiatry* **47**, 736-739 (2008).

975. Longstreth, W. T., Koepsell, T. D. & vanBelle, G. Clinical neuroepidemiology. *Arch Neurol* **44**, 1091-1099 (1987).

976. Lorber, J. & Priestley, B. L. Children with large heads: a practical approach to diagnosis in 557 children, with special reference to 109 children with megalencephaly. *Develop. Med. Child Neurol.* **23**, 494-504 (1981).

977. Lovejoy, D. W. *et al.* Neuropsychological performance of adults with attention deficit hyperactivity disorder (ADHD): diagnostic classification estimates for measures of frontal lobe/executive functioning. *J. Int. Neuropsychol. Soc.* **5**, 222-233 (1999).

978. Lowenstein, L. F. The etiology, diagnosis and treatment of the fire-setting behavior of children. *Child Psychiatry Hum. Dev.* **19**, 186-194 (1989).

979. Luborsky, L. & Barrett, M. S. The history and empirical status of key psychoanalytic concepts. *Annu. Rev. Clin. Psychol* **2**, 1-19 (2006).

980. Luborsky, L. *et al.* A context analysis of psychological states prior to petit mal EEF paroxysms. *J. Nerv. Ment. Dis.* **160**, 282-298 (1975).

981. Lue, T. F. Erectile dysfunction. *New Engl. J Med.* **342**, 1802-1813 (2000).

982. Lukman, Z. M. The Prevalence of Running Away from Home among Prostituted Children in Malaysia. *J. Soc. Sci.* **5**, 157-162 (2009).

983. Lynch, J. *et al.* Is income inequality a determinant of population health? Part 1. A systematic review. *Milbank Q* **82**, 5-99 (2004).

984. Lyon, H. M., Startup, M. & Bentall, R. P. Social cognition and the manic defense: Attributions, selective attention, and self-schema in bipolar affective disorder. *J. Abnorm. Psychol.* **108**, 273-282 (1999).

985. Lyon, M. & Robbins, T. W. The action of CNS stimulant drugs: A general theory concerning amphetamine effects. *Curr. Dev. Psychopharmacol.* **2**, 79-163 (1975).

986. Lytton, W. W. Computer modelling of epilepsy. *Nat Rev. Neurosci* **9**, 626-637 (2008).

987. Lyytinen, P., Eklund, K. & Lyytinen, H. Language development and literacy skills in late-talking toddlers with and without familial risk for dyslexia. *Annals of dyslexia* **55**, 166-192 (2005).

988. MacAllister, W. S., Boyd, J. R., Holland, N. J., Milazzo, M. C. & Krupp, L. B. The psychosocial consequences of pediatric multiple sclerosis. *Neurology* **68**, S66-S69 (2007).

989. MacCorquodale, K. & Meehl, P. E. On a distinction between hypothetical constructs and intervening variables. *Psychol Rev.* **55**, 95-107 (1948).

990. Mackay, S., Paglia-Boak, A., Henderson, J., Marton, P. & Adlaf, E. Epidemiology of firesetting in adolescents: mental health and substance use correlates. *J Child Psychol Psychiatry* **50**, 1282-1290 (2009).

991. Maggio, V. & Wheless, J. Dietary treatment of seizures from a hypothalamic hamartoma in Schmidt, D. & Schachter, S. C. (eds.), *Puzzling cases of epilepsy*.pp. 350-354 (Elsevier, New York,2008).

992. Magnus, J. R., Polterovich, V. M., Danilov, D. L. & Savvateev, A. V. Tolerance of cheating: An analysis across countries. *J. Econ. Educ.* **33**, 125-135 (2002).

993. Mahone, E. M., Bridges, D., Prahme, C. & Singer, H. S. Repetitive arm and hand movements (complex motor stereotypies) in children. *J Pediatr.* **145**, 391-395 (2004).

994. Mahr, G. Psychogenic communication disorders in Johnson, A. F. & Jacobson, B. H. (eds.), *Medical Speech-Language Pathology: A Practitioner's Guide*.pp. 655-666 (Thieme Medical, New York,1998).

995. Malfait, F., Hakim, A. J., De, P. A. & Grahame, R. The genetic basis of the joint hypermobility syndromes. *Rheumatology (Oxford)* **45**, 502-507 (2006).

996. Malik, S. My brother the bomber. *Prospect Magazine* **Issue 135**, (2007).

997. Malm, D. & Nilssen, O. Alpha-mannosidosis. *Orphanet J. Rare Dis.* **3**, 21-30 (2008).

998. Malm, G. & Mansson, J.-E. Mucopolysaccharidosis type III (Sanfilippo disease) in Sweden: clinical presentation of 22 children diagnosed during a 30-year period. *Acta Paediatr.* **(in press)**, (2010).

999. Malone, A. J. & Massler, M. Index of nailbiting in children. *J. Abnorm. Soc. Psychol.* **47**, 193-202 (1952).

1000. Maltsberger, J. T. Ecstatic suicide. *Arch. Suicide Res.* **3**, 283-301 (1997).

1001. Mandy, W. P. & Skuse, D. H. Research review: What is the association between the social-communication element of autism and repetitive interests, behaviours and activities? *J Child Psychol Psychiatry* **49**, 795-808 (2008).

1002. Manford, M. & Andermann, F. Complex visual hallucinations. Clinical and neurobiological insights. *Brain* **121 (Pt 10)**, 1819-1840 (1998).

1003. Manford, M. *et al.* Case study: neurological brain waves causing serious behavioral brainstorms. *J. Am. Acad. Child Adolesc. Psychiatry* **37**, 1085-1090 (1998).

1004. Mannerkoski, M. *et al.* Childhood growth and development associated with need for full-time special education at school age. *Eur. J. Paediatr. Neurol.* **14**, 62-68 (2009).

1005. Manners, P. J. Gender identity disorder in adolescence: a review of the literature. *Child Adolesc. Mental Health* **14**, 62-68 (2009).

1006. Manson, J. A. E. Prenatal exposure to sex steroid hormones and behavioral/cognitive outcomes. *Metabolism* **57**, S16-S21 (2008).

1007. Mantzicopoulos, P. Conflictual relationships between kindergarten children and their teachers: Associations with child and classroom context variables. *J. School Psychology* **43**, 425-442 (2005).

1008. Manusov, V. & Spitzberg, B. Attribution Theory in Baxter, L. A. & Braithwaite, D. O. (eds.), *Engaging theories in interpersonal communication: Multiple perspectives*.pp. 37-49 (Sage Publications, London,2008).

1009. Margolis, R. L. Psychiatry of the Cerebellum in Jeste, D. V. & Friedman, J. H. (eds.), *Psychiatry for neurologists*.pp. 241-255 (Humana Press, Totawa,2006).

1010. Marks, I. & Mataix-Cols, D. Diagnosis and classification of phobias: a review in Maj, M., Akiskal, H. S., Lopez-Ibor, J. J. & Okasha, A. (eds.), *Phobias*.pp. 1-32 (John Wiley & Sons, Ltd, New York,2004).

1011. Marks, I. & Tobena, A. What do the neurosciences tell us about anxiety disorders? A comment. *Psychol. Med.* **16**, 9-12 (1986).

1012. Marneros, A. Schizophrenic first-rank symptoms in organic mental disorders. *Br. J Psychiatry* **152**, 625-628 (1988).

1013. Marneros, A. Beyond the Kraepelinian dichotomy: acute and transient psychotic disorders and the necessity for clinical differentiation. *Br. J Psychiatry* **189**, 1-2 (2006).

1014. Maron, E., Hettema, J. M. & Shlik, J. Advances in molecular genetics of panic disorder. *Mol. Psychiatry* **15**, 681-701 (2010).

1015. Marshall, P. *et al.* Effectiveness of symptom validity measures in identifying cognitive and behavioral symptom exaggeration in adult attention deficit hyperactivity disorder. *The Clinical Neuropsychologist* **24**, 1204-1237 (2010).

1016. Marshall, W. A. & Tanner, J. M. Variations in the pattern of pubertal changes in boys. *Arch Dis Child* **45**, 13-23 (1970).

1017. Marshall, W. A. & Tanner, J. M. Variations in pattern of pubertal changes in girls. *Arch Dis Child* **44**, 291-303 (1969).

1018. Martens, M. A., Wilson, S. J. & Reutens, D. C. Research Review: Williams syndrome: a critical review of the cognitive, behavioral, and neuroanatomical phenotype *J Child Psychol Psychiatry* **49**, 576-608 (2008).

1019. Martin, J. R. & Arici, A. Fragile X and reproduction. *Curr. Opin. Obstet. Gynecol.* **20**, 216-220 (2008).

1020. Martins, A. M. *et al.* Guidelines to diagnosis and monitoring of Fabry disease and review of treatment experiences. *J Pediatr.* **155**, S19-S31 (2009).

1021. Marx, B. P., Forsyth, J. P., Gallup, G. G., Fuse, T. & Lexington, J. M. Tonic immobility as an evolved predator defense: Implications for sexual assault survivors. *Clinical Psychology: Science and Practice* **15**, 74-90 (2008).

1022. Masicampo, E. J. & Baumeister, R. F. Toward a physiology of dual-process reasoning and judgment: lemonade, willpower, and expensive rule-based analysis. *Psychol. Science* **19**, 255-260 (2008).

1023. Maskey, S. Obsessive-Compulsive Disorder in Skuse, D. (ed.), *Child Psychology and Psychiatry: An introduction*.pp. 95-100 (Medicine Publishing Company, Kidlington,2003).

1024. Maslow, A. H. Some theoretical consequences of basic need-gratification. *J. Personality* **16**, 402-416 (1948).

1025. Mason, S. J., Harris, G. & Blissett, J. Tube feeding in infancy: implications for the development of normal eating and drinking skills. *Dysphagia* **20**, 46-61 (2005).

1026. Mataix-Cols, D., Pertusa, A. & Snowdon, J. Neuropsychological and neural correlates of hoarding: a practice-friendly review. *J. Clin. Psychol: In session* **67**, 467-476 (2011).

1027. Matthews, W. & Wallis, D. N. Patterns of self-inflicted injury. *Trauma* **4**, 17-20 (2002).

1028. May, M., Emond, A. & Crawley, E. Phenotypes of chronic fatigue syndrome in children and young people. *Arch Dis Child* **95**, 245-249 (2010).

1029. Mazeh, D. *et al.* Itching in the psychiatric ward. *Acta Derm Venereol* **88**, 128-131 (2008).

1030. Mazur, A., Booth, A. & Dabbs, J. M. Testosterone and chess competition. *Soc. Psychol. Q.* **55**, 70-77 (1992).

1031. McAbee, G. N., Prieto, D. M., Kirby, J., Santilli, A. M. & Setty, R. Permanent Visual Loss Due to Dietary Vitamin A Deficiency in an Autistic Adolescent. *J. Child Neurol.* **24**, 1288-1289 (2009).

1032. McCann, D. *et al.* Food additives and hyperactive behaviour in 3-year-old and 8/9-year-old children in the community: a randomised, double-blinded, placebo-controlled trial. *Lancet* **370**, 1560-1567 (2007).

1033. McClellan, J. & Werry, J. Practice parameters for the assessment and treatment of children and adolescents with bipolar disorder. *J Am. Acad. Child Adolesc. Psychiatry* **36**, 157S-176S (1997).

1034. McClellan, J., Werry, J. & Work Group on Quality Issues Practice parameter for the assessment and treatment of children and adolescents with schizophrenia. *J. Am. Acad. Child Adolesc. Psychiatry* **40**, 4S-23S (2001).

1035. McCord, B. E., Iwata, B. A., Galensky, T. L., Ellingson, S. A. & Thomson, R. J. Functional analysis and treatment of problem behavior evoked by noise. *J. Appl. Behav. Anal.* **34**, 447-462 (2001).

1036. McCray, G. M. Excessive masturbation of childhood: a symptom of tactile deprivation? *Pediatrics* **62**, 277-279 (1978).

1037. McCurley, C. & National Ctr for Juvenile Justice *Self-Reported Law-Violating Behavior from Adolescence to Early Adulthood in a Modern Cohort*. Pittsburgh, PA: National Center for Juvenile Justice, (2007).

1038. McDougle, C. J. *et al.* Risperidone for the core symptom domains of autism: results from the study by the autism network of the research units on pediatric psychopharmacology. *Am. J. Psychiatry* **162**, 1142-1148 (2005).

1039. McDowell, M. A., Brody, D. J. & Hughes, J. P. Has age at menarche changed? Results from the National Health and Nutrition Examination Survey (NHANES) 1999-2004. *J. Adolesc. Health* **40**, 227-231 (2007).

1040. McEwen, B. S. & Wingfield, J. C. The concept of allostasis in biology and biomedicine. *Horm. Behav.* **43**, 2-15 (2003).

1041. McFarland, R., Taylor, R. W. & Turnbull, D. M. A neurological perspective on mitochondrial disease. *Lancet Neurol.* **9**, 829-840 (2010).

1042. McFarlane, J., Parker, B. & Soeken, K. Physical abuse, smoking, and substance use during pregnancy: Prevalence, interrelationships, and effects on birth weight. *J. Obstetric, Gynecologic, Neonatal Nursing* **25**, 313-320 (1996).

1043. McGaw, S. Parenting exceptional children in Hoghughi, M. & Long, N. (eds.), *Handbook of parenting*.pp. 213-236 (Sage, London,2004).

1044. McGee, M. C. The ideograph: A link between rhetoric and ideology. *Q. J. Speech* **66**, 1-16 (1980).

1045. McGee, R. & Stanton, W. R. Smoking in pregnancy and child development to age 9 years. *J. Paediatr. Child Health* **30**, 263-268 (1994).

1046. McGhee, P. E. *Humor: Its origin and development*. WH Freeman, San Francisco (1979).

1047. McGowan, P. O. *et al.* Epigenetic regulation of the glucocorticoid receptor in human brain associates with childhood abuse. *Nat Neurosci* **12**, 342-348 (2009).

1048. McGrath, P. A. The multidimensional nature of children's pain experiences in McGrath, P. A. (ed.), *Pain in children: Nature, assessment, and treatment*.pp. 1-40 (Guilford Press, New York,1990).

1049. McGuffin, P. & Martin, N. Science, medicine, and the future: Behaviour and genes. *Br. Med. J.* **319**, 37-40 (1999).

1050. McKenna, P. & Warrington, E. K. The analytical approach to neuropsychological assessment in Grant, I. & Adams, K. M. (eds.), *Neuropsychological Assessment of Neuropsychiatric and Neuromedical Disorders*.pp. 25-41 (Oxford University Press, New York,2009).

1051. McLoyd, V. C., Jayaratne, T. E., Ceballo, R. & Borquez, J. Unemployment and work interruption among African American single mothers: Effects on parenting and adolescent socioemotional functioning. *Child Dev.* **65**, 562-589 (1994).

1052. McManus, I. C., Porac, C., Bryden, M. P. & Boucher, R. Eye-dominance, writing hand, and throwing hand. *Laterality* **4**, 173-192 (1999).

1053. McPherson, G. E. Diary of a child musical prodigy, *International Symposium on Performance Science*.2007).

1054. McQuaid, E. L., Kopel, S. J. & Nassau, J. H. Behavioral adjustment in children with asthma: a meta-analysis. *J. Dev. Behav. Pediatr.* **22**, 430-439 (2001).

1055. Meador, K. J., Allen, M. E., Adams, R. J. & Loring, D. W. Allochiria vs Allesthesia: Is There a Misperception? *Arch. Neurol.* **48**, 546-549 (1991).

1056. Meilleur, A. A. & Fombonne, E. Regression of language and non-language skills in pervasive developmental disorders. *J. Intellect. Disabil. Res* **53**, 115-124 (2009).

1057. Meissner, W. W. Toward a Neuropsychological Reconstruction of Projective Identification. *J. Am. Psychoanal. Assoc.* **57**, 95-129 (2009).

1058. Meister, I. G. *et al.* Motor cortex hand area and speech: implications for the development of language. *Neuropsychologia* **41**, 401-406 (2003).

1059. Menezes-Filho, J. A., Bouchard, M., Sarcinelli, P. N. & Moreira, J. C. Manganese exposure and the neuropsychological effect on children and adolescents: a review. *Revista Panamericana de Salud P·blica* **26**, 541-548 (2009).

1060. Meng, L. F. The rate of handedness conversion and related factors in left-handed children. *Laterality.* **12**, 131-138 (2007).

1061. Mercuri, E., Pane, M., Messina, S. & Beradinelli, A. Mental retardation in patients with neuromuscular disorders in Riva, D., Bulgheroni, S. & Pantaleoni, C. (eds.), *Mental Retardation*.pp. 33-48 (John Libbey Eurotext, Montrouge, France,2007).

1062. Merlini, L. Marinesco Sjogren syndrome, Fanfare, and more. *Neuromuscul. Disord.* **18**, 185-188 (2008).

1063. Mertin, P. & Hertwig, S. Auditory hallucinations in nonpsychotic children: diagnostic considerations. *Child Adolesc. Mental Health* **9**, 9-14 (2004).

1064. Messer, S. The effect of anxiety over intellectual performance on reflection-impulsivity in children. *Child Dev* **41**, 723-735 (1970).

1065. Messiaen, L. *et al.* Clinical and mutational spectrum of neurofibromatosis type 1-like syndrome. *JAMA* **302**, 2111-2118 (2009).

1066. Meuret, A. E., Ritz, T., Wilhelm, F. H. & Roth, W. T. Voluntary hyperventilation in the treatment of panic disorder--functions of hyperventilation, their implications for breathing training, and recommendations for standardization. *Clin. Psychol Rev.* **25**, 285-306 (2005).

1067. Mevissen, L. & de, J. A. PTSD and its treatment in people with intellectual disabilities: A review of the literature. *Clin Psychol Rev.* **30**, 308-316 (2010).

1068. Meyer, A. *et al.* The Mutation p. Ser298Pro in the sulphamidase gene (SGSH) is associated with a slowly progressive clinical phenotype in mucopolysaccharidosis type IIIA (Sanfilippo A Syndrome). *Hum. Mutat.* **29**, 770-775 (2008).

1069. Meyer-Lindenberg, A. & Weinberger, D. R. Intermediate phenotypes and genetic mechanisms of psychiatric disorders. *Nat. Rev. Neurosci.* **7**, 818-827 (2006).

1070. Michael, T., Ehlers, A., Halligan, S. L. & Clark, D. M. Unwanted memories of assault: what intrusion characteristics are associated with PTSD? *Behav Res Ther.* **43**, 613-628 (2005).

1071. Michell, A. W., Lewis, S. J., Foltynie, T. & Barker, R. A. Biomarkers and Parkinson's disease. *Brain* **127**, 1693-1705 (2004).

1072. Migone, P. Expressed emotion and projective identification: a bridge between psychiatric and psychoanalytic concepts? *Contemporary Psychoanalysis* **31**, 617 (1995).

1073. Mikkelsson, M., Sourander, A., Piha, J. & Salminen, J. J. Psychiatric symptoms in preadolescents with musculoskeletal pain and fibromyalgia. *Pediatrics* **100**, 220-227 (1997).

1074. Milberg, W. P., Hebben, N. & Kaplan, E. The Boston Process approach to neuropsychological assessment in Grant, I. & Adams, K. M. (eds.), *Neuropsychological Assessment of Neuropsychiatric and Neuromedical Disorders*.pp. 42-65 (Oxford University Press, New York,2009).

1075. Milgram, S. Some conditions of obedience and disobedience to authority. *Int. J. Psychiatry* **6**, 259-276 (1968).

1076. Miller, C. Childhood animal cruelty and interpersonal violence. *Clin. Psychol Rev.* **21**, 735-749 (2001).

1077. Miller, G. A. The magical number seven plus or minus two: some limits on our capacity for processing information. *Psychol Rev.* **63**, 81-97 (1956).

1078. Miller, J. M., Singer, H. S., Bridges, D. D. & Waranch, H. R. Behavioral therapy for treatment of stereotypic movements in nonautistic children. *J. Child Neurol.* **21**, 119-125 (2006).

1079. Miller, N. R. Neuro-ophthalmologic manifestations of psychogenic disease. *Semin. Neurol* **26**, 310-320 (2006).

1080. Millichap, J. G. Etiologic classification of attention-deficit/hyperactivity disorder. *Pediatrics* **121**, e358-e365 (2008).

1081. Millichap, J. G. & Yee, M. M. The diet factor in pediatric and adolescent migraine. *Pediatr. Neurol.* **28**, 9-15 (2003).

1082. Mills, R. P., Albert, D. M. & Brain, C. E. Tinnitus in childhood. *Clin. Otolaryngol. Allied Sciences* **11**, 431-434 (1986).

1083. Milner, B., Squire, L. R. & Kandel, E. R. Cognitive neuroscience and the study of memory. *Neuron* **20**, 445-468 (1998).

1084. Milner, K. M. *et al.* Prader-Willi syndrome: intellectual abilities and behavioural features by genetic subtype. *J. Child Psychol Psychiatry* **46**, 1089-1096 (2005).

1085. Minderaa, R. B. *et al.* Brief report: Snout and visual rooting reflexes in infantile autism. *J. Autism Dev. Disord.* **15**, 409-416 (1985).

1086. Mineka, S. & Cook, M. Mechanisms involved in the observational conditioning of fear. *J Exp. Psychol Gen.* **122**, 23-38 (1993).

1087. Mineka, S. & Oehlberg, K. The relevance of recent developments in classical conditioning to understanding the etiology and maintenance of anxiety disorders. *Acta Psychol. (Amst)* **127**, 567-580 (2008).

1088. Minor, D. L., Jr. The neurobiologist's guide to structural biology: a primer on why macromolecular structure matters and how to evaluate structural data. *Neuron* **54**, 511-533 (2007).

1089. Mintz, M. *et al.* The underrecognized epilepsy spectrum: the effects of levetiracetam on neuropsychological functioning in relation to subclinical spike production. *J Child Neurol* **24**, 807-815 (2009).

1090. Minuchin, S. *Families and Family Therapy.* Tavistock Publications, London (1974).

1091. Minuchin, S. *et al.* A conceptual model of psychosomatic illness in children: Family organization and family therapy. *Arch. Gen. Psychiatry* **32**, 1031-1038 (1975).

1092. Mirastschijski, U., Altmann, S., Lenz-Scharf, O., Muschke, P. & Schneider, W. Syndromes with focal overgrowth in infancy: Diagnostic approach and surgical treatment. *Scand J Plast. Reconstr. Surg. Hand Surg.* **(in press)**, (2010).

1093. Mitchell, J. P., Nosek, B. A. & Banaji, M. R. Contextual variations in implicit evaluation. *J Exp Psychol Gen.* **132**, 455-469 (2003).

1094. Miyazaki, K., Miyazaki, K. & Doya, K. Activity of serotonergic neurons in the dorsal raphe nucleus of freely moving rats during reward and non-reward delay period. *Neurosci. Res.* **58**, 169 (2007).

1095. Mockford, K., Weston, M. & Subramaniam, R. Management of high-flow priapism in paediatric patients: A case report and review of the literature. *J Pediatr. Urol.* **3**, 404-412 (2007).

1096. Moffitt, T. E. *et al.* Research review: DSM-V conduct disorder: research needs for an evidence base. *J. Child Psychol Psychiatry* **49**, 3-33 (2008).

1097. Mohr, C., Bracha, H. S. & Brugger, P. Magical ideation modulates spatial behavior. *J. Neuropsychiatry Clin. Neurosci.* **15**, 168-174 (2003).

1098. Molina-Garrido, M. J., Guillen-Ponce, C., Martinez, S & Guirado-Risueno, M. Diagnosis and current treatment of neurological paraneoplastic syndromes. *Clin. Transl. Oncology* **8**, 796-801 (2006).

1099. Momjian-Mayor, I. & Baron, J. C. The pathophysiology of watershed infarction in internal carotid artery disease: review of cerebral perfusion studies. *Stroke* **36**, 567-577 (2005).

1100. Monack, D. M., Mueller, A. & Falkow, S. Persistent bacterial infections: the interface of the pathogen and the host immune system. *Nat. Rev. Microbiol.* **2**, 747-765 (2004).

1101. Monahan, J. & Steadman, H. J. *Violence and mental disorder: Developments in risk assessment.* University of Chicago Press, London (1994).

1102. Moncrieff, J. & Cohen, D. How do psychiatric drugs work? *Br. Med. J* **338**, b1963 (2009).

1103. Monrad-Krohn, G. H. Dysprosody or altered" melody of language.". *Brain* **70**, 405-415 (1947).

1104. Monroe, R. R. DSM-III style diagnoses of the episodic disorders. *J. Nerv. Ment. Dis.* **170**, 664-669 (1982).

1105. Montalto, M. *et al.* Classification of malabsorption syndromes. *Dig. Dis.* **26**, 104-111 (2008).

1106. Montell, C. Speculations on a privileged state of cognitive dissonance. *J. Theory Social Behav* **31**, 119-137 (2001).

1107. Moore, B. R. The evolution of learning. *Biol. Rev. Camb. Philos. Soc.* **79**, 301-335 (2004).

1108. Moore, M. M. Courtship signaling and adolescents. *J. Sex Res* **32**, 319-328 (1995).

1109. Moradi, A. R., Doost, H. T., Taghavi, M. R., Yule, W. & Dalgleish, T. Everyday memory deficits in children and adolescents with PTSD: performance on the Rivermead Behavioural Memory Test. *J Child Psychol Psychiatry* **40**, 357-361 (1999).

1110. Moreira-Almeida, A. Differentiating spiritual from psychotic experiences. *Br. J Psychiatry* **195**, 370-371 (2009).

1111. Morgan, J. F. & Lacey, J. H. Scratching and fasting: a study of pruritus and anorexia nervosa. *Br. J. Dermatol.* **140**, 453-456 (1999).

1112. Morgan, L., Wetherby, A. M. & Barber, A. Repetitive and stereotyped movements in children with autism spectrum disorders late in the second year of life. *J. Child Psychol Psychiatry* **49**, 826-837 (2008).

1113. Morita, S., Suzuki, M. & Iizuka, K. Non-organic hearing loss in childhood. *Int. J. Pediatr. Otorhinolaryngol.* **74**, 441-446 (2010).

1114. Morris, D. *Manwatching.* Triad/Panther Books, St Albans (1978).

1115. Morris, L. W. & Engle, W. B. Assessing various coping strategies and their effects on test performance and anxiety. *J. Clin. Psychol.* **37**, 165-171 (1981).

1116. Mortimer, J. G. Acute water intoxication as another unusual manifestation of child abuse. *Arch. Dis. Child.* **55**, 401-403 (1980).

1117. Moskowitz, A. K., Barker-Collo, S. & Ellson, L. Replication of dissociation-psychosis link in New Zealand students and inmates. *J. Nerv. Ment. Dis.* **193**, 722-727 (2005).

1118. Mottus, M., Indus, K. & Allik, J. Accuracy of only children stereotype. *J. Res. Personality* **42**, 1047-1052 (2008).

1119. Mouridsen, S. E., Rich, B., Isager, T. & Nedergaard, N. J. Pervasive developmental disorders and criminal behaviour: a case control study. *Int. J. Offender Therapy Comparative Criminology* **52**, 196-205 (2008).

1120. Mouridsen, S. E. & Sorensen, S. A. Psychological aspects of von Recklinghausen neurofibromatosis (NF1). *J. Med. Genet.* **32**, 921-924 (1995).

1121. Moyer, K. E. Kinds of aggression and their physiological basis. *Commun. Behavioral Biology* **2**, 65-87 (1968).

1122. Mularski, R. A., Grazer, R. E., Santoni, L., Strother, J. S. & Bizovi, K. E. Treatment advice on the internet leads to a life-threatening adverse reaction: hypotension associated with Niacin overdose. *Clin Toxicol. (Phila)* **44**, 81-84 (2006).

1123. Mullen, P. E. A modest proposal for another phenomenological approach to psychopathology. *Schizophr. Bull.* **33**, 113-121 (2007).
1124. Muris, P., Plessis, M. & Loxton, H. Origins of common fears in South African children. *J. Anxiety Disord.* **22**, 1510-1515 (2008).
1125. Murray, D., Lesser, M. & Lawson, W. Attention, monotropism and the diagnostic criteria for autism. *Autism* **9**, 139-156 (2005).
1126. Murray, J. The effects of imprisonment on families and children of prisoners in Liebling, A. & Maruna, S. (eds.), *The effects of imprisonment.* pp. 442-462 (Willan Publishing, Portland,2005).
1127. Murray, L. *et al.* The effect of cleft lip on socio-emotional functioning in school-aged children. *J Child Psychol Psychiatry* **51**, 94-103 (2010).
1128. Myers, K. A. & Farquhar, D. R. E. Does this patient have clubbing? *JAMA* **286**, 341-347 (2001).
1129. Myers, K. M. & Davis, M. Mechanisms of fear extinction. *Mol. Psychiatry* **12**, 120-150 (2007).
1130. Myers, W. C. Serial murder by children and adolescents. *Behavioral Sciences & the Law* **22**, 357-374 (2004).
1131. Myles, B. S. & Southwick, J. *Asperger syndrome and difficult moments*. Autism Asperger Publishing Company, Shawnee Mission, KS (2005).
1132. Nader, K., Pynoos, R., Fairbanks, L. & Frederick, C. Children's PTSD reactions one year after a sniper attack at their school. *Am. J. Psychiatry* **147**, 1526-1530 (1990).
1133. Naglieri, J. A. *Draw a person: a quantitative scoring system.* Psychological Corporation, San Antonio, TX (1988).
1134. Nair, P. S., Sobhakumar, S. & Kailas, L. Diagnostic Re-evaluation of Children with Congenital Hypothyroidism. *Indian Pediatr.* **47**, 753-754 (2010).
1135. Nakalawa, L., Musisi, S., Kinyanda, E. & Okello, E. S. Demon attack disease: a case report of mass hysteria after mass trauma in a primary school in Uganda. *African J. Traumatic Stress* **1**, 43-48 (2010).
1136. Nascimento, L. F. C., Rizol, P. M. S. R. & Abiuzi, L. B. Establishing the risk of neonatal mortality using a fuzzy predictive model. *Cadernos Saude Publica* **25**, 2043-2052 (2009).
1137. Nassogne, M. C., Heron, B., Touati, G., Rabier, D. & Saudubray, J. M. Urea cycle defects: management and outcome. *J Inherit. Metab Dis* **28**, 407-414 (2005).
1138. National collaborating centre for women's and children's health *NICE Clinical guideline 89: When to suspect child maltreatment: Quick reference guide.* NHS, National Institute for Health & Clinical Excellence, London (2009).
1139. Neisser, U. Five kinds of self-knowledge. *Philosophical psychology* **1**, 35-59 (1988).
1139a. Neligan, G. & Prudham, D. Norms for four standard developmental milestones by sex, social class and place in family. Dev. Med. Child Neurol. 11, 413-422 (1969).
1140. Nelson, K. B. & Lynch, J. K. Stroke in newborn infants. *Lancet Neurol.* **3**, 150-158 (2004).
1141. Nelson, T. D. & Aylward, B. S. Pediatric feeding disorders in Shaw, R. J. & DeMaso, D. R. (eds.), *Textbook of pediatric psychosomatic medicine.* pp. 173-184 (American Psychiatric Publishing, Arlington,2010).
1142. Neri, G. & Moscarda, M. Overgrowth syndromes: a classification. *Endocr. Dev* **14**, 53-60 (2009).
1143. Neubauer, B. A. *et al.* Photosensitivity: Genetics and clinical significance in Delgado-Escueta, A. V. *et al.* (eds.), *Adv.Neurol., vol.95: Myoclonic Epilepsies.* pp. 217-226 (Lippincott Williams & Wilkins, Philadelphia,2005).
1144. Newberger, E. *The men they will become: The nature and nurture of male character*. Da Capo Press, Cambridge, MA (2000).
1145. Newey, P. J. *et al.* Asymptomatic children with multiple endocrine neoplasia type 1 (MEN1) mutations may harbour non-functioning pancreatic neuroendocrine tumors. *J. Clin. Endocrinol. Metab* **94**, 3640-3646 (2009).
1146. Newson, A. J. Depression under stress: ethical issues in genetic testing. *Br. J. Psychiatry* **195**, 189-190 (2009).
1147. Newson, E., Le, M. K. & David, C. Pathological demand avoidance syndrome: a necessary distinction within the pervasive developmental disorders. *Arch Dis. Child* **88**, 595-600 (2003).
1148. Ng, F., Berk, M., Dean, O. & Bush, A. I. Oxidative stress in psychiatric disorders: evidence base and therapeutic implications. *Int. J. Neuropsychopharmacol.* **11**, 851-876 (2008).
1149. Nicholls, D. & Arcelus, J. Making eating disorders classification work in ICD-11. *Eur. Eat. Disord. Rev.* **18**, 247-250 (2010).
1150. Nicholls, D., Chater, R. & Lask, B. Children into DSM don't go: a comparison of classification systems for eating disorders in childhood and early adolescence. *Int. J. Eat. Disord.* **28**, 317-324 (2000).
1151. Nicholls, D. & Jaffa, T. Selective eating and other atypical eating problems in Jaffa, T. & McDermott, B. (eds.), *Eating disorders in children and adolescents.* pp. 144-157 (Cambridge Univ Pr, Cambridge,2007).
1152. Nichols, D. E. & Nichols, C. D. Serotonin receptors. *Chem. Rev.* **108**, 1614-1641 (2008).
1153. Nichols, M. P. & Schwartz, R. C. *Family Therapy: Concepts and Methods*. Allyn & Bacon, Boston (2004).
1154. Nichols, P. L. Familial mental retardation. *Behav. Genet.* **14**, 161-170 (1984).
1155. Nickman, S. L. *et al.* Children in adoptive families: overview and update. *J. Am. Acad. Child Adolesc. Psychiat* **44**, 987-995 (2005).
1156. Nico, D. & Daprati, E. The egocentric reference for visual exploration and orientation. *Brain Cogn* **69**, 227-235 (2009).
1157. Nico, D. *et al.* The role of the right parietal lobe in anorexia nervosa. *Psychol. Med.* **(in press)**, 1-9 (2010).
1158. Nicolson, R. I. & Fawcett, A. J. Procedural learning difficulties: reuniting the developmental disorders? *Trends Neurosci* **30**, 135-141 (2007).
1159. Nicpon, M. F., Wodrich, D. L. & Kurpius, S. E. Utilization behavior in boys with ADHD: a test of Barkley's theory. *Dev. Neuropsychol.* **26**, 735-751 (2004).
1160. Nielsen, T. A. *et al.* The typical dreams of Canadian university students. *Dreaming* **13**, 211-235 (2003).
1161. Nigg, J. T. Temperament and developmental psychopathology. *J Child Psychol Psychiatry* **47**, 395-422 (2006).
1162. Nigrovic, P. A., Fuhlbrigge, R. C. & Sundel, R. P. Raynaud's phenomenon in children: a retrospective review of 123 patients. *Pediatrics* **111**, 715-721 (2003).
1163. Nijs, J. *et al.* In the mind or in the brain? Scientific evidence for central sensitization in chronic fatigue syndrome. *Eur. J. Clin. Invest.*
1164. NIMH Life Charting. *Bipolar Network News* **8**, 1-15 (2002).
1165. Noachtar, S. & Peters, A. S. Semiology of epileptic seizures: a critical review. *Epilepsy Behav* **15**, 2-9 (2009).
1166. Noachtar, S. & Remi, J. The role of EEG in epilepsy: a critical review. *Epilepsy & Behavior* **15**, 22-33 (2009).
1167. Noble, J. M. C., Mandel, A. & Patterson, M. C. Scurvy and Rickets Masked by Chronic Neurologic Illness: Revisiting "Psychologic Malnutrition". *Pediatrics* **119**, e783-e790 (2007).
1168. Nokes, C., Grantham-McGregor, S. M., Sawyer, A. W., Cooper, E. S. & Bundy, D. A. Parasitic helminth infection and cognitive function in school children. *Proc. Biol. Sci.* **247**, 77-81 (1992).

1169. Nolano, M. *et al.* Absent innervation of skin and sweat glands in congenital insensitivity to pain with anhidrosis. *Clin. Neurophysiol.* **111**, 1596-1601 (2000).

1170. Norman, R. J., Dewailly, D., Legro, R. S. & Hickey, T. E. Polycystic ovary syndrome. *Lancet* **370**, 685-697 (2007).

1171. Northoff, G., Wenke, J. & Pflug, B. Increase of serum creatine phosphokinase in catatonia: an investigation in 32 acute catatonic patients. *Psychol. Med.* **26**, 547-553 (2009).

1172. Nunn, K., Nicholls, D. & Lask, B. A new taxonomy for child psychiatry. *Clin. Child Psychol. Psychiatry* **5**, 313-327 (2000).

1173. Nurcombe, B., Tramontana, M. & LaBarbera, J. D. Diagnostic evaluation in Ebert, M. H., Loosen, P. T. & Nurcombe, B. (eds.), *Current diagnosis & treatment in psychiatry.* pp. 502-519 (Lange Medical Books, New York, 2000).

1174. Nutt, D. J. & Sharpe, M. Uncritical positive regard? Issues in the efficacy and safety of psychotherapy. *J Psychopharmacol.* **22**, 3-6 (2008).

1175. Nyberg, G., Ekelund, U. & Marcus, C. Physical activity in children measured by accelerometry: stability over time. *Scand J Med Sci Sports* **19**, 30-35 (2009).

1176. O'Connor, T. G. Attachment disorders of infancy and childhood in Rutter, M. & Taylor, E. (eds.), *Child and adolescent psychiatry.* (Blackwell, Oxford, 2008).

1177. O'Hare, A. E., Bremner, L., Nash, M., Happe, F. & Pettigrew, L. M. A Clinical Assessment Tool for Advanced Theory of Mind Performance in 5 to 12 Year Olds. *J. Autism Dev. Disord.* **39**, 916-928 (2009).

1178. O'Reilly, R. C. Biologically based computational models of high-level cognition. *Science* **314**, 91-94 (2006).

1179. O'Reilly, R. C. Modeling integration and dissociation in brain and cognitive development in Munakata, Y. & Johnson, M. H. (eds.), *Processes of Change in Brain and Cognitive Development: Attention and Performance.* pp. 375-402 (OUP, New York, 2006).

1180. O'Sullivan, M. & O'Morain, C. Nutrition in inflammatory bowel disease. *Best Practice & Research Clinical Gastroenterology* **20**, 561-573 (2006).

1181. Ochsner, K. N. *et al.* Bottom-up and top-down processes in emotion generation. *Psychol. Science* **20**, 1322-1331 (2009).

1182. Odding, E., Roebroeck, M. E. & Stam, H. J. The epidemiology of cerebral palsy: incidence, impairments and risk factors. *Disabil. Rehabil.* **28**, 183-191 (2006).

1183. Ogden, T. E., Robert, F. & Carmichael, E. A. Some sensory syndromes in children: Indifference to pain and sensory neuropathy. *J. Neurol. Neurosurg. Psychiat.* **22**, 267-276 (1959).

1184. Ohry, A., Rattok, J. & Solomon, Z. Post-traumatic stress disorder in brain injury patients. *Brain Inj.* **10**, 687-695 (1996).

1185. Olafsson, R. F. & Johannsdottir, H. L. Coping with bullying in the workplace: the effect of gender, age and type of bullying. *Br. J. Guid. Counsel.* **32**, 319-333 (2004).

1186. Olden, K. W. & Chepyala, P. Functional nausea and vomiting. *Nat. Clin. Prac. Gastroenterol. Hepatol.* **5**, 202-208 (2008).

1187. Olds, D. D. Identification: psychoanalytic and biological perspectives. *J Am. Psychoanal. Assoc.* **54**, 17-46 (2006).

1188. Olincy, A. *et al.* Inhibition of the P50 cerebral evoked response to repeated auditory stimuli: Results from the Consortium on Genetics of Schizophrenia. *Schizophr. Res.* **119**, 175-182 (2010).

1189. Olincy, A. *et al.* Proof-of-concept trial of an alpha-7 nicotinic agonist in schizophrenia. *Arch. Gen. Psychiatry* **63**, 630-638 (2006).

1190. Oliver, C. *et al.* Self-injurious behaviour in Cornelia de Lange syndrome. Trident Communications, Coventry (2003).

1191. Olney, J. W. Excitotoxic amino acids and neuropsychiatric disorders. *Annu. Rev. Pharmacol. Toxicol.* **30**, 47-71 (1990).

1192. Olson, D. M., Howard, N. & Shaw, R. J. Hypnosis-provoked nonepileptic events in children. *Epilepsy & Behavior* **12**, 456-459 (2008).

1193. Olweus, D. *Bullying at school: What we know and what we can do.* Wiley-Blackwell, (1993).

1194. OPD Task Force & von der Tann, M. *Operationalized Psychodynamic Diagnosis OPD-2: Manual of Diagnosis and Treatment Planning.* Hogrefe & Huber, Cambridge, MA (2008).

1195. Ophoff, R. A. *et al.* Familial hemiplegic migraine and episodic ataxia type-2 are caused by mutations in the Ca 2 channel gene CACNL1A4. *Cell* **87**, 543-552 (1996).

1196. Orioli, I. M. & Castilla, E. E. Epidemiology of holoprosencephaly: Prevalence and risk factors. *Am. J Med Genet. C Semin. Med Genet.* **154C**, 13-21 (2010).

1197. Ornoy, A. Valproic acid in pregnancy: How much are we endangering the embryo and fetus? *Reprod. Toxicol.* **28**, 1-10 (2009).

1198. Osterhues, A., Holzgreve, W. & Michels, K. B. Shall we put the world on folate? *Lancet* **374**, 959-961 (2009).

1199. Ostrow, L. W. & Llinas, R. H. Eastchester clapping sign: a novel test of parietal neglect. *Ann. Neurol.* **66**, 114-117 (2009).

1200. Otter, M. X-chromosome abnormality and schizophrenia. *Br. J. Psychiatry* **190**, 450 (2007).

1201. Otter, M., Schrander-Stumpel, C. T. & Curfs, L. M. Triple X syndrome: a review of the literature. *Eur. J Hum. Genet.* (2009).

1202. Owens, J. A. The ADHD and sleep conundrum: a review. *J. Dev. Behav. Pediatr.* **26**, 312-322 (2005).

1203. Owens, J. A. Sleep in children: cross-cultural perspectives. *Sleep and Biological Rhythms* **2**, 165-173 (2004).

1204. Oza, R. K. Puberphonia and voice training. *Ind. J. Otolaryngol. Head Neck Surgery* **19**, 22-24 (1967).

1205. Ozonoff, S., South, M. & Miller, J. N. DSM-IV defined Asperger syndrome: cognitive, behavioral and early history differentiation from high-functioning autism. *Autism* **4**, 29-46 (2000).

1206. Pacan, P., Grzesiak, M., Reich, A. & Szepietowski, J. C. Onychophagia as a Spectrum of Obsessive-compulsive Disorder. *Acta Derm. Venereol.* **89**, 278-280 (2009).

1207. Paciorkowski, A. R. & Fang, M. Chromosomal microarray interpretation: what is a child neurologist to do? *Pediatr. Neurol* **41**, 391-398 (2009).

1208. Pack, R. P., Wallander, J. L. & Browne, D. Health risk behaviors of African American adolescents with mild mental retardation: prevalence depends on measurement method. *Am. J. Ment. Retard.* **102**, 409-420 (1997).

1209. Packman, A. & Kuhn, L. Looking at stuttering through the lens of complexity. *Int. J. Speech-Language Pathol.* **11**, 77-82 (2009).

1210. Paediatric Accident and Emergency Research Group *The management of a child with a decreased conscious level.* University of Nottingham, Nottingham (2005).

1211. Page, L. A., Hajat, S. & Kovats, R. S. Relationship between daily suicide counts and temperature in England and Wales. *Br. J. Psychiatry* **191**, 106-112 (2007).

1212. Page, L. A. *et al.* Frequency and Predictors of Mass Psychogenic Illness. *Epidemiology* **21**, 744-747 (2010).

1213. Palmer, B. & Frimberger, D. Successful treatment of idiopathic priapism in a 13-year-old boy. *J Pediatr. Urol.* **5**, 145-146 (2009).

1214. Panagariya, A., Sharma, B., Tripathi, G., Kumar, H. & Agarwal, V. Gelastic epilepsy associated with lesions other than hypothalamic hamartoma. *Ann. Indian Acad. Neurol* **10**, 105-108 (2007).

1215. Panayiotopoulos, C. P., Michael, M., Sanders, S., Valeta, T. & Koutroumanidis, M. Benign childhood focal epilepsies: assessment of established and newly recognized syndromes. *Brain* **131**, 2264-2286 (2008).

1216. Paracchini, S., Scerri, T. & Monaco, A. P. The genetic lexicon of dyslexia. *Annu. Rev. Genomics Hum. Genet.* **8**, 57-79 (2007).

1217. Parens, E. & Johnston, J. Controversies concerning the diagnosis and treatment of bipolar disorder in children. *Child Adolesc. Psychiatry Ment Health* **4**, 9 (2010).

1218. Parent, A. S. *et al.* The timing of normal puberty and the age limits of sexual precocity: variations around the world, secular trends, and changes after migration. *Endocr. Rev.* **24**, 668-693 (2003).

1219. Pareyson, D. & Marchesi, C. Diagnosis, natural history, and management of Charcot-Marie-Tooth disease. *Lancet Neurol.* **8**, 654-667 (2009).

1220. Parkes, J. *et al.* Psychological problems in children with cerebral palsy: a cross-sectional European study. *J. Child Psychol. Psychiatry* **49**, 405-413 (2008).

1221. Parra, J., Kalitzin, S. N. & Lopes da Silva, F. H. Photosensitivity and visually induced seizures: review. *Curr. Opin. Neurol.* **18**, 155-159 (2005).

1222. Parsons, T. Illness and the role of the physician: a sociological perspective. *Am. J. Orthopsychiatry* **21**, 452-460 (1951).

1223. Parton, A., Malhotra, P. & Husain, M. Hemispatial neglect. *J. Neurol. Neurosurg. Psychiatry* **75**, 13-21 (2004).

1224. Pasquini, M. *et al.* Bradykinesia in patients with obsessive-compulsive disorder. *European Psychiatry* **(in press)**, (2010).

1225. Passolunghi, M. C., Cornoldi, C. & De Liberto, S. Working memory and intrusions of irrelevant information in a group of specific poor problem solvers. *Memory & Cognition* **27**, 779-790 (1999).

1226. Patel, K., Roskrow, T., Davis, J. S. & Heckmatt, J. Z. Dopa responsive dystonia. *Arch Dis Child* **73**, 256-257 (1995).

1227. Patel, V. Crying behavior and psychiatric disorder in adults: A review. *Compr. Psychiatry* **34**, 206-211 (1993).

1228. Patterson, C. J. Children of lesbian and gay parents. *Current directions in psychological science* **15**, 241-244 (2006).

1229. Patton, N. Self-inflicted eye injuries: a review. *Eye* **18**, 867-872 (2004).

1230. Paul, L. K. *et al.* Agenesis of the corpus callosum: genetic, developmental and functional aspects of connectivity. *Nat. Rev. Neurosci.* **8**, 287-299 (2007).

1231. Paul, R., Augustyn, A., Klin, A. & Volkmar, F. R. Perception and production of prosody by speakers with autism spectrum disorders. *J. Autism Dev. Disord.* **35**, 205-220 (2005).

1232. Paus, T. *et al.* Structural maturation of neural pathways in children and adolescents: in vivo study. *Science* **283**, 1908-1911 (1999).

1233. Pavuluri, M. N., Henry, D. B., Devineni, B., Carbray, J. A. & Birmaher, B. Child mania rating scale: development, reliability, and validity. *J. Am. Acad. Child Adolesc. Psychiatry* **45**, 550-560 (2006).

1234. Pearl, J. *Causality: Models, reasoning, and inference*. Cambridge Univ.Press, Cambridge (2000).

1235. Pearl, P. L., Capp, P. K., Novotny, E. J. & Gibson, K. M. Inherited disorders of neurotransmitters in children and adults. *Clin. Biochem.* **38**, 1051-1058 (2005).

1236. Pearl, P. L., Weiss, R. E. & Stein, M. A. Medical mimics. Medical and neurological conditions simulating ADHD. *Ann. N. Y. Acad. Sci.* **931**, 97-112 (2001).

1237. Pearson, D. A. *et al.* Treatment effects of methylphenidate on cognitive functioning in children with mental retardation and ADHD. *J. Am. Acad. Child Adolesc. Psychiat.* **43**, 677-685 (2004).

1238. Pellegrini, A. D. Practitioner review: The role of direct observation in the assessment of young children. *J Child Psychol Psychiatry* **42**, 861-869 (2001).

1239. Peltz, E. *et al.* Functional connectivity of the human insular cortex during noxious and innocuous thermal stimulation. *Neuroimage* **15**, 1324-1335 (2011).

1240. Pennington, B. F. & Bishop, D. V. Relations among speech, language, and reading disorders. *Annu. Rev. Psychol.* **60**, 283-306 (2009).

1241. Penry, J. K., Porter, R. J. & Dreifuss, R. E. Simultaneous recording of absence seizures with video tape and electroencephalography. A study of 374 seizures in 48 patients. *Brain* **98**, 427-440 (1975).

1242. Peppe, S., McCann, J., Gibbon, F., O'Hare, A. & Rutherford, M. Receptive and expressive prosodic ability in children with high-functioning autism. *J Speech Lang Hear. Res* **50**, 1015-1028 (2007).

1243. Pepperberg, I. M. *Alex & me: How a scientist and a parrot uncovered a hidden world of animal intelligence - and formed a deep bond in the process*. Collins, New York (2008).

1244. Peralta, V. & Cuesta, M. J. Cycloid psychosis. *Int. Rev. Psychiatry* **17**, 53-62 (2005).

1245. Perquin, C. W. *et al.* Pain in children and adolescents: a common experience. *Pain* **87**, 51-58 (2000).

1246. Perry, B. D. The neurodevelopmental impact of violence in childhood in Schetky, D. & Benedek, E. (eds.), *Textbook of child and adolescent forensic psychiatry*.pp. 221-238 (American Psychiatric Press, Washington DC,2001).

1247. Perry, J. C. & Lanni, F. F. Observer-rated measures of defense mechanisms. *J. Pers.* **66**, 993-1024 (1998).

1248. Peters, B. R., Atkins, M. S. & McKay, M. M. Adopted children's behavior problems: a review of five explanatory models. *Clin Psychol Rev.* **19**, 297-328 (1999).

1249. Peters, T. E., Parvin, M., Petersen, C., Faulk, V. C. & Levine, R. L. A case report of Wernicke's encephalopathy in a pediatric patient with anorexia nervosa-Restricting type. *J. Adolesc. Health* **40**, 376-383 (2007).

1250. Petitclerc, A., Boivin, M., Dionne, G., Zoccolillo, M. & Tremblay, R. E. Disregard for rules: the early development and predictors of a specific dimension of disruptive behavior disorders. *J Child Psychol Psychiatry* **50**, 1477-1484 (2009).

1251. Petreska, B., Adriani, M., Blanke, O. & Billard, A. G. Apraxia: a review. *Prog. Brain Res.* **164**, 61-83 (2007).

1252. Pfeifer, S. Belief in demons and exorcism in psychiatric patients in Switzerland. *Br. J. Med. Psychol.* **67**, 247-258 (1994).

1253. Pfeiffer, S. I. The gifted: clinical challenges for child psychiatry. *J Am. Acad. Child Adolesc. Psychiatry* **48**, 787-790 (2009).

1254. Pickles, A. *et al.* Child psychiatric symptoms and psychosocial impairment: relationship and prognostic significance. *Br. J. Psychiatry* **179**, 230-235 (2001).

1255. Pierson, M. H. *Dark Horses and Black Beauties: Animals, Women, A Passion*. W.W.Norton & Company, New York (2000).

1256. Pinker, S. *How the mind works*. W.W. Norton, New York (1997).

1257. Piper, A. & Merskey, H. The persistence of folly: critical examination of dissociative identity disorder. Part II. The defence and decline of multiple personality or dissociative identity disorder. *Can. J Psychiatry* **49**, 678-683 (2004).

1258. Pittock, S. J. *et al.* Glutamic acid decarboxylase autoimmunity with brainstem, extrapyramidal, and spinal cord dysfunction. *Mayo Clin. Proc.* **81**, 1207-1214 (2006).

1259. Plotkin, S. A. & Rubin, S. Mumps vaccine in Plotkin, S. A., Orenstein, W. A. & Offit, P. A. (eds.), *Vaccines*.pp. 436-465 (Elsevier Saunders, Philadelphia,2008).

1260. Pluess, M. *et al.* Serotonin transporter polymorphism moderates effects of prenatal maternal anxiety on infant negative emotionality. *Biol Psychiatry* **69**, 520-525 (2011).

1261. Polak-Toste, C. P. & Gunnar, M. R. Temperamental exuberance: Correlates and consequences in Marshall, P. J. & Fox, N. A. (eds.), *The development of social engagement: Neurobiological perspectives*.pp. 19-45 (OUP, Oxford,2006).

1262. Polatajko, H. J. & Cantin, N. Developmental coordination disorder (dyspraxia): an overview of the state of the art. *Semin. Pediatr. Neurol.* **12**, 250-258 (2006).

1263. Polit, D. F. & Falbo, T. The intellectual achievement of only children. *J. Biosoc. Sci.* **20**, 275-286 (1988).

1264. Pollak, S. D., Messner, M., Kistler, D. J. & Cohn, J. F. Development of perceptual expertise in emotion recognition. *Cognition* **110**, 242-247 (2009).

1265. Pope Jr, H. G., Gruber, A. J., Choi, P., Olivardia, R. & Phillips, K. A. Muscle dysmorphia. An underrecognized form of body dysmorphic disorder. *Psychosomatics* **38**, 548-557 (1997).

1266. Pope, H. G., Jr., Kouri, E. M. & Hudson, J. I. Effects of supraphysiologic doses of testosterone on mood and aggression in normal men: a randomized controlled trial. *Arch Gen. Psychiatry* **57**, 133-140 (2000).

1267. Pope, H. G., Poliakoff, M. B., Parker, M. P., Boynes, M. & Hudson, J. I. Is dissociative amnesia a culture-bound syndrome? Findings from a survey of historical literature. *Psychol. Med.* **37**, 225-233 (2007).

1268. Porcerelli, J. H. & Sandler, B. A. Anabolic-androgenic steroid abuse and psychopathology. *Psychiatr. Clin. North Am.* **21**, 829-833 (1998).

1269. Porter, G. & Kakabadse, N. K. HRM perspectives on addiction to technology and work. *J. Management Development* **25**, 535-560 (2006).

1270. Posner, J. B., Saper, C. B., Schiff, N. & Plum, F. *Plum and Posner's diagnosis of stupor and coma.* Oxford University Press, USA, (2007).

1271. Postle, N., McMahon, K. L., Ashton, R., Meredith, M. & de Zubicaray, G. I. Action word meaning representations in cytoarchitectonically defined primary and premotor cortices. *Neuroimage.* **43**, 634-644 (2008).

1272. Potegal, M. *et al.* The behavioral organization, temporal characteristics, and diagnostic concomitants of rage outbursts in child psychiatric inpatients. *Curr. Psychiatry Rep.* **11**, 127-133 (2009).

1273. Potter, N. N. What is manipulative behavior, anyway? *J Pers. Disord.* **20**, 139-156 (2006).

1274. Poulin, F. & Chan, A. Friendship stability and change in childhood and adolescence. *Dev. Rev.* **30**, 257-272 (2010).

1275. Powsner, S. & Kennedy, R. S. Internet filtering and psychiatric investigation. *Psychosomatics* **50**, 639 (2009).

1276. Prasad, A., Prasad, C. & Jog, M. S. Ataxia with Identified Genetic and Biochemical Defects. *eMedicine* (2009).

1277. Prashanth, L. K., Taly, A. B., Sinha, S. & Ravi, V. Subacute sclerosing panencephalitis (SSPE): an insight into the diagnostic errors from a tertiary care university hospital. *J. Child Neurol.* **22**, 683-688 (2007).

1278. Prendergast, M. Types of psychiatric treatment. Drug treatment. *Arch. Dis. Child.* **67**, 1488-1494 (1992).

1279. Preston, R. The Possessed (Lesch-Nyhan Syndrome). *New Yorker* (2007).

1280. Priano, L. *et al.* On the origin of sensory impairment and altered pain perception in Prader-Willi syndrome: a neurophysiological study. *Eur. J. Pain* **13**, 829-835 (2009).

1281. Price, C. S. *et al.* Prenatal and Infant Exposure to Thimerosal From Vaccines and Immunoglobulins and Risk of Autism. *Pediatrics* **(in press)**, (2010).

1282. Price, J., Cole, V. & Goodwin, G. M. Emotional side-effects of selective serotonin reuptake inhibitors: qualitative study. *Br. J. Psychiatry* **195**, 211-217 (2009).

1283. Prizant, B. M. & Rydell, P. J. Analysis of functions of delayed echolalia in autistic children. *J. Speech Hear. Res.* **27**, 183-192 (1984).

1284. Procopio, M. & Marriott, P. Intrauterine hormonal environment and risk of developing anorexia nervosa. *Arch. Gen. Psychiatry* **64**, 1402-1407 (2007).

1285. Pulvermuller, F. Brain mechanisms linking language and action. *Nat. Rev. Neurosci.* **6**, 576-582 (2005).

1286. Purselle, D. C. & Nemeroff, C. B. Serotonin transporter: a potential substrate in the biology of suicide. *Neuropsychopharmacology* **28**, 613-619 (2003).

1287. Putnam, F. W. Development of dissociative disorders in Cicchetti, D. & Cohen, D. J. (eds.), *Developmental Psychopathology*.pp. 581-608 (John Wiley, New York,1995).

1288. Quinn, D. *et al.* Comparative pharmacodynamics and plasma concentrations of d-threo-methylphenidate hydrochloride after single doses of d-threo-methylphenidate hydrochloride and d,l-threo-methylphenidate hydrochloride in a double-blind, placebo-controlled, crossover laboratory school study in children with attention-deficit/hyperactivity disorder. *J. Am. Acad. Child Adolesc. Psychiatry* **43**, 1422-1429 (2004).

1289. Quinn, N. P. Dopa-responsive dystonia. *Dev Med Child Neurol* **33**, 750 (1991).

1290. Quint, E. H. Menstrual issues in adolescents with physical and developmental disabilities. *Ann. N. Y. Acad. Sci.* **1135**, 230-236 (2008).

1291. Raafat, R. M., Chater, N. & Frith, C. Herding in humans. *Trends Cogn Sci.* **13**, 420-428 (2009).

1292. Rachman, S. Primary obsessional slowness. *Behav. Res. Ther.* **12**, 9-18 (1974).

1293. Rachman, S. & De Silva, P. Abnormal and normal obsessions. *Behav. Res. Ther.* **16**, 233-248 (1978).

1294. Raff, M. L. & Byers, P. H. Joint hypermobility syndromes. *Curr. Opin. Rheumatol.* **8**, 459-466 (1996).

1295. Rahman, Q. & Wilson, G. D. Born gay? The psychobiology of human sexual orientation. *Personality and individual differences* **34**, 1337-1382 (2003).

1296. Rai, R. & Regan, L. Recurrent miscarriage. *Lancet* **368**, 601-611 (2006).

1297. Rajagopal, S. Catatonia. *Adv. Psychiat. Treat.* **13**, 51-59 (2007).

1298. Ramachandran, V. S. & Hubbard, E. M. Synaesthesia--a window into perception, thought and language. *J. Consciousness Studies* **8**, 3-34 (2001).

1299. Ramakrishnan, U. Prevalence of micronutrient malnutrition worldwide. *Nutr. Rev.* **60**, S46-S52 (2002).

1300. Ramus, F. Neurobiology of dyslexia: a reinterpretation of the data. *Trends Neurosci.* **27**, 720-726 (2004).

1301. Ramus, F. *et al.* Theories of developmental dyslexia: insights from a multiple case study of dyslexic adults. *Brain* **126**, 841-865 (2003).

1302. Rao, V. Bullying in schools. *Br. Med. J.* **310**, 1065-1066 (1995).

1303. Rapa, A. *et al.* Subclinical hypothyroidism in children and adolescents: a wide range of clinical, biochemical, and genetic factors involved. *J Clin Endocrinol. Metab* **94**, 2414-2420 (2009).

1304. Rapee, R. M., Schniering, C. A. & Hudson, J. I. Anxiety Disorders During Childhood and Adolescence: Origins and Treatment. *Annu. Rev. Clin. Psychol* (2009).

1305. Rapoport, J., Chavez, A., Greenstein, D., Addington, A. & Gogtay, N. Autism-Spectrum Disorders and Childhood Onset Schizophrenia: Clinical and Biological Contributions to a Relationship Revisited. *J. Am. Acad. Child Adolesc. Psychiatry* **48**, 10-18 (2009).

1306. Rapoport, J. L. *et al.* Dextroamphetamine: cognitive and behavioral effects in normal prepubertal boys. *Science* **199**, 560-563 (1978).

1307. Rapoport, J. L. & Inoff-Germain, G. Responses to methylphenidate in Attention-Deficit/Hyperactivity Disorder and normal children: update 2002. *J. Atten. Disord.* **6 Suppl 1**, S57-S60 (2002).

1308. Rashid, A., Squire, R., Stringer, M. D. & McClean, P. Meckel's Diverticulum as a Rare Cause of Chronic Screaming: The Importance of Clinical Examination During Anaesthesia. *J. Pediatr. Gastroenterol. Nutr.* **28**, 346-347 (1999).

1309. Rask-Andersen, M., Olszewski, P. K., Levine, A. S. & Schioth, H. B. Molecular mechanisms underlying anorexia nervosa: Focus on human gene association studies and systems controlling food intake. *Brain research reviews* **62**, 147-164 (2010).

1310. Rass, U., Ahel, I., West, S. C., Connelly, J. C. & Leach, D. R. F. Defective DNA repair and neurodegenerative disease. *Cell* **130**, 991-1004 (2007).

1311. Rassin, E., Merckelbach, H., Muris, P. & Spaan, V. Thought-action fusion as a causal factor in the development of intrusions. *Behav Res Ther.* **37**, 231-237 (1999).

1312. Ravelli, G. P., Stein, Z. A. & Susser, M. W. Obesity in young men after famine exposure in utero and early infancy. *N. Engl. J. Med.* **295**, 349-353 (1976).

1313. Ray, P., Zia Ul, H. M. & Nizamie, S. H. Aripiprazole-induced hiccups: a case report. *Gen. Hosp. Psychiatry* **31**, 382-384 (2009).

1314. Rayman, M. P. The importance of selenium to human health. *Lancet* **356**, 233-241 (2000).

1315. RCPCH *Evidence based guideline for the management of CFS/ME in children and young people.* Royal College of Paediatrics and Child Health, London (2004).

1316. Reading, R., Langford, I. H., Haynes, R. & Lovett, A. Accidents to preschool children: comparing family and neighbourhood risk factors. *Social Science & Medicine* **48**, 321-330 (1999).

1317. Reaven, J. & Hepburn, S. Cognitive-behavioral treatment of obsessive-compulsive disorder in a child with Asperger syndrome: a case report. *Autism* **7**, 145-164 (2003).

1318. Rechlin, T., Loew, T. H. & Joraschky, P. Pseudoseizure "status". *J. Psychosom. Res* **42**, 495-498 (1997).

1319. Reddi, B. A. & Carpenter, R. H. The influence of urgency on decision time. *Nat Neurosci* **3**, 827-830 (2000).

1320. Reeb-Sutherland, B. C. *et al.* Startle response in behaviorally inhibited adolescents with a lifetime occurrence of anxiety disorders. *J. Am. Acad. Child Adolesc. Psychiatry* **48**, 610-617 (2009).

1321. Regnerus, M. D. Religion and positive adolescent outcomes: A review of research and theory. *Review of Religious Research* **44**, 394-413 (2003).

1322. Rehman, H. U. Classic diseases revisited: Fish odour syndrome. *Br. Med. J.* **75**, 451-452 (1999).

1323. Reichborn-Kjennerud, T. *et al.* The relationship between avoidant personality disorder and social phobia: a population-based twin study. *Am. J. Psychiatry* **164**, 1722-1728 (2007).

1324. Reichle, E. D., Rayner, K. & Pollatsek, A. The EZ Reader model of eye-movement control in reading: Comparisons to other models. *Behavioral and Brain Sciences* **26**, 445-476 (2003).

1325. Reilly, C. Autism spectrum disorders in Down syndrome: a review. *Res. Autism Spectrum Dis* **3**, 829-839 (2009).

1326. Reiss, A. L. Childhood developmental disorders: an academic and clinical convergence point for psychiatry, neurology, psychology and pediatrics. *J. Child Psychol Psychiatry* **50**, 87-98 (2009).

1327. Reiss, H. E. Foetal asphyxia associated with umbilical cord around the neck. *Br. Med. J.* **5084**, 1394-1395 (1958).

1328. Reiss, S. Multifaceted nature of intrinsic motivation: The theory of 16 basic desires. *Rev. Gen. Psychol.* **8**, 179-193 (2004).

1329. Reitan, R. M. & Wolfson, D. A selective and critical review of neuropsychological deficits and the frontal lobes. *Neuropsychol. Rev.* **4**, 161-198 (1994).

1330. Remington, G. & Kapur, S. Antipsychotic Dosing: How Much but also How Often? *Schizophr. Bull.* **36**, 900-903 (2010).

1331. Repka, M. X. Pseudotumor Cerebri in Singer, H. S., Kossoff, E. H., Hartman, A. L. & Crawford, T. O. (eds.), *Treatment of Pediatric Neurologic Disorders.*pp. 237-242 (Taylor & Francis Group, Boca Raton,2005).

1332. Rescorla, L. Age 17 language and reading outcomes in late-talking toddlers: support for a dimensional perspective on language delay. *J Speech Lang Hear. Res* **52**, 16-30 (2009).

1333. Resnick, P. J. & Knoll, J. Faking it: How to detect malingered psychosis. *J. Family Practice* **4**, (2005).

1334. Reynell, J. Developmental patterns of visually handicapped children. *Child Care Health Dev.* **4**, 291-303 (1978).

1335. Ribai, P. *et al.* Psychiatric and cognitive difficulties as indicators of juvenile Huntington disease onset in 29 patients. *Arch. Neurol.* **64**, 813-819 (2007).

1336. Rice, M. L., Redmond, S. M. & Hoffman, L. Mean length of utterance in children with specific language impairment and in younger control children shows concurrent validity and stable and parallel growth trajectories. *J. Speech, Language, Hearing Research* **49**, 793-808 (2006).

1337. Rich, J. Types of stealing. *Lancet* **270**, 496-498 (1956).

1338. Richards, H. & Goodman, R. Are only children different? A study of child psychiatric referrals. A research note. *J. Child Psychol Psychiatry* **37**, 753-757 (1996).

1339. Richardson, A. J. & Montgomery, P. The Oxford-Durham study: a randomized, controlled trial of dietary supplementation with fatty acids in children with developmental coordination disorder. *Pediatrics* **115**, 1360-1366 (2005).

1139a. Neligan, G. & Prudham, D. Norms for four standard developmental milestones by sex, social class and place in family. Dev. Med. Child Neurol. 11, 413-422 (1969).

1340. Richardson, J. & Lelliott, P. Mental health of looked after children. *Adv. Psychiat. Treat.* **9**, 249-256 (2003).

1341. Richman, N. & Lansdown, R. *Problems of preschool children.* WileyBlackwell, Chichester (1988).

1342. Richman, N., Stevenson, J. E. & Graham, P. J. Prevalence of behaviour problems in 3-year-old children: an epidemiological study in a London borough. *J. Child Psychol. Psychiatry* **16**, 277-287 (1975).

1343. Richter, S. *et al.* Behavioral and affective changes in children and adolescents with chronic cerebellar lesions. *Neurosci. Lett.* **381**, 102-107 (2005).

1344. Ridley, R. M. The psychology of perserverative and stereotyped behaviour. *Prog. Neurobiol.* **44**, 221-231 (1994).

1345. Riela, A. R. & Roach, E. S. Etiology of stroke in children. *J Child Neurol* **8**, 201-220 (1993).

1346. Rietveld, S. & van Beest, I. Rollercoaster asthma: when positive emotional stress interferes with dyspnea perception. *Behav. Res. Ther.* **45**, 977-987 (2007).

1347. Rimbaux, S. *et al.* Adult onset ornithine transcarbamylase deficiency: an unusual cause of semantic disorders. *J. Neurol. Neurosurg. Psychiatry* **75**, 1073-1075 (2004).

1348. Risch, N. *et al.* Interaction between the serotonin transporter gene (5-HTTLPR), stressful life events, and risk of depression: a meta-analysis. *JAMA* **301**, 2462-2471 (2009).

1349. Rivinus, T. M., Jamison, D. L. & Graham, P. J. Childhood organic neurological disease presenting as psychiatric disorder. *Arch. Dis. Child* **50**, 115-119 (1975).

1350. Rizzo, M. & Barton, J. Central disorders of visual function in Miller, N. R. & Newman, N. J. (eds.), *Walsh & Hoyt's Clinical neuro-ophthalmology.*pp. 575-648 (Lippincott Williams & Wilkins, Philadelphia,2004).

1351. Robbins, T. W. Shifting and stopping: fronto-striatal substrates, neurochemical modulation and clinical implications. *Phil. Trans. Royal Society B: Biological Sciences* **362**, 917-932 (2007).

1352. Robbins, T. W. The 5-choice serial reaction time task: behavioural pharmacology and functional neurochemistry. *Psychopharmacology (Berl)* **163**, 362-380 (2002).

1353. Roberts, C. G. P. & Ladenson, P. W. Hypothyroidism. *Lancet* **363**, 793-803 (2004).
1354. Roberts, M. W. Enforcing chair timeouts with room timeouts. *Behav Modif.* **12**, 353-370 (1988).
1355. Robertson, C. Review of M.N.Wangila's "Female Circumcision". *NWSA Journal* **20**, 234-235 (2008).
1356. Robinson, B. E. Workaholic children in Chase, N. D. (ed.), *Burdened children*.pp. 56-74 (Sage Publications, Thousand Oaks, CA,2009).
1357. Robinson, T. E. & Berridge, K. C. The neural basis of drug craving: an incentive-sensitization theory of addiction. *Brain research reviews* **18**, 247-291 (1993).
1358. Robinson, T. E. & Berridge, K. C. The incentive sensitization theory of addiction: some current issues. *Phil. Trans. R. Soc. B* **363**, 3137-3146 (2008).
1359. Rodin, E. A. Psychomotor epilepsy and aggressive behavior. *Arch Gen. Psychiatry* **28**, 210-213 (1973).
1360. Rodkin, P. C., Farmer, T. W., Pearl, R. & Van Acker, R. They're cool: Social status and peer group supports for aggressive boys and girls. *Soc. Develop.* **15**, 175-204 (2006).
1361. Roediger, H. L., III Relativity of remembering: why the laws of memory vanished. *Annu. Rev. Psychol* **59**, 225-254 (2008).
1362. Rogers, C. R. Empathic: An unappreciated way of being. *The counseling psychologist* **5**, 2-10 (1975).
1363. Rogers, R. Detection strategies for malingering and defensiveness in Rogers, R. (ed.), *Clinical assessment of malingering and deception*. (Guilford Press, New York,2008).
1364. Rogers, S. J. & Ozonoff, S. Annotation: what do we know about sensory dysfunction in autism? A critical review of the empirical evidence. *J. Child Psychol Psychiatry* **46**, 1255-1268 (2005).
1365. Rogers, S. J., Ozonoff, S. & Maslin-Cole, C. A comparative study of attachment behavior in young children with autism or other psychiatric disorders. *J. Am. Acad. Child Adolesc. Psychiatry* **30**, 483-488 (1991).
1366. Rogers, S. J., Ozonoff, S. & Maslin-Cole, C. Developmental aspects of attachment behavior in young children with pervasive developmental disorders. *J. Am. Acad. Child Adolesc. Psychiatry* **32**, 1274-1282 (1993).
1367. Rokem, A. & Ahissar, M. Interactions of cognitive and auditory abilities in congenitally blind individuals. *Neuropsychologia* **47**, 843-848 (2009).
1368. Rollins, N., Lord, J. P., Walsh, E. & Weil, G. R. Some roles children play in their families: Scapegoat, baby, pet, and peacemaker. *J. Am. Acad. Child Adolesc. Psychiat.* **12**, 511-530 (1973).
1369. Rolls, E. T., Loh, M. & Deco, G. An attractor hypothesis of obsessive-compulsive disorder. *Eur. J. Neurosci.* **28**, 782-793 (2008).
1370. Rommel, N., De Meyer, A. M., Feenstra, L. & Veereman-Wauters, G. The complexity of feeding problems in 700 infants and young children presenting to a tertiary care institution. *J Pediatr. Gastroenterol. Nutr* **37**, 75-84 (2003).
1371. Ronald, A. *et al.* Genetic heterogeneity between the three components of the autism spectrum: a twin study. *J. Am. Acad. Child Adolesc. Psychiatry* **45**, 691-699 (2006).
1372. Roozendaal, B., Okuda, S., Van der Zee, E. A. & McGaugh, J. L. Glucocorticoid enhancement of memory requires arousal-induced noradrenergic activation in the basolateral amygdala. *Proc. Natl. Acad. Sci. U. S. A* **103**, 6741-6746 (2006).
1373. Ropper, A. H. & Brown, R. H. Disorders of smell and taste, *Adams & Victor's Principles of Neurology*.pp. 195-2022005).
1374. Rose, S. J. & Meezan, W. Variations in perceptions of child neglect. *Child Welfare* **75**, 139-160 (1996).
1375. Rosebush, P. I. & Mazurek, M. F. Catatonia and its treatment. *Schizophr. Bull.* **36**, 239-242 (2010).
1376. Rosenbaum, S., Abramson, S. & MacTaggart, P. Health information law in the context of minors. *Pediatrics* **123**, S116-S121 (2009).
1377. Rosenberg, L. B., Gibson, K. & Shulman, J. F. When cultures collide: Female genital cutting and US obstetric practice. *Obstet. Gynecol.* **113**, 931-934 (2009).
1378. Rosser, R. A., Ensing, S. S., Glider, P. J. & Lane, S. An information-processing analysis of children's accuracy in predicting the appearance of rotated stimuli. *Child Dev* **55**, 2204-2211 (1984).
1379. Rossor, M. Snouting, pouting and rooting. *Pract. Neurol.* **1**, 119-121 (2001).
1380. Rotenstein, O. H. *et al.* The validity of DSM-IV passive-aggressive (negativistic) personality disorder. *J. Personality Dis.* **21**, 28-41 (2007).
1381. Roth-Isigkeit, A., Thyen, U., Stoven, H., Schwarzenberger, J. & Schmucker, P. Pain among children and adolescents: restrictions in daily living and triggering factors. *Pediatrics* **115**, e152-e162 (2005).
1382. Rothner, A. D. & Dunn, D. Headaches in children and adolescents in Walker, A. M., Kaufman, D. M., Pfeffer, C. R. & Solomon, G. E. (eds.), *Child and Adolescent Neurology for.Psychiatrists*.pp. 151-170 (Lippincott Williams & Wilkins, Philadelphia,2008).
1383. Rotton, J. & Cohn, E. G. Outdoor temperature, climate control, and criminal assault. *Environ. Behavior* **36**, 276-306 (2004).
1384. Roubertoux, P. L. & Carlier, M. Neurogenetic Analysis and Cognitive Functions in Trisomy 21 in Kim, Y.-K. (ed.), *Handbook of Behavior Genetics*.pp. 175-185 (Springer, New York,2009).
1385. Rourke, B. P. *Syndrome of nonverbal learning disabilities*. The Guilford Press, New York (1995).
1386. Rouw, R. & Scholte, H. S. Increased structural connectivity in grapheme-color synesthesia. *Nat. Neurosci.* **10**, 792-797 (2007).
1387. Rowe, R., Maughan, B., Worthman, C. M., Costello, E. J. & Angold, A. Testosterone, antisocial behavior, and social dominance in boys: Pubertal development and biosocial interaction. *Biol. Psychiatry* **55**, 546-552 (2004).
1388. Roy, T. & Chatterjee, S. C. The experiences of adolescents with thalassemia in West Bengal, India. *Qual. Health Res.* **17**, 85-93 (2007).
1389. Royal Australasian College of Physicians *Australian Guidelines on ADHD*. RACP, (2009).
1390. Roze, E. *et al.* Neuropsychiatric disturbances in presumed late-onset cobalamin C disease. *Arch. Neurol.* **60**, 1457-1462 (2003).
1391. Rozen, T. D. Cluster headache: diagnosis and treatment. *Curr. Neurol Neurosci Rep.* **5**, 99-104 (2005).
1392. Rubin, G. J., Hahn, G., Everitt, B. S., Cleare, A. J. & Wessely, S. Are some people sensitive to mobile phone signals? Within participants double blind randomised provocation study. *Br. Med. J.* **332**, 886-891 (2006).
1393. Rubin, K. H., Fein, G. G. & Vandenberg, B. Playpp. 693-774 (John Wiley and Sons, New York,1983).
1394. Rumsey, J. M., Rapoport, J. L. & Sceery, W. R. Autistic children as adults: psychiatric, social, and behavioral outcomes. *J Am. Acad. Child Psychiatry* **24**, 465-473 (1985).
1395. Russell, A. J., Mataix-Cols, D., Anson, M. & Murphy, D. G. Obsessions and compulsions in Asperger syndrome and high-functioning autism. *Br. J Psychiatry* **186**, 525-528 (2005).
1396. Russell, P. S. Self-injurious behavior to the lower extremities among children with atypical development: a diagnostic and treatment algorithm. *Int. J. Low Extrem. Wounds.* **5**, 10-17 (2006).
1397. Rutter, M. Incidence of autism spectrum disorders: changes over time and their meaning. *Acta Paediatr.* **94**, 2-15 (2005).
1398. Rutter, M. The development of infantile autism. *Psychol Med* **4**, 147-163 (1974).
1399. Rutter, M. Clinical implications of attachment concepts: retrospect and prospect. *J. Child Psychol Psychiatry* **36**, 549-571 (1995).
1400. Rutter, M. *et al.* Early adolescent outcomes of institutionally deprived and non-deprived adoptees. III. Quasi-autism. *J. Child Psychol. Psychiatry* **48**, 1200-1207 (2007).

1401. Rutter, M. & O'Connor, T. G. Are there biological programming effects for psychological development? Findings from a study of Romanian adoptees. *Dev Psychol* **40**, 81-94 (2004).
1402. Rutter, M. & Quinton, D. Parental psychiatric disorder: Effects on children. *Psychol. Med.* **14**, 853-880 (1984).
1403. Rutter, M., Thapar, A. & Pickles, A. Gene-environment interactions: biologically valid pathway or artifact? *Arch Gen. Psychiatry* **66**, 1287-1289 (2009).
1404. Ruuhela, R., Hiltunen, L., Venalainen, A., Pirinen, P. & Partonen, T. Climate impact on suicide rates in Finland from 1971 to 2003. *Int. J. Biometeorol.* **53**, 167-175 (2009).
1405. Ryan, A. M., Pintrich, P. R. & Midgley, C. Avoiding seeking help in the classroom: Who and why? *Educ. Psychol. Rev.* **13**, 93-114 (2001).
1406. Ryan, G., Miyoshi, T. J., Metzner, J. L., Krugman, R. D. & Fryer, G. E. Trends in a national sample of sexually abusive youths. *J Am. Acad. Child Adolesc. Psychiatry* **35**, 17-25 (1996).
1407. Ryle, A. Projective identification: a particular form of reciprocal role procedure. *Br. J. Med. Psychol* **67**, 107-114 (1994).
1408. Sabin, T. D. An approach to chronic fatigue syndrome in adults. *Neurologist.* **9**, 28-34 (2003).
1409. Sachdev, P. S. Alternating and postictal psychoses: review and a unifying hypothesis. *Schizophr. Bull.* **33**, 1029-1037 (2007).
1410. Sacks, O. A walking Grove in Sacks, O. (ed.), *The man who mistook his wife for a hat.*pp. 178-184 (Pan Books, London,1986).
1411. Sacks, O. Hands in Sacks, O. (ed.), *The man who mistook his wife for a hat.*pp. 56-62 (Pan Books, London,1986).
1412. Sacks, O. Witty Ticcy Ray in Sacks, O. (ed.), *The man who mistook his wife for a hat.*pp. 87-96 (Pan Books, London,1986).
1413. Sacks, O. The man who mistook his wife for a hat in Sacks, O. (ed.), *The man who mistook his wife for a hat.*pp. 7-21 (Pan Books, London,1986).
1414. Sacks, O. Neurological dreams in Barrett, D. (ed.), *Trauma and dreams.*pp. 212-216 (Harvard University Press, Boston,2001).
1415. Sadleir, L. G. *et al.* Factors influencing clinical features of absence seizures. *Epilepsia* **49**, 2100-2107 (2008).
1416. Sadleir, L. G., Scheffer, I. E., Smith, S., Connolly, M. B. & Farrell, K. Automatisms in absence seizures in children with idiopathic generalized epilepsy. *Arch Neurol.* **66**, 729-734 (2009).
1417. Saint-Marc Girardin, M. F. *et al.* Computer-aided selection of diagnostic tests in jaundiced patients. *Gut* **26**, 961-967 (1985).
1418. Salekin, R. T., Kubak, F. A. & Lee, Z. Deception in children and adolescents in Rogers, R. (ed.), *Clinical assessment of malingering and deception.* (Guilford Press, New York,2008).
1419. Sallee, F. R., DeVane, C. L. & Ferrell, R. E. Fluoxetine-related death in a child with cytochrome P-450 2D6 genetic deficiency. *J. Child Adolesc. Psychopharmacol.* **10**, 27-34 (2000).
1420. Sallustro, F. & Atwell, C. W. Body rocking, head banging, and head rolling in normal children. *J Pediatr.* **93**, 704-708 (1978).
1421. Salmivalli, C., Lagerspetz, K., Bj¬rkqvist, K., Ísterman, K. & Kaukiainen, A. Bullying as a group process: Participant roles and their relations to social status within the group. *Aggress. Behav.* **22**, 1-15 (1996).
1422. Samaha, A. N., Seeman, P., Stewart, J., Rajabi, H. & Kapur, S. "Breakthrough" Dopamine Supersensitivity during Ongoing Antipsychotic Treatment Leads to Treatment Failure over Time. *J. Neurosci.* **27**, 2979-2986 (2007).
1423. Samuel, A. G. Organizational vs retrieval factors in the development of digit span. *J. Exp. Child Psychol.* **26**, 308-319 (1978).
1424. Sanberg, P. R., Bunsey, M. D., Giordano, M. & Norman, A. B. The catalepsy test: its ups and downs. *Behav Neurosci* **102**, 748-759 (1988).
1425. Sandson, J. & Albert, M. L. Varieties of perseveration. *Neuropsychologia* **22**, 715-732 (1984).
1426. Sanislow, C. A. & Carson, R. C. Schizophrenia: A critical examination in Adams, H. E. (ed.), *Comprehensive handbook of psychopathology.*pp. 403-441 (Springer, Berlin,2001).
1427. Sapolsky, R. M. *A Primate's Memoir.* Scribner, New York (2001).
1428. Sarason, I. G., Sarason, B. R., Keefe, D. E., Hayes, B. E. & Shearin, E. N. Cognitive interference: Situational determinants and traitlike characteristics. *J. Pers. Soc. Psychol.* **51**, 215-226 (1986).
1429. Savino, F. Focus on infantile colic. *Acta Paediatr.* **96**, 1259-1264 (2007).
1430. Savitz, D. A. & Pastore, L. M. Causes of prematurity in McCormick, M. C. & Siegel, J. E. (eds.), *Prenatal care: effectiveness and implementation.*pp. 63-104 (Cambridge Univ Press, Cambridge,1999).
1431. Sawyer, M. G. *et al.* *Mental health of young people in Australia.* Commonwealth Dept of Health and Aged Care, Canberra (2000).
1432. Schachter, S. & Singer, J. E. Cognitive, social and physiological determinants of emotional state. *Psychol. Rev.* **69**, 379-399 (1962).
1433. Schaefer, G. B. Genetics considerations in cerebral palsy. *Semin. Pediatr. Neurol.* **15**, 21-26 (2008).
1434. Schattmann, L. & Sherwin, B. B. Effects of the pharmacologic manipulation of testosterone on cognitive functioning in women with polycystic ovary syndrome: a randomized, placebo-controlled treatment study. *Horm. Behav* **51**, 579-586 (2007).
1435. Schempf, A. H. Illicit drug use and neonatal outcomes: a critical review. *Obstet. Gynecol. Survey* **62**, 749-757 (2007).
1436. Schepis, C., Failla, P., Siragusa, M. & Romano, C. Skin-picking: the best cutaneous feature in the recognition of Prader-Willi syndrome. *Int. J. Dermatol.* **33**, 866-867 (1994).
1437. Schmahmann, J. D., Weilburg, J. B. & Sherman, J. C. The neuropsychiatry of the cerebellum: Insights from the clinic. *Cerebellum* **6**, 254-267 (2007).
1438. Schneider, W., Klauer, T. & Freyberger, H. J. Operationalized psychodynamic diagnosis in planning and evaluating the psychotherapeutic process. *Eur. Arch. Psychiatry Clin. Neurosci.* **258**, 86-91 (2008).
1439. Schoentjes, E., Deboutte, D. & Friedrich, W. Child sexual behavior inventory: A Dutch-speaking normative sample. *Pediatrics* **104**, 885-893 (1999).
1440. Schott, G. D. Exploring the visual hallucinations of migraine aura: the tacit contribution of illustration. *Brain* **130**, 1690-1703 (2007).
1441. Schott, J. M. & Rossor, M. N. The grasp and other primitive reflexes. *J. Neurol. Neurosurg. Psychiatry* **74**, 558-560 (2003).
1442. Schrag, A., Quinn, N. P., Bhatia, K. P. & Marsden, C. D. Benign hereditary chorea-entity or syndrome? *Mov. Disord.* **15**, 280-288 (2000).
1443. Schreck, K. A., Williams, K. & Smith, A. F. A comparison of eating behaviors between children with and without autism. *J Autism Dev Disord.* **34**, 433-438 (2004).
1444. Schreier, H. A. Hallucinations in nonpsychotic children: more common than we think? *J. Am. Acad. Child Adolesc. Psychiatry* **38**, 623-625 (1999).
1445. Schultz, P. W. & Searleman, A. Rigidity of thought and behavior: 100 years of research. *Genet Soc. Gen. Psychol Monogr* **128**, 165-207 (2002).
1446. Scott, S. Integrating attachment theory with other approaches to developmental psychopathology. *Attach. Hum. Dev.* **5**, 307-312 (2003).
1447. Scott, S. & Dadds, M. R. Practitioner review: When parent training doesn't work: theory-driven clinical strategies. *J Child Psychol Psychiatry* **50**, 1441-1450 (2009).

1448. Sedel, F., Baumann, N., Lyon-Caen, O., Saudubray, J. M. & Cohen, D. Psychiatric manifestations revealing inborn errors of metabolism in adolescents and adults. *J Inherit. Metab Dis* 1-11 (2007).

1449. Seligman, L. D. & Ollendick, T. H. Comorbidity of anxiety and depression in children and adolescents: An integrative review. *Clin. Child Family Psychol. Rev.* **1**, 125-144 (1998).

1450. Sell, A., Tooby, J. & Cosmides, L. Formidability and the logic of human anger. *PNAS* **106**, 15073-15078 (2009).

1451. Sellers, J. G., Mehl, M. R. & Josephs, R. A. Hormones and personality: Testosterone as a marker of individual differences. *J. Res. Personality* **41**, 126-138 (2007).

1452. Semrud-Clikeman, M. & Glass, K. Comprehension of humor in children with nonverbal learning disabilities, reading disabilities, and without learning disabilities. *Ann. Dyslexia* **58**, 163-180 (2008).

1453. Sent, D. & Van der Gaag, L. C. Automated test selection in decision-support systems: a case study in oncology. *Stud. Health Technol. Inform.* **124**, 491-496 (2006).

1454. Serra, L., Montagna, P., Mignot, E., Lugaresi, E. & Plazzi, G. Cataplexy features in childhood narcolepsy. *Mov Disord.* **23**, 858-865 (2008).

1455. Serrano, M. *et al.* Neuropsychiatric Manifestations in Late-Onset Urea Cycle Disorder Patients. *J. Child Neurol.* **25**, 352-358 (2010).

1456. Sevecke, K., Pukrop, R., Kosson, D. S. & Krischer, M. K. Factor structure of the Hare Psychopathy Checklist: Youth version in German female and male detainees and community adolescents. *Psychol. Assess.* **21**, 45-56 (2009).

1457. Seyfarth, R. M., Cheney, D. L. & Bergman, T. J. Primate social cognition and the origins of language. *Trends Cogn Sci.* **9**, 264-266 (2005).

1458. Shadley, M. L. Critical incidents: Life events for experienced family therapists. *Contemp. Fam. Therapy* **12**, 253-262 (1990).

1459. Shanks, G. D., Hay, S. I. & Bradley, D. J. Malaria's indirect contribution to all-cause mortality in the Andaman Islands during the colonial era. *Lancet Infect. Dis* **8**, 564-570 (2008).

1460. Shannon, M. Ingestion of toxic substances by children. *N. Engl. J. Med.* **342**, 186-191 (2000).

1461. Shapiro, E. G., Lockman, L. A., Balthazor, M. & Krivit, W. Neuropsychological outcomes of several storage diseases with and without bone marrow transplantation. *J. Inherit. Metab. Dis.* **18**, 413-429 (1995).

1462. Shapiro, S. M. Definition of the clinical spectrum of kernicterus and bilirubin-induced neurologic dysfunction (BIND). *J. Perinatol.* **25**, 54-59 (2005).

1463. Sharpe, M. *et al.* Neurology out-patients with symptoms unexplained by disease: illness beliefs and financial benefits predict 1-year outcome. *Psychol Med.* 1-10 (2009).

1464. Shawyer, F. *et al.* Acting on harmful command hallucinations in psychotic disorders: An integrative approach. *J. Nerv. Ment. Dis.* **196**, 390-398 (2008).

1465. Shayer, M. & Adey, P. *Towards a science of science teaching.* Heinemann Educational Books, London (1981).

1466. Sheehan, W. & Thurber, S. Review of two years of experiences with SPECT among psychiatric patients in a rural hospital setting. *J Psychiatr. Pract.* **14**, 318-323 (2008).

1467. Shekhar, A. *et al.* Selective muscarinic receptor agonist xanomeline as a novel treatment approach for schizophrenia. *Am. J Psychiatry* **165**, 1033-1039 (2008).

1468. Sheldrake, R. The sense of being stared at. Part 1: Is it real or illusory? *J. Consciousness Studies* **12**, 10-31 (2005).

1469. Sheldrick, C. The assessment and management of risk in adolescents. *J. Child Psychol Psychiatry* **40**, 507-518 (1999).

1470. Shepherd, J. Activities of daily living and adaptation for independent living in Case-Smith, J. (ed.), *Occupational Therapy for Children.* (Elsevier-Mosby, St Louis,MO,2005).

1471. Sherif, M. A study of some social factors in perception. *Arch. Psychol.* **187**, 1-60 (1935).

1472. Shermer, M. *Why people believe weird things.* W.H.Freeman, New York (1998).

1473. Shevtsov, V. A. *et al.* A randomized trial of two different doses of a SHR-5 Rhodiola rosea extract versus placebo and control of capacity for mental work. *Phytomedicine* **10**, 95-105 (2003).

1474. Shinn, L. K. & O'Brien, M. Parent-child conversational styles in middle childhood: gender and social class differences. *Sex Roles* **59**, 61-67 (2008).

1475. Ship, J. A. & Chavez, E. M. Special senses: Disorders of taste and smell in Silverman, S., Eversole, L. R. & Truelove, E. L. (eds.), *Essentials of oral medicine.*pp. 277-288 (BC Decker Inc, Hamilton, Ontario,2002).

1476. Shirtcliff, E. A., Dahl, R. E. & Pollak, S. D. Pubertal development: Correspondence between hormonal and physical development. *Child Dev.* **80**, 327-337 (2009).

1477. Siebelink, B. M., Bakker, D. J., Binnie, C. D. & Kasteleijn-Nolst Trenite, D. G. Psychological effects of subclinical epileptiform EEG discharges in children. II. General intelligence tests. *Epilepsy Res.* **2**, 117-121 (1988).

1478. Siegel, D. H. Cutaneous mosaicism: a molecular and clinical review. *Adv. Dermatol.* **24**, 223-244 (2008).

1479. Siegel, J. M. Narcolepsy: a key role for hypocretins (orexins). *Cell* **98**, 409-412 (1999).

1480. Siegel, K. & Schrimshaw, E. W. Reasons and justifications for considering pregnancy among women living with HIV/AIDS. *Psychol. Women Q* **25**, 112-123 (2001).

1481. Simner, J. *et al.* Synaesthesia: The prevalence of atypical cross-modal experiences. *Perception* **35**, 1024-1033 (2006).

1482. Simon, H. B. Hyperthermia. *New Engl. J. Med.* **329**, 483-487 (1993).

1483. Simon, T. J. Cognitive characteristics of children with genetic syndromes. *Child Adolesc. Psychiatr. Clin N. Am.* **16**, 599-616 (2007).

1484. Simonoff, E. *et al.* The Croydon Assessment of Learning Study: prevalence and educational identification of mild mental retardation. *J Child Psychol Psychiatry* **47**, 828-839 (2006).

1485. Simonoff, E., Pickles, A., Wood, N., Gringras, P. & Chadwick, O. ADHD symptoms in children with mild intellectual disability. *J Am. Acad. Child Adolesc. Psychiatry* **46**, 591-600 (2007).

1486. Simpson, G. M., Lee, J. H., Zoubok, B. & Gardos, G. A rating scale for tardive dyskinesia. *Psychopharmacology (Berl)* **64**, 171-179 (1979).

1487. Sims, A. *Symptoms in the mind.* Elsevier, Philadelphia (2003).

1488. Sjolund, M. & Schaefer, C. E. The Erica method of sand play diagnosis and assessment in O'Connor, K. J. & Schaefer, C. E. (eds.), *Handbook of Play Therapy.*pp. 231-252 (Wiley, New York,1994).

1489. Skovbjerg, S., Zachariae, R., Rasmussen, A., Johansen, J. D. & Elberling, J. Attention to bodily sensations and symptom perception in individuals with idiopathic environmental intolerance. *Environ. Health Prevent. Med.* **15**, 141-150 (2010).

1490. Skuse, D. Epidemiological and definitional issues in failure to thrive. *Child Adolesc. Psychiatr. Clin. N. Am.* **2**, 37-59 (1993).

1491. Skuse, D. *et al.* Risk factors for development of sexually abusive behaviour in sexually victimised adolescent boys: cross sectional study. *Br. Med. J.* **317**, 175-179 (1998).

1492. Slater, M. *et al.* A virtual reprise of the Stanley Milgram obedience experiments. *PLoS ONE.* **1**, e39 (2006).

1493. Slee, P. T. & Rigby, K. Australian school children's self appraisal of interpersonal relations: the bullying experience. *Child Psychiat. Hum. Dev.* **23**, 273-282 (1993).

1494. Slee, P. T. & Rigby, K. The relationship of Eysenck's personality factors and self-esteem to bully-victim behaviour in Australian schoolboys. *Personality Individual Differences* **14**, 371-373 (1993).

1495. Slocombe, K. E., Townsend, S. W. & Zuberbuhler, K. Wild chimpanzees (Pan troglodytes schweinfurthii) distinguish between different scream types: evidence from a playback study. *Anim Cogn* **12**, 441-449 (2009).

1496. Slocombe, K. E. & Zuberbuhler, K. Agonistic screams in wild chimpanzees (Pan troglodytes schweinfurthii) vary as a function of social role. *J. Comp. Psychol.* **119**, 67 (2005).

1497. Smith, A. H. & Steinmaus, C. M. Health effects of arsenic and chromium in drinking water: recent human findings. *Annu. Rev. Public Health* **30**, 107-122 (2009).

1498. Smith, C., Denton, M. L., Faris, R. & Regnerus, M. Mapping American adolescent religious participation. *J. Sci. Study Religion* **41**, 597-612 (2002).

1499. Smith, C. I. E., Ochs, H. D. & Puck, J. M. Genetically determined immunodeficiency diseases: a perspective in Ochs, H. D., Smith, C. I. E. & Puck, J. M. (eds.), *Primary immunodeficiency diseases: A molecular and genetic approach. Second Edition.* pp. 3-15 (Oxford University Press, New York,2007).

1500. Smith, D. J. *A Culture of corruption: Everyday deception and popular discontent in Nigeria.* Princeton Univ Press, (2006).

1501. Smith, M. J., Breitbart, W. S. & Platt, M. M. A critique of instruments and methods to detect, diagnose, and rate delirium. *J. Pain Symptom. Manage.* **10**, 35-77 (1995).

1502. Smith, M. L. Atypical psychosis. *Psychiatr. Clin North Am.* **21**, 895-904 (1998).

1503. Smith, S. D. Genes, language development, and language disorders. *Mental Ret. Devel. Disab. Res. Rev* **13**, 96-105 (2007).

1504. Snowling, M. J. Specific disorders and broader phenotypes: the case of dyslexia. *Q. J Exp Psychol (Colchester.)* **61**, 142-156 (2008).

1505. Snyder, S. H. & Ferris, C. D. Novel neurotransmitters and their neuropsychiatric relevance. *Am. J Psychiatry* **157**, 1738-1751 (2000).

1506. Snyder, S. M. & Hall, J. R. A meta-analysis of quantitative EEG power associated with attention-deficit hyperactivity disorder. *J. Clin. Neurophysiol.* **23**, 441-456 (2006).

1507. Soares, J. B. & Leite-Moreira, A. F. Ghrelin, des-acyl ghrelin and obestatin: three pieces of the same puzzle. *Peptides* **29**, 1255-1270 (2008).

1508. Soderlund, G., Sikstrom, S. & Smart, A. Listen to the noise: noise is beneficial for cognitive performance in ADHD. *J. Child Psychol. Psychiatry* **48**, 840-847 (2007).

1509. Soderstrom, H., Nilsson, T., Sjodin, A. K., Carlstedt, A. & Forsman, A. The childhood-onset neuropsychiatric background to adulthood psychopathic traits and personality disorders. *Compr. Psychiatry* **46**, 111-116 (2005).

1510. Sokol, R. I., Webster, K. L., Thompson, N. S. & Stevens, D. A. Whining as mother-directed speech. *Infant Child Devel* **14**, 478-490 (2005).

1511. Solnick, J. V., Rincover, A. & Peterson, C. R. Some determinants of the reinforcing and punishing effects of timeout. *J Appl. Behav Anal.* **10**, 415-424 (1977).

1512. Solomon, B. D. *et al.* Analysis of genotype-phenotype correlations in human holoprosencephaly. *Am. J. Med. Genet. C: Sem. Med. Genet.* **154**, 133-141 (2010).

1513. Solomon, S. *et al.* Impairment of memory function by antihypertensive medication. *Arch Gen. Psychiatry* **40**, 1109-1112 (1983).

1514. Soni, S. *et al.* The phenomenology and diagnosis of psychiatric illness in people with Prader-Willi syndrome. *Psychol Med.* **38**, 1505-1514 (2008).

1515. Sontag, S. *Notes on "Camp".* (1964).

1516. Sonuga-Barke, E. J. S. *et al.* Does parental expressed emotion moderate genetic effects in ADHD? An exploration using a genome wide association scan. *Am. J. Med. Genet. B: Neuropsychiat. Genet.* **147**, 1359-1368 (2008).

1517. Sorensen, T. L., Mortzos, P. & Ogard, C. Social impairment due to extreme photophobia. *Acta Paediatr.* **98**, 1707-1708 and 1856 (2009).

1518. Sorrells, S. F., Caso, J. R., Munhoz, C. D. & Sapolsky, R. M. The stressed CNS: When glucocorticoids aggravate inflammation. *Neuron* **64**, 33-39 (2009).

1519. Sotres-Bayon, F., Bush, D. E. & LeDoux, J. E. Emotional perseveration: an update on prefrontal-amygdala interactions in fear extinction. *Learn. Mem.* **11**, 525-535 (2004).

1520. Souter, A. & Kraemer, S. "Given up hope of dying": A child protection approach to deliberate self harm in adolescents admitted to a paediatric ward. *Child & Family Social Work* **9**, 259-264 (2004).

1521. Spacks, P. M. *Boredom.* University of Chicago Press, Chicago (1995).

1522. Sparrow, S. S., Balla, D. A. & Cicchetti, D. V. *Vineland Adaptive Behavior Scales.* American Guidance Service, Circle Pines, Minnesota (1984).

1523. Spence, S. H., Rapee, R., McDonald, C. & Ingram, M. The structure of anxiety symptoms among preschoolers. *Behav Res Ther.* **39**, 1293-1316 (2001).

1524. Spence, S. J. & Schneider, M. T. The role of epilepsy and epileptiform EEGs in autism spectrum disorders. *Pediatr. Res* **65**, 599-606 (2009).

1525. Spencer, D. A. Consultants in mental handicap and adults with severe learning difficulty/multiple handicaps. *Psychiat. Bull.* **14**, 241 (1990).

1526. Spicknall, K. E., Zirwas, M. J. & English III, J. C. Clubbing: an update on diagnosis, differential diagnosis, pathophysiology, and clinical relevance. *J. Am. Acad. Dermatol.* **52**, 1020-1028 (2005).

1527. Squier, R. W. A model of empathic understanding and adherence to treatment regimens in practitioner-patient relationships. *Soc. Sci. Med.* **30**, 325-339 (1990).

1528. Squire, L. R. & Wixted, J. T. The cognitive neuroscience of human memory since H.M. *Annu. Rev Neurosci* **34**, 259-288 (2011).

1529. Srivastava, A. & Grube, M. Does intuition have a role in psychiatric diagnosis? *Psychiatr. Q.* **80**, 99-106 (2009).

1530. Staddon, J. E. R. A note on the evolutionary significance of" supernormal" stimuli. *Am. Naturalist* **109**, 541-545 (1975).

1531. Stadtler, A. C., Gorski, P. A. & Brazelton, T. B. Toilet training methods, clinical interventions, and recommendations. *Pediatrics* **103**, 1359-1361 (1999).

1532. Stagoll, B. Gregory Bateson (1904-1980): a reappraisal. *Aust. N. Z. J. Psychiatry* **39**, 1036-1045 (2005).

1533. Stander, S. *et al.* Clinical classification of itch: a position paper of the International Forum for the Study of Itch. *Acta Derm Venereol* **87**, 291-294 (2007).

1534. Stankiewicz, P. & Lupski, J. R. Structural variation in the human genome and its role in disease. *Ann. Rev. Med.* **61**, 437-455 (2010).

1535. Stauffer, W. & Fischer, P. R. Diagnosis and treatment of malaria in children. *Clin Infect. Dis* **37**, 1340-1348 (2003).

1536. Stayer, C. *et al.* Looking for childhood schizophrenia: case series of false positives. *J. Am. Acad. Child Adolesc. Psychiatry* **43**, 1026-1029 (2004).

1537. Stearns, D. M. Multiple hypotheses for chromium (III) biochemistry: Why the essentiality of chromium (III) is still questioned, *The nutritional biochemistry of chromium (III).* pp. 57-70 (Elsevier Science Ltd,2007).

1538. Stefanatos, G. A. Regression in autistic spectrum disorders. *Neuropsychol. Rev.* **18**, 305-319 (2008).

1539. Stefanatos, G. A., Kinsbourne, M. & Wasserstein, J. Acquired epileptiform aphasia: a dimensional view of Landau-Kleffner syndrome and the relation to regressive autistic spectrum disorders. *Child Neuropsychol.* **8**, 195-228 (2002).

1540. Steil, R. & Ehlers, A. Dysfunctional meaning of posttraumatic intrusions in chronic PTSD. *Behav Res Ther.* **38**, 537-558 (2000).

1541. Stein, M. A. *et al.* Dopamine transporter genotype and methylphenidate dose response in children with ADHD. *Neuropsychopharmacology* **30**, 1374-1382 (2005).

1542. Stein, M. T. *et al.* Self-injury and mental retardation in a 7-year-old boy. *J. Dev. Behav. Pediatr.* **26**, 241-245 (2005).

1543. Stephens, R., Atkins, J. & Kingston, A. Swearing as a response to pain. *Neuroreport* **20**, 1056-1060 (2009).

1544. Stevens, D. L., Lee, M. R. & Padua, Y. Olanzapine-associated neuroleptic malignant syndrome in a patient receiving concomitant rivastigmine therapy. *Pharmacotherapy* **28**, 403-405 (2008).

1545. Stevenson, J., McCann, D., Watkin, P., Worsfold, S. & Kennedy, C. The relationship between language development and behaviour problems in children with hearing loss. *J Child Psychol Psychiatry* **51**, 77-83 (2010).

1546. Stokes, S. J., Saylor, C. F., Swenson, C. C. & Daugherty, T. K. A comparison of children's behaviors following three types of stressors. *Child Psychiatry Hum. Dev.* **26**, 113-123 (1995).

1547. Stolman, L. P. In hyperhidrosis (excess sweating), look for a pattern and cause. *Cleve. Clin. J. Med.* **70**, 896-898 (2003).

1548. Stolorow, R. D., Orange, D. M. & Atwood, G. E. Projective identification begone! Commentary on paper by Susan H. Sands. *Psychoanalytic Dialogues* **8**, 719-725 (1998).

1549. Stone, J. *et al.* What should we call pseudoseizures? The patient's perspective. *Seizure.* **12**, 568-572 (2003).

1550. Storch, E. A. *et al.* Compulsive hoarding in children. *J. Clin. Psychol: In session* **67**, 507-516 (2011).

1551. Stores, G. Practitioner review: Recognition of pseudoseizures in children and adolescents. *J. Child Psychol Psychiatry* **40**, 851-857 (1999).

1552. Storr, A. *Freud.* Oxford University Press, Oxford (1989).

1553. Stout, A. U. & Borchert, M. Etiology of eyelid retraction in children: a retrospective study. *J. Pediatr. Ophthalmol. Strabismus* **30**, 96-99 (1993).

1554. Strahm, B. & Malkin, D. Hereditary cancer predisposition in children: genetic basis and clinical implications. *Int. J. Cancer* **119**, 2001-2006 (2006).

1555. Strakowski, S. M. & Sax, K. W. Secondary mania in Soares, J. C. & Gershon, S. (eds.), *Bipolar disorders: Basic mechanisms and therapeutic implications.*pp. 13-30 (Marcel Decker, Inc., New York,2000).

1556. Stravynski, A. Behavioral treatment of psychogenic vomiting in the context of social phobia. *J Nerv Ment Dis* **171**, 448-451 (1983).

1557. Strick, P. L., Dum, R. P. & Fiez, J. A. Cerebellum and nonmotor function. *Annu. Rev. Neurosci* **32**, 413-434 (2009).

1558. Stringaris, A. & Goodman, R. Longitudinal outcome of youth oppositionality: irritable, headstrong, and hurtful behaviors have distinctive predictions. *J. Am. Acad. Child Adolesc. Psychiatry* **48**, 404-412 (2009).

1559. Strohle, A. Physical activity, exercise, depression and anxiety disorders. *J. Neural Transm.* **116**, 777-784 (2009).

1560. Sturmey, P. *Functional analysis in clinical treatment.* Academic Press, London (2007).

1561. Sturzenegger, C. & Bassetti, C. L. The clinical spectrum of narcolepsy with cataplexy: a reappraisal. *J Sleep Res* **13**, 395-406 (2004).

1562. Styne, D. M. Disorders of puberty in Molitch, M. E. (ed.), *Challenging cases in endocrinology.*pp. 349-374 (Humana Press, Totowa,NJ,2002).

1563. Sullivan, P. F., Neale, M. C. & Kendler, K. S. Genetic epidemiology of major depression: review and meta-analysis. *Am. J. Psychiatry* **157**, 1552-1562 (2000).

1564. Sulloway, F. J. Birth order and sibling competition in Dunbar, R. & Barrett, L. (eds.), *Handbook of evolutionary psychology.*pp. 297-311 (Oxford University Press, Oxford,2007).

1565. Sulloway, F. J. & coles, R. *Born to rebel: Birth order, family dynamics, and creative lives.* Pantheon Books, New York (1996).

1566. Sumer, M. M., Atik, L., Unal, A., Emre, U. & Atasoy, H. T. Frontal lobe epilepsy presented as ictal aggression. *Neurol. Sci.* **28**, 48-51 (2007).

1567. Sun, S. S. *et al.* National estimates of the timing of sexual maturation and racial differences among US children. *Pediatrics* **110**, 911-919 (2002).

1568. Superti-Furga, A. & Unger, S. Nosology and classification of genetic skeletal disorders: 2006 revision. *Am J Med Genet A* **143**, 1-18 (2007).

1569. Suresh, P. A., Sebastian, S., George, A. & Radhakrishnan, K. Subclinical hyperthyroidism and hyperkinetic behavior in children. *Pediatr. Neurol.* **20**, 192-194 (1999).

1570. Surtees, R., Mills, P. & Clayton, P. Inborn errors affecting vitamin B6 metabolism. *Future Neurol.* **1**, 615-620 (2006).

1571. Susman, E. J. *et al.* Longitudinal development of secondary sexual characteristics in girls and boys between ages 91/2 and 151/2 years. *Arch Pediatr. Adolesc. Med* **164**, 166-173 (2010).

1572. Sussman, S. Teen sexual addiction in Essau, C. A. (ed.), *Adolescent Addiction.*pp. 269-296 (Academic Press, London,2008).

1573. Suzuki, K. *et al.* Neuronal and glial accumulation of -and -synucleins in human lipidoses. *Acta Neuropathol. (Berl).* **114**, 481-489 (2007).

1574. Swedo, S. & Rapoport, J. L. Phenomenology and differential diagnosis of obsessive-compulsive disorder in children and adolescents in Rapoport, J. L. (ed.), *Obsessive-compulsive disorder in children and adolescents.*pp. 13-32 (American Psychiatric Press, Washington,D.C.,1989).

1575. Swedo, S. E. *et al.* Pediatric autoimmune neuropsychiatric disorders associated with streptococcal infections: clinical description of the first 50 cases. *Am. J. Psychiatry* **155**, 264-271 (1998).

1576. Symons, F. J. *et al.* Evidence of altered epidermal nerve fiber morphology in adults with self-injurious behavior and neurodevelopmental disorders. *Pain* **134**, 232-237 (2008).

1577. Szasz, T. S. Power and Psychiatry in Henslin, J. M. (ed.), *Deviance in American Life.*pp. 53-60 (Rutgers State University, Piscataway, NJ,1989).

1578. Szatmari, P. & Taylor, D. C. Overflow movements and behavior problems: scoring and using a modification of Fogs' test. *Dev. Med. Child Neurol.* **26**, 297-310 (1984).

1579. Taber, K. H., Hurley, R. A. & Yudofsky, S. C. Diagnosis and treatment of neuropsychiatric disorders. *Annu. Rev. Med* **61**, 121-133 (2010).

1580. Tager-Flusberg, H. Evaluating the theory of mind hypothesis of autism. *Curr. Direc. Psychol Sci.* **16**, 311-315 (2007).

1581. Takeuchi, T. *et al.* Primary obsessional slowness: long-term findings. *Behav. Res. Ther.* **35**, 445-449 (1997).

1582. Talley, J. L. Memory in learning disabled children: Digit span and the Rey Auditory Verbal Learning Test. *Arch. Clin. Neuropsychol.* **1**, 315-322 (1986).

1583. Tambs, K. *et al.* Structure of genetic and environmental risk factors for dimensional representations of DSM-IV anxiety disorders. *Br. J. Psychiatry* **195**, 301-307 (2009).

1584. Tannen, D. Toward a theory of conversational style: the machine-gun question. Sociolinguistic Working Paper Number 73. 1980. Austin, Texas, SW Educational Development Laboratory. Ref Type: Report

1585. Tannock, R., Schachar, R. & Logan, G. Methylphenidate and cognitive flexibility: dissociated dose effects in hyperactive children. *J. Abnorm. Child Psychol.* **23**, 235-266 (1995).

1586.   Taylor, D. C., Powell, R. P., Cherland, E. E. & Vaughan, C. M. Overflow movements and cognitive, motor and behavioural disturbance: a normative study of girls. *Dev Med Child Neurol* **30**, 759-768 (1988).
1587.   Taylor, E. Dysfunctions of attention in Cicchetti, D. & Cohen, D. (eds.), *Developmental psychopathology Volume 2. Risk, disorder, and adaptation*.pp. 243-273 (Wiley, New York,1995).
1588.   Taylor, E. & Rogers, J. W. Practitioner review: early adversity and developmental disorders. *J. Child Psychol. Psychiatry* **46**, 451-467 (2005).
1589.   Taylor, E. *et al.* Which boys respond to stimulant medication? A controlled trial of methylphenidate in boys with disruptive behaviour. *Psychol. Med.* **17**, 121-143 (1987).
1590.   Taylor, J., Spencer, N. & Baldwin, N. Social, economic, and political context of parenting. *Arch Dis Child* **82**, 113-120 (2000).
1591.   Taylor, J. C. & Carr, E. G. Severe problem behaviors related to social interaction. 2: A systems analysis. *Behav. Modif.* **16**, 336-371 (1992).
1592.   Taylor, M. A. & Fink, M. Restoring melancholia in the classification of mood disorders. *J. Affect. Disord.* **105**, 1-14 (2008).
1593.   Teasdale, G. & Jennett, B. Assessment of coma and impaired consciousness. A practical scale. *Lancet* **2**, 81-84 (1974).
1594.   Teasdale, T. W. & Owen, D. R. Secular declines in cognitive test scores: A reversal of the Flynn Effect. *Intelligence* **36**, 121-126 (2008).
1595.   Teese, R. *et al.* Early school leaving: A review of the literature. Australian National Training Authority, Brisbane (2000).
1596.   Temudo, T. *et al.* Stereotypies in Rett syndrome: analysis of 83 patients with and without detected MECP2 mutations. *Neurology* **68**, 1183-1187 (2007).
1597.   Tepper, B. J. Nutritional implications of genetic taste variation: the role of PROP sensitivity and other taste phenotypes. *Annu. Rev. Nutr* **28**, 367-388 (2008).
1598.   Terr, L. C. *et al.* When formulation outweighs diagnosis: 13 "moments" in psychotherapy. *J. Am. Acad. Child Adolesc. Psychiatry* **45**, 1252-1263 (2006).
1599.   Thaler, V. *et al.* Different behavioral and eye movement patterns of dyslexic readers with and without attentional deficits during single word reading. *Neuropsychologia* **47**, 2436-2445 (2009).
1600.   Thomaes, S., Bushman, B. J., Stegge, H. & Olthof, T. Trumping shame by blasts of noise: narcissism, self-esteem, shame, and aggression in young adolescents. *Child Dev.* **79**, 1792-1801 (2008).
1601.   Thomas, A. & Chess, S. *Temperament and development.* Brunner/Mazel, New York (1977).
1602.   Thomas, J. E., Rooke, E. D. & Kvale, W. F. The neurologist's experience with pheochromocytoma. A review of 100 cases. *JAMA* **197**, 754-758 (1966).
1603.   Thomas, K. B. General practice consultations: is there any point in being positive? *Br. Med J (Clin Res Ed)* **294**, 1200-1202 (1987).
1604.   Thompson, D. F. & Pierce, D. R. Drug-induced nightmares. *Ann. Pharmacother.* **33**, 93-98 (1999).
1605.   Thorburn, D. R. Mitochondrial disorders: prevalence, myths and advances. *J. Inherit. Metab. Dis.* **27**, 349-362 (2004).
1606.   Thrane, L. E. & X.Chen Impact of running away on girls' sexual onset. *J. Adolesc. Health* **46**, 32-36 (2010).
1607.   Thwaites, G. *et al.* British Infection Society guidelines for the diagnosis and treatment of tuberculosis of the central nervous system in adults and children. *J. Infect.* **59**, 167-187 (2009).
1608.   Tiedens, L. Z. Powerful emotions: The vicious cycle of social status positions and emotions in Ashkanasy, N. M., Hartel, C. E. J. & Zerbe, W. K. (eds.), *Emotions in the workplace: Research, theory, and practice*.pp. 72-81 (Quorum Books, Westport, CT,2000).
1609.   Tierney, E. P., Sage, R. J. & Shwayder, T. Kwashiorkor from a severe dietary restriction in an 8-month infant in suburban Detroit, Michigan: case report and review of the literature. *Int. J Dermatol.* **49**, 500-506 (2010).
1610.   Tiihonen, J. *et al.* Antidepressants and the risk of suicide, attempted suicide, and overall mortality in a nationwide cohort. *Arch Gen. Psychiatry* **63**, 1358-1367 (2006).
1611.   Tinbergen, N. Social releasers and the experimental method required for their study. *Wilson Bulletin* **60**, 6-51 (1948).
1612.   Tinbergen, N. & Perdeck, A. C. On the stimulus situation releasing the begging response in the newly hatched Herring Gull chick. *Behaviour* **3**, 1-39 (1950).
1613.   Tong, K. A. *et al.* Susceptibility-weighted MR imaging: a review of clinical applications in children. *Am J Neuroradiol.* **29**, 9-17 (2008).
1614.   Tordjman, S. *et al.* Pain reactivity and plasma beta-endorphin in children and adolescents with autistic disorder. *PLoS. One.* **4**, 1-10 (2009).
1615.   Torgersen, S., Kringlen, E. & Cramer, V. The prevalence of personality disorders in a community sample. *Arch. Gen. Psychiatry* **58**, 590-596 (2001).
1616.   Torkelson, R. D., Leibrock, L. G., Gustavson, J. L. & Sundell, R. R. Neurological and neuropsychological effects of cerebral spinal fluid shunting in children with assumed arrested ("normal pressure") hydrocephalus. *J. Neurol. Neurosurg. Psychiat.* **48**, 799-806 (1985).
1617.   Toufexis, M. & Gieron-Korthals, M. Early testing for Huntington Disease in children: pros and cons. *J. Child Neurol.* **25**, 482-484 (2010).
1618.   Traber, M. G., Frei, B. & Beckman, J. S. Vitamin E revisited: do new data validate benefits for chronic disease prevention? *Curr. Opin. Lipidol.* **19**, 30-38 (2008).
1619.   Trahair, J. F., DeBarro, T. M., Robinson, J. S. & Owens, J. A. Restriction of nutrition in utero selectively inhibits gastrointestinal growth in fetal sheep. *J. Nutr.* **127**, 637-641 (1997).
1620.   Tranel, D. The Iowa-Benton school of neuropsychological assessment in Grant, I. & Adams, K. M. (eds.), *Neuropsychological Assessment of Neuropsychiatric and Neuromedical Disorders*.pp. 66-83 (Oxford University Press, New York,2009).
1621.   Tremblay, R. E. The development of aggressive behaviour during childhood: What have we learned in the past century? *International Journal of Behavioral Development* **24**, 129-141 (2000).
1622.   Trimble, M., Kanner, A. & Schmitz, B. Postictal psychosis. *Epilepsy & Behavior* **19**, 159-161 (2010).
1623.   Tsao, D. Y. & Livingstone, M. S. Mechanisms of face perception. *Annu. Rev. Neurosci.* **31**, 411-437 (2008).
1624.   Tsoi, W. F. The Ganser syndrome in Singapore: a report on ten cases. *Br. J. Psychiatry* **123**, 567-572 (1973).
1625.   Tu, Y. R. *et al.* Epidemiological survey of primary palmar hyperhidrosis in adolescent in Fuzhou of People's Republic of China. *Eur. J. Cardiothorac. Surg.* **31**, 737-739 (2007).
1626.   Tucker, D. M., Luu, P. & Pribram, K. H. Social and emotional self-regulation. *Annals- New York Acad. Sciences* **769**, 213-239 (1995).
1627.   Tupes, E. C. & Christal, R. E. *Recurrent personality factors based on trait ratings.* US Air Force, Lackland Air Force Base, Texas (1961).
1628.   Turk, J. Behavioural phenotypes: their applicability to children and young people who have learning disabilities. *Advances in Mental Health and Learning Disabilities* **1**, 4-13 (2007).
1629.   Turki, I. *et al.* Polyneuropathy in 8 glue-sniffers. *Neuromuscul. Disord.* **7**, 456 (1997).
1630.   Turner Ellis, S. A., Miles, T. R. & Wheeler, T. J. Extraneous bodily movements and irrelevant vocalizations by dyslexic and non-dyslexic boys during calculation tasks. *Dyslexia.* **15**, 156-163 (2009).
1631.   Turner, M. Annotation: Repetitive behaviour in autism: a review of psychological research. *J. Child Psychol Psychiatry* **40**, 839-849 (1999).

1632.   Tyler, K. A. & Bersani, B. E. A longitudinal study of early adolescent precursors of running away. *J. Early Adolesc.* **28**, 230-251 (2008).

1633.   Tyrka, A. R. *et al.* Interaction of childhood maltreatment with the corticotropin-releasing hormone receptor gene: effects on hypothalamic-pituitary-adrenal axis reactivity. *Biol. Psychiatry* **66**, 681-685 (2009).

1634.   Ucar, S. K. *et al.* Clinical overview of children with mucopolysaccharidosis type III A and effect of Risperidone treatment on children and their mothers psychological status. *Brain Dev.* **32**, 156-161 (2010).

1635.   Ucles, P., Mendez, M. & Garay, J. Low-level defective processing of non-verbal sounds in dyslexic children. *Dyslexia.* **15**, 72-85 (2009).

1636.   Uher, R., Heyman, I., Turner, C. M. & Shafran, R. Self-, parent-report and interview measures of obsessive-compulsive disorder in children and adolescents. *J Anxiety Disord.* **22**, 979-990 (2008).

1637.   Ullrich, N. J. Neurologic sequelae of brain tumors in children. *J Child Neurol* **24**, 1446-1454 (2009).

1638.   Ungvari, G. S., Chiu, H. F., Chow, L. Y., Lau, B. S. & Tang, W. K. Lorazepam for chronic catatonia: a randomized, double-blind, placebo-controlled cross-over study. *Psychopharmacology (Berl)* **142**, 393-398 (1999).

1639.   Unnikrishnan, A. G. & Rajaratnam, S. A young man with seizures, abusive behaviour, and drowsiness. *Postgrad. Med. J* **77**, 54-59 (2001).

1640.   Uziel, Y. & Hashkes, P. J. Growing pains in children. *Pediatr. Rheumatol. Online J* **5**, 5-8 (2007).

1641.   Vahter, M. Health effects of early life exposure to arsenic. *Basic Clin. Pharmacol. Toxicol.* **102**, 204-211 (2008).

1642.   Vaidya, G., Chalhoub, N. & Newing, J. Stalking in adolescence: A case report. *Child Adolesc. Mental Health* **10**, 23-25 (2005).

1643.   Vaillant, G. E. *Ego mechanisms of defense: a guide for clinicans and researchers.* American Psychiatric Press Inc, Washington DC (1992).

1644.   Valentino, K., Cicchetti, D., Rogosch, F. A. & Toth, S. L. True and false recall and dissociation among maltreated children: The role of self-schema. *Dev. Psychopathol.* **20**, 213-232 (2008).

1645.   Valois, R. F., MacDonald, J. M., Bretous, L., Fischer, M. A. & Drane, J. W. Risk factors and behaviors associated with adolescent violence and aggression. *American Journal of Health Behaviour* **26**, 454-464 (2002).

1646.   Van Borsel, J. *et al.* Prevalence of stuttering in regular and special school populations in Belgium based on teacher perceptions. *Folia Phoniatrica et Logopaedica* **58**, 289-302 (2006).

1647.   Van Borsel, J. & Tetnowski, J. A. Fluency disorders in genetic syndromes. *J. Fluency Dis.* **32**, 279-296 (2007).

1648.   Van Cleve, S. N., Cannon, S. & Cohen, W. I. Part II: Clinical Practice Guidelines for adolescents and young adults with Down Syndrome: 12 to 21 Years. *J Pediatr. Health Care* **20**, 198-205 (2006).

1649.   van der Lely, H. K. J., Rosen, S. & McClelland, A. Evidence for a grammar-specific deficit in children. *Curr. Biol.* **8**, 1253-1258 (1998).

1650.   Van Egmond, J. J. Multiple meanings of secondary gain. *Am. J. Psychoanalysis* **63**, 137-147 (2003).

1651.   van Ewijk, R. *Discussion Paper No 926 Long-Term Health Effects on the Next Generation of Ramadan Fasting During Pregnancy.* Centre for Economic Performance, LSE, (2009).

1652.   van Gelder, M. M. H. J. *et al.* Maternal periconceptional illicit drug use and the risk of congenital malformations. *Epidemiology* **20**, 60-66 (2009).

1653.   Van Hove, J. L. *et al.* Expanded motor and psychiatric phenotype in autosomal dominant Segawa syndrome due to GTP cyclohydrolase deficiency. *J Neurol Neurosurg. Psychiatry* **77**, 18-23 (2006).

1654.   van Ijzendoorn, M. H. & Juffer, F. The Emanuel Miller Memorial Lecture 2006: adoption as intervention. Meta-analytic evidence for massive catch-up and plasticity in physical, socio-emotional, and cognitive development. *J. Child Psychol. Psychiatry* **47**, 1228-1245 (2006).

1655.   Van Koppen, M. V., De Poot, C. J., Kleemans, E. R. & Nieuwbeerta, P. Criminal trajectories in organized crime. *Br. J. Criminology* **50**, 102-123 (2010).

1656.   Van Lancker Sidtis, D., Pachana, N., Cummings, J. L. & Sidtis, J. J. Dysprosodic speech following basal ganglia insult: Toward a conceptual framework for the study of the cerebral representation of prosody. *Brain Lang.* **97**, 135-153 (2006).

1657.   van Loon, A. M., Koch, T. & Kralik, D. Care for female survivors of child sexual abuse in emergency departments. *Accid. Emerg. Nurs.* **12**, 208-214 (2004).

1658.   Van Oosterwijk, J. *et al.* Pain inhibition and postexertional malaise in myalgic encephalomyelitis/chronic fatigue syndrome: An experimental study. *J. Intern. Med.* **268**, 265-278 (2010).

1659.   Vanderver, A. Tools for diagnosis of leukodystrophies and other disorders presenting with white matter disease. *Curr. Neurol. Neurosci. Rep.* **5**, 110-118 (2005).

1660.   Vanheule, S. Challenges for alexithymia research. *J. Clin. Psychol.* **64**, 332-337 (2008).

1661.   VanMeter, L., Fein, D., Morris, R., Waterhouse, L. & Allen, D. Delay versus deviance in autistic social behavior. *J. Autism Dev. Disord.* **27**, 557-569 (1997).

1662.   VanRie, A., Mupuala, A. & Dow, A. Impact of the HIV/AIDS epidemic on the neurodevelopment of preschool-aged children in Kinshasa, Democratic Republic of the Congo. *Pediatrics* **122**, e123-e128 (2008).

1663.   VanTongerloo, A. & DePaepe A. Psychosocial adaptation in adolescents and young adults with Marfan syndrome: an exploratory study. *J. Med. Genet.* **35**, 405-409 (1998).

1664.   Vargha-Khadem, F., Gadian, D. G., Copp, A. & Mishkin, M. FOXP2 and the neuroanatomy of speech and language. *Nat Rev. Neurosci* **6**, 131-138 (2005).

1665.   Vargha-Khadem, F. *et al.* Differential effects of early hippocampal pathology on episodic and semantic memory. *Science* **277**, 376-380 (1997).

1666.   Veale, D. Body dysmorphic disorder. *Postgrad. Med. J.* **80**, 67-71 (2004).

1667.   Ventura, S. J., Abma, J. C., Mosher, W. D. & Henshaw, S. K. Estimated pregnancy rates by outcome for the United States, 1990-2004. *Natl. Vital Stat. Rep.* **56**, 1-25, 28 (2008).

1668.   Verhoef, M. *et al.* Secondary impairments in young adults with spina bifida. *Dev. Med. Child Neurol.* **46**, 420-427 (2004).

1669.   Verhoeven, E. W. *et al.* Biopsychosocial mechanisms of chronic itch in patients with skin diseases: a review. *Acta Derm. Venereol.* **88**, 211-218 (2008).

1670.   Verhoeven, W., Egger, J. & Tuinier, S. Thoughts on the behavioural phenotypes in Prader-Willi syndrome and velo-cardio-facial syndrome. *Acta Neuropsychiatrica* **19**, 244-250 (2007).

1671.   Verhoeven, W. M. & Tuinier, S. Prader-Willi syndrome: atypical psychoses and motor dysfunctions. *Int. Rev. Neurobiol.* **72**, 119-130 (2006).

1672.   Verhoeven, W. M. A., Egger, J. I. M., Gunning, W. B., Bevers, M. & de Pont, B. J. H. B. Recurrent schizophrenia-like psychosis as first manifestation of epilepsy: a diagnostic challenge in neuropsychiatry. *Neuropsychiatric Dis. Treat.* **6**, 227-231 (2010).

1673.   Vernes, S. C. *et al.* A functional genetic link between distinct developmental language disorders. *N. Engl. J. Med.* **359**, 2337-2345 (2008).

1674.   Vickerman, K. A. & Margolin, G. Rape treatment outcome research: empirical findings and state of the literature. *Clin. Psychol Rev.* **29**, 431-448 (2009).

1675.   Vider, S. Rethinking Crowd Violence: Self Categorization Theory and the Woodstock 1999 Riot. *Journal for the theory of social behaviour* **34**, 141-166 (2004).

1676.   Vidyasagar, T. R. & Pammer, K. Dyslexia: a deficit in visuo-spatial attention, not in phonological processing. *Trends Cog. Sci.* **14**, 57-63 (2010).

1677. Vieira, T. *et al.* Mucopolysaccharidoses in Brazil. *Am. J. Med. Genet. A* **146A**, 1741-1747 (2008).
1678. Visser, J. Developmental coordination disorder: a review of research on subtypes and comorbidities. *Hum. Mov Sci.* **22**, 479-493 (2003).
1679. Vitek, L. Is there really a link between hyperbilirubinemia and schizophrenia? *Prog. Neuropsychopharmacol. Biol. Psychiatry* **33**, 914-916 (2009).
1680. Vitiello, B. & Stoff, D. M. Subtypes of aggression and their relevance to child psychiatry. *J Am. Acad. Child Adolesc. Psychiatry* **36**, 307-315 (1997).
1681. Vitiello, B. & Stoff, D. M. Subtypes of aggression and their relevance to child psychiatry. *J. Am. Acad. Child Adolesc. Psychiatry* **36**, 307-315 (1997).
1682. Vodanovich, S. J., Wallace, J. C. & Kass, S. J. A confirmatory approach to the factor structure of the Boredom Proneness Scale: evidence for a two-factor short form. *J. Pers. Assess.* **85**, 295-303 (2005).
1683. Volden, J. Nonverbal learning disability: a tutorial for speech-language pathologists. *Am. J Speech Lang Pathol.* **13**, 128-141 (2004).
1684. Volkmar, F. R., State, M. & Klin, A. Autism and autistic spectrum disorders: diagnostic issues for the coming decade. *J. Child Psychol Psychiatry* **50**, 108-115 (2009).
1685. Volkow, N. D., Gatley, S. J., Fowler, J. S., Wang, G. J. & Swanson, J. Serotonin and the therapeutic effects of ritalin. *Science* **288**, 11 (2000).
1686. Volkow, N. D. *et al.* Dopamine transporter occupancies in the human brain induced by therapeutic doses of oral methylphenidate. *Am. J. Psychiatry* **155**, 1325-1331 (1998).
1687. Volkow, N. D. *et al.* Evidence that methylphenidate enhances the saliency of a mathematical task by increasing dopamine in the human brain. *Am. J. Psychiatry* **161**, 1173-1180 (2004).
1688. Volkow, N. D. *et al.* Evaluating dopamine reward pathway in ADHD: clinical implications. *JAMA* **302**, 1084-1091 (2009).
1689. Vollm, B., Jamieson, L. & Taylor, P. J. What's in a name? Reasons for changing names among English high security hospital patients. *J. Forensic Psychiat. Psychol.* **17**, 37-52 (2006).
1690. Vollmer, T. R., Sloman, K. N. & Borrero, C. S. W. Behavioral assessment of self-injury in Matson, J. L. (ed.), *Assessing childhood psychopathology and developmental disabilities*.pp. 341-369 (Springer, London,2009).
1691. von Aster, M. G. & Shalev, R. S. Number development and developmental dyscalculia. *Dev. Med. Child Neurol* **49**, 868-873 (2007).
1692. Vorstman, J. A. *et al.* The 22q11.2 deletion in children: high rate of autistic disorders and early onset of psychotic symptoms. *J. Am. Acad. Child Adolesc. Psychiatry* **45**, 1104-1113 (2006).
1693. Vulliemoz, S., Raineteau, O. & Jabaudon, D. Reaching beyond the midline: why are human brains cross wired? *Lancet Neurol.* **4**, 87-99 (2005).
1694. Wachtel, L. E., Hartshorne, T. S. & Dailor, A. N. Psychiatric diagnoses and psychotropic medications in CHARGE syndrome: A pediatric survey. *J. Dev. Phys. Disabil.* **19**, 471-483 (2007).
1695. Waddell, G., Main, C. J., Morris, E. W., Di, P. M. & Gray, I. C. Chronic low-back pain, psychologic distress, and illness behavior. *Spine (Phila Pa 1976.)* **9**, 209-213 (1984).
1696. Wade, C. H., Wilfond, B. S. & McBride, C. M. Effects of genetic risk information on children's psychosocial wellbeing: A systematic review of the literature. *Genetics in Medicine* **(in press)** (2010).
1697. Wagner, A. *et al.* Altered insula response to taste stimuli in individuals recovered from restricting-type anorexia nervosa. *Neuropsychopharmacology* **33**, 513-523 (2008).
1698. Waites, C. L. & Garner, C. C. Presynaptic function in health and disease. *Trends Neurosci* **34**, 326-337 (2011).
1699. Wakefield, J. C., Horwitz, A. V. & Schmitz, M. F. Are we overpathologizing the socially anxious? Social phobia from a harmful dysfunction perspective. *Can. J. Psychiatry* **50**, 317-319 (2005).
1700. Wakschlag, L. S. *et al.* A developmental framework for distinguishing disruptive behavior from normative misbehavior in preschool children. *J. Child Psychol Psychiatry* **48**, 976-987 (2007).
1701. Walker, E. *et al.* Relationship of chronic pelvic pain to psychiatric diagnoses and childhood sexual abuse. *Am. J. Psychiatry* **145**, 75-80 (1988).
1702. Walker, J. R. & Casale, A. J. Prolonged penile erection in the newborn. *Urology* **50**, 796-799 (1997).
1703. Walker, R. H. *et al.* Developments in neuroacanthocytosis: expanding the spectrum of choreatic syndromes. *Movement Dis.* **21**, 1794-1805 (2006).
1704. Walker, R. H. *et al.* Neurologic phenotypes associated with acanthocytosis. *Neurology* **68**, 92-98 (2007).
1705. Walker, S. P. *et al.* Child development: risk factors for adverse outcomes in developing countries. *Lancet* **369**, 145-157 (2007).
1706. Wallace, M. T. & Stein, B. E. Early experience determines how the senses will interact. *J. Neurophysiol.* **97**, 921-926 (2007).
1707. Walpurger, V., Hebing-Lennartz, G., Denecke, H. & Pietrowsky, R. Habituation deficit in auditory event-related potentials in tinnitus complainers. *Hear. Res.* **181**, 57-64 (2003).
1708. Walterfang, M. *et al.* Gender dimorphism in siblings with schizophrenia-like psychosis due to Niemann-Pick disease type C. *J. Inher. Metab. Dis.* **(in press)**, (2009).
1709. Walters, G. D., Berry, D. T., Rogers, R., Payne, J. W. & Granacher, R. P., Jr. Feigned neurocognitive deficit: taxon or dimension? *J. Clin. Exp. Neuropsychol.* **31**, 584-593 (2009).
1710. Wang, D. *et al.* The molecular basis of pyruvate carboxylase deficiency: Mosaicism correlates with prolonged survival. *Mol. Genet. Metab.* **95**, 31-38 (2008).
1711. Wang, P. P. & Bellugi, U. Evidence from two genetic syndromes for a dissociation between verbal and visual-spatial short-term memory. *J. Clin. Exp. Neuropsychol.* **16**, 317-322 (1994).
1712. Warby, S. C. *et al.* CAG expansion in the Huntington disease gene is associated with a specific and targetable predisposing haplogroup. *Am. J. Hum. Genet.* **84**, 351-366 (2009).
1713. Warneken, F. & Tomasello, M. Extrinsic rewards undermine altruistic tendencies in 20-month-olds. *Dev. Psychol.* **44**, 1785-1788 (2008).
1714. Wasserman, L. I. & Trifonova, E. A. Diabetes mellitus as a model of psychosomatic and somatopsychic interrelationships. *Span. J. Psychol* **9**, 75-85 (2006).
1715. Waterlow, J. C. Classification and definition of protein-calorie malnutrition. *Br. Med. J.* **3**, 566 (1972).
1716. Waters, E. & Deane, K. E. Defining and assessing individual differences in attachment relationships: Q-methodology. *Mon. Soc. Res. Child Devel.* **50**, 41-65 (1985).
1717. Watson, C., Hoeft, F., Garrett, A. S., Hall, S. S. & Reiss, A. L. Aberrant brain activation during gaze processing in boys with fragile X syndrome. *Arch. Gen. Psychiatry* **65**, 1315-1323 (2008).
1718. Watson, M. *et al.* Factors associated with emotional and behavioural problems among school age children of breast cancer patients. *Br. J. Cancer* **94**, 43-50 (2006).
1719. Watson, N. V. & Kimura, D. Nontrivial sex differences in throwing and intercepting: relation to psychometrically-defined spatial functions. *Personality and individual differences* **12**, 375-385 (1991).
1720. Watts, D. J. & Strogatz, S. H. Collective dynamics of 'small-world' networks. *Nature* **393**, 440-442 (1998).
1721. Weaver, I. C. G. *et al.* Epigenetic programming by maternal behavior. *Nat. Neurosci.* **7**, 847-854 (2004).
1722. Webb, E., Shankleman, J., Evans, M. R. & Brooks, R. The health of children in refuges for women victims of domestic violence: cross sectional descriptive survey. *Br. Med. J.* **323**, 210-213 (2001).
1723. Webb, E. A. & Dattani, M. T. Septo-optic dysplasia. *Eur. J. Hum. Genet.* **18**, 393-397 (2010).

1724. Webb, N. B. *Helping bereaved children: A handbook for practitioners.* The Guilford Press, New York (2010).

1725. Weber, C. & Obermayer, K. Emergence of modularity within one sheet of neurons: a model comparison in Wermter, S., Austin, J. & Willshaw, D. (eds.), *Emergent Neural Computational Architectures.* pp. 53-67 (Springer, Berlin,2001).

1726. Webster, D. M., Richter, L. & Kruglanski, A. W. On leaping to conclusions when feeling tired. *J. Exp. Soc. Psychol.* **32**, 181-195 (1996).

1727. Webster, J., Chandler, J. & Battistutta, D. Pregnancy outcomes and health care use: effects of abuse. *Am. J Obstet. Gynecol.* **174**, 760-767 (1996).

1728. Wedig, M. M. & Nock, M. K. Parental expressed emotion and adolescent self-injury. *J. Am. Acad. Child Adolesc. Psychia* **46**, 1171-1178 (2007).

1729. Wegner, D. M., Schneider, D. J., Carter, S. R., III & White, T. L. Paradoxical effects of thought suppression. *J Pers. Soc. Psychol* **53**, 5-13 (1987).

1730. Weir, K. Clinical advice to courts on children's contact with their parents following parental separation. *Child Adolesc. Mental Health* **11**, 40-46 (2006).

1731. Weisbrot, D. M. Prelude to a school shooting? Assessing threatening behaviors in childhood and adolescence. *J. Am. Acad. Child Adolesc. Psychiatry* **47**, 847-852 (2008).

1732. Weisbrot, D. M. *et al.* Psychiatric comorbidity in pediatric patients with demyelinating disorders. *J Child Neurol* **25**, 192-202 (2010).

1733. Weiss, H. B., Songer, T. J. & Fabio, A. Fetal deaths related to maternal injury. *JAMA* **286**, 1863-1868 (2001).

1734. Weissenberger, A. A. *et al.* Aggression and psychiatric comorbidity in children with hypothalamic hamartomas and their unaffected siblings. *J. Am. Acad. Child Adolesc. Psychiatry* **40**, 696-703 (2001).

1735. Weissman, D. E. & Haddox, J. D. Opioid pseudoaddiction--an iatrogenic syndrome. *Pain* **36**, 363-366 (1989).

1736. Weitoft, G. R., Hjern, A., Haglund, B. & Rosen, M. Mortality, severe morbidity, and injury in children living with single parents in Sweden: a population-based study. *Lancet* **361**, 289-295 (2003).

1737. Wells, S. J., Fluke, J. D. & Brown, C. H. The decision to investigate: Child protection practice in 12 local agencies. *Children Youth Services Review* **17**, 523-546 (1995).

1738. Wermter, A. K. *et al.* Evidence for the involvement of genetic variation in the oxytocin receptor gene (OXTR) in the etiology of autistic disorders on high-functioning level. *Am. J. Med. Genet. B Neuropsychiatr. Genet.* **153B**, 629-639 (2010).

1739. Werner, E. & Dawson, G. Validation of the phenomenon of autistic regression using home videotapes. *Arch. Gen. Psychiatry* **62**, 889-895 (2005).

1740. Wernicke, J. F. *et al.* Cardiovascular effects of atomoxetine in children, adolescents, and adults. *Drug Saf* **26**, 729-740 (2003).

1741. Wessa, M. & Flor, H. Failure of extinction of fear responses in posttraumatic stress disorder: evidence from second-order conditioning. *Am. J. Psychiatry* **164**, 1684-1692 (2007).

1742. Wessely, S. Risk, psychiatry and the military. *Br. J. Psychiatry* **186**, 459-466 (2005).

1743. Westermeyer, J. Working with an interpreter in psychiatric assessment and treatment. *J. Nerv. Ment. Dis.* **178**, 745-749 (1990).

1744. Wheatley, M., Plant, J., Reader, H., Brown, G. & Cahill, C. Clozapine treatment of adolescents with posttraumatic stress disorder and psychotic symptoms. *J. Clin. Psychopharmacol.* **24**, 167-173 (2004).

1745. White, B. Children, work and 'child labour': changing responses to the employment of children. *Development and Change* **25**, 849-878 (1994).

1746. White, S. W., Oswald, D., Ollendick, T. & Scahill, L. Anxiety in children and adolescents with autism spectrum disorders. *Child Psychol. Review* **29**, 216-229 (2009).

1747. White, T., Anjum, A. & Schulz, S. C. The schizophrenia prodrome. *Am. J. Psychiatry* **163**, 376-380 (2006).

1748. White, T., Miller, J., Smith, G. L. & McMahon, W. M. Adherence and psychopathology in children and adolescents with cystic fibrosis. *Eur. Child Adolesc. Psychiatry* **18**, 96-104 (2009).

1749. White, T. & Schultz, S. K. Naltrexone treatment for a 3-year-old boy with self-injurious behavior. *Am. J. Psychiatry* **157**, 1574-1582 (2000).

1750. Whitehead, W. E., Palsson, O. & Jones, K. R. Systematic review of the comorbidity of irritable bowel syndrome with other disorders: What are the causes and implications?**. *Gastroenterology* **122**, 1140-1156 (2002).

1751. Whitehouse, W. P. Breath holding spells. *J. Pediatr. Neurol.* **8**, 49-50 (2010).

1752. Whitehouse, W. P. Reflex anoxic seizures. *J. Pediatr. Neurol.* **8**, 51-53 (2010).

1753. Whitney, I., Smith, P. K. & Thompson, D. Bullying and children with special educational needs in Smith, P. K. & Sharp, S. (eds.), *School Bullying.* pp. 213-240 (Routledge, New York,1994).

1754. Whittle, C. L., Fakharzadeh, S., Eades, J. & Preti, G. Human breath odors and their use in diagnosis. *Ann. N. Y. Acad. Sci.* **1098**, 252-266 (2007).

1755. Whooley, M. A., Avins, A. L., Miranda, J. & Browner, W. S. Case-Finding Instruments for Depression: Two Questions Are as Good as Many. *J. Gen. Intern. Med.* **12**, 439-445 (1997).

1756. Wicherts, J. M., Dolan, C. V., Carlson, J. S. & van der Maas, H. L. J. Raven's test performance of sub-Saharan Africans: Average performance, psychometric properties, and the Flynn Effect. *Learn. Individ. Dif.* **20**, 135-151 (2010).

1757. Wichstrom, L. & Hegna, K. Sexual orientation and suicide attempt: a longitudinal study of the general Norwegian adolescent population. *J. Abnorm. Psychol* **112**, 144-151 (2003).

1758. Wickel, E. E. *et al.* Do children take the same number of steps every day? *Am. J Hum. Biol.* **19**, 537-543 (2007).

1759. Wigal, S. B. *et al.* Catecholamine response to exercise in children with attention deficit hyperactivity disorder. *Pediatr. Res.* **53**, 756-761 (2003).

1760. Wigal, T. *et al.* Stimulant medications for the treatment of ADHD: Efficacy and limitations. *Ment. Retard. Dev. Disabil. Res. Rev.* **5**, 215-224 (1999).

1761. Wigren, M. & Heimann, M. Excessive picking in Prader-Willi syndrome: a pilot study of phenomenological aspects and comorbid symptoms. *Int. J. Disabil. Devel. Educ.* **48**, 129-142 (2001).

1762. Wilens, T. E., Faraone, S. V., Biederman, J. & Gunawardene, S. Does stimulant therapy of attention-deficit/hyperactivity disorder beget later substance abuse? A meta-analytic review of the literature. *Pediatrics* **111**, 179-185 (2003).

1763. Wiley, S. D. Deception and detection in psychiatric diagnosis. *Psychiatr. Clin North Am.* **21**, 869-893 (1998).

1764. Wilhelm, S. *et al.* Self-injurious skin picking: clinical characteristics and comorbidity. *J. Clin. Psychiatry* **60**, 454-459 (1999).

1765. Wilkin, T. J., Mallam, K. M., Metcalf, B. S., Jeffery, A. N. & Voss, L. D. Variation in physical activity lies with the child, not his environment: evidence for an 'activitystat' in young children (EarlyBird 16). *Int. J Obes.* **30**, 1050-1055 (2006).

1766. Wilkinson, L. S., Davies, W. & Isles, A. R. Genomic imprinting effects on brain development and function. *Nat. Rev. Neurosci.* **8**, 832-843 (2007).

1767. Wilkinson, P. O. & Goodyer, I. M. Attention difficulties and mood-related ruminative response style in adolescents with unipolar depression. *J Child Psychol Psychiatry* **47**, 1284-1291 (2006).

1768. Wilkinson, R. G. Socioeconomic determinants of health. Health inequalities: relative or absolute material standards? *Br. Med. J.* **314**, 591-595 (1997).

1769. Williams, D. A. & Clauw, D. J. Understanding fibromyalgia: Lessons from the broader pain research community. *J. Pain* **10**, 777-791 (2009).
1770. Williams, J. Discounting and ADHD: Multiple minor traits and states in Madden, G. J., Bickel, W. K. & Critchfield, T. S. (eds.), *Impulsivity: Theory, Science, and Neuroscience of Discounting*. (APA Books,2008).
1771. Williams, J. & Taylor, E. Dopamine appetite and cognitive impairment in attention deficit/hyperactivity disorder. *Neural Plast.* **11**, 115-132 (2004).
1772. Williams, J. & Taylor, E. The evolution of hyperactivity, impulsivity, and behavioural diversity. *J. Roy. Soc. Int* **3**, 399-413 (2005).
1773. Williams, J. G., Higgins, J. P. & Brayne, C. E. Systematic review of prevalence studies of autism spectrum disorders. *Arch Dis Child* **91**, 8-15 (2006).
1774. Williams, N. For all posterity. *Curr. Biol.* **18**, 138-139 (2008).
1775. Williams, S. K. *et al.* Risperidone and adaptive behavior in children with autism. *J. Am. Acad. Child Adolesc. Psychiatry* **45**, 431-439 (2006).
1776. Williams, V. C. *et al.* Neurofibromatosis type 1 revisited. *Pediatrics* **123**, 124-133 (2009).
1777. Wilson, B. A., Ivani-Chalian, R., Besag, F. M. C. & Bryant, T. Adapting the Rivermead Behavioural Memory Test for use with children aged 5 to 10 years. *J. Clin. Exp. Neuropsychol.* **15**, 474-486 (1993).
1778. Wilson, N. R., Sun, R. & Mathews, R. C. A motivationally-based simulation of performance degradation under pressure. *Neural Netw.* **22**, 502-508 (2009).
1779. Wilson, T. D., Lindsey, S. & Schooler, T. Y. A model of dual attitudes. *Psychol Rev.* **107**, 101-126 (2000).
1780. Wilson, T. D. & Nisbett, R. E. The accuracy of verbal reports about the effects of stimuli on emotions and behavior. *Soc. Psychol.* **41**, 118-131 (1978).
1781. Winchel, R. M. & Stanley, M. Self-injurious behavior: a review of the behavior and biology of self-mutilation. *Am. J. Psychiatry* **148**, 306-317 (1991).
1782. Wing, L. & Wing, J. K. Multiple impairments in early childhood autism. *J Autism Child Schizophr.* **1**, 256-266 (1971).
1783. Winnicott, D. W. *Through paediatrics to psycho-analysis: collected papers*. Basic Books, New York (1958).
1784. Wittchen, H. U., Stein, M. B. & Kessler, R. C. Social fears and social phobia in a community sample of adolescents and young adults: prevalence, risk factors and co-morbidity. *Psychol Med.* **29**, 309-323 (1999).
1785. Wolff, S. & Smith, A. M. C. Children who kill. *Br. Med. J.* **322**, 61-62 (2001).
1786. Wolfish, N. M., Pivik, R. T. & Busby, K. A. Elevated sleep arousal thresholds in enuretic boys: clinical implications. *Acta Paediatr.* **86**, 381-384 (1997).
1787. Wong, B. L. Management of the child with weakness. *Semin. Pediatr. Neurol.* **13**, 271-278 (2006).
1788. Wong, F. K. & Hagg, U. An update on the aetiology of orofacial clefts. *Hong Kong Med. J.* **10**, 331-336 (2004).
1789. Wong, L. J. C. Diagnostic challenges of mitochondrial DNA disorders. *Mitochondrion* **7**, 45-52 (2007).
1790. Wong, V., Chen, W. X. & Wong, K. Y. Short- and long-term outcome of severe neonatal nonhemolytic hyperbilirubinemia. *J. Child Neurol* **21**, 309-315 (2006).
1791. Woodbury, M. M., DeMaso, D. R. & Goldman, S. J. An integrated medical and psychiatric approach to conversion symptoms in a four-year-old. *J. Am. Acad. Child Adolesc. Psychiatry* **31**, 1095-1097 (1992).
1792. Woodward, L., Dowdney, L. & Taylor, E. Child and family factors influencing the clinical referral of children with hyperactivity: a research note. *J. Child Psychol. Psychiatry* **38**, 479-485 (1997).
1793. Woolf, C. J. Central sensitization: Implications for the diagnosis and treatment of pain. *Pain* **152**, S2-S15 (2011).
1794. Wordsworth, S. *et al.* Diagnosing idiopathic learning disability: a cost-effectiveness analysis of microarray technology in the National Health Service of the United Kingdom. *Genomic Med* **1**, 35-45 (2007).
1795. World Health Organisation *WHO Child Growth Standards: Growth reference data for 5-19 years*. http://www.who.int/growthref/who2007_bmi_for_age/en/index.html (2007).
1796. World Health Organization *Schedules for Clinical Assessment in Neuropsychiatry (SCAN): Version 2 - Glossary*. American Psychiatric Press, Arlington (2009).
1797. World Health Organization *The ICD-10 classification of mental and behavioural disorders: Clinical descriptions and diagnostic guidelines*. WHO, Geneva (1992).
1798. Worrall-Davies, A., Kiernan, K., Barrett, J. & Marino-Francis, F. *Evaluation of primary care CAMH consultation and referral*. University of Leeds, (2005).
1799. Wrennall, L. Misdiagnosis of child abuse related to delay in diagnosing a paediatric brain tumour. *Clin. Med: Pediatrics* **1**, 1-12 (2008).
1800. Wright, M. H. Burkeian and Freudian theories of identification. *Commun. Q* **42**, 301-310 (1994).
1801. Wu, C. S. *et al.* Health of children born to mothers who had preeclampsia: a population-based cohort study. *Am. J. Obstet. Gynecol.* **201**, 269-270 (2009).
1802. Wu, G. Amino acids: metabolism, functions, and nutrition. *Amino. Acids* **37**, 1-17 (2009).
1803. Wu, M. F. *et al.* Locus coeruleus neurons: cessation of activity during cataplexy. *Neurosci* **91**, 1389-1399 (1999).
1804. Xuei, X. *et al.* GABRR1 and GABRR2, encoding the GABA-A receptor subunits rho1 and rho2, are associated with alcohol dependence. *Am. J. Med. Genet. B Neuropsychiatr. Genet.* **153B**, 418-427 (2010).
1805. Yakovlev, P. I. & Lecours, A. R. The myelogenetic cycles of regional maturation of the brain in Minkowski, A. (ed.), *Regional development of the brain in early life*.pp. 3-70 (Blackwell Scientific, Oxford & Edinburgh,1967).
1806. Yamada, T., Koguchi, Y. & Hirayama, K. Juvenile parkinsonism with marked diurnal fluctuation. *Jpn. J Psychiatry Neurol* **43**, 205-212 (1989).
1807. Yang, M. L., Fullwood, E., Goldstein, J. & Mink, J. W. Masturbation in infancy and early childhood presenting as a movement disorder: 12 cases and a review of the literature. *Pediatrics* **116**, 1427-1432 (2005).
1808. Yerkes, R. M. & Dodson, J. D. The relation of strength of stimulus to rapidity of habit-formation. *J. Comp. Neurol. Psychol.* **18**, 459-482 (1908).
1809. Yirmiya, N., Kasari, C., Sigman, M. & Mundy, P. Facial expressions of affect in autistic, mentally retarded and normal children. *J. Child Psychol Psychiatry* **30**, 725-735 (1989).
1810. Yoo, J. H., Valdovinos, M. G. & Williams, D. C. Relevance of donepezil in enhancing learning and memory in special populations: a review of the literature. *J Autism Dev Disord.* **37**, 1883-1901 (2007).
1811. Young, R., Sweeting, H. & West, P. Prevalence of deliberate self harm and attempted suicide within contemporary Goth youth subculture: longitudinal cohort study. *Br. Med. J.* **332**, 1058-1061 (2006).
1812. Young, S. E. *et al.* Substance use, abuse and dependence in adolescence: prevalence, symptom profiles and correlates. *Drug Alcohol Depend.* **68**, 309-322 (2002).
1813. Yu, A. J. & Dayan, P. Uncertainty, neuromodulation, and attention. *Neuron* **46**, 681-692 (2005).
1814. Zachar, P. & Kendler, K. S. Psychiatric disorders: A conceptual taxonomy. *Am. J. Psychiatry* **164**, 557-565 (2007).

1815. Zadra, A. & Donderi, D. C. Threat perceptions and avoidance in recurrent dreams. *Behav. Brain Sci.* **23**, 1017-1018 (2000).

1816. Zametkin, A. J., Zoon, C. K., Klein, H. W. & Munson, S. Psychiatric aspects of child and adolescent obesity: a review of the past 10 years. *J. Am. Acad. Child Adolesc. Psychiatry* **43**, 134-150 (2004).

1817. Zarkowski, P., Pasic, J., Russo, J. & Roy-Byrne, P. "Excessive tears": a diagnostic sign for cocaine-induced mood disorder? *Compr. Psychiatry* **48**, 252-256 (2007).

1818. Zeanah, C. H. Beyond insecurity: a reconceptualization of attachment disorders of infancy. *J. Consult Clin. Psychol* **64**, 42-52 (1996).

1819. Zelnik, M., Kim, Y. J. & Kantner, J. F. Probabilities of intercourse and conception among U.S. teenage women, 1971 and 1976. *Fam. Plann. Perspect.* **11**, 177-183 (1979).

1820. Zelnik, N., Pacht, A., Obeid, R. & Lerner, A. Range of neurologic disorders in patients with celiac disease. *Pediatrics* **113**, 1672-1676 (2004).

1821. Zempleni, J., Wijeratne, S. S. & Hassan, Y. I. Biotin. *Biofactors* **35**, 36-46 (2009).

1822. Zimmermann, M. B. Iodine requirements and the risks and benefits of correcting iodine deficiency in populations. *J. Trace Elem. Med. Biol.* **22**, 81-92 (2008).

1823. Zimmermann, M. B. Iodine deficiency in industrialised countries. *Proc. Nutr. Soc.* **69**, 133-143 (2009).

1824. Zipursky, R. B., Meyer, J. H. & Verhoeff, N. P. PET and SPECT imaging in psychiatric disorders. *Can. J. Psychiat.* **52**, 146-157 (2007).

1825. Zola, I. K. Self, identity and the naming question: Reflections on the language of disability. *Soc. Sci. Med.* **36**, 167-173 (1993).

1826. Zuccoli, G., Siddiqui, N., Bailey, A. & Bartoletti, S. C. Neuroimaging findings in pediatric Wernicke encephalopathy: a review. *Neuroradiology* **52**, 523-529 (2010).

rec. Apr. 22, 2014